The King and Di

The True Story

Howard Hodgson

Howard Hodgson

All rights reserved. No part of this publication may be reproduced, stored in a retrieval system, or in any form or by any means, without the prior permission in writing of the publisher, nor be otherwise circulated in any form of binding or cover other than that in which it is published and without a similar condition including this condition being imposed on the subsequent publisher.

Published by
Chipmunka Publishing
PO Box 6872
Brentwood
Essex CM13 1ZT
United Kingdom

ISBN 978-1-84747-674-6

© Text copyright Howard Hodgson 2009
Cover image Getty Images
Proof read Barbra Bagnall

Every attempt has been made to contact the relevant copyright-holders, but some were unobtainable. We would be grateful if the appropriate people could contact us.

Dedication

To Christine

Howard Hodgson

Foreword

Howard Hodgson's biography of Princess Diana and Prince Charles is a refreshing approach to the urban myth of two of the most well known and revered public figures of the late twentieth and early twenty first century. Hodgson reveals how Prince Charles cared for Diana in her time of need and how family members support the suffering of their loved ones.

Hodgson writes with sensitivity, honesty and pathos. He shows how Prince Charles and his family are loving people that have sometimes been misrepresented by the world's media.

Few of us can imagine the mental pressure that results in being destined to be King. Prince Charles is a heroic figure that cares about the world and acts in people's best interests.

Hodgson explores the mental frailty of Princess Diana and his view of her having Borderline Personality Disorder. Chipmunka Publishing supports Howard's book as we realise that many public figures have mental health issues and caring issues to deal with. Princess Diana as sufferer and Prince Charles as carer are no exception.

Jason Pelger
CEO Chipmunka Publishing Ltd

Howard Hodgson

Preface

HRH the Prince of Wales is one of the most recognized men in the world. He is, after all, next in line to sit on the world's most famous throne. He didn't always enjoy his school days but overcame his shyness, lack of self-confidence and low self-esteem to become known by the press as 'Action Man' in the 1970s. He served in both the Royal Navy and Royal Air Force before retiring to concentrate on raising money for his many interests – all of which strive to help create a peaceful world where there is religious harmony, a protected environment and increased opportunity for the young, especially those from deprived backgrounds. Such interests include British heritage, the well-being of the armed services, education, the environment, architecture, inner-city deprivation, the jobless, world poverty and putting the Great back into Britain.

His work has caused him to be viewed by some as a 'saintly' man; by others as a man who has wrongly stepped over the constitutional line, who believe that it is not the monarchy's job to involve themselves in political issues which might court controversy.

Such controversy has thus made him enemies within various vested interest groups and republican circles alike. In the 1980s they labeled him 'the loony Prince' - a tag that was happily seized upon by Britain's cruel tabloid press. In the 1990s an unfair and largely untrue account of his marriage further damaged his image as his late wife sought to rip a page out of British history and replace it with her own version of such events. Nevertheless, he pushed forward with dogged determination, believing that the implementation of his goals was his mission in life while waiting to become King Charles III. Today, he sits at the head of nineteen charities – one of which, the Prince's Trust, is one of Britain's most successful, and heralded around the world. As the following quotations testify, it is not unfair to claim that the Prince of Wales has done more to assist young people to help themselves towards a better future than any British politician since the Second World War. Moreover, in a world in which politicians fall over themselves to show their green credentials, nobody is pointing Prince Charles out as a loony any longer.

During his life he has enjoyed and endured in some cases many fascinating relationships; with his parents; his grandmother; his mentor Lord Mountbatten who adored him, as do his children. Friends and staff are very fond of him while also being fiercely loyal in their protection of him. In addition, there have also been his marriages to Diana Princess of Wales and Camilla the Duchess of Cornwall and his interesting associations with various British politicians and world leaders, including an intriguing relationship with Margaret Thatcher which was originally founded on mutual mistrust but ended with a grudging mutual respect.

To some, Prince Charles is a self-pitying adulterer, to others he has overcome a lack of self-esteem and self-confidence to become Britain's most enlightened Prince of Wales ever. Of course he is not perfect. He does lack self-esteem and on occasion can be self-pitying. But on the other hand, he is a kind and caring man and a wonderful father; never the horrid husband that certain tabloids and books would have us believe. Like all of us he has his failings but he is essentially a good man and there are thousands of young people across the globe who can bear testament to that and do so gladly as they sing 'God Bless the Prince of Wales'.

The Prince's Trust

If you look at The Prince's Trust, it's probably one of the most successful voluntary sector organizations in the world, never mind in this country.
Tony Blair

I love The Prince's Trust. I love the foresight it has, knowing that every young person is special and different, and if encouraged and supported that person will give back tenfold and have a happier life.
Joanna Lumley OBE, Prince's Trust Ambassador.

The Prince's Trust has been a friend to young people in Britain for almost 30 years. I became involved because I saw, at first hand, that it makes a difference and improves lives.
Jools Holland

The Prince's Trust isn't afraid to take risks, and trusts in young people who society have given up on.
Pierce Brosnan

The King and Di

The Prince's Trust does invaluable work in helping young people to pursue their ambitions and aspirations. Without the financial support of The Trust, these people would have few opportunities to make something of their lives.
Sir David Garrard

The Prince's Trust listened and gave me choices I never knew about. They knew about my background but they supported me anyway. They gave me the chance to show who I am and what I can do.
Andy Bowley, reformed teenager

If the Prince of Wales hadn't been born to be King of England, then his work would have seen him made a saint instead.
Melvyn Bragg

As heir to the throne, he is committed to making a difference for the better, in this country and internationally, and to using his position to draw attention to and foster the nation's talents and traditions.
St James's Palace Mission Statement:

Prince Charles is a self-pitying moaner.
Sir Max Hastings

Howard Hodgson

Acknowledgements

It is hard to know where to start when acknowledging the help and unselfish efforts of others who have helped me compile the background information that has lead to this portrait of the man who will be the next King of the United Kingdom of Great Britain and Northern Ireland. Over the last five years I have encountered literally hundreds of people who have either directly or indirectly helped construct the true picture of who HRH the Prince of Wales really is, while dispelling the myths created by numerous publications, long accepted by magazines, newspapers and television the world over as accurate, resulting in a largely unfair and inaccurate picture of the Prince. I truly hope that with the help of these people this book will achieve its aim of correcting these widely-held fictions and replace them with a balanced and faithful portrait.

Therefore, I wholeheartedly thank those contributors who were happy to be named and those who refused out of loyalty to either the Prince or late Princess of Wales but nevertheless provided invaluable information. In a number of cases, these people are still in royal employment and have helped me on the strict understanding that they remain completely anonymous. Wherever it has been possible for me to name my sources, I have done so; whenever my sources have asked me to respect their anonymity, I have been scrupulous in honouring their wishes. Nevertheless, my thanks are due to the many people without whose unique insight into the life of Charles and Diana this book could never have been written. I would also acknowledge the works of the scores of journalists and writers who have written articles and books on this subject and have thus provided useful reference points.

My family has always been most loving and supportive of me during the research and writing of my previous books but not more than on this occasion when they all cut out articles or recorded television programmes and even made appointments for me to see various contributors. In particular, I would like to thank my wife Christine, for her hours of proof reading and attempts to temper explosions of rage and indignation that I might have otherwise committed to the page without her sensible advice.

Lastly, I would like to thank my subject for being a man whose good character, warts and all, is worthy of revision, and Andrew

Howard Hodgson

Morton whose book *Diana – Her True Story* inspired me to write this book in the first place.

Contents

Part One – The Childhood and Adolescent Years
Chapter One: Charles: His Early Years (1948–62)   23
Chapter Two: Diana: Her Early Years (1961–77)   47
Chapter Three: The Making of a Prince (1962–70)   66
Chapter Four: Charles Meets the Navy and Camilla (1970–76)   103
Chapter Five: The Prince Gains a Mission (1977–79)   153

Part Two – The Preparation of a Princess
Chapter Six: The Preparation of a Princess (1977–81)   185
Chapter Seven: The Waiting, the Wedding Day and the Honeymoon (1981)   227

Part Three – The Birth of Children, and of an Icon
Chapter Eight: It Wasn't Always Bad (1981–86)   279
Chapter Nine: Affairs of State (1986–92)   320
Chapter Ten: Affairs of the Heart (1984–92)   366
Chapter Eleven: Charles and Diana at Close Quarters (1991–96)   415

Part Four – Separation, Divorce and Death
Chapter Twelve: The Children (1982–96)   431
Chapter Thirteen: The Greatest Deception (1991–92)   443
Chapter Fourteen: The Separation (1992)   486
Chapter Fifteen: The Divorce (1993–96)   498
Chapter Sixteen: The Dynasty and the Destiny (1996–97)   562
Chapter Seventeen: The Last Summer (1997)   598
Chapter Eighteen: The Funeral (1997)   632

Conclusion: 'They who would rule in this kingdom'   651
Bibliography   664

Howard Hodgson

The King and Di

Introduction

The history of the British Isles is peppered with myths, inaccuracies and out-and-out lies that were usually created for a particular reason: Richard III was almost certainly not born with a full head of hair, a mouthful of teeth, a withered hand and a horribly deformed hump on his back; Bloody Mary burned fewer Protestants than her half-sister, Elizabeth I, burned Catholics; there was so much more to Charles II than wine, women and song; and Captain Bligh was a first-rate seaman and a most capable navigator, whereas Fletcher Christian was more of an idle fop and womaniser than a humanitarian. However, in all these cases the public perception is quite different to the truth.

Why? Because spin wasn't invented by Bill Clinton or Tony Blair. It has been around as long as man. Henry Tudor – Richard III's enemy and the man who stole his crown – had his aides put about a story of frightening deformity that suggested to the masses that his predecessor was thoroughly evil, in order to strengthen his claim to the throne. As a Protestant nation we have been encouraged to forget about Elizabeth I's appalling acts of cruelty, but to be horrified by those of her Catholic sister. It was a Hanoverian Protestant government in England that needed to play down the virtues of the most successful Stuart king as his Catholic descendants attempted to regain the throne. And Fletcher Christian's family was rich: they published pamphlets for mass distribution that were designed to gain public support for the pardoning of Christian for leading a mutiny against the largely invented cruelty of Bligh, when the real – and unpardonable – reason for the mutiny was Christian's love of Polynesian women.

The rich and powerful have been rewriting history for their own benefit long before Hollywood or British tabloid newspapers caught on to how lucrative it could be for them. The name of the game has always been the same: if the truth doesn't suit, write a story that does. But if the lie isn't corrected at an early stage, it often becomes accepted as historical fact. It was very easy, in the days of illiteracy and slow communication, for Henry VII to rewrite history in order to strengthen his very questionable right to the English throne. In the reign of his son, Henry VIII, Sir Thomas More adopted this point of view in his *History of King Richard III*, which in turn became a source for Shakespeare's play and one of the most famous stage villains of all time: an evil-looking man with a withered hand and a hunchback – gripping stuff, but mostly myth built on spin. And yet this is how today's schoolchildren imagine Richard III, as did their parents and grandparents before them.

One might be forgiven for thinking that, while this sort of thing was possible more than five hundred years ago, surely in our world of twenty-four-hour media the truth will always come out. Quite wrong. Today the dark art of spin, the media's appetite for making a quick buck and the insatiable desire of a shallow and greedy public to devour celebrity gossip and stick with a lie they like, rather than be confronted with a truth they don't, means that the public often ends up believing very inaccurate stories. Future historians may well have to unravel these tales in order to reveal the truth to future generations, but by that time the damage will have been done.

The story of Britain's future king and his late wife is a case in point. Much has been written about Charles, Prince of Wales and the widely mourned Diana, Princess of Wales. They were, after all, the star attraction in the world's most famous monarchy for nearly two decades. And much has also been written about the kingdom in which they lived – a little island in the North Atlantic that built the world's largest and most powerful empire before retreating, bankrupt, by the cost of winning two world wars.

In the eyes of many – especially in America – Great Britain had become a nation that was morally magnificent but financially ruined. Delusions of grandeur by successive British governments dictated that the country should continue to be America's best friend and strongest ally so that, by riding on the coat-tails of the new world leader, it could still pretend to be a great world power. And as it flattered to deceive in order to be something that it wasn't on the world stage, so it became something that it never intended to be at home.

Nevertheless, people across the world have long looked with affection and perhaps even a little respect upon a nation so steeped in such a rich and wonderful history. Even that theatre of dreams Hollywood has come to draw upon it time and again for inspiration. America may have grown into the world's leading power – prosperous, fashionable and powerful – but there is still something to admire about the British, those quaint, old-fashioned people who, according to Hollywood, either speak with a cockney accent or with a cut-glass voice from Oxford. Such folks might not be as rich as their American cousins, but they possess a different kind of historical wealth with their

The King and Di

legends and histories: King Arthur, Richard the Lionheart, Robin Hood, Lord Nelson, Winston Churchill and hundreds of other real or imaginary heroes and heroines.

Moreover, the British still have a real Royal Family, and have done for more than a thousand years. In 1981, this Royal Family put on a real royal wedding that joined together an authentic, handsome and dashing young prince with a beautiful, innocent, shy and even younger aristocratic girl. The whole world was enchanted. They watched in their millions and saw the ceremony being acted out on their television screens, amazed that the stars were actually playing themselves. That was where the attraction lay: this was a real fairy tale, not one dreamed up by Hollywood or adapted from a children's book. If it had been, of course, the words 'And they all lived happily ever after' would have appeared before the final credits; but this wasn't a film. Life went on and they did not live happily ever after. Indeed, the 'War of the Waleses' became one of the biggest media sagas of the twentieth century, fuelled as it was by love affairs, scandals, divorce and an awful and untimely death. Their story was to fill newspapers and magazines around the world, and it spawned many books. However, a very high proportion of what was written about the Prince, the Princess and many of the supporting characters in this tale might just as well have been written by a Hollywood scriptwriter as it was shallow, simplistic, inaccurate and all too often simply not true.

Equally – and perhaps because the United Kingdom has recently loyally supported its closest ally in Kosovo, Afghanistan and Iraq – the British people continue to be seen by many Americans, if not the rest of the world, as a reliable, good and law-abiding race of respected and respectful people who play cricket, prefer tea to coffee and drink warm beer.

This image is also inaccurate. Since the end of the Second World War the British nation has experienced an amazing and most unfortunate change of character. The United Kingdom is sadly no longer the same country that I grew up in. It has become a society that has experienced more domestic wealth than ever before, only to become obsessed by the shallow and the worthless; a world where all that glitters is taken to be gold; a place where the people would seem to favour the exaggerated and sensational outpourings of a vicious press above reasonable behaviour towards their fellow man and reasonable deference towards legitimate authority; a nation where too many people have become couch potatoes happy to watch talentless 'celebrities' on television, rather than trouble themselves to set examples for their children, who in turn are growing up poorer as a result. It has become in too many places a quite horrid, violent, lawless and disrespectful island; this, as much as anything else, has become a major cause of the monarchy's current problems. The hypocrisy of a delinquent nation that expects perfection from its fairy-tale monarchy has made the royals' job almost impossible for mere mortals.

As many Third World countries continue to battle against famine, pestilence and plague, Britain, instead of being concerned for them or even simply grateful for its own prosperity, now battles against self-indulgence, obesity, drug addiction, child abuse and domestic and street violence where the weak and the elderly are too often the victims; it has become a place where religion, moral values and decency have all too often been replaced by greed, self-interest and cruelty; its people, having lost their national identity and self-respect in a changing world, now seek to blame anybody but themselves, obsessed as they are with a compensation culture. The story of Charles and Diana, therefore, cannot just be one of monarchy, but also of a nation searching for the self-destruct button with one hand while pointing the finger of blame with the other.

I was born in 1950, and am proud to be British. I grew up in the United Kingdom and have often seen its Royal Family at close quarters. I remain fiercely patriotic. Moreover, I believe in the importance of opinions based on the truth. In the real world there can only ever be one starting point, and that is the evidence; an opinion based on a falsehood is worthless. Consequently, I have made the gathering of facts the basis of this book. Where there is doubt, I report the facts and leave the reader to draw their own conclusions. If you think that the argument of hard evidence is a foundation upon which to base your opinion, I believe you will find this book interesting. On the other hand, if you do not wish your opinion to be altered by the evidence, this account may be distressing. Either way I hope you find it compelling.

This book has taken years to research and write. In the course of its creation I have spoken to many politicians, courtiers and members of the public who have encountered the Prince and Princess of Wales in their daily lives and so can attempt to bring clarity to certain events. I have also read scores of books about the couple. In the main I have found that the people who knew them tend to be more fair and objective than those who have written about them. Perhaps this is because the latter tend to have a hidden agenda. They seem to fall into three categories. Some seek fame and fortune by repeating stories that first appeared in the early 1990s courtesy of Andrew Morton's 'unofficial' biography *Diana: Her True Story*; these people often back these stories up by unidentified, untraceable and in certain instances, I suspect, invented quotes in order to exploit Diana's memory for personal gain. Others are driven by a desire to hijack the tragic elements of the Princess's story for the promotion of political or even feminist dogma. The third, often people who were actually part of her working life, make very damning claims against the Princess, but fail to take a balanced view of her whole life; their snapshots, while not perhaps being untrue, do not necessarily reflect the real princess, or how she became that person. Very few of these publications give the reader the opportunity to study the whole picture or put this period of British monarchical history into its proper perspective.

There is of course an argument that quite enough has been written about the couple. Perhaps it is time that the memory of the Princess is laid to rest so that her sons, as well as her ex-husband (who has incidentally done more than anyone to protect her memory) are left to remember her in peace. My view is that this cannot happen until a page of British history that was ripped out and falsely replaced has been corrected. I believe that no one has the right to hijack our history, and that any society willing to accept fiction in place of fact is flirting with immense danger.

My sincere desire, therefore, has been to tell the true story of their lives. In the final analysis, it is a story of two similar people who came from very similar backgrounds and yet came to stand for totally different things. It is a tale of a very different boy and girl to the ones the public believe they know. It is the true story of Charles and Diana. It is based on fact – the fiction has been stripped away – but this makes it no less interesting. Indeed, it is in many ways more beautiful as an accurate celebration of real people who are much more complex than the two-dimensional cardboard cut-outs that the tabloid press has painted hitherto ...

Howard Hodgson

Howard Hodgson

The King and Di

Part One
The Childhood and Adolescent Years

Howard Hodgson

Chapter One
Charles: His Early Years (1948–62)

Prince Charles was born at 9.14 p.m. on 14 November 1948. A crowd of more than 3,000 braved the cold night air and sang into the early hours outside Buckingham Palace; the fountains in Trafalgar Square flowed blue for a boy; the next morning, Union Jacks appeared in the streets, and warships of His Majesty's various fleets, on station across the globe, fired a royal birthday salute as church bells rang out in every city, town and village in the land. In the United States of America, a republic with more than a passing interest in the British monarchy, radio programmes were interrupted to make the announcement that a future king of England had been born. The story was blazoned across every front page of an adoring American press.

Such was the majesty of the British Monarchy, seen at home and abroad as having played a vital role in the dark hours of the Second World War. At one time only a defiant Britain and her far-flung empire had stood alone, battered but not bowed against the forces of Nazism. The quiet fortitude of George VI, his wife Queen Elizabeth and their two daughters in refusing to quit London during the Blitz had helped inspire a patriotic nation to fight on, united behind the wonderful oratory of that pugnacious British bulldog Winston Churchill.

However, the truth was that Britain had been seriously holed beneath the waterline by the gigantic price of the First World War. Now, victorious once more, its moral standing throughout the world was never higher; but it was facing bankruptcy – or at least a harsh financial future. The debts that had been collected in pursuit of victory on behalf of a grateful world had to be repaid, and Britain was not to be granted the huge cash injections that the US poured into Germany and Japan in order to kick-start their obliterated economies. On the contrary, Britain would have to repay America all of its war debt, along with the accumulated interest. As a result, it now faced supporting an empire it could no longer afford. At the time of Prince Charles's birth, his grandfather still presided over 800 million subjects. To protect them, he headed armed forces totalling nearly one and a half million.

In 1945, a nation more concerned about creating a socialist 'land fit for heroes' than rewarding its victorious prime minister with another term in office elected a radical Labour government under the leadership of Clement Attlee. It meant well, but was too ideologically obsessed and was never up to halting the nation's downward economic spiral. Food rationing was every bit as bad as it had been during the war, and basic commodity imports were cut by the government to minimum levels. For example, timber imports were squeezed to the point where national newspapers were cut back to four pages a day. Even worse, the basic petrol ration was abolished, although there was a supplementary allowance introduced for those living more than two miles from the nearest form of public transport. The government even urged the public to smoke cigarettes to the butt, adding that it might be good for your health.

All of this had about as much effect as moving the deck chairs around on the *Titanic*, and so failed to halt the slide in sterling. In 1949, a newly appointed chancellor of the exchequer, Sir Stafford Cripps, was forced to devalue the pound from $4.025 to $2.80, amid cries of 'national humiliation'. Indeed, it would take the Labour Party many years to lose the 'party of devaluation' tag that it gained as a result – although there was, in fairness, no alternative.

Surveying the state of this once great nation, the London correspondent of the *New York Times* wrote that Britain had become an 'impoverished second rate power, morally magnificent but economically bankrupt'. He wasn't far wrong. While on the surface Britain might still have appeared a major player on the world stage, the economic reality was somewhat different. Following the Second World War, both Europe and Japan lay devastated; the United States was hovering between world involvement and a return to isolationism, and Britain – with most of its huge empire still intact and sterling a reserve currency – was still a leading player on the world stage along with the USSR and America. The hard facts behind this façade, however, were different. Britain had lost £7 billion, one quarter of its entire wealth, during the war, and in 1947, after the first of a seemingly endless series of sterling crises, the pound had been devalued against the dollar.

Between autumn 1945 and summer 1947, six measures of public ownership were carried through Parliament: the Bank of England, cable and wireless, civil aviation, local electricity and road and rail transportation. Gas, iron and steel followed in 1950. This wholesale nationalization was the Labour government's answer to what they saw as the greedy exploitation by the bosses of the country's workers. Thirty years later, as Margaret Thatcher's government sold all but the Bank of England back to the people, not even the Labour Party raised much of a protest, confining itself to criticising the government over the giveaway prices. Back in the 1940s, however, the cradle-to-the-grave interference and protection by the state had as few critics as it has defenders today.

In the 1951 election, a tired Labour government was beaten and replaced by a Conservative administration more inclined to leave matters to the market. Rationing, which had been imposed on all staples, was gradually abandoned, and for most of the next ten years the country steadily became prosperous. Elizabeth II was crowned in 1953, and at times – usually when the balance of payments was in surplus – there was talk of a second Elizabethan Age. Harold Macmillan was able to tell voters, who returned yet another Tory administration to power in 1959, 'You've never had it so good.'

But back in 1948 the country was still circled by dark economic clouds. The previous year had been dubbed an 'annus horrendus' by the then chancellor Hugh Dalton. The atrocious weather of 1947 had brought Britain to a virtual standstill for three months. Coal shortages forced the closure of power stations and unemployment leaped to more than two million as the nation shivered in misery. Food rationing included meat, cheese, butter, margarine, cooking fat, sugar, milk and eggs. Minute amounts of each were exchanged weekly for coupons. The economy was stricken and seemed to be deteriorating by the day. The land fit for heroes had turned into a nightmare of a cold and hungry nation.

Churchill, now growling from the opposition's side of the house, was angered by the government's obsession with nationalization and commented that they had taken a 'burglar's jemmy to crack the capitalist crib'. But the government was not to be diverted and so, despite economic failure, their own exhaustion and the nation's obvious misery, continued wearily on the same path.

To make matters worse, in the middle of these harsh realities there was a surge in delinquency. In the decade leading up to 1948, crime had doubled, inclining the *Recorder of London* to comment on 'this distemper of dishonesty which has swept over the country in the last few years until people have lost sight of the difference between right and wrong.'

So it is possible to see how the birth of a boy born to be king was a welcome distraction from the dull and hard life that had followed years of war. In a world that seemed to ration every luxury or pleasure, however slight, and had done so for so long, this was just the excuse needed for a party and a celebration of monarchy and empire. The nation could cheer itself up and remember, with some pride, who it was. The British press was keen to reflect the mood of the nation, and headlines echoed the popular rejoicing. *The Times*, which considered itself in those pre-Murdoch days to be the nation's chronicle, sought to record the moment for history. Its editorial read: 'The birth of a child to the Heiress-Presumptive is a national and imperial event which can for a moment divert the people's thoughts from the acrimonies of domestic argument and the anxieties of the international scene. All can be united in rejoicing as the guns salute and the bells peal. Every newborn child represents to some family the thought and image of the future towards which it moves; this child from the moment of his birth becomes the symbol of their common aspirations for an even more splendid realm and Commonwealth than have been handed down to them by the virtue and prowess of their ancestors ...'

My goodness, it might be unjust to lay such burden of expectation upon a small baby whose characteristics are not yet known; but don't these words just perfectly capture the values of the time as well as the mood? It is hard to imagine *The Times* of today recording a similar event with such well-measured, thoughtful and deferential prose.

A month after his birth, the second in line to the world's most celebrated throne was baptized Charles Philip Arthur George in the music room at Buckingham Palace by the Archbishop of Canterbury with water from the Jordan. In attendance were his parents and eight godparents who included his grandparents – the king and queen themselves. Prince Charles was admitted to the Church of England, the rites of which he would be obliged, as the future sovereign, to pledge to defend, and which he could never deny without seriously jeopardizing his claim to the throne. It was a short service, not so different from those that had water splashing in the eyes of millions of other babies across Britain; but for Charles, it was the first bond to be attached to this dutiful prince for the rest of his life.

He was by all accounts a bonny baby. The queen's sister, Lady Granville, reported that, 'He could not be more angelic looking. He is golden-haired and has the most beautiful complexion, as well as amazingly delicate features for so young a baby.' His mother, Princess Elizabeth, observed that his hands were 'rather large but fine with long fingers – quite unlike mine and certainly not like his father's. It will be interesting to see what they become.'

So here was a nation – indeed an empire – rejoicing in the birth of a son to the next in line to the throne, who guaranteed the succession for years. But such an event, however joyous, could only be but a single happy moment in Britain's troubled post-war history. At this time, however, deference to the Establishment was still the order of the day and therefore the public, who didn't have a disrespectful tabloid press to whip up resentment, didn't really complain; where complaints were heard, they were directed at the civil servants and bureaucrats who were seen as stifling initiative and enterprise with their restrictions and red tape. The main pillars of the Establishment, such as the Church, the law and parliament, were still held in respect. The monarchy commanded a kind of awe: in those days it was thought that it should set the nation's moral tone, and popular affection for the monarchy and its individual members was fervent. Not to love the Royal Family was seen at the very least to be most unpatriotic; at worst it was seen as treason. For at least fifty years, this family had been totally secure in the knowledge that, even when the chips were down, loyalty to the Crown was automatic and almost religious.

Having withstood some domestic hostility and avoided the violent uprisings that occurred throughout much of Europe in Queen Victoria's reign, her son Edward VII passed on an untarnished and perfectly secure crown to his son, George V. It was during George's reign that the final transformation of the monarch from political leader to constitutional head of state took place. He had come to represent, in the person of the sovereign, not so much the embodiment of the age, as the values and the moral tone of its generation. As a result, in the public's mind, the distinction between the monarchy and the Royal Family became so blurred that the king remarked in 1935, when moved by the enthusiasm of a large East End crowd during a Silver Jubilee visit, 'I am beginning to think that they must like me for myself.' They did, and this was how the new monarchy proceeded despite the years of recession and the growing fear that the nation would once again be engulfed in a world war.

Upon his death, there was an outbreak of genuine public grief as the man in the street somehow felt that he had lost a personal friend as well as a king, demonstrating how effectively the intimate and the mystical had combined to great effect in his person. His eldest son,

Edward VIII, followed him. David, as his family knew him, looked to be a good bet. He was the best-established sex symbol of his day, a world-famous star. It was Edward's photograph that appeared in the frame on the bedside tables of half the young ladies of Britain and America, as perhaps he would have appeared on a bedroom-wall poster today. He was, in 1933, as Paul McCartney was in 1963 or David Beckham in 2003. Moreover, in addition to his charm and good looks, he had a social conscience. The distress at the plight of the unemployed in the valleys of south Wales during the recession had made him make the now famous public pronouncement, 'Something must be done to find them work.' This did nothing to endear him to the Conservative government of the day as they saw it as an act of monstrous political interference, but it made him very popular with those people who would never forgive Winston Churchill for sending the troops in against the miners.

Understandably, years later, comparisons were to be drawn between this Prince of Wales and the current one. Indeed, the latter's mentor, Lord Louis Mountbatten, who had also been a great friend of the former, was keen that Charles should learn from his great-uncle's mistakes. On superficial inspection there appear to be some similarities. Both had fathers who were disappointed with and disapproving of them and, as a result, were harsh with them. They were both dashing and fearless 'action men' in their teens. They both went on to become immensely successful representatives of the monarch on foreign tours and state visits. As a result, both became very popular throughout the Commonwealth and beyond. And both served their country in the armed forces.

But upon closer inspection the similarities are perhaps more down to the fact that the two men shared the same role, rather than the same characteristics. Indeed, in many ways Great-uncle David was more like Diana than Charles. Both were huge, worldwide icons, whose actions, rather than words, seemed to touch the common people almost effortlessly with a type of charisma never really possessed by Charles. And both could – and indeed usually did – put self-interest before the rigors of public life in a way that the dutiful Charles would never contemplate.

In the case of Edward VIII, the test of self-interest versus public duty was to bring about the abdication crisis. He had come to the throne enjoying mass support, but before he could be crowned he opted for the love of the twice-married American divorcee Wallis Simpson in favour of the throne, once he had realized that he could not have both. It was a sharp reminder of the fragility of the relationship between sovereign and subject: it was considered by the ruling classes of Britain, the Empire and the Commonwealth that in choosing to put self-interest before duty, Edward was committing a serious betrayal of the sacred trust of the Church, his subjects' governments and indeed his subjects. To put his love for this woman before his duty to the peoples of the Empire would not only ruin his own image, it would also seriously damage the collective image of his subjects.

At that time, such behaviour by a member of the Royal Family, especially one born to be king, was considered to be shocking and quite incompatible with the role of monarch. Nevertheless, the affair with Wallis Simpson was well known by Fleet Street for months, its exposure blocked by the press barons in the national interest. Can you imagine that happening in the midst of today's cut-throat circulation wars? What was the same then as now, however, was that the personality of royalty had become so entwined with the institution of the monarchy that for a time – as was the case in the days immediately following Diana's death – the very institution was exposed, if not actually under threat. There was a slight hint of republicanism in the air, and a certain coolness displayed to the new king, George VI, who was actually seen as a pale replacement for his previously popular brother. This moved Stanley Baldwin, the prime minister who had had to deal with the abdication crisis, to reassure his sovereign, 'If I may say so, you have no need to fear for the future. The whole country is behind you with deep and understanding sympathy.' This was clearly not the case, as the shy and retiring George stammered his way into the role.

However, supported by a strong queen and two attractive and appealing daughters, he soon made a favourable impression on the public. Here was a good man of family virtue. He was not dashing, charismatic and charming like his elder brother, but he was reliable, and suddenly that was seen to be important. He was a man of good moral standing who would always put duty first and not desert his subjects as his brother had. It was even felt, in some quarters, that perhaps the country had experienced a lucky escape, rather than suffer a crisis.

The restoration of the monarch as a family man in the image of his father became popular and was even enhanced further by the Royal Family's contribution to the war effort. In his biography of Prince Charles, Jonathan Dimbleby noted that, 'The King had a limited gift for rhetoric and inspiration (although his voice easily touched the listener), but he was at least seen to share the dangers and care about the suffering. By no means of the people, he was most assuredly with them and for them. As a survivor of the Coventry blitz recorded later, "We suddenly felt that if the King was there everything was alright and the rest of England was behind us."' In visiting the scene of devastation, the King echoed the empathy of the "rest of England", symbolizing their empathy as well as offering his own compassion. 'Though not everyone shared the attitude – some were indifferent, a few even hostile – for most people George VI and his family had become emblematic of the trials which they had to endure and the victory which they finally secured. By the end of the war, the consolidation of the familial monarchy had been accomplished.'

Anyone who has watched footage of Winston Churchill on the balcony of Buckingham Palace with the king and his family during the VE celebrations knows that Dimbleby is spot on. Additionally, it also proves that, while we might admire the bright star of charisma as displayed by Edward VIII and later the Princess of Wales, there comes a time when the less glamorous discipline of duty is vital, both for the nation and the monarchy itself.

After the war, in 1947, the marriage of the king's eldest daughter Princess Elizabeth to a young naval officer called Philip Mountbatten offered a momentary reprieve from the cheerless life of rationed Britain. The Princess was young, attractive and very popular, her suitor tall, dashing and noble. There was some doubt about having an opulent wedding during such an austere climate, but on the day the decision seemed to be right, as the whole nation appeared to take pleasure in the occasion. Thousands packed the route, and millions more gathered around wireless sets at home or in factories. The following day, a lifelong socialist recorded her thoughts in *Mass Observation* – a sort of precursor to opinion polls that published national comment as opposed to attempting to judge the national mood by establishing percentage opinion. This woman was astonished to discover that she couldn't find a newspaper to buy anywhere. Every copy had been sold. She added, 'I think the Royal Family is very popular. Were they to disappear, the people would be very upset.' The statement would have been received

The King and Di

by the readers as stating the bleeding obvious at the time, but it nevertheless describes a totally different sentiment to the prevailing atmosphere of a decade earlier, when the cold winds of abdication were blowing through the corridors of Buckingham Palace.

When Charles was born the following year, *The Times*, carried along on this wave of national pride and with re-established respect for the monarchy, described the sovereign as the nation's 'supreme representative', which 'in modern times is a more royal function than any duty of state,' affirming that, 'The representative monarchy has made every one of its subjects feel friend and neighbour to the Royal Family; and so it is that the simple joy which the coming of this child has brought to them is shared by all.'

This was an impossible dream. Re-establishing the monarchy in the hearts and minds of the nation by virtuous example now meant that there had developed a determined failure to distinguish the institute of monarchy and the character of the Royal Family: the sovereign was the supreme symbol of the realm as well as a model neighbour and a great friend. In the decades ahead, such a contradiction in function was to set the monarchy impossible targets.

But those problems were for the future and therefore, amid the euphoria of royal enthusiasm surrounding the birth of Prince Charles, even the radical socialist George Bernard Shaw wrote that the king stood 'for the future and the past, for posterity that has no vote and the tradition that never had any … For the great abstractions: for conscience and virtue; for the eternal against the expedient; for the evolutionary appetite against the day's gluttony; for intellectual integrity, for humanity.' These fine words might have been written with the future battles of the current Prince of Wales with respect to the protection of our environment, architecture, history and traditions in mind; but most people would also have applauded them then. Nobody would have considered the danger that would be presented if the Royal Family failed to live up to them.

In 1949, the Prince and Princess (Philip had been granted the title of prince upon his marriage to Elizabeth) moved themselves and their baby son out of their apartment in Buckingham Palace and into Clarence House, which had been used by the Red Cross during the war but was now refurbished as a new home for the royal couple. There, a nursery was established, along with a fairly standard routine – all supervised by two nannies, Helen Lightbody and Mabel Anderson. In addition, a plain-clothes constable from the Metropolitan Police permanently guarded their royal charge. Such an upbringing, police guard excepted, was not unusual in houses where the wealthy could afford such staff. Moreover, in the case of Prince Charles, his parents' busy lives didn't leave much time for childcare. Prince Philip was still a serving officer in the Royal Navy, while Princess Elizabeth was increasingly occupied with her role as heiress-presumptive, although when at home she did make a point of attending bath time, and would stay to read the young Prince a bedtime story.

In August 1950, Princess Anne was born and joined in her royal brother's daily routine. By now, however, it was clear that the king was ailing and that Princess Elizabeth would not only have to perform the many public engagements that proved too much for his stamina, she would also have to prepare herself to become sovereign upon his death. Inevitably, this meant that she didn't see as much of her children as she would have liked. It was their nannies who assisted their first steps and taught them how to play, paint, write their names and share things; it was their nannies who scolded bad behaviour or rewarded good; they who kissed a grazed knee better or soothed a bruised ego; they who listened to the excited happy chatter of expectation or consoled tears of disappointment. This, coupled with the normal emotional reserve of the period (seen as an attribute by the high-minded and definitely practiced by Princess Elizabeth and her husband) meant that the young Prince would form a bond with his nannies as close – and in the case of Mabel Anderson as enduring – as he would with his parents.

Soon after the Prince's second birthday, his mother flew off to join his father in Malta, where he had been promoted to command a frigate, so the couple could spend Christmas together. In those days, it was unthinkable that small children would accompany their parents on such a trip. So Prince Charles and his tiny four-month-old sister were sent to Sandringham to spend Christmas with their grandparents, the king and queen. Perhaps Princess Anne was a little too young to warrant a lot of attention from their Royal Highnesses, but a letter written from the king to his daughter at that time makes it clear that they both doted on their grandson and would 'enjoy having him'.

The future Prince of Wales had been taught, on entering the room, to bow to the king and kiss the queen's hand before jumping into her lap for a cuddle and a story. This is perhaps from where the mutual love, admiration and deep affection first sprung between the Prince and his grandmother. It was to provide Charles with essential praise and encouragement, which his frail ego sometimes needed, throughout his life until her death. This, the most successful and enduring relationship Prince Charles was to experience with the close members of his family, also worked for her. He was to become, without doubt, her favourite grandchild: she admired in him the sensitivity, care, kindness and sense of duty that reminded her of her husband. Conversely, she was unable to forgive her late brother-in-law, Edward VIII, for causing the abdication crisis that brought her husband to the throne and, by her way of thinking, led to his early death.

Charles's third birthday saw his parents abroad again, this time on a state visit to Canada, and he and his sister were once again billeted with their grandparents. Jonathan Dimbleby writes of a photograph of the Prince sitting with his grandfather to mark the occasion. 'The King had recently endured the latest of three operations in as many years, and it was known in the royal household that his death from cancer could not be long delayed. In the photograph, the drawn face of the sovereign looks down tenderly on the chubby boy, who was to hold that moment as his only personal memory of George VI.'

The family was reunited for Christmas that year. A month later, the dying king waved his daughter off on a Commonwealth tour that he had been forced to postpone four years earlier and certainly could not undertake now. Princess Elizabeth was not to see her father alive again. On 6 February, George VI died peacefully in his bed at Sandringham.

Although his death had been anticipated, when it came it caused shock, sorrow and provoked an outburst of immense national grief. His relationship with his subjects might have been remote – a voice on the wireless or an image on the newsreels – but he had become their friend and neighbour as well as their monarch. He had stood by them throughout the war and now, in the hour of his death, the sense of loss was very intimate. A drinker who had declared that the King was 'only shit and soil now like everyone else' had to be removed from the premises for his own safety.

Princess Elizabeth, whose Commonwealth tour had reached Africa, returned home. Her accession was formally proclaimed on 8 February by the Earl Marshall from four places in London: 'The High and Mighty Princess Elizabeth Alexandra Mary is now, by the Death of Our late Sovereign of Happy Memory, become Queen Elizabeth the

Second, by the Grace of God Queen of this Realm and all Her other Realms and Territories, Head of the Commonwealth, Defender of the Faith, to whom her lieges do acknowledge all faith and consistent Obedience …'

In accordance with tradition, the king lay in state in Westminster Hall, as his wife would fifty years later. His coffin was guarded in silent vigil as it lay upon the catafalque beneath the Royal Standard and the Imperial Crown in which the exquisite ruby, said to have been worn by Henry V at Agincourt, is set. Thousands and thousands of people slowly filed passed to pay homage. The silent line snaked from St Thomas's Hospital, across Westminster Bridge and along the Embankment before entering the hall. The queue moved so slowly the mourners spent many hours in bitterly cold weather before they reached and then passed through the candlelit hall. This was a sombre mark of respect and affection for a good king.

The celebrated BBC commentator and presenter Richard Dimbleby watched the mourners patiently make their way to Westminster Hall. He observed a dark stream of human beings, waiting patiently under a white canopy that crosses the pavement at the great doors of Westminster Hall. 'They speak very little these people, but their footsteps sound faintly as they cross the yard and go through the gates, back into the night from which they came … No one knows from where they came or where they go, but they are the people, and to watch them pass is to see the nation pass.'

Dimbleby, so famous for finding the words to express the nation's feelings, was of course right: as one mourner was to remark, 'It's a great tribute to him and it's a great tribute to us. Because George VI is us. He is us and we are him. He is the British people, all that is best in us, and we all know it.' It was a wonderful tribute, but a dangerous one, condemning the monarchy with near-sanctity.

Upon the king's death, his three-year-old grandson became Duke of Cornwall. But this must have been no consolation to the young Prince Charles, who was now destined to see even less of his mother as she was burdened by the awesome work of her responsibilities and was determined to fulfil such duties in front of any other demands on her time. At Easter, with the court still in official mourning, the young Queen moved her family back to Buckingham Palace, the official residence of the monarch. And a little over a year after the death of the king, the four-year-old Charles was in attendance at Westminster

Abbey to see his mother crowned – the first coronation to be shown on television. The cameras also captured a bored little boy tugging at the sleeve of his grandmother, perhaps wondering when he would be allowed to go home. Later he was brought out on to the balcony of Buckingham Palace as the newly anointed Queen acknowledged the roars of the vast crowd below.

By now Charles was starting to understand that his lot in life was very different to that of other children. However, at about this time, the *Sunday Pictorial* described him as 'The eldest child of a typical British family.' The paper was only stating what had become the progression of conventional wisdom that 'they are no longer distant, aloof, majestic puppets' but 'the number one family in a nation of families and a family of nations.' It was a lovely idea, but quite lunatic, even dangerous. Certainly it was an ideal that was totally impossible for any family to fulfil even in a conservative world, let alone one that was to spiral out of spiritual and moral control over the next fifty years. The idea must have been as confusing for Charles as it was dangerous for the monarchy. The Royal Family had gone from political autocrats to constitutional monarchs quite sedately; but they were now jumping from being the supreme symbol of the realm to 'a typical British family' in a matter of months. If the Royal Family was to be viewed in this way, it would only be a matter of time before the public turned on them: the nation did not want a typical British family; it wanted a special family that maintained a certain aloofness, distance and majesty. How different this expectation was from what was to come. The problems that were so exasperated by the arrival of Lady Diana Spencer and Sarah Ferguson were not entirely of those two young ladies' making. The origins of these faults can be found as far back as 1945, and the seeds of fertilization were well sown by 1952, not so much by the Royal Family itself, but by the public perception of what a 'new and socialist' Britain thought the 'new and socialist' Royal Family should be.

As an adult, Charles was to discover self-deprecation as a useful form of protection. He would claim with sincerity, 'I am just an ordinary person in an extraordinary position.' However, as a shy little boy who was yet to discover this form of self- protection and understood very little of what was expected of him, he stayed quietly in the background as his younger sister in this 'typical' family delighted in making the sentries at Buckingham Palace present arms repeatedly by marching to and fro in front of them.

Prince Philip delighted in his daughter's boldness, while being frustrated by his son's timidity. He might have wished to swap their personalities around, if that had been possible, believing the boisterous Anne was better suited to the role of monarch. That would have been a mistake, as Prince Charles, armed with a sense of duty, a compassion for his future subjects and the need to do good, overcame much of his childhood shyness. Bolstered by self-deprecation and the understanding and encouragement of his grandmother and his great-uncle and mentor Lord Mountbatten, he was to go on to become probably the country's most dedicated and hard-working Prince of Wales.

However, the Duke of Edinburgh was not to know that at the time, and so was very hard on his son in an attempt to toughen him up. A close friend of the Duke's told Richard Dimbleby that, 'Philip was trying to bring up a son who would be able to take over as king in a tough world. Certainly Charles was no crybaby, but he was terribly sensitive. Prince Philip didn't quite realise how sensitive he was. Another child might not have noticed, but Charles used to curl up ... he just shrank.' And so the Duke's efforts to shape Prince Charles into his own idea of kingship were to put the relationship between father and son to the greatest of tests, with anger and impatience on the one side, trepidation and a resulting low self-esteem on the other.

But despite this bullying, Charles continued to love and respect his father and today, to his credit, has as many fond memories of model-making and country rambles as he does of being told off by him. It was Prince Philip who gave him his love of the outdoor life and the pursuit of country sports that has been passed on to his own sons.

To this day, however, while the Prince of Wales undoubtedly loves both of his parents, he finds communication with them difficult. It is very probable that the Queen's long absences from his childhood and her very reserved and non-maternal attitude, along with Prince Philip's intimidation of him, left their mark and were responsible for this.

Shortly before Charles's fifth birthday, one of the rooms of the nursery was converted to a classroom and Catherine Peebles, who had previously taught Prince Michael and Princess Alexandra of Kent, was engaged to teach the heir to the throne some primary-school skills. Mispy, as she became known, soon discovered that the way to get the best out this polite and serious little boy with a fragile ego was to be gentle and encouraging. Sometime later she said, 'He was very responsive to kindness, but if you raised your voice to him he would draw back into his shell and for a time you would be able to do nothing with him.' He duly worked hard, but was not, at this point, to show any of the intellectual curiosity that would later distinguish him in adulthood. However, by using the opposite tactics to Prince Philip, Mispy was able to get very reasonable results and quite soon Prince Charles could write his name, read and especially draw with more than normal competence. He also enjoyed singing.

Unfortunately his parents were to witness little of this early education. They decided to stay in Sandringham while Prince Charles spent his fifth birthday at Buckingham Palace. Nine days later they left Britain on an official tour of ten Commonwealth countries. They would be away for six months. Prince Charles traced their progress on the globe in his classroom. He was not to see them again until the following spring. Thank goodness there was always his grandmother to provide that bond which is special to blood relatives, and which was also a source of comfort to the widowed Queen Mother.

On 14 April 1954, Prince Charles and his sister were driven to Portsmouth and placed aboard the Royal Yacht *Britannia* bound for Malta; in order to join their parents for the official visit there before continuing on to Gibraltar. Seven days later, *Britannia* entered the magnificent harbour at Valetta. This remains today one of the most beautiful waterfronts in the world: ancient cities tumble down the slopes to the deep-water harbour's edge, and high away to the left stands what was then the Mediterranean headquarters of the Royal Navy. The harbour was full of aircraft carriers, cruisers, destroyers, frigates and submarines, all flying the white ensign in an ominous display of power. The whole place bustled with activity. Picket boats steamed up and down ferrying supplies or men, and smart-looking officers in neatly pressed white uniform saluted each other as they went about their business.

A few days later the entire fleet, under the command of Lord Louis Mountbatten, was to steam past the Royal Yacht with thousands and thousands of naval ratings lining their decks and saluting Her Majesty the Queen. The empire might have been in its twilight years, but old habits die hard, and navies can't just disappear overnight.

Malta might only be a small Mediterranean island, but throughout its history it has always been of tremendous strategic value and played a vital role as a naval and supply base during the Second World War. Without Malta harbouring the Royal Navy and thus helping to supply the North African campaign, victory there would have been virtually impossible; and defeating the Germans in North Africa was not only an important morale-booster, it ensured that the British had access to oil while the enemy went without.

The Germans had also realised the importance of the island, and subjected it to some of the most severe bombing of the Second World War. As a result the Maltese suffered dreadful hardship, but their loyalty was repaid. The island was awarded, collectively, the George Cross, the highest award that can be granted to a civilian; and after the war, despite its own precarious financial position, Britain invested heavily in Malta to help rebuild the island and create work for its people. A bond between the British and Maltese survives today as a result.

But back in 1954, this splendid sight of majestic naval power displaying homage to his mother was to be indelibly marked upon Charles's memory; he would later recall it with a shiver of national pride and patriotism. Perhaps this is where Charles first started to grasp what was going to be expected of him, and began to understand the need to develop some defences in order to see the job through.

This first foreign visit by Prince Charles was deemed a success. The *Guardian* reported that at the end of one military parade attended by the royal children, 'The Duke of Cornwall took his sister's hand as she patted down the steps, shepherded her carefully into the car, and turned to wave a little shyly to the photographers and reporters who formed a polite scrum around the car. "Enchanting, quite enchanting, bless them," said a Maltese government official who had been watching.' A *Guardian* reporter writing in a similar positive fashion today would probably have his or her laptop thrown out of the window. However, in those days the press were more open-minded and concerned with reporting what they actually saw. Their compliant nature may be judged by a letter sent by Sir Richard Colville, the Queen's press secretary, in 1955 to the Newspaper Proprietors Association, seeking their cooperation concerning the next stage of Prince Charles's education. 'I am commanded by the Queen to say that her Majesty and the Duke of Edinburgh have decided that their son has reached the stage when he should take part in more grown-up educational pursuits with other children.

'In consequence, a certain amount of the Duke of Cornwall's instruction will take place outside his home; for example he will visit museums and other places of interest. The Queen trusts, therefore, that His Royal Highness will be able to enjoy this in the same way as other children without the embarrassment of constant publicity …

'I would be grateful if you would communicate this to your members and seek their co-operation in this matter, informing them at the same time that they are at liberty to publish this letter if they so wish.'

The clear authority of this letter places it firmly in the 1950s, miles away from today. It was obeyed to the letter by the deferential press of the time, and the Prince duly got to visit all the museums and galleries that Miss Peebles felt important for his education without the attention of Fleet Street. So it was that the Prince started his love affair with history and art. He was artistic by nature and history was largely one long and illustrious story of kings and queens and battles and victories with his family in most of the starring roles. Not surprisingly, he was to become most adept at both subjects.

On 7 November, a week before his eighth birthday, Prince Charles, accompanied by Miss Peebles, was driven to Hill House, a pre-preparatory school in West London. It is still there today and remains conspicuous by the baggy, rust-coloured knee breeches that its pupils have to wear. Going to school, as opposed to school going to you, was something new for the royals – a break with tradition that was driven as much by a need to be like the 'typical British family' as by the Queen's desire to save her son some of the frustrations she had experienced by home education.

Of course, this attempt to give the future king a 'normal' education with other children of his own age was largely doomed from the outset: it was impossible to achieve simply because he wasn't a normal child, but the heir to the throne. Nevertheless, he did get to play sports with other boys, got to see and use money and even travelled on public transport. All round the experiment wasn't a bad one. The Prince was shy but polite and kind. He mixed with the other pupils quietly, and seemed quite happy. He also made reasonable progress with his studies, with the exception of maths, a subject that was to torment him throughout his schooldays and beyond. His school report for the Lent term of 1957 read: 'Reading – very good indeed. Good expression. Writing – Good. Firm, clear well formed. Arithmetic – Below form average. Careful but slow – not very keen. Scripture – shows keen interest. Geography – good. History – loves this subject. French – shows promise. Latin – made a fair start. Art – Good, and simply loves drawing and painting. Singing – A sweet voice, especially in the lower register. Football – enjoying the game. Gymnastics – Good. Henry Townend, Headmaster.'

This report is testimony to the knowledge Colonel Townend displayed about his royal pupil as it is to the consistency of the Prince: it was those subjects of art, history and scripture that were already arousing his interest. The imagination and intelligence were there, but they were as yet submerged under a cloud of low self-confidence, which was not helped by the fact that he was frequently away from school due to colds, flu and, on one occasion, in the spring of 1957, the need to have his tonsils removed. The young Prince, following his operation, was presented with his now detached tonsils in a jar and insisted on taking them everywhere with him. Dimbleby reports that, 'At Windsor he had conceived affection for the little chapel which lay between the Grand Corridor and St George's Hall. There, alone, he would stand in the pulpit delivering sermons to an imaginary but rapt congregation.' So taken by his own performance on one occasion, the Prince swept out into the Grand Corridor – forgetting that he had left his tonsils on the pulpit.

So his early education was to show cautious progress rather than the scholastic vigour of some of his ancestors such as Henry VIII or Edward VI. If not born to be king, I rather think, this prince might have wished to enter the church, and could have been quite successful. His tenderness, spiritualism and desire to help his fellow man would have stood him in good stead. On the other hand, the 'Camillagate' tapes might have rocked the Church of England somewhat!

At the age of eight, the heir to the throne was quietly settling into school life, while experiencing an extraordinary home existence by most other boys' standards. The weekdays were spent at Buckingham Palace, weekends, in term time, at Windsor Castle and the holidays at either Sandringham in the winter or Balmoral in the summer. And in a more carefree age, with few fears of attack from terrorists, kidnappers or intrusion from the press, the young Prince was free to explore these great houses and their grounds, which he did with much enthusiasm.

Balmoral was to become his favourite. He, like Queen Victoria before him, found it almost impossible to tear himself away from a place that, despite its vastness, he came to know so well that he could picture every tree and brook for miles around. He quickly came to love this intimacy with nature, something a city dweller might find impossible, as Diana later did, to understand as being anything other than solitude and boring loneliness. It was here that he was most happy – playing football in the yard behind the pantry, cycling to the village shop with only a discreet policeman in the background, picnicking with his parents and their guests and even playing games with them. Once the family had departed the royal train at Ballater Station and smiled and waved at the photographers, they were but minutes away from the seclusion of this royal estate, and a holiday atmosphere would break over the whole household in a fashion not repeated in any of the other royal residences.

Taught to shoot and fish by his father, he was to grow up steeped in these rural pursuits and see them as quite natural. It also allowed him a much needed chance to get a little closer to his father and attempt to please a demanding man, who could still so easily destroy his sensitive son's fragile confidence. For the Duke of Edinburgh continued to be most concerned about the contrast in his children's personalities. Princess Anne was noisy, wilful and fearless, as second children often are, while Prince Charles was kind, caring and withdrawn. The duke's rough and rude attempts to mould the boy into his idea of a son to be proud of only served to make matters worse, because it drove Charles away from his father and the obvious benefits of a warm relationship with him, and further into his shell.

However, instead of realising this, the implacable duke chose to blame one of the children's nannies, Helen Lightbody, for undermining his preferred regime for the young Prince. He became of the opinion that she was the main impediment to the Prince's development. He perceived that she favoured the Prince over the Princess and rewarded his gentle nature, while punishing his daughter for displaying the boisterous spirit he longed to see in his son. There was an inevitable disagreement between the two and, naturally, it was Miss Lightbody who departed.

But this summer of 1957 at Balmoral was a marvellous and immensely happy time for the young Prince. He not only got to join the shooting parties for the first time, but also grew close to the keepers, gillies and foresters who cared for the place so professionally. For their part they discovered that the heir to the throne was a keen pupil and a country boy at heart. He was to learn from them about grouse, red deer and salmon as well as other creatures and the environment in which they lived.

He was also happy because a place can seem so special and a time so happy when one is aware of gathering storm clouds. The young Duke of Cornwall would have to leave Balmoral in September to go to boarding school, and it was a thought that filled the shy little boy with much trepidation. Cheam School in Berkshire housed some eighty boys between the ages of eight and fourteen. The school had been founded in the seventeenth century for the education of the sons of the aristocracy. It became known in the nineteenth century by the nickname of 'The Little House of Lords' and boasted Lord Randolph Churchill, father of Winston, among its pupils. In 1930, an exiled Greek prince living in Paris was sent to the school as a nine-year-old. Prince Philip of Greece (as the Duke of Edinburgh was known at that time) arrived knowing little English and little about the British. Cheam had served him well and helped turn him into the tough character he was now. It was therefore deemed by him to be ideal for his son. Some time later he was to write, 'Children may be indulged at home, but school is expected to be a Spartan and disciplined experience in the process of developing into self-controlled, considerate and independent adults. The system may have its eccentricities, but there can be little doubt that these are far outweighed by its values.'

The headmaster Peter Beck had written to all parents to inform them of the 'great honour' that had been conferred on the school by its being entrusted with the education of the Prince, but he assured everyone that Prince Charles was to be treated just like any other boy. At the start of the third week of September, the Queen and Prince Philip accompanied the heir to the throne to the school, where the headmaster, his wife and business partner were standing outside to greet them as the royal car squeezed through a drive full of police, parents, boys, villagers, reporters and cameramen flashing away like crazy. Treated like any other boy? Well, tomorrow perhaps.

His parents stayed long enough to see where Prince Charles would sleep, but then, after an exchange of a few brief courtesies, the royal car disappeared down the drive and the eight-year-old Prince was left alone. To be so young, in a strange place, with so many unfamiliar older boys who all seem to know each other and the place so well – and who were not always kind to new boys – would have been daunting for any small boy. Many of us have fallen victim to this nineteenth-century British middle-class obsession with banishing little boys from home at an early age and not permitting them back again until they are adult. There is an initial feeling of total despair that can take away the appetite and even cause vomiting, and one wondering why one's parents could do this to you. It is ridiculously referred to, by those who have never experienced it, as homesickness.

The Prince manfully struggled through the early days, keenly reminding himself of who he was while stifling his tears into his pillow at night, lest anyone should hear his dismay.

As a shy boy of little self-confidence, he found it hard to mix, and would paint a lonely image in the playground as he wandered alone while the rest of the school formed into gangs and played happily around him, not noticing his misery. Years later, the Prince would recall that, 'It was not easy to make large numbers of friends ... I'm not a gregarious person so I've always had a horror of gangs ... I have always preferred my own company or just a one to one.'

Even though by today's standards the press were then better mannered and less intrusive, their fascination with the young Prince was a twenty-four-hours-a-day affair and caused the school major problems. The headmaster had to become a public-relations expert overnight but, as he couldn't possibly supply personal details regarding any pupil, let alone Prince Charles, the tabloids took to making up stories. One, concerning the Prince having to sell some of his own personal possessions in order to pay his corner at the end-of-term midnight feast, due to the small amounts of cash sent to him by the Queen, got as far as the US. Delegates of the Retail Candy Stores Institute of America then in conference in San Francisco, passed a resolution to help him out and duly sent him forty-eight tins of candy. They were donated to the Red Cross.

The press attention was thought to be intolerable. Action was called for and so Richard Colville summoned the editors to Buckingham Palace. There, headmaster Beck restated the school's need for privacy, and Colville's warning that unless the press desisted, the Queen would have no alternative but to remove Prince Charles and have him educated in private reinforced this. He told the editors that she had concluded that this would be as much in the interests of the other boys as it was for the Duke of Cornwall. The move was successful, and peace once more descended upon the school.

Like the other boys, the Prince was obliged to write home once a week. Dimbleby reports that most of his letters were 'dutiful'. However, there was one that not only displayed a more selfish objective, it also marked the early years of a relationship that was to become one of the most important in shaping the Prince's future. On 12 October 1957, he wrote to Mountbatten, 'Do you think I could not have the silly-putty for my birthday but please can I have a bicycle if you can.' The First Sea Lord duly obliged and even carefully chose the model personally. His card to the Prince in celebration of his ninth birthday read: 'Your birthday bicycle will be delivered at Xmas. About your birthday present: I don't mind changing the silly-putty for a bicycle, but as a bicycle is much more expensive, it will have to do as a combined birthday and Christmas present from Aunt Edwina and me.'

Clearly this royal prince was not spoiled, and interestingly a major present like a bicycle was politely demanded of a great-uncle rather than his parents. Although this probably reflects more on the fact that this was a different period and since then our wealth and values have changed, it has to be said that the Royal Family hardly ever spoil each other with what they consider to be extravagant presents. For example, Princess Anne once gave her older brother a toilet seat for Christmas.

Before the Prince had been thrown in at the deep end of life at a boys' boarding school, someone had had the presence of mind to think that the heir to the throne might need to be able to protect himself. He had been taught to wrestle and box and could look after himself adequately. If things became physical, he didn't back off. As a result of scrapping he was to be confined to the classroom, ordered to weed the cricket pitch and was twice beaten. I only hope he remembered to tell his father, who would no doubt have been delighted. He was to comment years later, 'I am one of those people for whom corporal punishment actually worked ... We had two headmasters when I was there, which was odd ... They took turns at beating us ... I didn't do it again.'

These were the twilight years of the empire, and Victorian values still ruled in fee-paying, middle-class preparatory schools such as Cheam. This was how things were done there and it was just part of an everyday routine.   The Cheam routine started daily at 7.15 a.m. with the clanging of the school bell. Once washed and dressed, the boys presented themselves individually to the matron who ensured each was clean and tidy. Next came morning prayers, after which the boys, on their way into breakfast, filed past the two headmasters and shook their hands while directly looking them in the eye. This was considered to be part of their character-building programme: it was meant to encourage honesty, openness and confidence. Charles did not need to be taught this. It had been instilled in him from an early age that 'good manners' dictated direct eye contact at all times and, despite his natural shyness, he made sure that he always did it. The habit remains with him today.

One Saturday afternoon during the summer term of 1958, headmaster Beck summoned a group of boys to his study. The Prince was among them. It was the last day of the Empire and Commonwealth Games in Cardiff. The boys were to watch the closing ceremony on television. It was announced that while the Queen was unable to attend in person due to an attack of sinusitis, she would address both the packed stadium and the television audience in a recorded message. Charles's mother appeared on the screen with a simple message: 'The British Empire and Commonwealth Games in the capital ... have made this a memorable year for the Principality. I have therefore decided to mark it further by an act, which will, I hope, give much pleasure to all Welshmen as it does to me. I intend to create my son Charles Prince of Wales today ... When he is grown up, I will present him to you at Caernarfon.'

His chums (despite his introversion, he now had friends in good supply) offered their congratulations – much to his embarrassment. Now there could never be any turning back. He had become His Royal Highness Prince Charles Philip Arthur George, Prince of Wales and Earl of Chester, Duke of Cornwall, Duke of Rothesay, Earl of Carrick, Lord of the Isles and Baron of Renfrew and Great Steward of Scotland. At a later date, Knight Companion of the Most Noble Order of the Garter was also added. The newspapers were most enthusiastic about the Queen's decision, and this appeared to be echoed throughout the land and especially in Wales where his Great-uncle David had been very popular as the last Prince of Wales.

A fortnight later, the Royal Family visited Anglesey in the Royal Yacht en route for Scotland. Once ashore, the Prince was greeted with great enthusiasm. Cheering crowds broke through the police cordons. An excited dog nearly knocked the heir to the throne to the ground. The Prince kept his composure and patted the dog. Prince Philip put a reassuring arm around his son's shoulder in an act of paternal care and both father and son waved to the crowd. The Principality had a new prince, and it was clearly delighted.

In the autumn it was back to school. Prince of a great Welsh nation he might have become, but he was still only nine years of age. Although never very happy at Cheam – he has been quoted as saying that he 'loathed' his time there – he nevertheless went on to do better than most. He had discovered a liking for acting, and was thought to be good at it, his shyness disappearing on stage. He also captained the school's first eleven at soccer and played in the first eleven at cricket (which he liked) and in the first fifteen at rugger (which he didn't). In 1962, after five years at Cheam, he was made head boy. Was this honour bestowed on him because he was the Prince of Wales? Well, it is true that he wasn't the dashing schoolboy hero of a nineteenth-century novel – the academic, sports and leadership qualities that were to come through eventually hadn't really been recognised by this time. But, on the other hand, he was gentle, kind and unusually thoughtful of others – a good example for all and not a bad foundation on which to develop the character of a future king of England. That in itself probably justified the decision.

So, all in all, it had been a steady start, if not a truly brilliant one, for the boy who was born to be king. Even Prince Philip could not complain too much about a son who was in his school's first team at soccer, cricket and rugby and who completed his time there as head boy. However, the immediate future was not looking too bright. His next school, Gordonstoun, where his father had also been as boy, was to prove to be a far more daunting prospect than Cheam. The young heir to the throne would endure many bleak and unhappy terms there.

Chapter Two
Diana: Her Early Years (1961–77)

The story of Diana, Princess of Wales is extraordinary and complex. It is the story of a noisy and chubby little tomboy who grew into a truly beautiful woman. It is the story of a teenage girl who dreamed of marrying the world's most eligible bachelor, did, and as a result stood to become the future queen of England. It is a story of a girl who discovered in her teens that she could bring amazing comfort to the handicapped, the ill and the dying and, to her eternal credit, she did so to very great effect throughout her life. It is a story of a girl who was sometimes unhappily married and whose life was to end far too soon.

However, it is also a story where dark secrets have been concealed, where the truth has been hidden and where the general public's grasp of the real story remains amazingly weak, mainly due to a barrage of inaccurate press reporting. In addition, a host of lurid allegations have been made by authors purporting to support the Princess, before depicting her as a dishonest, mad woman who lived for intrigue, deceit and the wrecking of other women's marriages. They then excuse such behaviour by vilifying others. What has been written by her biographer and butler, to name but two, not only do her a disservice, but also is at times inaccurate and contains much hearsay. The Princess's life, especially that period from the time of her engagement to her death, is worthy of better explanation.

Diana Spencer was born into an aristocratic family. The first Lord Spencer bought his peerage from an impoverished James I nearly 400 years ago. He had made his fortune in the wool trade and then went on to capture the London meat contracts. This made him one of the wealthiest men in the land, so he could easily afford to buy a genealogy from the College of Heralds that apparently traced his line back via the French de Spencers to William the Conqueror. It was not until 1901 that the de Spencer coat of arms was declared to be a fraud and the Spencer pedigree to be false. But by that time the Spencers had been a leading British family for generations, and had played a major role in the affairs of state for more than 100 years before the German relations of the present Royal Family arrived in England.

It was the Spencers who helped put William III on the throne by delivering the support of the nobles who had fought on the parliamentarian side during the Civil War. In return, the new king had to accept a limitation on his powers that his uncle by marriage, Charles II, had fought so hard to re-establish following the restoration of the monarchy in 1660. When William's successor Queen Anne died in 1714, having outlived her seventeen children and thus failing to produce a Protestant heir, it was the Spencers who were among the 'great and the good' who imported the Elector of Hanover from Germany to become George I. Thus the Spencers perceived themselves as being just as great a family as the Windsors and, while being loyal and respectful in public, were anything but in private. The Windsors were 'Germans' that the English aristocracy, with the Spencers at its head, had placed on the throne.

Diana grew up conscious of this history and attitude: she would come to refer to the Royal Family as 'the Germans', a term that she had become familiar with during her childhood. Moreover, the Spencers also had blue blood running through their veins. The family had acquired, by marriage, a descending line from Henry VII and James I; more importantly they were directly related to Charles II. Indeed, Prince Charles, Princess Diana, Sarah, Duchess of York and Camilla Parker Bowles are all distantly related via the Merry Monarch – Charles legitimately and his wife, sister-in-law and second wife illegitimately. As a result, all four were born into a small and elite society of grand and mainly landed families, but only one was to be held to account by accepting the responsibility of kingship. The public looks to love and respect its Royal Family; it does not look to the other families of the court for such a relationship. As a result, those families have always enjoyed much of the privilege without having to accept any of the responsibility. Courtiers have always been able to bask in reflected glory by being close to the Royal Family while living the most comfortable and carefree lifestyle of the landed gentry – a life that, if adopted by the Royal Family, would no doubt lead to calls of 'parasite'.

However, the Spencers, who had never been weighed down by the Windsors' duties of state or need to set a good example, were nevertheless pretty weighed down by their own finances. The sixth Earl of Spencer, Diana's great-grandfather, was a senior courtier. He was lord chamberlain and so helped organise the coronation of George V, but his devotion to the Crown came at the considerable personal cost of neglecting his own affairs. Upon his death in 1922, his son Albert Edward John became the seventh earl and the first for several generations not to attend court. The reason was that, although the House of Spencer appeared to be very rich, the young earl soon realised that if he did not act to save his neglected and decaying heritage, it could disappear under a mountain of debt, mortgages and death duties. Worse, the palace of Althorp in Northamptonshire and the palazzo called Spencer House in St James's Place, which acted as collateral against such debt, were falling into disrepair by the month. Urgent action was called for.

Luckily for Jack, as the seventh earl was known, he had one or two valuable pieces of art in the family. He quickly raised £300,000 (more than £8 million at today's prices) by selling six masterpieces by Reynolds, Gainsborough, van Dyck and Frans Hals to buyers in the United States. This literally stopped the rot. During the war, the major remaining pieces at Spencer House were moved to Althorp to avoid being destroyed by German bombers. This meant that the palace had a stunning art collection. The public was to benefit by this from 1957 onwards when the Earl accepted a government grant and opened his home to them to save the house from dry rot and death-watch beetle.

But even though Jack was preoccupied with saving the Spencer fortune, his wife, Lady Cynthia, kept up ties with the Windsors. In 1936 she was made a Woman of the Bedchamber, and she was later to become a lady-in-waiting to the present Queen. She was still a courtier when Diana, her granddaughter, was born in 1961.

Diana's first home was in the grounds of Sandringham. Park House had been leased from George VI by Lord Fermoy, Diana's maternal grandfather, in the 1930s when he and his wife started a family. Lord Fermoy was a great friend of the king, as was his wife, Ruth, to the queen. Indeed, the friendship between the two women was to remain close for more than sixty years until Lady Fermoy's death. Later Park House was to pass on to the Fermoys' daughter, Frances Roche, Diana's mother.

So in a way Diana was to grow up as the girl next door to the future king of England. However, she would not have been too noticeable as the youngest of three girls: in the minds of the relevant adults she would have been paired off as a possible future bride for Prince Edward or possibly Andrew, leaving them to debate which of her elder sisters would make the better bride for the main catch – the heir to the throne.

Diana's father Johnnie Spencer, Viscount Althorp (so titled as the eldest son of the earl) was educated at Eton, went on to Sandhurst and, as an officer in the Royal Scots Guards, fought with some distinction in Normandy in 1944. Following the war, he was appointed an equerry to the king and held the same post in Elizabeth II's household following her father's death in 1952. In 1953, as a most eligible twenty-nine-year-old bachelor, he met the bright and pretty, if somewhat self-obsessed, Frances Roche on a visit to Sandringham. She was just seventeen and twelve years his junior – ironically the same age difference that separated Prince Charles and Princess Diana. She was clearly swept off her feet by this man with both position and wealth, as was he by her youth, beauty and family background. After a whirlwind romance, the couple were married on 1 June 1954. The service took place in Westminster Abbey – a special honour – and it was attended by 1,700 guests, including nine members of the Royal Family, among whom were the Queen, Prince Philip and the Queen Mother. It was deemed to be the wedding of the year by the press, and the Queen even allowed St James's Palace to be used for the reception.

As would have been expected in those days, the couple immediately set about starting a family, the main objective being the production of a son and heir. However, as sometimes happens, this proved to be easier said than done. In 1955 Frances produced a daughter, Sarah. In 1957 she was blessed with another girl, Jane. The third child was a boy, John, but he was to die within hours of his birth on 12 January 1960. This served to put the marriage under pressure: Johnnie could hardly conceal his disappointment, while Frances was most resentful of being packed off to see obstetricians by her mother and mother-in-law in the belief that there must be something wrong with her. Jack Spencer had built a large bonfire at Althorp to celebrate the birth of a grandson and heir on the occasion of each pregnancy. The next one was to be no different but, instead of a boy, Diana was delivered in 1961. Years later she was to tell Andrew Morton that she was to grow up feeling inadequate as she had come into the world unwanted. This was fanciful thinking by the Princess. Indeed her mother believed that the idea was put into Diana's head by the army of therapists she was to engage in later life. Frances pointed out that Diana was only three when a son and heir was finally produced on 20 May 1964: she had no time to develop any realisation of such feelings within the family, and after the birth of Charles Spencer, the problem disappeared.

However, what Diana could have picked up on was that the production of a son did not cure the tension at Park House. Her mother and father had drifted apart. There were arguments and tales of drink and violence from Frances's friends, and tales of selfish and neurotic behaviour by Frances from the Spencers, some of which were to be supported by her own family. They pointed out that a good wife and mother should be running the family home, whereas Frances seemed only to be concerned with her own happiness, which seemed to be found by leaving the family behind in Norfolk and spending more and more time in London.

So either Frances was a selfish woman and a poor mother and wife, or she was a sensible young woman who found her husband a bore and occasionally violent; having done her duty by producing a son, she had a right to look to her own happiness. And given that her husband was rich and she was financially independent herself, why shouldn't she? More likely, the truth lies somewhere between these two extremes: there are always two sides to every story. What is evident, though, is that the atmosphere at home in Diana's early years might have contributed to her insecurities in later life.

In 1966 Frances met Peter Shand Kydd. He was the heir to a very successful wallpaper business, although not quite as successful as perhaps thought at the time. He was adventurous and intelligent and soon Frances, having made friends with Peter's wife Janet, was able to ensure that the Spencers and the Shand Kydds were seeing each other socially and even holidaying together. Soon it became apparent that Frances and Peter felt a strong attraction for each other. Eventually Peter left his wife and met Frances secretly during her visits to London. She was later to say, 'We realised it was an impossible situation, but what could we do?' Her husband found out and, after some violent confrontations, he seemed to understand that his wife wouldn't give Shand Kydd up and offered her the option of what amounted to an open marriage. She refused, explaining, 'If Johnnie and I had had a better marriage, it wouldn't have happened. But our marriage was not working out. Suddenly, here I was with a chance of real happiness. I made my decision and left.'

So, in September 1967, the Spencers also split up and Frances took the two younger children to London, where she had found a flat in Cadogan Place; but it was unlikely that the children knew about the separation at this point as their father visited at weekends. At

Christmas, when Diana's two elder sisters were home from boarding school, the whole family converged on Park House for the celebrations. However, when the festivities were over, Johnnie refused to allow the children to return to London and so Frances left alone. It is perhaps at this moment that Diana felt the real sense of maternal rejection that she was to claim made her childhood so miserable.

In April 1968 Mrs Shand Kydd sued her husband for divorce on the grounds of her husband's adultery with Frances. In September Frances went to court in an attempt to win custody of her children. Her mother, Lady Fermoy, gave evidence against her and she lost. Johnnie's friends claimed that this was a clear sign that even her own mother did not believe Frances to be a good mother, while Frances's allies countered that her mother loved the Spencer association more than her daughter and was horrified that Frances had run off with a mere tradesman. Johnnie cross-petitioned in court and cited Frances's already proven adultery. He duly won the case and gained custody of the children.

Lady Fermoy was now the villain of the piece to Frances's friends, who claimed that she had betrayed her own daughter in an outdated act of snobbish behaviour that typified her repressed and sinister generation. Diana, having learned this opinion at her mother's knee, used it without compunction in later life. She was to identify the Royal Family with this kind of cynical action while she attempted to portray her own behaviour as classless and sensitive. She sought to cast herself as a caring modern girl who was only a victim of the wicked dark forces of the snooty old order, just as her Bohemian mother had been some thirty years earlier. But might this not be just a case of the old 1960s trick of claiming the moral high ground by association with a classless society, while attacking your enemies for being elitist snobs and relying on the fact that such snobs wouldn't hit back – and thus the truth could remain a secret?

Most of Diana's many biographers have bought into Frances's account and Lady Fermoy went to her grave, without her side of the story being told, a damned woman who was not to be forgiven for the unhappiness that she had brought about for her daughter and grandchildren. Like the Royal Family, she hadn't hit back and therefore was an easy target.

As a result of this bitter divorce and custody battle, Lady Fermoy and her daughter were to experience years of strain. Diana was to grow up blaming her grandmother (rather than the custody battle) for the divorce and her relationship with Lady Fermoy wasn't made any easier by the fact that Diana's charm did not work on the old lady, who believed that she could see through Diana and wasn't afraid to tell her so. But the real question that remains is whether all this domestic upheaval was a reason or just an excuse for some of Diana's more erratic behaviour in later life.

It had been a nasty divorce; but Diana saw lots of both of her parents and was made to feel loved and wanted by them. In June 1969 Frances married Peter Shand Kydd and the children were shuffled between their parents' homes at weekends during term time, while school holidays were divided up equally. The children were also materially spoiled, as often happens in well-off families when parents vie for a position in their children's hearts, and so it is fair to say that every effort was made to give them both love and stability.

Johnnie was probably more successful in this department. His emotions appeared to be more controlled and whatever his inner mood he was consistent in his dealings with the children. However, tapes made by Peter Settelen, Diana's voice coach, in 1992/3 reveal that the Princess thought her father was cold, distant and that he never told her that he loved her. Nevertheless, it must be remembered, as we shall see later on, that these tapes were made at the lowest point in the Princess's life, when she was clearly mentally unwell and her recollections about this period, as with all others, were inconsistent with the facts and also the memories of others. Those who knew the Spencer family during this time remember clearly that the earl loved all of his children, and was a well-balanced parent.

Frances found the situation harder, and although she would speak to the children on the telephone daily and saw them most weekends, this could have a negative effect: on occasion she would sometimes burst into tears and spend time pouring out her problems to them. This had the effect of giving out unpredictable doses of love or stress, and it clearly made an impression on the dramatic side of Diana's character: Diana was to put Prince William through the same experience at an equally young age.

Frances was not to live happily ever after. Not only was she to become a 'semi-detached' mother to her children, but a distance appeared in her second marriage as the passion that she had put so much store by ebbed away. Peter Shand Kydd was to spend more and more time travelling, while Frances preferred to stay in Scotland. In 1988, the couple separated. Frances claimed that she was 'devastated'. Her friends were to explain that the split was at her instigation because she needed more time to herself after she had discovered that he had found another woman. Shand Kydd eventually married a third time, in 1991, to a French woman named Marie-Pierre Palmer. However, his winters were to be spent in Australia with Frances, and she often admitted that he came alone to stay with her in Scotland. By this time Frances had a serious drink problem, which saw her convicted for drink-driving; she was also suffering from an eating disorder.

Theirs was a love affair that had caused much disruption, chaos and heartbreak to everyone it touched. It was to become Diana's self-justification for her own failings. Yet right until the end of her life in 2004, Frances was steadfastly to refuse to accept any blame for what she had done, and insisted that she had no regrets about putting her own happiness ahead of the welfare of her children. Not even during her final illness would she shake her belief that she would not have done anything differently. In her mind she had done the right thing. Her self-justification for everything and her responsibility for nothing were remarkably similar stands to those made by her daughter.

As her childhood progressed, Diana appears to have been a lot happier than she was later to make out. Most remember her as a tomboy who loved animals, climbing trees, eating and swimming (at which she shone), and hated wearing dresses and doing school work (at which she didn't). She was known to be a bit spoiled, and at times attention-seeking, but nothing too serious. However, as she got older some less pleasant elements of her personality began to display themselves more openly. Penny Junor reports in her book *Charles: Victim or Villain* of a local family who didn't think their daughter's friendship with Diana was having a good effect on her: 'A very senior member of the Royal Household, who had a daughter at Riddlesworth Hall prep school with Diana until the age of twelve, volunteered long before things became bad with the Princess that he had made specific enquiries about where Diana would next be going to school, so that he could choose somewhere different for his daughter.'

Indeed, during her first term at her next school, West Heath, Diana was, by her own admission, to delight in the bullying of smaller girls. There is apparently no shortage of her contemporaries who claim to have been reduced to tears by her. In her second year she got some of her own medicine from a number of the older girls. She reacted to this interestingly and bravely by becoming a daring heroine in an attempt to court popularity. She led nocturnal raids on the school's kitchen, or expeditions to enjoy secret midnight swims.

All innocent fun? Perhaps, but such behaviour, which was probably motivated by attention-seeking and an insatiable desire to be loved, was quite disruptive for the staff and a worry for the parents of other girls. As a result the headmistress almost expelled her for such acts, especially as her school work was poor and her teachers found her to be a very different kettle of fish to her more academically bright and better-behaved sisters who had been there before her.

Diana, while being an excellent swimmer and showing a keen interest in ballet, where progress was to be denied by her size, was rather lacklustre at most other disciplines. She apparently added to her disappointing absence of any academic skill by lacking any ambition in the classroom: she showed no desire to improve her position and had great difficulty in concentrating for any length of time. In addition she could also throw violent tantrums if thwarted in her desires. One of her contemporaries at the school enthralled a Knightsbridge dinner party that I attended in 1992 with such tales, explaining how she had even been restrained and locked in her dormitory on one occasion.

This problem was not addressed successfully and was to become increasingly present in her adult life. One exclusive and much respected doctor from London's Sloane Street told me, on the strict understanding that he remained anonymous for obvious professional reasons, that both he and one of his colleagues had been called to attend to the Princess of Wales on more than one occasion following violent tantrums where valuable china, priceless ornaments and even her own person were flung about in a fit of uncontrollable rage. At Highgrove, she had once had to be physically restrained before she could be sedated.

On the other hand her teachers have never reported, as far as I am aware, scenes of such a serious nature; they claim that much of her behaviour could be put down to the usual things that happen to young girls: her sisters were a hard act to follow, she had come to the school late when coursework had already started and she really wasn't interested in obtaining an academic education anyway. Instead of laying all of her problems at the door of a troubled home life, most believe that it was a combination of all these factors and that for much of her time at the school she appeared to be a happy girl, even if at times somewhat disruptive.

This is in stark contrast to what Diana was later to recall when dictating her story to Andrew Morton. At thirty she was to tell him that her childhood was both lonely and extremely unhappy. This version stands alone and is opposed by her teachers, friends and family. There are bound to be unhappy days in all childhoods, perhaps more so if you come from a broken home, and Diana was certainly not short of traumatic days when faced with her mother's emotion. But it is the clear exaggeration of it all in Diana's version of events that stands out.

By the time Diana Spencer was entering her teens there were signs of her being difficult and somewhat manipulative; some say that at times she was quite violent and cruel. She had to explain this to herself as much as find a defence against those who knew of such problems – and such problems were well known within the family circle. Diana's grandmother, Lady Fermoy, described her granddaughter as a 'dishonest and difficult girl' and, during the last weeks of her life in 1993, admitted that she should have shown the courage to warn the Prince of Wales about Diana's character before he married her. In addition, Diana's father, who died in 1991 and who loved his daughter deeply as she did him, also said that he had been wrong not to have made Diana's mental difficulties clear to the heir to the throne.

Then why didn't they? Well, blood is thicker than water, and perhaps they believed that on becoming Princess of Wales – her declared dream and goal in life as well as being a great honour – she would simply be cured and things would get better. Perhaps most of us would have done the same if placed in this position. Here is a beautiful girl and dearly loved daughter who suddenly has the chance of becoming the future queen of England. This is something that the Spencers had wanted and felt that they had deserved for generations, and about which the Fermoys could only have dreamed until then. Who would have wished to deny her the chance?

In April 1975 Jack Spencer died at the age of eighty-three. Johnnie Spencer was now the eighth earl, and Althorp was his. He was naturally saddened by his father's death, but by inheriting his father's title, his children were automatically elevated to their own titles of lord or lady, and understandably the young Diana was delighted by the news. She had already acquired the nickname 'Duch' – her brother Charles explained that this was short for 'Duchess' after the leading cat in Disney's *The Aristocats* – and she had always been most conscious that one day she would be titled. She was not particularly snobbish about it, just delighted to have been born an aristocrat in a romantic sort of way. Penny Walker, Diana's music teacher, remembers her hearing the news of her grandfather's death at school: 'She rushed along the corridor with her dressing gown billowing out behind her, saying, "I'm a lady, I'm *Lady* Diana now." She was so excited.'

Norfolk was soon abandoned in favour of the Northamptonshire stately home which boasted 121 rooms and 13,000 acres of good-quality farmland. And, as his father had over fifty years before him, the new earl was forced to raid the art collection in order to settle the death duties which arose as a result of his father's death. Tax planning was obviously not the boom industry that it is today, and with the Labour Chancellor Denis Healey talking of 'squeezing the rich until the pips squeaked', two van Dycks had to be sold to deal with the £4 million pounds of tax that became due.

This was to be a period of change in Diana's life. On the positive side she was now Lady Diana Spencer and her family lived in one of the finest houses in England; on the other hand she was to learn that she was going to have to share this wonderful new home with daddy's new girlfriend. The earl had met Raine, Countess of Dartmouth and daughter of the famous and prolific *grande dame* of romantic novels, Barbara Cartland, while she was working on a book herself entitled *What Is Our Heritage?* They soon began an affair. Lord Dartmouth divorced his wife in 1975 and in July 1976 Johnnie married her, making her Countess Spencer. As a result Raine was part of the move to Althorp and got to get her feet under the table there at the same time as Diana and her siblings. Given her strength of character, it wasn't long before she was organising both the house and the estate.

The earl seemed pleased by this, relieved and somewhat grateful. Diana, her brother and sisters were exactly the opposite. They hated Raine from day one. They resented her hold over their father, her iron will, her undoubted ability that put her beyond criticism and the fact that, now that it was at last their turn to be lords and ladies of their own palace, Raine had come into their life and they were little more than pawns in her grand scheme of things. Raine is said to have complained on more than one occasion that, 'Those children made my life hell on earth.' A family friend agreed and added that, 'Their capacity for hatred was frightening.'

Diana's sister Sarah seemed to sum up her siblings' position when she announced, 'I would sooner take up residence in Lenin's tomb, cuddling his corpse for warmth, than have Raine Dartmouth for my stepmother.' Little by little the children became more distant from their father, and this only served to strengthen Raine's position within the household. Diana and her younger brother were away at school and only spent a part of their holidays at Althorp, and Jane and Sarah seemed to visit less and less. None of them were ever to make any effort to conceal their dislike of this formidable woman who had stolen their father's affections and so much of his expenditure budget. Upon the earl's own death in 1991, his son and heir Charles Spencer, now the ninth earl, and his youngest sister, the Princess of Wales, are reported to have gathered up Raine's clothes, put them into large black bin bags, taken them to the top of Althorp and thrown them down the giant stairwell.

Their treatment of Raine was not an act of support for their mother, as Lady Sarah Spencer-Churchill, daughter of the Duke of Marlborough and cousin of Sir Winston Churchill, pointed out to Lady Colin Campbell in *The Real Diana*: 'Close as they were to their mother, Diana and Charles never had the sympathy for Frances that they should have. Especially when you stop to consider that she was an abused wife… It struck me that she [Diana] didn't want the emotional burden of a distressed mother. Diana could be very hard-hearted when her own feelings were at stake. Very self-protective. In that respect, the woman remained very much the sort of person the little girl had been.'

Sarah Spencer-Churchill knew the Spencer children very well, and, with the possible exception of Jane, thought that on occasion they could be selfish, cruel and vengeful.

Now well into her teens and still doing poorly in class, Diana's teachers were delighted to discover a sphere in which she excelled. West Heath had agreed to send a group of girls to Darenth Park, a large hospital for the mentally and physically handicapped. Diana was among the first to volunteer. As a result she became part of a team of girls who would regularly visit this huge, daunting, Victorian Gothic building isolated in lonely countryside and surrounded by imposing walls. Once through the giant main doors, they came face to face with the patients, often severely handicapped, who would be waiting there for them, their excited voices echoing around the great hall.

Everybody quickly understood that Diana was special and excelled in communicating with these people. She never had to be reminded that physical contact was important and so, when dancing with those in wheelchairs, Diana would naturally use her undoubted dancing skills to bend down and, having taken the wheelchair's arms in her hands, would proceed to dance backwards in order that she could face the person in the chair. Other girls just tended to wheel the chairs around from the back to the rhythm of the music, which was a less satisfying experience for the patient. All the girls were attempting to do something good, but Diana clearly had a natural talent for communication with the ill and so, as she freely gave, she seemed to receive a warm contentment herself, which was richly deserved.

Years later she would make similar visits to other such establishments, motivated by a desire to give and receive instant emotional contact. She could immediately understand a total stranger's innermost feelings, and both she and the stranger would appear to draw strength from that moment; and then she was gone, having left behind a warm glow of human kindness. It has been claimed by some journalists that this was little more than a ghoulish desire to satisfy her morbid curiosity. But there is no evidence to support this unfair notion, and in any case both parties were to benefit from these visits greatly, not just Diana.

In 1995, in that unfortunate *Panorama* interview, Diana said, 'I know I can give love for a minute, for half an hour, for a day, for a month, and I want to do that.' There were those who immediately doubted that a wilful and spoiled girl from a very privileged background could do any such thing. They were quite wrong: she could, and had a very real need to.

Diana suffered from low self-esteem and, as a result, at times from an acute inferiority complex. This was not helped by the fact that she failed every one of her O level exams, despite having taken them all twice. This would have been an extremely poor performance for an under-privileged child attending some violent inner-city ghetto school; for a girl enjoying Diana's standard of private education, it was nothing short of pitiful, and Diana was most conscious of the failure. She became all the more aware of it once she was surrounded by the well-read and highly educated members of the court, palace employees and in particular Prince Charles's friends. They were shocked by how little she knew, while she, now feeling the pressure, started to believe that they were laughing at her dimness. As it happens, there is no evidence that they were, especially as Charles's robust defence of his wife forbade any such behaviour in the early years of their marriage. But telling Diana so would have been of no consequence in her state of mind.

The chronically ill, the poor and the dying were not going to laugh at her. They loved her, admired her and she could give to them and they were always so very grateful. She didn't feel inferior and self-conscious with them. She wanted to give and they wanted to take and she was uplifted by the emotional experience that often seemed to free her from her mind's self-imposed shackles. It recharged her emotional batteries and eased her pain almost like a desperately needed drug. And whatever else the Princess of Wales was about, she can never be charged with anything but the highest praise possible for the comfort and pleasure that she bought to people who needed a cuddle and a little human warmth during their time of trial. Nothing that she did in her private life should ever be allowed to detract from that, and for confirmation of this one has only to turn to the relatives of those she visited or the members of the medical world or charities with whom she worked.

Years later, during the lowest point of her mental discomfort, she was to recall on tape the occasion when she first met the Prince of Wales, who was dating her sister Sarah at the time: 'I remember meeting him and feeling desperately sorry for him ... That my sister was wrapped around his neck, 'cause she's quite, um, a tough old thing – if she had blinkers on she'd get what she wanted ... I couldn't care two hoots who Charles was. I thought, Poor old thing. But I wasn't impressed with anything around him.'

Like so many of Diana's other recollections, this simply was not true. As the dormitory walls of her year at West Heath saw horses replaced by pop stars, Lady Diana's pin-up wasn't a singer or an actor but Charles, Prince of Wales.

There was nothing so very strange about this. In late 1970s this man in his late twenties was widely regarded as the most eligible bachelor in the world. His image was dashing, athletic and daring. The tabloids, who were then fattening him up with praise for a slow twenty-year roasting later, called him 'Action Man'. He had served in the RAF, the Royal Navy and the Fleet Air Arm, and had put himself through their toughest training courses often in double-quick time. He rode horses competitively, played polo like a cavalry officer, dived with killer whales and occasionally threw himself out of aeroplanes. As a result, he was often seen on the nation's television screens or in the newspapers dressed, in all the uniforms needed for these pursuits, like the military toy doll from which the press had derived his nickname. He was also a good skier and immediately took up windsurfing when the sport was first introduced to the UK at that time.

He cut a dark, handsome, tanned and muscular figure, and was more often than not seen with a glamorous woman on his arm – pop singers, actresses, models and of course the best that the British aristocracy could muster, including the Duke of Wellington's descendent Lady Jane Wellesley and the extremely beautiful Davina Sheffield.

Property developer Peter Palumbo has known the Prince of Wales since they were teenagers. They played polo together at Windsor, and he went on to become a close friend and confidante of the Princess of Wales and was most supportive of her during her difficult times following the couple's separation and divorce. He told Tim Clayton and Phil Craig for their book *Diana: Story of a Princess* that, 'He had all the aces – he had everything. He was the future King of England, he was wealthy, he was good looking, he was intelligent, he was sporting, he was a man of action, and he was a very considerable person. He was immensely eligible. I thought the Prince of Wales was quite wonderful. I mean, he was funny, he was obviously full of his responsibility in terms of public duty, but he was amusing and he was kind.' The press and society speculated wildly about whom he might marry, and with every passing year as a bachelor the speculation became even more fevered.

This description, which is undoubtedly true, is in direct contrast to the image of the shy little lad at Cheam. The change is a measure of how far his own determination had propelled him forward, and it is also an indication how his own frailty, coupled with a constant barrage of unfair media criticism, could throw him back again during the worst years of his marriage. For these were the golden years of Prince Charles's image in the media. His was to go on from here and do much excellent work, but following his marriage most of it would either go unnoticed or be ridiculed by the press.

But then his star was in the ascendancy, and the teenage Diana was not alone in her crush: many girls from her year at West Heath remember discussing the future and whom they might marry. They all expected to marry well, but it was totally understood that the greatest catch from every perspective was Charles Windsor, the handsome Action Man who would be king of England.

Diana could already claim with total justification that there were close ties between her family and his. But during the summer of 1977, while she was busy – or perhaps not so busy – failing her O levels, her hero became a close friend to her sister Sarah. This was not such a romantic attachment as has previously been suggested: the Prince was helping Sarah get over the break-up of her relationship with Gerald Grosvenor, and it is doubtful that he ever contemplated more than friendship. However, from Diana's point of view the exciting thing was that the Prince of Wales was actually dating her sister, and as a result she might get to meet her hero. In the autumn, Charles accepted an invitation to stay at Althorp for a shooting weekend. It was November, and the sixteen-year-old Diana was now resitting all her previously failed exams. However, revising would have to wait – she wasn't going to pass up on this chance, and she made sure she was back at home for the weekend.

The couple's first meeting was in a ploughed field near the village of Nobottle. He almost certainly would not have thought of her in romantic terms on that first meeting, but he did notice her. He later commented that she was 'jolly' and 'bouncy', and was impressed by how easily she had chatted away to him. She was still, understandably, a noisy and slightly plump teenager who lacked the level of maturity a twenty-nine-year-old would have been looking for, and no doubt at that time he hadn't noticed the legs that would go on to sexually motivate the future king of England. Many, many years later – not too long before her death – Diana was to comment, in answer to a question from Patrick Jephson, her private secretary, on why she looked so happy, 'Charles has just told me that he'd forgotten how wonderfully long my legs were.'

As Lady Diana was growing up and Prince Charles was enduring his miserable time at Gordonstoun, before enjoying mainly better times at university and in the services, the kingdom was busy discarding an empire abroad while welcoming social change at home under the dark clouds of one economic crisis after another. The 'new Elizabethan age' of 1950s recovery was long forgotten by the mid-1960s.

Having won the Second World War, it now seemed certain that

Britain was to lose the peace. It seemed incapable of competing with its overseas competitors on the grounds that it paid itself too much to do too little. One factor that prevented Britain from competing effectively with its overseas rivals was the entrenched position of the trade unions, which had been given unique legal privileges in the Trade Disputes Act of 1906, and had used them regularly ever since. The incoming government in 1951 spoke of dealing sternly with the unions and of repealing the 1906 Act. (The Heath Government in 1970 and the Thatcher Government of 1979 also campaigned with the same ideals.) In the end, however, the Tories backed off from confrontation. The Minister of Labour, Sir Walter Monckton, took on a role that meant maintaining close relationships with the TUC, and setting up many more courts of inquiry that usually gave the unions whatever they were asking for. As a result the British disease of inflationary pay settlements with little advance in productivity became entrenched. By the 1960s, Britain's uncompetitiveness was beginning to cause ever more frequent sterling crises, as foreign holders of sterling worried alternatively about inflation, balance of payment deficits, and wildcat strikes.

The new Labour Administration of 1964, heralded in Prime Minister Harold Wilson's promise of a 'white-hot technological revolution', adopted the same weak approach, with strikes being settled – always in the union's favour – informally over beer and sandwiches at Number Ten.

For every business inflation had become the norm, although during the 1950s and 1960s it averaged 4 and 5%, apart from two bad years early in the 1950s when the Korean War caused an explosion in the price of commodities and pushed the rate up to over 9%. Nevertheless, the overall effect was corrosive. By 1970, the 1950 pound was worth less than ten shillings, or 50p as it would become with decimalisation. Anything needing replacing would cost twice as much, in some cases more, and wage rates had risen much faster than the retail price index. Therefore when business was renewing capital equipment it needed a great deal more profit to do so.

By 1966, and after only eighteen months in power, Wilson, who hardly had a workable majority in the House of Commons, cut and ran for the polling stations. He was rewarded with a large majority and thanked the electorate by imposing swingeing public expenditure cuts and tax increases in July of that year. However, the British economy failed to improve and was hit by another sterling crisis in the autumn of 1967 – partly brought about by the closing of the Suez Canal in the Six-Day War between Egypt and Israel. This forced the Labour government to devalue the pound from $2.80 to $2.40, and confirmed them in the mind of the electorate once more as the 'party of devaluation'. It was seen as a major national humiliation, made worse by Wilson talking on national television as though it was some kind of victory for common sense. He was to regret bitterly making his now famous 'this doesn't affect the pound in your pocket' statement.

Moreover, it could only have ever been a victory of any sort if the necessary action was to be taken to restrain wage rises and improve managerial efficiency by allowing market forces to rule without the interference of government. Unfortunately, Britain was to wait many more years and suffer many more crises and humiliations before those conditions necessary for economic success were to be brought about by Margaret Thatcher.

In the meantime, Britain was not ready for any such harsh realities. The Windsors, and to a lesser extent the Spencers, might not have been participating, but most of the rest of the country had decided to have a 'love-in' led by the now all-powerful baby boomers. The 1960s was a time of youthful rebellion. In place of the staid teenagers of the 1940s and the tough Teddy-boy thugs of the 1950s, the predominant theme of the 1960s was that of more (on face value at least) tolerant mods, who became notorious for their clashes with the more raucous rockers at seaside resorts each bank holiday. Then the 'flower people' took over: clothing became wild and bohemian, and for girls much more daring with skirts getting shorter and shorter. 'Free love' became the new slogan as the pill became widely available.

The new heroes and heroines of the day were rebellious and, above all, young. The old were considered to be staid, unsexy, snobbish and had been responsible for nothing but war after war. There was no more powerful symbol than the Beatles, with Paul McCartney then considered to be the most talented (as opposed to John Lennon following the latter's death) and his Beckham-like effeminate appearance appealing to boys and girls alike. Permissiveness was the rage and self-expression the god. Traditional disciplines, conveyed by parents, policemen, church leaders, school teachers, employers and any other symbol of authority, were to be disobeyed and derided. The country has never recaptured those pre-1960s values and disciplines, despite the fact that opinion polls continually tell us that a majority of people wish it could.

In 1966, England won the football World Cup and soon the new enthusiasm for the game saw the mods and rockers turn into football supporters: soccer violence was born as a new kind of tribal warfare, and welcomed by a generation brought up with few real wars to fight. The British achieved world-leader status in football violence – as they did in most things decadent during the 1960s – and became deservedly famous for it.

The Beatles, the Rolling Stones, free love, pot, flower power, Carnaby Street and the King's Road made Twiggy's mini-skirted London the swinging capital of the world. Bonnie and Clyde turned up on the cinema screens and became a cult as anti-heroes. Even the good guys became more ruthless and violent, with Clint Eastwood leading the way as America tried to catch up. *Hair* arrived on stage, boasting full-frontal nudity as the kids of the day were rushing towards rebellion, tearing down accepted standards, mocking tradition and saying 'no' to everything their parents were a part of.

And revelling in this newfound permissive society, keen to learn how to exploit it by constantly striving to find the seediest side to anything and so plunging their profession into new depths of immorality, were the editors of the tabloid press. Little did they know that the matching of the boy born to be king with an aristocratic girl who would come to be seen the world over as a beautiful version of Mother Theresa would present them with so many opportunities for mischief ...

Chapter Three
The Making of a Prince (1962–70)

As Prince Charles's days at Cheam were drawing to a close, there was no shortage of advice coming from all quarters as to where the future king of England should be educated next. Indeed, it became a source of constant speculation in the press. The popular choice was Eton, often the first choice of British aristocrats, Conservative politicians and those from home or abroad who wished to have their children network with the crème de la crème of British society.

But it was only idle speculation: Prince Philip had already decided where his eldest son was to go to school next. As usual the Queen had left the decision to her husband, and it was no surprise to anyone who knew him that his choice was Gordonstoun, the school he himself had attended after Cheam. It had, after all made him who he was today, and no doubt its style would toughen up 'the boy'.

Such a decision might not have surprised anyone who knew the Royal Family, but it did take the rest of the world by surprise. Journalist Peregrine Worsthorne had to explain to his American readers, 'What is unique about Eton is not the way it teaches Latin or maths but the fact that virtually all its pupils come from the upper class or upper middle class ... Thus the significance of the decision not to send Prince Charles there, and not to have him educated by private tutors, but to send him instead to Gordonstoun is ... that he will be the first monarch to be educated in an institution which is fundamentally classless.'

This statement not only reflects wonderfully the thinking behind the 1960s passive revolution, it is also complete nonsense. It would be true to say that Gordonstoun students were distinguished by diversity as opposed to uniformity as in the case of Eton, but the fees at Gordonstoun were higher and thus the students were just as upper class or upper middle class as those at Eton or Harrow. The major difference was that Gordonstoun attracted a different sort of boy, and that was largely because it had different aims.

Eton, Harrow and other public schools were there to provide an excellent academic education and give the sons of those who could afford the fees the chance to grow up with people who would be useful to them in later life – a sort of disciplined 'old boys' network' that would stand a chap in good stead throughout life, provided that he

The King and Di

learned to play by the rules. Discipline was thought to be essential and, until the 1970s, many of these schools were run like the Royal Navy at the time of Lord Nelson. Form and rules were supposed to turn out very uniform young men to run the Empire. This idea had really been the brainchild of the eighteenth-century emerging middle classes as opposed to the aristocracy, and was born on the back of those clean-living Protestant family values that were to become so popular in the nineteenth century and so very unpopular during the second half of the twentieth. Team games were thought to be important, and the needs of the team were always perceived to be greater than those of the individual. Self-sacrifice for God, king, country and colleagues was the order of the day. This is where the British 'stiff upper lip' was born and put to good effect during the Empire years. However, the gentlemen these establishments turned out so well for the Empire found it harder to adapt to the new demands of managing a poorly performing British economy during the post-war years, and this in itself played a part in giving rise to the Thatcher meritocracy.

On the other hand, Gordonstoun and its more expensive and even harsher unofficial Swiss offspring Aiglon, which had the misfortune to educate me, were founded on very different principles and expected to get very different results. The individual was most important. He must learn to respect other team members, but above all he must be true to himself and God. Character-building and high individual principles were sought rather than academic qualifications, although of course exams were sat. The result was that Gordonstoun tended to attract boys whose fathers were resistant to the British public-school system, or who were perhaps not well enough developed academically to enter those schools and would thus benefit from the opportunity provided to develop strong character traits of leadership brought about by the tough, Spartan life.

As a result, individual boys, poorly behaved boys, boys not blessed with academic genius or good health were sent from all over the world to either Gordonstoun or Aiglon and more often than not had but one thing in common: their fathers were extremely rich. When I was at Aiglon at about the same time as Prince Charles was at Gordonstoun, my friends' fathers ran and owned much of Cadbury Chocolates, Burton Tailors and Singer Sewing Machines, while others were the sons of famous actors, Hollywood directors, US politicians and even five-star generals. I was quite famous with my peers for having a mysterious father – the mystery being that nobody had ever heard of him.

So the social class of a boy at Gordonstoun was the same as at Eton, but the breed very different. As a result Worsthorne wasn't so very far from the mark when he reflected in the same article, 'there is clearly a strong case for his not growing up exclusively in the company of an upper class which has long ceased to fulfil its proper function'. Social change was bound to accelerate as a result of a doomed empire and its order being overtaken by the flower-power generation. At Gordonstoun they were still all upper class, but at least they were individuals and not the clones turned out at that time by the more usual British public school, catering for an empire that no longer existed.

Prince Charles was to admit many years later that he did benefit from a regime that took a tremendous amount of his parents' money each term in order to treat him like a prisoner in a cold and damp camp. After all, the school produced at the end of it a tougher young man than those of his peers who had ended up at Eton. Aiglon did the same for me. But like him, it took me years to admit it; such was our misery at the time.

Gordonstoun was established on the shores of the Moray Firth in northeast Scotland in 1934 by Dr Kurt Hahn, a refugee from Nazi Germany. He modelled the school on one founded in 1919 at Salem in southern Germany by Prince Max of Baden as a result of Germany's collapse at the end of the First World War. Prince Max had appointed Hahn headmaster and charged him to 'build up the imagination of the boy of decision and the will-power of the dreamer so that in future wise men will have the nerve to lead and men of action will have the vision to imagine the consequences of their decisions.'

Kurt Hahn, like his former employer, was inspired by Plato. He believed that good and wise government could only occur when philosophers became rulers or rulers became philosophers. This could only be achieved by education – not just academic education, but also moral and physical training of the mind, the body and in particular the character. Hahn knew that it was most unlikely that he could change the world enough to appreciate his point of view. However, he believed that if he could establish his ideals in the minds of the fee-paying students at his school who came from the elite of their generation, he might construct an egalitarian society free from internal hierarchies other than merit and a character built on self-reliance and self-discipline. As a result he would be able to send his graduates into the world in order to change it for the better. In this way he could believe that the accident of birth into financial privilege should not inhibit a commitment to social equality. Indeed, as his pupils were mainly from the ruling classes, he came to see their privileged position as an advantage because if he was successful in converting them to his way of thinking, it made future change in the world order more likely.

Although the Prince of Wales was to experience the unhappiest years of his life at Gordonstoun, it is easy to see that some of his future attitudes, habits and even philosophies owe more than a little to the Gordonstoun experience. Indeed, if Kurt Hahn were alive today, I rather think that he would have been very proud of a philosopher prince who had the courage of his convictions and yet retained a kindly attitude to his fellow man.

Prince Charles was delivered into this Spartan world by his father, allocated to Windmill Lodge, one of seven houses scattered through the grounds, and abandoned to his fate. Like the other houses, Windmill Lodge was a wooden hut that had been acquired from the RAF as temporary accommodation years before, but never replaced. At night the windows were kept open by order, and if a student was unlucky enough to have been allocated a bed near to one, if the weather was poor, which it often was, he awoke to a rain-soaked bed in the summer or one covered in snow in the winter. Prince Charles was one of the unlucky ones: his first bed was directly beneath a window. There were fourteen boys crammed into a dormitory, all having to sleep on the crudest of wooden beds. There was no time or space for privacy. This proved to be a bigger burden upon the shy Prince of Wales than on some of his more outgoing colleagues.

The Gordonstoun day began, irrespective of season or weather, with early-morning physical training, followed by a two-minute cold shower. At Aiglon, having done ten minutes' PT in a blizzard at 4,000 feet in the Alps, the obligatory two-minute freezing shower seemed to last forever. I expect it was just as bad, if not worse, at Gordonstoun as the chill, damp sea mist blew in from the Moray Firth. Initially, the daily routine had been organised around an elaborate structure of self-supervision with boys monitoring their own PT, cold showers and personal hygiene. It was believed that this led to self-reliance and that a boy should learn that to cheat the system was to cheat himself. However, by the time Prince Charles arrived at the school nearly thirty years later, it had been recognised that self-supervision works much better if it is itself supervised!

By 1962 the reigns at Gordonstoun had been passed on to Robert Chew, who had taught at Salem and had been chosen to keep the 'good work' going upon Hahn's retirement. He shared Hahn's beliefs but, as a remote and even awkward man, he slowly became more and more removed from the school's pulse. As a result, 'God's purpose' at Gordonstoun had somewhat gone awry. A contemporary of Prince Charles, the author William Boyd, was later to write: 'We were not so much members of different houses as of different tribes ... My house, at least when I first joined it, was very hard.' Once the housemasters had retired for the night, the dormitories would erupt into an orgy of brutality that would have had Kurt Hahn spinning over and over in his grave. Gangs of thugs preyed upon the smaller boys, beating them up, stealing their money, eating their tuck and taking their belongings in an atmosphere of real terror.

If a pupil was unlucky enough to be sent with a message from his house to another, he could expect at best humiliation by ridicule upon his arrival, or more likely violent physical assault. The journalist Ross Benson was another contemporary of Prince Charles. He has recorded that new boys were usually greeted 'by taking a pair of pliers to their arms and twisting until the flesh tore open. In all houses boys were regularly trussed up in one of the wicker laundry baskets and left under the cold shower, sometimes for hours.'

This was the quite terrifying prospect that faced any thirteen-year-old boy entering Gordonstoun for the first time. However, Charles, Prince of Wales was not just any boy, and this was to make his predicament a thousand times worse. When he arrived, his housemaster warned the other boys that to be caught bullying the heir to the throne would risk expulsion. This had, unsurprisingly in such a lawless environment, exactly the opposite effect: according to a fellow new boy, Charles was picked upon at once, 'maliciously, cruelly and without respite'.

As Dimbleby observes, a prince – let alone a shy and insecure prince – would have found it hard enough to befriend his peers, but to break through the barrier, which the boys at Gordonstoun had immediately erected around him, was virtually impossible. 'Even to open a conversation with the heir to the throne was to court humiliation, to face the charge of "sucking up" and to hear the collective "slurping" noises that denoted a toady and a sycophant.' And because he was a shy boy, burdened with the responsibility of royalty, he did not feel able to win over his tormentors in the way Lady Diana would do, by being more badly behaved than they were.

Naturally the sports field became the perfect place to take a swing at the heir to the throne. William Boyd would remember overhearing, 'We did him over. We just punched the future king of England.' The Prince took this thuggery on the chin, without complaint and apparently without nurturing enmity. He was far too proud, brave and disciplined to let it show and therefore let his parents down. However, the real extent of his despair can be judged by his letters home. In the middle of his third term he wrote, 'I hate coming back here and leaving everyone at home ... Papa rushed me so much on Monday when I had to go, that I hardly had time to say goodbye to Mabel and June properly ... I've been in bed for the last week suffering from a cold or 'flu, I'm not sure, but I came out on Thursday morning worst luck! It was much nicer in bed. I hardly get any sleep at the House because I snore and get hit on the head the whole time. It's absolute hell.'

In the same letter he writes longingly for his parents' return from an official tour of Australia, of a comforting phone call from 'Granny' and of his desire to see his brother Andrew, before continuing, 'Oh dear it's Monday tomorrow. However, one Monday more means one less, there are only six and a half weeks now. I hope it goes quickly ... I don't like it much here. I simply dread going to bed as I get hit all night long ... I can't stand being hit on the head by a pillow now.'

However, the Prince never dreamed of writing in such a fashion to his parents, or of complaining to his housemaster or anyone one else in authority, so the torment continued unabated well past his second year. Prince Philip did notice that the boy had become more withdrawn, which was the opposite effect to the one he had desired, but decided that it was not his place to interfere, believing that, if given the time, the school would accomplish the job for which he was paying them. He was sadly quite unaware that his son was now at a school where the name and place were the only things in common with the school he had himself attended some thirty years earlier. Prince Philip's Gordonstoun had been a bracing and uplifting experience where the pupils believed in Hahn's ideals and were self-consciously upright in thought, word and deed. Now, smoking and drinking were commonplace, joyriding in stolen cars was not unheard of and shoplifting was a most popular school sport. As the school lurched into the swinging sixties, sex raised its inviting head. An illicit trade in pornographic magazines thrived, and boys graduated from masturbating over these to having sex with consenting part-time kitchen maids by the time they reached the sixth form. The school rules were still the same, but in Philip's day they were to be honoured; in Charles's, the honour with one's peers seemed to come from breaking as many as possible.

The lack of religious retreat was a further hindrance. The young Prince had grown up in the knowledge that his mother was the head of the Church of England and that he would follow her in that role one day. In such an atmosphere, it was natural for him to develop a strong loyalty to God, queen and country and to understand his duty and deference to all three. Consequently, he had developed a strong sense of right and wrong built on Christian principles, as well as a devout belief in God. This seems to have been completely at odds with the vast majority of his peers at the school, who thought that to express any form of religious belief marked you down as a wet. They preferred to worship the Beatles, Bob Dylan and the Rolling Stones. As a result, the Prince was a loner in this regard and was dismayed at what he saw as a pagan atmosphere, which was not helped by the lack of a proper school chapel. He wrote at the time: 'There's hardly any religion … And you should see where we have to have church. It's a sort of hall which is used for films and assemblies and plays, sometimes for football or gymnastics if the weather is too foul for going outside during break. And then one is expected to worship there. It's hopeless, there's no atmosphere of the mysterious that a church gives one …' It must have seemed to him a million miles away from St George's Chapel at Windsor.

Ironically, the Prince's letter also gives a wonderful insight into how poor the facilities were at Gordonstoun. The Queen was paying for one of the most expensive educations that money could buy at the time and yet, unlike most public schools, it did not boast a chapel or theatre; worse, unlike any state school, there wasn't even a gymnasium.

As Charles grew older, and his peers became more mature, so things began to improve. His school life was still not to his liking, but neither was it all misery. One of the strengths of Hahn's doctrine was the belief that every individual has a special talent if nurtured. As a result there was an unusually wide range of extra-curricular activities to choose from. This allowed Prince Charles to spend many happy hours in the art room painting, or at the potter's wheel, or swimming, which like his future wife he was very good at – so good, in fact, that he acquired a life-saving certificate at the public baths in Elgin and took his place in the school's surf-rescue unit. He also became so proficient in a canoe that he could paddle from Hopeman Beach to Findhorn Bay – a distance of some twelve miles but about double that when allowing for wind and tide. In poor weather the trip took the entire day, but the Prince was flushed as much by his achievement as by the sheer exhaustion at its end. He also joined the Coastguard Service and took his turn at the lookout point on top of the cliffs.

In his second year, he joined the crew of *Pinta*, one of two ketches owned by the school. On his first trip in the summer of 1963, he sailed into Stornoway Harbour on the Isle of Lewis. He and four other boys were given shore leave to have dinner and then see a film. Naturally, the four were accompanied by the Prince's detective, Donald Green. As they walked towards the Crown Hotel they began to attract a small crowd. By the time they were in the lounge a larger crowd had gathered outside the main window and flash bulbs were going off as folk jostled to get a photograph. Embarrassed by all the attention, Prince Charles retreated from the room and, followed by his detective, found himself in the public bar. Thirty years later he was to explain to Dimbleby how bewildered being alone in a bar was. 'Everybody was looking at me. And I thought, I must have a drink – that's what you are supposed to do in a bar. I went and sat down at the bar and the barman said, "What do you want to drink?" I thought that you had to have an alcohol in a bar, so I said, "Cherry brandy."' At that very moment a female journalist walked into the bar and so the incident was to become headline news.

At first, the Palace denied the story was true. But it wouldn't go away. Two days later the Palace was forced to withdraw its denial with Richard Colville claiming that the Prince's detective had initially misled him and so he sincerely regretted giving the newspapers incorrect information. The consequences of this were serious for both the Prince and Donald Green. Once back at school, Charles was sent for by the headmaster and was demoted a rank in the school system. This affected his privileges, pocket money and status and was thus humiliating. But all of this paled into insignificance when he discovered what had been meted out to Green. He had been removed from royal duty by the Metropolitan Police. The Prince was horrified and still smoulders about the decision today: 'I have never been able to forgive them for doing that because he defended me in the most marvellous way and he was the most wonderful, loyal splendid man ... I thought it was atrocious what they did.'

Exposed by the media, horrified by Green's sacking and humiliated by his own demotion, the Prince thought that this brush with the press was the end of the world. In reality it was nothing compared to the frenzy that he would have to endure from them in the years to come. The slide from deference to cynicism in the attitude of the media towards the monarchy, and the change from suspicion to complete contempt by Prince Charles towards the media, was a slow process, and there was no one instance when everything changed on both sides. However, the 'cherry brandy affair' undoubtedly played a part.

Despite this ridiculously over-exposed incident, life at Gordonstoun had to go on. The Prince found comfort in improving his pottery and painting skills and he took to music, which, with the exception of his grandmother who could sing a little and his Aunt Margaret who could play the piano after a fashion, was most unusual for a Windsor. He mastered the trumpet well enough to perform in a public recital in Edinburgh when he was fifteen and again when, a year later, he performed in Handel's *Messiah*. He also sang in the choir at Elgin Town Hall, later commenting, 'It was a wonderful thing ... and I'm so glad I did it. There were about 150 to 200 people in the chorus and four soloists from London who were very good. It [Handel's *Messiah*] lasts for two and a half hours and it became unbelievably hot; I, as usual, came out looking like a beetroot. People remarked upon my condition volubly.'

However, it was the cello that became his preferred instrument. Lady Fermoy, Diana's grandmother and an excellent pianist in her own right, recalled after hearing the heir to the throne give an impromptu performance at her home near Sandringham that, 'He could have been a very good cellist because he's such a sensitive musician and he made a lovely sound.' The Prince's opinion of the same recital was summed up in two words: 'I'm hopeless.' This wasn't false modesty, but a genuine feeling of inadequacy that was heightened by his Gordonstoun experiences, the demands of his father and the general failure of his family, with the exception of his grandmother, to offer congratulation or encouragement. As he grew older, he would realise that his great-uncle Dickie Mountbatten was the man to whom he could turn for advice, praise, encouragement and constructive criticism; as a result his fragile confidence would improve. But for now it remained low, and so he developed self-deprecation as a form of self-defence. Despite his own low opinion of his musical ability, however, he was soon playing in weekly concerts at the school.

In 1964 a talented young graduate was recruited by the school to teach English. He was also charged by the headmaster to resuscitate the school play in an attempt to regain the initiative and steer the school back in the right direction. Eric Anderson, who in later life would become headmaster of Eton between 1980 and 1994, set about his task with gusto and decided to put on Shakespeare's *Henry V*. He asked for volunteer actors and Prince Charles applied. Anderson quickly came to the opinion that the Prince was not only the most able reader but probably the best actor as well. However, he did not want to be seen to be favouring the heir to the throne, and was also fearful of what a failure might do to the boy's frail ego. So instead of casting Charles in the lead role, he gave him the part of Exeter. The play was a success, but the audience of local people insisted that it was a pity that the best actor was playing Exeter instead of Henry.

Encouraged by this, Anderson persuaded the headmaster that there should be a winter play as well. In November, a production of *Macbeth* was hastily planned and the Prince of Wales was offered the title role. A few weeks later he was to write, 'We're doing *Macbeth* this term for the school play. Mr Anderson, the producer, only decided to do it after about two weeks of term, so we've had five weeks of rehearsal. I was asked to play *Macbeth* and of course I said "yes". I wasn't going to miss a chance like that. Tomorrow is the first performance – Thursday – and Mummy and Papa are coming to see the third one on Saturday night ... I shall see them on Saturday and Sunday which is marvellous. I do hope they'll enjoy it ... I had a large number of lines to learn, but it's been great fun and it will be VERY sad when it's all over as it will be all too quickly I'm afraid. The costumes are quite good and I have a splendid beard, moustache and bushy eyebrows, the remains of which I've been trying to pick out of my eyebrows and temples since lunch ... I shall be quaking in my boots before I go on stage tomorrow at 8 o'clock.'

He needn't have worried – his performance was sensitive, regal and convincing and amazed the producer, the staff, the pupils and even Papa. Like many other introverted souls, Charles had discovered that once on the stage he could lose himself inside the character he was playing and all self-doubt disappeared.

Once the curtain came down on the last performance, the Prince had to turn his attention to the more tedious task of retaking his Maths O level. In the summer term of 1964 he had worked hard enough to pass his GCE exams in Latin, French, History, English Language and English Literature. This was, by his contemporaries' standards at Gordonstoun, a commendable performance and he had no need to feel any sense of intellectual inferiority. However, Maths, a subject that he had always hated and found difficult, had beaten him again and now had to be re-sat. Once the exam was out of the way, he had the Christmas holidays to look forward to and after that he was to be sent on a sabbatical term to a school in Australia. The Prince seemed uncharacteristically optimistic about the future, possibly because this guaranteed him a longer holiday, or more likely because it took him away from Gordonstoun. He wrote, 'I'm rather looking forward to it, though one doesn't know what to expect ... It is an awful long way away and I shall hate leaving everyone for so long, especially Edward (who was a baby) and Mabel. I hope he isn't too big when I get back. The term begins on 1st February, which gives me slightly longer holidays, although I expect I shall be going several days earlier. I also hope to see something of Australia before I come back.'

He did, and he liked what he saw.

The Duke of Edinburgh, having totally failed to realise that the Gordonstoun he had attended was not the same school to which he had committed his son, began to accept that Charles had not responded to what he mistakenly believed to be the spirit of the school, so it was thought that a spell in Australia might benefit the boy. The impatient Duke of Edinburgh was still determined to mould the romantic, dreaming Prince into his own image. Sir Robert Menzies, the Australian prime minister and a strong anglophile and monarchist, was consulted during an autumn 1965 visit to Balmoral. Menzies recommended a grammar school in Victoria.

As a result, arrangements were made for the headmaster; one Thomas Garnett of the Geelong Church of England Grammar School, to come to England and advise the Duke on what might best suit the young Prince. The duke devoted much time to telling Garnett about his son's personality and what was needed.

Garnett recommended Timbertop, an outback offshoot of the main school in the foothills of the Great Dividing Range. The purpose of the school was 'to develop initiative and self-reliance'; the Duke was pleased as this was obviously just what was needed – an Australian version of Gordonstoun. The same thought had occurred to Prince Charles who was obviously less pleased by the prospect, but he kept his opinions to himself for fear of disappointing his father.

The Prince was to be accompanied by Squadron Leader David Checketts, the Duke's own equerry, in the unofficial role of private secretary and adviser. He was to be treated as a normal student, and the visit was to be private and not official. This was to cause a sharp exchange of letters between Buckingham Palace and Government House in Canberra, who understandably wanted to show off the seventeen-year-old Prince to the Australian people. After all, the Prince was heir to *their* throne, and there was much interest in and affection for him 'down under'. But despite Canberra's sensible case for just one speech in Victoria, the Palace stood its ground and permission was refused.

This refusal played right into the hands of the small but growing anti-monarchical and anti-British group that had found a standard-bearer in the Murdoch press. However, some sanity prevailed and it was decided that a deal would be struck with the media that gave them many photo opportunities in the first week in exchange for privacy thereafter. Accordingly, no fewer than 320 pressmen and women were waiting to cover his arrival. It was a baptism of fire. No member of the Royal Family had ever before been required to deal with such a barrage at such a young age and by this time, in the second half of the 1960s, the old respect and deference of the media, was giving way to a less reverent way of reporting. This was especially the case with the Murdoch media.

The morning was humid and sullen when Charles' plane touched down and he was greeted by a large welcoming party, including the governor general and the prime minister, as well as hordes of men and women with flashguns and notepads. Apart from a short skiing holiday, this was the first time the Prince had been abroad since his trip to Malta as a five-year-old. He wrote to Mountbatten: 'I was getting nervous by the time I got off the plane at Sydney, having been kept on the plane for five or ten minutes watching the goings on outside and the people being lined up at the foot of the steps. However I did nothing as foolish to fall down the steps and land on my face at the bottom. I'm dreading the day when I do that!'

The party then flew on to Canberra, where it was raining. Charles was amazed by the fact that, despite the rain, people had braved the weather to go to the airport to greet him, and even stood sodden along the route to Government House. They all seemed so very pleased that he was there. The Prince was about to discover that, while he might have a fairly low opinion of himself, he clearly mattered to these people. He was most encouraged, and at last a little self-confidence flowed through him.

Prince Charles had worried that Timbertop was going to be another hellhole like Gordonstoun; indeed it had been founded on Hahnian principles, but was designed to be even tougher. The idea was that the 'spotty year' (boys between the ages of fourteen and fifteen) would go from the main school in Victoria to Timbertop to learn self-reliance. They would have to prepare their own food, cut wood for heating and go off on long expeditions into the hills that surrounded the school. There were about 140 'spotties', and they were supervised by a skeleton staff that was supported by a small gang of older boys that included the Prince of Wales. In his capacity as a quasi-NCO, he had charge of three compounds, a total of forty-five boys.

At first the Prince feared the worst, but to his amazement he found the boys and masters friendly, got on very well with his room-mate, enjoyed talking to the chaplain and benefited from the 'beautiful chapel' which was 'made in the shape of a very steep roof going right down to the ground with a window behind the altar reaching also to the ground with a lovely view over the treetops and hills.' More importantly, Timbertop was what Gordonstoun had been when his father had attended, not what it had become during Prince Charles's period. As a result, the benefits that the Duke had wished to bestow on his son by an education at Gordonstoun were at last received, and for the first time Charles started to enjoy school life without being stricken by fearful bouts of homesickness.

Moreover, his new responsibilities helped his newfound self-confidence to flower. His letters home were very different. They told of what he was up to, rather than expressing the bitter pain of missing his family. Not long after arriving, he reported, 'Yesterday we all staggered up Mount Timbertop behind the school. It was very steep and very hot and very thick in places. Coming down was even worse and I think I had blisters on both my big toes. On Friday we also did a cross-country run, which nearly killed me. We have to do two a week and then an expedition each weekend for four weeks, and then it's not compulsory ... In a short time I shall have to go and chop logs and see that no-one cuts off their toes or someone else's head!'

A few weeks later he was to walk seventy miles through the hills in three days, fried by a baking sun in the day and shivering his way through freezing nights as ice formed on his tent. He led the younger boys by fine example and even the Duke must have been pleased by the way his son had adapted so quickly to this new life.

In between these adventures, Prince Charles was expected to teach himself A-level French and History. This he did, but he often found it more congenial to go trout fishing in a nearby stream. After he had completed his four expeditions, he was allowed to spend his weekends visiting the Checketts family, who had taken a small farm in the village of Coldstream just outside the market town of Lillydale, some hundred or so miles away from the school. The Prince adopted the Checketts as his 'Australian family', formed a strong bond with the squadron leader that was to flourish for more than a decade and very much enjoyed the company of his wife Leila and their three children. And they liked having him around, too: David and Leila were much touched by the tenderness with which the Prince treated their children. He would play with them in the garden, read to them at bedtime, amuse them with made-up stories and even comfort them when they were distressed. On one occasion, the Checketts were awoken in the middle of the night by their son Simon, who had a severe attack of croup. They rushed into his bedroom to find the heir to the throne already there – having got the boy upright, he was gently patting his back while softly comforting him. This incident would remind the squadron leader, in years to come when he and the Prince would fall out over something or other, that behind the man throwing a tantrum at that moment was a very kind and tender personality – one that was obviously quite different to that which Diana would describe years later. Moreover, the Prince made them all laugh frequently and sometimes hysterically. On his first visit to the farm, he and Checketts were testing a boomerang. With his first throw, Charles hit himself on the head and fell into a cowpat. Checketts waited for his reaction and was delighted when he discovered that the heir to the throne couldn't speak as he was convulsed by uncontrollable laughter. Prince Charles's shyness and low confidence had helped him develop acting and mimicking skills. It was sometimes easier to hide behind another character than have to play himself. He was also a great fan of the British comedy troop the Goons, and could impersonate Peter Sellers, Spike Milligan and Harry Secombe to perfection. He often converted some piece of pompous behaviour he had witnessed into 'Goon speak', which would have all the Checketts 'reduced to dribbling hysterics'.

The Duke of Edinburgh had wanted his son to stay at Timbertop for two terms. However, given the Prince's diffidence, he had decided to allow Charles to choose whether he should stay for one or two; it was much to his surprise and pleasure when Charles opted for the latter. He felt much more comfortable in the hot and tough Australian outback than he did among the goings-on at Gordonstoun; after only six weeks of being in Australia, his mind was made up. Another consideration had helped him to reach the decision. The school was planning a trip to Papua New Guinea, and if he stayed on he would get to go.

On arriving in New Guinea, the party had a long launch trip around the coast to a place called Dogura where there was a cathedral and an Anglican mission. For several days before the party arrived in the village of Wadu, which adjoined the mission, the drums had been beaten in anticipation of this royal visit, and on the night before Prince Charles arrived, their greeting beat out throughout the night without pause. As the launch approached the beach, the Prince and his companions could see a great crowd had gathered to greet their royal guest. One of his friends wrote, 'There was an absolute silence as the boat drew to the wharf. As the boat came we drew away from the Prince so that the people could see him. He was dressed in a yellow open-necked shirt and khaki Bombay shorts. Then suddenly the crowd saw and recognised the Prince and there was a mighty shout of "Egaulau" (Wedau for greeting).' The Prince did not shrink from the crowd and walked happily and freely among them. Pushed on by his own determination and encouraged by the people's enthusiasm, he was at last winning his private war with his own self-doubt and shyness.

He loved the country and its people, and was most impressed by the cathedral, recording that, 'Everyone was so eager to take part in the services, and the singing was almost deafening. One felt it might be almost the original Church. Where Christianity is new, it must be much easier to enter into the whole spirit of it wholeheartedly, and it is rather wonderful to go somewhere where this strikes you.'

He was fascinated by the faith healing; the witch doctors, the spiritualism and the Papuan folk art and customs that he feared would die out if the younger generation did not take more care to preserve them. The future defender of the faith was already respectful of and interested in other faiths, and his religious curiosity was already leading him way beyond the stuffy confines of Anglican tradition. For four days he feasted, danced, threw spears and openly enjoyed the carnival atmosphere that existed because he had come to visit these marvellous people. And the Papuan folk were as impressed with their guest as he was with them. An Anglican sister at the mission was to write later, 'We loved his natural goodness, his thoughtfulness for others, and he was so very interested in many things; and he has a wonderful smile which resembles that of his mother ... In any company he is outstanding. It was grand to see him walking around Dogura – walking alone with no gaping crowds waiting for him ... I do not suppose there are many opportunities for such times in his life. One of the ordinands, when taking prayers before lessons the other morning, gave thanks for the Prince's visit and then went on to give thanks for the one who had come amongst them as if in a cage and how before their eyes he had become free.'

During his stay in Australia, the Prince got to play polo, shear sheep, waterski, chop wood for war widows, muster cattle on horseback, surf, go deep-sea fishing and pan for gold. He taught fly-fishing in his first term at Timbertop and became a ski instructor during his second. Checketts was later to comment that he had gone out to Australia with a boy and had returned home with a man. He now looked leaner, stronger and more mature. He was more disciplined, made decisions on his own and was no longer frightened to venture his opinions. Perhaps some of these changes would have naturally occurred as a part of growing up. On the other hand, free from the awful torment of Gordonstoun, away from the harsh words of his father, the preying eyes of the British press and the prison of royal life, he had been presented with an opportunity at Timbertop, and he had gratefully accepted it with both hands.

Prince Charles left Australia with sadness. In a statement he thanked the Australian people for 'a marvellous and worthwhile experience' and for their kindness, adding that he was very sorry to be leaving. He meant it. He has loved Australia even since.

The Prince did not look forward to returning to Gordonstoun. He sat on the Balmoral lawn, clutching his Labrador for comfort while drinking in the view for the last time for months. However, and much to his relief, after overcoming the first few days of homesickness, he settled down to the Gordonstoun regime more easily than before. After all, he was now approaching eighteen, had travelled across the world, had discovered a new self-confidence in Australia and, much to his surprise and his parents' amazement, Robert Chew had appointed him head boy. The Prince of Wales may not have been the best rugby player or brightest academic in the school, but the appointment was worthy. He had gained a lot of experience and self-reliance on his Timbertop adventure, which his peers lacked, and he had picked up a range of skills at which he was competent and even one or two where he excelled. In addition, he was kind and humane and had just been to a school where the Kurt Hahn way was working.

As head boy he was presented with the opportunity to do what he could to reform the brutal Gordonstoun society and banish some of its barbaric bullying. He hoped to prevent new boys coming to the school experiencing the cruel and unhappy tortures that he had been forced to endure and had done so, for the sake of queen and family honour, in silence. He was allowed his own room, which was next to the art teacher, Robert Waddell. Waddell had always encouraged Charles's painting and pottery, and would comment that the Prince would have been able to earn a living from the sales of either; such was the quality of his work. Now he was to encourage him to improve his appreciation of art and literature. The Prince of Wales had received no such encouragement previously – neither his father nor his mother had any interest in either of these subjects, and the Queen Mother's was only vague. Waddell, who saw Charles as a prince among philistines at the school, delighted in the teaching as the heir to the throne did in the learning.

The Prince and Waddell took to playing duets of classical music together, Charles on the cello and Waddell on the piano. They even entertained the local great houses with their talents, but on occasion failed to reach the standard that they might have wished to achieve. Nevertheless, everyone seemed to enjoy his or her recitals. Charles also started devouring literature, poetry and art with the gluttony of a man starved of such things all his life. But his main enthusiasm remained for music and, in February 1967, he was to appear in a recital at St Giles Cathedral in Edinburgh. He wrote, 'I shall play the cello in about two things, including I hope the sixth movement from Handel's Water Music which is such bliss to play on the cello, 'tho' rather fast. I'm also supposed to play the trumpet and sing, so I shall have to be carried home! All the same I adore it and wouldn't miss it for anything. At least it's something that gives me great enjoyment and also relaxation, which I feel is really quite important. It's misery having to sit down at a desk all day and you can't even play it!!'

He went on to participate in other concerts and was to sing with semi-professional singers in Bach's *Mass in B-minor*. His own ability in the arts and appreciation of others' work in these fields snowballed. Waddell had given Charles an introduction to Vivaldi, Mozart, great literature and even some philosophy, and the Prince had consumed all with the appetite of one most keen to learn. In return, the Prince introduced his art teacher to the Goons – or more accurately his own highly amusing mimicry of them. Waddell was often reduced to tears of laughter, just as the Checketts had been before him. It was a happy time, despite the fact that he was in a place where he did not feel at home.

Waddell, who had watched the heir to the throne from his first day at Gordonstoun, had always been impressed by how different he was from his contemporaries. This was not because he was a prince and they weren't; it was because he was more aesthetic, thoughtful and kind. He delighted in talking as an adult might about music, literature, art and religion, and did so with the enthusiasm that only immense curiosity and commitment bring.

It is fair to say that the Prince seems to have had his adolescence condensed into six months in Australia and that the school there was an excellent experience for him. As Checketts would later say he went out there with a boy and yet within months brought home a man. On the other hand Gordonstoun was not at all suitable for a young artistic and gentle boy like Prince Charles. The Duke of Edinburgh had behaved like a bull in a china shop and things could have gone horribly wrong.

In July 1967, Prince Charles became the first heir to the throne openly to test his own academic ability by sitting his A-level examinations for university. He received a commendable grade B in History and a satisfactory grade C in French. He also took a special paper in History, designed for high-flyers to test their judgement, initiative and acumen. According to the secretary of the examining board, he had shone. He went on to say that the Prince's performance 'was extraordinary, especially when you consider he was digging about in Australia and that kind of thing. He has so many things to do; he must have worked like a demon.' The secretary's comments may have been coloured somewhat by the fact that the student he was referring to was the heir to the throne – only he would know – but there can be no disputing that to come in the top 240 out of 4,000 candidates speaks for itself: the Prince of Wales had done his 'mum and dad' proud and thoroughly deserved his seat at university.

And so ended the most testing chapter of the young Prince's early years. Gordonstoun had been endured, if not conquered, Australia had made a man of him, and he had achieved public acclaim in his exams and driven away many of the demons of self-doubt. He was now to enter a more civilised adult world and would be all the happier for it. He left Gordonstoun with absolutely no desire to return, and made a promise to himself that his children would never have to endure the place. They didn't.

Just before Christmas 1965, the Queen organised a dinner party at Buckingham Palace with the view to forming a committee to be chaired by the Duke of Edinburgh for the purpose of deciding which university the Prince of Wales should attend. The members included the prime minister of the day Harold Wilson, the Archbishop of Canterbury Michael Ramsey, the chief of the defence staff Lord Mountbatten, the dean of Windsor Robin Woods and Sir Charles Wilson, chairman of the Committee of Vice Chancellors (of British universities) – quite an impressive list of gentlemen to be able to call upon in order to decide the further education of one's son. The opinion of the Prince himself was not sought. Moreover, he really didn't seem to mind as long as he didn't have to attend a modern 'red-brick' university and could read the subjects he wanted.

The prime minister wanted Oxford, the archbishop Cambridge and Mountbatten neither. He insisted that his great-nephew be sent straight to the Royal Naval College at Dartmouth. It was decided that the Prince should attend university first and then serve in one or more of the armed forces. But which university? After nine months of discussion it was eventually decided to go for Cambridge. This was probably because the Dean of Windsor swung his vote behind the Archbishop and the Queen and Prince Philip, neither of whom had attended university, trusted his opinion.

The King and Di

It was perhaps ironic that the first British prince ever to attend university in the proper sense of attendance was to be dispatched to 'republican' Cambridge as opposed to 'royalist' Oxford. On the other hand, maybe that was precisely why it was chosen. Trinity was selected as the college, and then other questions had to be addressed. What should he study? Where should he live? Who should be his advisors, who his friends? Where would his detective stay? Where would he eat? What clubs should he join and how should the press be dealt with?

With regard to his studies, it was decided by Prince Philip, the Dean of Windsor and the former Chancellor of the Exchequer Lord Butler, who was now the master of the college, that Prince Charles read a course especially tailored for him. It would include anthropology and archaeology, but would also include history, economics, constitutional law and a modern language. In February 1967, the dean was sent to Gordonstoun to inform the Prince what had been selected for him. To everyone's surprise the Prince, now growing in confidence, dismissed the suggestion outright. He insisted that he only wanted to read anthropology and archaeology, wanted to do so via a standard, full, three-year tripos, and would thus be judged entirely on his own abilities. He demanded to be listened to, and he won.

The Prince arrived at university having won his first battle with the palace officials. He was now not in a mood to retreat, but it was to take some time for the officials to realise that he was no longer going to comply with their advice automatically. The palace became disconcerted that the heir to the throne was now actually becoming what his father had always wanted – a stronger and much more stubborn individual. And as he continued to assert his own identity against them, they came to view him as rather truculent. Actually, he was only behaving like most teenage boys who are discovering manhood, except he was doing so more politely, I dare say, than most of us did.

Nevertheless, this newfound determination with people he knew was not extended to those whom he didn't, and to them he still appeared to be very much a solitary character. He had become friendly with the Dean of Windsor's second son Edward Woods, who was in the year at Trinity College and was even reading the same tripos. Edward's cousin and room-mate, James Buxton, became another close friend, and these two then slowly built a court of acquaintances with which the Prince felt comfortable. But outside this circle he remained very shy.

Characteristically he blamed himself for this shortcoming, writing at the time, '... when I come here and try to go around with people, it is pretence and the awful thing is that I feel they can feel it. However, I must try to improve myself.'

Moreover, this reliance on people from his own hunting and shooting background was not at all approved of by Lord Butler, who made the mistake of complaining to a highly opinionated journalist by the name of Ann Leslie that the Prince was not surrounding himself with a broad enough cross-section of the college. Miss Leslie shared this with her readers, and when the Prince read the article he was enraged enough to comment, 'Most of what Rab Butler says is preposterous and a reflection of some curious desire to be seen as my constitutional and philosophical tutor without whom I would still be a semi-moron.'

But in time, the Prince's circle was to expand as he gained confidence both in himself and in those whom he came to know as he went about his business. Lucia Santa Cruz, daughter to the Chilean ambassador, became a friend and would remain one for several years; and then the Prince, by his own standards, struck up a most unusual friendship.

Hywel Jones was a scholarship boy from Wales, a rock musician, a bright economist and a socialist – perhaps the first real socialist that Prince Charles had ever met for long enough to discuss issues with. Having met on the stairs by the Prince's room and struck up a conversation, they quickly found out that they had both been excited by the idea of Cambridge, but fearful of coming. This seemed to make each of them sympathetic to the other, and an immediate friendship was formed. Thereafter they would often sit up late into the night discussing the economic decline of Britain, the merits of the Labour and Conservative parties and who they stood for, and the point and direction of the Vietnam War.

The Prince, who could hardly have failed to notice the student riots all over western Europe at that time, was stirred into political thought and began to take a greater interest in the social and political revolution that his generation was demanding and agitating for across the world. He didn't seem to share any of its spirit or many of its beliefs, perhaps because its ultimate aim might be to destroy his family, but maybe also because he was more thoughtful and mature than most of his contemporaries and thus could see his way past it to the awful mess that lay beyond.

Prince Charles discovered that Jones was a member of the Labour Club as well as the Conservative Association and even the Marxist Society. When asked why, Jones explained that it was the only way to attend all of the meetings and actually get to see it all. The heir to the throne wondered whether, if he himself also belonged to all the various political associations, he could really be accused of political bias. He asked Lord Butler, who advised that to attempt such a course of action would be highly dangerous. The Prince of Wales took his advice and so turned back to theological inquiry.

Charles attended a set of lectures delivered by the Reverend Harry Williams. Williams was a charismatic preacher with an unorthodox line of theological inquiry that he mingled with the works of Freud and Jung and a fascination with the 'inner self' of man. His teachings shocked traditionalists and fundamentalists alike, but inspired the young Prince. Reverend Williams was also dean of chapel at Trinity, and as such was able to build on the successful first meeting he had with the Prince, who soon began to dine with him on a regular basis so that they might attempt to push back the frontiers of radical theological inquiry.

Williams not only became impressed by the Prince's modesty and academic and spiritual zeal, he was also surprised on occasion by his acuity: in response to a question about the Archbishop of Canterbury he had replied, 'I thought he was a very deep man, but I couldn't get very far down.'

Williams would later comment on the Prince's depth. 'He had an interest in the deeper things of life, in the source of life, an openness of mind, a readiness to evaluate ideas, not taking things off the peg but thinking them out for himself ... It may sound absurd but I always thought he had the makings of a saint when he was young: he had the grace, the humility and the desire to help other people.'

Despite these new interests, the Prince buckled down to his studies, conscious that the national spotlight would be shone on his end-of-year results and he knew only too well that there would be those from the press waiting and hoping for a poor set of results in order to sneer. He achieved an upper second and was delighted that the press received the achievement with warm praise. He wrote to Checketts, 'I have achieved my desire anyway, and shown them, in some small way at least, that I am not totally ignorant or incompetent!' However, this was touched by a tinge of cynicism towards a press which he mistrusted when he added, 'The tables will now be turned and I will be envisaged as a princely swot.'

At eighteen, Prince Charles had become a Counsellor of State; one of the four members of the Royal Family authorised to act for the Queen when she is ill or abroad. He mingled with heads of state that included an exhausted US president Lyndon Johnson, whose health was being damaged by overwork and the ongoing poor conduct of the war in Vietnam. In 1967 he attended the state opening of Parliament for the first time, and later that year he attended the funeral of the Australian Prime Minister Harold Holt as his first royal visit on behalf of the Queen.

He had travelled out to Australia with the British Prime Minister Harold Wilson and the Conservative leader Edward Heath and noted that the two men only spoke to each other on the return trip. He observed, slightly cynically, 'I don't know how sincere these politicians are in their statements, but Mr Wilson made all sorts, mostly about himself.' Nevertheless, the Prince had been most encouraged by the reception he had received in Australia. He wrote to Mountbatten, 'The Australians seem relieved and very grateful that we'd come out. I think it is so important to show them that we care about them, because they are some of the finest people ... They were incredibly friendly and a large crowd was waiting at the airport. I only hope that politicians realise how loyal they are and don't leave them in the lurch ...'

The following June, the Prince became a knight of the garter, and in July he attended his first garden party at Buckingham Palace and made an official visit to Malta where he was deemed to be a success. Indeed, one who met him there was inspired to write to Mountbatten, 'This is a young man who reminds me very much of you; he's immensely interested in humanity and the details of human suffering ... Anyone can have brains but a warm heart is rare among the young today.'

While in Malta, there was also an opportunity for the Prince to show off his polo skills. He had become a passionate and tough polo player, and quite good enough to win a half blue at Cambridge. Now he had been invited to play in the centenary match of the All Malta Polo Club, of which Mountbatten was president. The Prince duly won the Prince Louis Cup and wrote to his great-uncle both to thank him for arranging for him to play, and to express his feeling of honour at winning his great-uncle's trophy. He also mentioned that on his last night on the island he had been taken to dinner in a restaurant 'in the middle of the most beautiful and complete mediaeval walled town where the streets are very narrow and the houses crowd together above you. It is dead quiet, and many of the houses are late Roman in design and quite beautiful.'

The Prince was writing about the silent city of Mdina, the capital of Malta prior to the Knights of St John building Valetta in the sixteenth century. When Charles went there for dinner it was as it had been for hundreds of years, and it remains exactly the same today. The houses, palaces, chapels, churches and cathedral all evoke that ancient mystique that the Prince has always craved in his quest to create an environment where man can both find and come to terms with himself.

After spending the rest of the summer at his beloved Balmoral, the future king returned to Cambridge having decided that history would be the subject for his part-two tripos. He also applied to join the Dryden Society, Trinity's drama group. The producers invited him to an audition, worried in case he was pretty awful and they were forced to reject the heir to the throne, and the Prince subjected himself to a public test of his talent. Nobody should have worried: Charles proved to be a huge hit with the two producers. One of them, Christian Bailey, was later to recall, 'We were rolling round on the floor he was so funny.'

He was offered the part of a padre in a revue. The news soon leaked out that he was to appear and the college was swamped with requests for tickets from the national press, international journalists, famous actors and actresses and even dons and their families who had previously shown no interest in attending the society's productions.

Prince Charles secretly modelled his part on the character of the then Archbishop of Canterbury, Michael Ramsey. Cameras were banned, but somehow the French publication *Paris Match* was able to get its photographer to take some 'exclusive' shots, which were then featured in a four-page article and were duly reproduced around the world – except in the British press, which continued to respect the embargo. Can you imagine that occurring today?

The following year, in an attempt to stall any repetition, the Palace made arrangements with the society for a special press review in advance of the first night. Prince Charles appeared in several skits, including one he had written himself as a monologue delivered by a weather forecaster: 'By morning promiscuity will be widespread, but it will lift, and may give way to some hill snog … Virility will at first be poor … A manic depression over Ireland … A warm front followed by a cold back.' Not brilliant, but pleasingly normal – the sort of stuff you might expect from a 1960s undergraduate. The Prince, performing in front of a poker-faced audience of pressmen, fluffed one phrase, which was duly pounced upon by the front-page reports the following morning. Despite this, however, most of what was written was supportive and even grudgingly complimentary of a young man who had faced a cold posse of hard-bitten journalists hoping for a poor performance, as that was much more newsworthy, and hadn't obliged them.

After four terms at Trinity, the Prince was sent to the University College of Wales at Aberystwyth in order to learn Welsh before his formal investiture as Prince of Wales. This was a political decision rather than a cultural outing. In the late sixties, as the conventional political parties struggled to establish confidence among the electorate that they could halt the British decline, so a rash of nationalism broke out in Scotland and Wales.

Both the Scottish and Welsh nationalist parties had won by-elections in 1967 as, following the pound's devaluation a year earlier, Harold Wilson's Labour government felt the anger of Labour strongholds in both countries. This might have been very bad for the Labour Party, but could be considered quite pleasing news for the Conservatives, who had long since ceased to count on such areas for support and who could only benefit from Labour's embarrassment.

More seriously, however, a bunch of crazy fanatics had formed the Free Wales Army and become a minor irritant to the police; they became much more than that when an RAF warrant officer was seriously injured by a gang of extremists. Then a bomb destroyed the Temple of Peace in Cardiff and another was found in the lost-luggage department of the railway station. It was a miracle that no one had been maimed or killed at either location. Nobody had claimed responsibility, but it was anonymously announced that the Prince of Wales was on the target list.

Just before his departure for Aberystwyth, the Prince recorded his first radio interview and, not surprisingly, he was asked about his attitude towards the hostility he was bound to face from Welsh extremists in the Principality. He replied, 'It would be unnatural, I think, if one didn't feel any apprehension about it. One always wonders what's going to happen ... As long as I don't get covered in too much egg and tomato I'll be all right. But I don't blame people demonstrating like that. They've never seen me before. They don't know what I'm like. I've hardly been to Wales, and you can't really expect people to be over-zealous about the fact of having a so-called English prince to come amongst them ...'

The decision to send him to Aberystwyth had been made in 1967 following representations from Labour's Welsh secretary of state for Wales, George Thomas, who saw it as a popular move that would benefit the Welsh Labour Party. But by 1969 the decision looked to be potentially dangerous. Things were then further whipped up by four students going on hunger strike. However, to cancel the term in Wales would provide a massive PR success for the extremists and a serious loss of face for the government and the Prince of Wales himself, who would be seen to be unpopular in the Principality and afraid to go there. The Prince believed that he would have to face a serious demonstration against his presence upon his arrival, but nevertheless headed off to Wales with much fortitude, telling himself that this would, after all, be nothing compared to the torment dished up at Gordonstoun.

However, upon his arrival at Pantycelyn Hall, where he was to share accommodation with 250 other students, he encountered a crowd of some 500 who could hardly contain their pleasure at seeing him. He was very touched and openly pleased, while being secretly much relieved by this reception – as, no doubt, were the government, the Queen and Prince Philip, who were all watching from the safety of London.

The Prince of Wales continued to be well treated by the people of Aberystwyth, who made his strolls around its streets enjoyable by their unbridled pleasure of seeing him there. And he experienced an incident-free – if somewhat lonely – existence at the university itself. He got on with his task without complaint, his only comment being that he missed Cambridge and now realised how lucky he had been to be sent there. However, this is not to say that the Prince did not develop a genuine sympathy for the people of the Principality. He wrote to a friend at Cambridge at the time, 'I'm sure speaking to these people sympathetically is the best one can do. So many people in the Government seem to dismiss them as bogeymen and I feel that is fatal.

If I've learned anything during the last eight weeks, it's been about Wales ... they feel so strongly about Wales as a nation, and it means something to them, and they are depressed by what might happen to it if they don't try and preserve the language and the culture, which is unique and special to Wales, and if something is unique and special, I see it as well worth preserving.'

The Prince of Wales has never had the politician's skill of disguising his feelings. Sometimes, in the years that were to follow, this would prove to be a serious disadvantage, especially when coming up against the silky manipulating skills and brilliant cunning possessed by his wife, but such honest opinions so sincerely expressed back in the late 1960s had a marked impact on public opinion in Wales – just as the government had hoped it would.

At the end of his eight-week term he was invited to close the Urdd National Eisteddfod – the annual Welsh youth festival for poetry, drama and music – before an audience of some 6,000 people all crammed into a large marquee. This was not only to be his first public speech of any significance; it was to be made in Welsh, a language that he had studied for just two months. On top of this, Welsh militants had declared their intention to infiltrate the proceedings and prevent him from speaking.

He made light of the threat, writing to a friend, 'It should be highly exciting and if I make a linguistic blunder I expect they will hurl the bardic harps and druidic oaths at me.' True to their word, as he got to his feet the demonstrators got to theirs and screamed abuse at the Prince. He stood his ground and just stared back at them without displaying any other emotion. The natural sympathy of the rest of the 6,000 was aroused and mayhem broke out as the crowd, many of whom were old ladies brandishing handbags, manhandled the militants and drove them from the marquee. The police were needed to restore order. The Prince was to record in his diary that night, 'It was extraordinarily warming to have so many people applauding and cheering and as a result my nerves were dissipated by the time that I was allowed to get anywhere near the microphone.'

The end of his speech was greeted by a roar of approval and a standing ovation. After just eight weeks, he had made a speech in a new tongue with passable pronunciation and apparently some command of the actual language, but it was the courage that he had displayed that had endeared him to the people and defeated his detractors. The government had wanted the Prince to go to Wales to quell the flames of separatism, the Palace as a preparation for the coming investiture. As the investiture was to demonstrate not long afterwards, the Prince had done a great job for Queen and country. Both missions were accomplished.

By now William Heseltine had replaced Richard Colville as the Queen's press secretary. Heseltine, an Australian, was not of the usual mould, and although he showed all the correct decorum, he was determined to move the Royal Family from their remote and mysterious world into the bright glare of the media. As the 1960s had progressed and attitudes to just about everything had changed, it is perhaps easy to see why he was determined to bring the Queen and her family closer to the people in this way: everything else was modernising so the monarchy must not be left behind. The Royal Family, in its new role of 'first national family', must be seen to be as 'with it' as any other modern family.

It was to prove a monumental error and the start of the slippery slope that was to propel the Royal Family into a goldfish bowl of over-exposure that not even the greatest politicians or celebrities have ever been able to withstand. Heseltine had thought that there was no alternative to removing the veils of mystique, and believed that he and his successors could always protect the Queen and her family by their ability to grant or deny access to them. He also assumed that the media, if granted more access, would nevertheless still respect the royals' right to have a private life. He was completely wrong on all counts.

Nevertheless, this was to be the policy, and just as Charles had been the pawn in the Welsh game, now he was to become the guinea pig for this media experiment in the lead-up to his investiture at Caernarfon Castle. This was to be the Prince of Wales's big 'coming-out' day. Not only would the Queen present her son to the Welsh people, the world media would be there to record it; thereafter he would emerge as a public figure with official duties and responsibilities.

Heseltine and Checketts believed that there was an element of the press that suspected the Prince was a bit of a wimp. They knew this was not true, and indeed that the young gentleman could be spirited and even arrogant as well as very courageous. However, they believed that in the absence of any evidence of this, the impression might grow and unfairly stick to the heir to throne. The public had never heard the

Prince utter a word until his 1969 radio interview, so it was decided to go on the offensive with an almost election-type media campaign to let everybody see what sort of a chap he really was.

Checketts was most confident. Of course he was aware that the Prince was shy and introverted, but he was also intelligent and alert and his self-deprecation and ability to laugh at himself were totally disarming – a very powerful weapon when reaching out for a mass audience. The fact that his radio-interview performance had been so good that the written media had produced large chunks of it unedited the next day, along with rave reviews, gave Heseltine the confidence to declare that in the heir apparent he had 'marvellous material to work on' and 'here was a young man who was both sensitive and witty and with a tremendous sense of the history of the institution of which he was part.'

The Prince himself was rather less pleased at the prospect of such a media blitz, commenting, 'I am myself convinced that everyone will be sick to death with seeing, hearing and reading about me in such over-concentrated doses, but the press office think otherwise.' Having said that, the Prince agreed to play his role and launched himself on the heavy media schedule with gusto. It was a huge success, but it started a new and quite different relationship with the media from which he would find it quite impossible to retreat.

The date of the investiture had been set for 1 July 1969. It had always been seen that this event, which was to be set in the mystical atmosphere of a mediaeval castle, was tailor-made for a worldwide television audience. On the Investiture Committee was the unofficial producer of this grand production, the Earl of Snowden. This pleased Charles, as Princess Margaret's husband was not only very artistic and a world-renowned photographer, he was extremely fond of the Prince and shared his sense of humour. Snowden was to oversee a pageant that was to be modern but historical and could entertain the worldwide television audience as well as the 3,500 invited guests without giving offence to anyone, while keeping security watertight as the Queen and her heir would be within inches of each other.

While all of these plans were being laid, the rumbling threats of the militant nationalists were heard like ever-present thunder in the distance. Perhaps they weren't quite what the PLO or the IRA would become, but they had to be taken seriously and nothing could be left to chance. As one republican wag was to put it, 'It would be sad if the boy was shot but highly embarrassing, for the Labour Government, if he was to be so in front of a worldwide TV audience.'

Three weeks before the event, after a military ceremony in Cardiff to inaugurate the newly formed Royal Regiment of Wales, the Prince, as its first colonel-in-chief, made a word-perfect speech in Welsh calling for tolerance and understanding that an increasing number of people were taking an interest in the Welsh language and culture. As we now know, these local passions and interests were to calm and virtually disappear, but back then it was a tense time, and this speech delivered by a non-political constitutional prince with genuine sincerity did the trick. The crowd took to him as one of their own, even if most Welsh people present didn't speak a word of the language and therefore failed to understand what he had said. They roared with pleasure as he accepted the freedom of the city of Cardiff on behalf of the new regiment.

As the final preparations for the investiture were being attended to, William Heseltine, ever keen to push his royal celebrities forward into the public's sitting rooms, came up with a programme, entitled *Royal Family*, that would treat her Majesty's subjects to the first ever glimpse of the royals at home. It was a documentary that followed the Queen and her family around while 'off duty'. It was this show that launched a thousand disasters as over the coming years the Royal Family were turned into a soap opera cast, giving rise directly to Prince Charles's television interview with Jonathan Dimbleby, which unfortunately mentioned his adultery, and Diana's historic and catastrophic *Panorama* interview. But no one could foresee this, and when *Royal Family* was first shown, it was universally applauded.

Eventually, 1 July arrived. On the eve of the investiture, the Prince, in the company of his parents, grandmother and the usual courtiers, boarded the royal train bound for Wales. All were very nervous. They knew that the pageant had to be flawless and capture the moment perfectly. They hoped the crowds would be large and enthusiastic. And above all they hoped that sound security would prevent any member of the public or even, God forbid, the Queen or her heir from being killed or maimed by a small minority of insane militants. Bombs had already exploded in north Wales, and more were promised for Caernarfon on the actual day.

Such nerves were relieved in true Windsor fashion by joking and horseplay. A television had been set up in the train's main compartment so that the royal party could watch an ancient recording of the last investiture back in 1911, when Great-uncle David had officially taken office. It was then that the Queen Mother caused much amusement with a typical prank. As the Prince entered the compartment halfway through the programme, his grandmother told him that, due to the security situation, it had been decided to proceed with the investiture early and with a stand-in. So far, she explained as she watched the screen, things seemed to be going rather well.

On the day itself, the Prince was driven through the streets of Caernarfon in an open carriage on his way to the castle. The crowd was huge and the cheering deafening. There were no missiles thrown at him, although he was later to note that one 'idiot threw a banana skin in front of the Household Cavalry'. As the guests and choir sang 'God Bless the Prince of Wales' he was conducted to the dais and knelt before the Queen. He later wrote, 'For me by far the most moving and meaningful moment came when I put my hands between Mummy's and swore to be her liege man of life and limb and to live and die against all manner of folks – such magnificent mediaeval, appropriate words, even if they were never adhered to in those old days.' This gives us yet another image of the young Prince searching for honour and inner strength from the mystique of ancient words in ancient surroundings. It was the same young man who commented in disbelief, when presented by the Queen to the crowds at Queen Eleanor's Gate after the ceremony that the castle precincts 'looked straight down on the local conveniences'

The Queen then presented the Prince to the crowd at Eagle Gate and at the lower ward to the sound of magnificent fanfares, which were largely drowned out by the cheers of an enormous and enthusiastic crowd. After that he was again paraded through the streets of the town to the delight of the people, before retiring aboard the Royal Yacht at Holyhead for a well-deserved dinner, an emotionally exhausted but very happy prince.

The next day he set off without the rest of the family to undertake a weeklong whistle-stop tour of the Principality. The investiture was deemed by all but the separatists to have been a great success and everywhere he went, through villages, market towns or cities, the response of the people was the same. They turned out in large numbers and cheered their prince. He was 'utterly amazed' by their reaction, especially at how the children 'seemed to go wild and broke ranks to run along behind the car'.

Indeed, as the tour progressed south, the crowds grew even bigger as media coverage whipped up the people's desire to join in. Eventually he arrived in the mining communities of south Wales and was most touched by how the people had 'lovingly decorated [their towns] with flags and flowers and pictures – even the streets I did not go down were decorated – which made the grim streets look unnaturally colourful and bearable.'

At every stop all the local dignitaries turned out to greet His Royal Highness. There was one notable exception: in Ebbw Vale, the local MP and extreme left-winger Michael Foot was most noticeable by his absence. Michael Foot was a highly intelligent man, who should have been bigger than this small-minded demonstration showed him to be. The Prince had been warned that this might happen and took it as a snub against himself; nevertheless, he was not resentful – rather he was disappointed as he had sincerely been looking forward to meeting Foot, whom he knew had a genuine care for his constituents.

At the end of the week, the Prince arrived exhausted but much motivated back at Windsor Castle, bursting to share his experiences with his family. However, he was to discover that neither his father nor his sister had bothered to wait up for him, while his mother had remained at Buckingham Palace as she was recovering from a cold. With a tinge of disappointment he retired to write up his diary, 'Last week has been an incredible one in my life and it now seems very odd not to have to wave to hundreds of people. The air seems so silent now, since the cheering and clapping has ceased abruptly and the handshaking has stopped too. I now seem to have a great deal to live up to and I hope I can be of assistance to Wales in constructive ways. To know that somebody is interested in them is the very least I can do at the moment.'

Even if his immediate family had taken his success for granted – and given the harsh criticism that the Duke had handed out in the face of perceived failure, a word of congratulation from him might not have gone amiss at this point – there were hundreds of letters of congratulation which flooded into the Prince's private office. Among them one stood out.

[

Howard Hodgson

My Dear Charles,

Confidential reports on Naval officers are summarised by numbers ... pretty poor 2 or 3, very good 7 or 8. Once in a while an officer achieves 9 – your father did it ... your performance since you went with Fleet coverage to Wales rates you at 9 in my opinion ... I'm sure that you will keep your head. Realise how fickle public support can be – it has to be earned over again every year. Your Uncle David had such popularity that he thought he could flout the Government and the Church and make a twice-divorced woman Queen. His popularity disappeared overnight. I am sure yours never will provided you keep your feet firmly on the ground. Well done and keep it up,

Your affectionate and admiring Uncle.

Mountbatten's letter to his great-nephew was not only what Prince Charles deserved but, given his still frail confidence, what he needed. This letter was the first of a sustained correspondence that would continue for a decade and would reflect a deepening affection as Mountbatten came to be the greatest influence of any over the Prince during those important years. This was not only because his great-uncle stood for and believed in everything that Prince Charles had been taught that he must uphold, but because he was kind, caring, encouraging and a man that the Prince could confide in. Indeed, he was a sort of surrogate father that the Prince had always had need of given his relationship with his natural father.

In reply, the Prince wrote, 'I, myself, cannot believe that I have really had an effect on people, particularly young ones, but several people have been writing recently saying very flattering things. The immediate problem is to remain sane and sensible and I try hard to do that. As long as I do not take myself too seriously I should not be too badly off. I thoroughly appreciate all you say in your letter and realise the fickleness of the public. The trouble is, they may expect too much of me, but I shall certainly do my best even if they do.'

Given the Prince's recent exam results at Cambridge, the fortitude he had shown at Aberystwyth, the courage in the face of protestors in the marquee at the Eisteddfod, the political skill in Cardiff, the success of the investiture and his Welsh tour, it is amazing that his letter remains fraught with self-doubt. But it is, and that is why his relationship with Mountbatten was to become so important to him and therefore to his future subjects.

It had been seven months since he had been at Cambridge, but despite writing to friends while he was in Wales to say how much he missed the place, he was to moan like mad about it on his return. This is one of the less attractive aspects of the Prince's personality. He can moan about quite trivial things and become most self-pitying over other matters that you and I would expect him to take in his stride. This seems to be a safety valve, like his explosive temper, because despite the moans, the pity and the occasional explosion, he steers the same constant course towards his goals, almost never expecting to get there but knowing that he must die in the effort or he will have let the nation, the Queen and himself down.

In November of that year he made a speech to 5,000 Indians at a meeting in London to celebrate the centenary of the birth of Mahatma Gandhi. He shared the stage with Mountbatten and delivered his speech in the presence of the prime minister who, following the success of the investiture, was urging the Queen to allow the Prince to take on more public engagements. He told his audience, 'I myself have discovered in a small way that it is perseverance that counts, even if you are frustrated ten or twenty times over ... The consequent sense of achievement is overwhelming ... The only trouble about this is that it requires effort, willpower and discipline. Some would have us believe that these are out-of-date concepts, but as long as man has an ounce of humanity left, they will survive.'

This tells us a lot: firstly, that his security blanket of hiding behind self-deprecation had now become a permanent part of any public pronouncement; secondly, that effort, willpower and discipline are qualities that he has been taught to think of as essential virtues, and that he has come to believe in them as their application, in the absence of more dashing qualities, had turned the introverted and complex boy into a popular prince; and thirdly, that his own personal virtue is already out of line with a worsening national character. Moreover, it also raises the following question: if, in post-millennium Britain it is accepted that willpower and discipline are in decline, has British society finally run out of its last ounce of humanity? Travelling through some of the ghetto housing estates of this once great country I am convinced that there are places that have.

So, when not studying at university, the Prince found himself increasingly attending state functions, opening some new building or bridge or making speeches. A lot of this he found a trifle boring, but did his job without complaint, as this was his duty, even, as he saw it, his *raison d'être*. For enjoyment he relied on shooting 'other people's pheasants' and playing polo with a courage and a passion that proved to all that now nobody should ever consider His Royal Highness to be a wimp.

In February 1970, the Prince was introduced to the House of Lords. Prince Philip could only be admitted to the House as one of his son's supporters if he took the Oath of Allegiance in that Parliament. He hadn't done so, and then discovered that he was due to leave the country on the intended date. He explained to his son that he could not change his plans at a mere four weeks' notice, and so missed another opportunity to bond with a son who had done so much to try and make his father proud of him.

The Prince was to record the occasion in his diary: 'Quite awe-inspiring to progress slowly into the Chamber and make the obeisances and take the oath to the accompanying pregnant silence and occasional baronial cough or ducal splutter. However I was determined not to be overawed and didn't feel too nervous. I took my seat on the right of the throne, placed the cocked hat on my head and sat there blinking for a few excruciating seconds and then rose to shake the Lord Chancellor's hand to the accompaniment of a low roar of "hear! hear!" … It has a relaxed atmosphere and an air of great dignity and civility. It is really like a large club … One day I intend to make a speech if I find something reasonable and non-controversial to interest myself in sufficiently. In some ways I think I ought to take my membership fairly seriously.'

However, most things that took his interest over the coming years, such as organic farming, inner-city poverty and deprivation, the environment, the Church and architecture, were to prove to be very controversial and would anger politicians, professionals and priests alike. So much so that if he *had* taken his membership seriously and turned up weekly with a new speech, a constitutional crisis may well have occurred. The speeches he did make angered many who thought it not his role to do so; to have made them in the Upper House would have amounted to spitting in the eye of Parliament.

Three weeks later, and only three months before his finals, he flew to Australia, Hong Kong, New Zealand and Japan for official visits. In

Australia he felt happy to be 'in a long-lost and loved home ... the people are so welcoming.' In New Zealand he joined the Queen and Prince Philip for the state opening of Parliament and made a speech from the throne there. Then it was off to Hong Kong, which totally captivated him as 'one of the old-style colonies', before moving on to Japan to attend the international trade fair Expo '70. He was the honoured guest of Emperor Hirohito and was forced to endure many formal meetings and meals where no English was spoken by his guests and Japanese-style proceedings must have seemed incredibly dull to a twenty-year-old. But he had been born to the job, and willpower, discipline and a sense of duty were to see him through.

By May he was back in Cambridge to face the moment of truth with his History finals. Had the countless distractions of monarchy taken their toll on him? Lord Butler, who believed the Prince to be 'really very clever', thought that they would. He had advised against the term in Aberystwyth and was horrified by how the Palace had expected a student in his final year to fulfil so many royal engagements. Prince Charles recalled in his diary that, 'although I have been hating the idea of these monstrous tests of scholastic knowledge, I was relieved when they finally began and some of the tension could subside.' And in answer to a good luck telegram that told him to 'beat the examiners', he replied with his usual sense of humour, 'your message has worked wonders. Several battered examiners in hospital.' Again the Prince came through this examination with flying colours. He was awarded a lower second-class degree, which, given all the disruption to his studies, was hailed as a major achievement by the college and this was echoed by the national press, which was most generous in its praise.

The Prince of Wales finished his academic education a very different person to the shy and introverted teenager who had been so very unhappy at Gordonstoun some eight years earlier. He had been through much and had never been found to be wanting. He still preferred solitude to gangs, and his confidence was still a little fragile, as it always would be; but with the encouragement of his grandmother and great-uncle, and mainly by his own grim determination to face every situation and do his very best, he had won through and had proved what can be achieved by willpower, discipline and effort.

He had looked for praise from his father, but when it was not forthcoming he had still put his best foot forward and done so without resentment. He had never sought to blame the Duke or anyone else for his own shortcomings. Even though he was now accomplished at many sports, he hadn't lost his compassion for people or his love of music and the arts. Indeed, he was now discovering a passion for great literature: he read *Anna Karenina* on his way to Australia on that last trip, and wrote that until then he had 'never realised to what extent words could move me. I've been experiencing the same sensations from this that I have from beautiful and stirring pieces of music. I'm sure it does the soul immense good.'

And he had genuinely kept faith with his religious conviction, constantly searching for his inner soul at a time when most teenagers of his age thought that 'soul' was a form of music. He was an apt person one day to become head of the Church of England.

He had been put through a time of lengthy trial and had not been found wanting. It had been a period of immense importance in the life of Charles, Prince of Wales, and one that he could look back on with pride.

Chapter Four
Charles Meets the Navy and Camilla (1970–76)

The Prince attended the May Ball at Trinity before leaving for Windsor and 'four days of glorious weather, marvellous company, delicious food [and] good polo'. The rest of the country was perhaps more concerned with the general election that took place on the Thursday. Mr Wilson had privately told the Prince that he would love to do what only Lord Liverpool had done before and win three elections running. He rather expected to. The economy had been growing quite well since the squeeze imposed by his chancellor Roy Jenkins in 1968, and he appeared to be comfortably ahead in the polls.

But pride was to come before a fall: on the Friday morning, Harold Wilson was on his way out of Downing Street having been defeated by Edward Heath, leader of the Conservative Party. That evening, much to the Prince's amazement, the new prime minister was honoured by a last-minute invitation to attend the joint seventieth birthday party for the Queen Mother, Mountbatten, Princess Alice and the Duke of Beaufort, to be held at Windsor Castle and attended by some 800 guests. The Prince was to note that the atmosphere was 'light-hearted and heady. Beaming, jolly faces peered from behind bubbling champagne glasses and people hobbled up to each other to express their amazement at the day's events ... Heath looked shattered (but happy) ... bemused by all the attention and congratulations ... It could so easily have been the other way round and he would probably been out of the leadership fairly rapidly.'

No doubt the Prince's comments were right, and as a result perhaps it was a good job that they were only confined to his diary: the Royal Family is supposed to be politically neutral, and while there is no expression here of his own feelings or those of his family, it is quite clear that their guests found it impossible to disguise their delight at the surprise news that a much-hated Labour Government had been defeated. Perhaps now the moral decline over which it had presided would come to an end. The ruling classes were overjoyed, believing that, now the party of law and order and sound economic management was back in power, things would get back on track.

This new confidence in the future was to be entirely misplaced. In the coming three years, in the face of collapsing business confidence and two possible major corporate catastrophes at Rolls Royce and

Upper Clyde Shipbuilders, Mr Heath performed a U-turn on his intended policies, saved lame-duck companies with government money and eased credit in the economy as a whole. The aim was to encourage investment in British manufacturing, but the result was speculation in financial instruments and in residential and commercial property. It was all to end in a spectacular bust at the end of 1973 after the chancellor, Anthony Barber, had not only printed money like paper, but had also embarked on his phase one, two and three incomes policies that fuelled inflation dreadfully as the government ran scared in the face of apparently unstoppable trade-union power.

Lord Barber, as he was to become, created what was to be known as the 'Barber Boom' by pumping money into the British economy in 1971 and 1972. Unfortunately, the whole of the developed world was booming together, largely on the back of an inflationary boom in the United States. This was caused by both the Johnson and Nixon administrations paying for the increasingly expensive involvement of the US in Vietnam not by raising taxes but by printing money.

In 1971 the United States turned from being an exporter of oil to an importer. In 1973, the Yom Kippur War broke out and the Arab oil producers decided to use oil as a weapon. They chose to quadruple its price and cut production. The effect on world trade was disastrous. Both industry and consumers had become extremely profligate in their use of oil, which had been getting cheaper and cheaper over the previous decade. Suddenly it was very expensive and, some believed, in short supply. The result was both panic and speculation, and so the price of oil rocketed. It was as though the whole world had received a massive increase in its taxes. Tens of billions of pounds, dollars, Deutschmarks, francs, yen and lira were taken out of the world economy and put into the Arabian Desert. Until this money could be recycled into the system, the world was going to suffer.

And suffer it did. Britain, because of its continuing structural weakness, suffered more than most of the western world. The 'Barber Boom' had not worked. British manufacturers had not invested as much as hoped, and the two main results of the expansion in credit had been an explosion in property prices and a rapid increase in inflation. In these pre-Thatcher years, home ownership was vastly lower than today, and only about six per cent of the public owned stocks and shares. As a result the majority of people failed to benefit from the rising property and stock-market prices, but had to pay the increased prices in the shops. This caused much resentment and in some quarters fuelled support for militant trade unions, which were keen to take on and get rid of a Conservative government.

And so, with the baby-boomer influence of the 1960s still favouring socialism as the way forward, Heath was pushed down a left road in order to retain support just as Tony Blair would be pushed down a right road in order to get elected some twenty-five years later. The government attempted to reduce resentment among the wage-earning classes by choking off inflation. However, unfortunately and in true socialist style, Heath and Barber, who had been elected to bring back market forces and sound money, only attempted to tackle the symptoms – rising prices, dividends and earnings – without tackling the real cause – too much money washing around in the economy.

In the autumn of 1973, just before the oil crisis was to blow up, the government introduced phase one of an incomes policy that could have been written by the old left-wing Labour Party. It allowed index-linked rises if inflation rose above seven per cent. Thanks to the oil-price hike, inflation rose quickly to that level, and automatic pay rises produced a ratchet effect, pushing it higher and higher.

The National Union of Mineworkers (NUM) saw its opportunity to wield political power. It had learned the lesson of craven collapses when faced with union pressure by both the main parties since the war and especially of the present government when faced with their own demands in the early part of 1972. It could smell blood and sensed it had the government on the run. It duly submitted a large pay claim and imposed an overtime ban on 8 November 1973. Heath panicked and declared a state of emergency on 13 November. A month later he declared a three-day week in order to preserve fuel. Although negotiations with both the Arab states and the NUM continued, the only results were the continuation of high oil prices, the miners' strike and the misery caused to millions by a three-day week when, by order of the government, the television stations were cut off at 10.30 p.m. in order to save power supplies.

Initially, the people swung behind Mr Heath and the government's standing rose in the opinion polls. It seemed as if a majority of the public was resentful that a union was dictating to the rest of the nation and holding it to ransom. But Heath delayed too long in asking them to confirm their support – probably by as much as three weeks. By the time he eventually called an election with the implied question 'Who runs the country, the elected government or the unions?', the electorate wasn't sure who should govern the country – the Tories, who had at long last shown some signs of standing up to the unions, or the Labour Party, who might at least get the miners back to work. In the end the nation polarised into class, and neither party gained an overall majority. The Tories won more votes but Labour won more seats: neither could form a government outright.

Heath tried to form a coalition with the Liberals, but their leader Jeremy Thorpe would not play. Labour claimed it would govern alone, which turned out not to be entirely correct as it was to come to rely on the Liberal–Labour pact for most of the 1970s. Heath stepped down in order that Wilson could form his third administration after all, and so Britain's moral and economic decline were once more in Wilson's safe hands: he had hardly been hurt by the worst Conservative government of the twentieth century.

What had gone before paled into insignificance when the new administration got its act together. Labour immediately gave in to the NUM, and so the rest of the union movement made a rush for the same sort of inflationary pay claim. As a result, inflation rose in their first year in office to twenty-five per cent, with thirty or even forty per cent on the cards for the following year, and yet productivity fell by over four per cent. Even the most idealistic and economically ridiculous observer knows that nobody can pay themselves twenty-five per cent more for doing four per cent less, and so British economic suicide was being committed.

Worse still, while the nation scrambled to grab ever more insane salary increases in order to keep up with this hyperinflation, financial institutions and to a lesser extent manufacturing businesses were still suffering severely from the financial squeeze imposed by Barber in the autumn of 1973. Nearly all the secondary banks went into liquidation or had to be rescued by the main banks. Even the high-street bank National Westminster was forced to make a formal denial that it was in trouble. If the new chancellor, Denis Healey, had not introduced a corporate tax-saving measure called 'stock relief', many manufacturing businesses would have collapsed too.

In view of this repeated economic mismanagement, it was hardly surprising that prices on the London Stock Exchange fell throughout 1974 and the *Financial Times* thirty-share index, which had been over 500 as long ago as 1968, crashed to 147 in January 1975, bringing with it much misery for retired people living off their savings.

As if giving in to every pay demand between March 1974 and the summer of 1975 wasn't madness enough, the Labour government also decided to give the unions enormous privileges, which would prove to be extremely costly to the nation throughout the rest of the decade and the start of the 1980s. It was the unions' abuse of these privileges as much as Labour's continued economic failure that was to sweep the Tories, under the leadership of Margaret Thatcher, to power again in 1979.

The Trade Union and Labour Relations Act of 1975 was masterminded by the left-wing Michael Foot – he who had failed to turn up to greet the Prince of Wales in Ebbw Vale in 1969 and who was to become, much to the delight of the Tories, a leader of the Labour Party, doing much to ensure that they remained in opposition for years. It granted the unions privileges not enjoyed by any institution since the Church before the Reformation. For example, this law meant that unions would no longer be liable for damage inflicted as a result of an industrial 'dispute' – even where the victim had nothing to do with the dispute. This idea of putting powerful institutions who were your friends and party funders above laws that were to be obeyed by the man in the street was not only economic suicide, it was wrong, immoral and gave a completely inappropriate message to the nation, and especially the nation's young. It is not a matter of right or wrong, this act seemed to say, but a case of how much clout you have. The message might as well have come straight out of George Orwell's *Animal Farm*, and the impression it gave was not to be lost upon future generations.

As the 1970s progressed, the government's fortunes and the economy were to sink so low that people feared it was to go into absolute decline. Inflation continued at an alarming rate in 1974 and 1975, with a forty per cent annual target becoming some unions' objective. Then, happily for Britain, help arrived from a most unexpected figure. Jack Jones, the general secretary of the Transport and General Workers' Union and the TUC and a very powerful man in this union-dominated country, suddenly realised that the party was over and something must be done. Jones knew this pay-rise tornado must stop or the lives of ordinary working people would be ruined. Although he had been hopelessly misguided in understanding how economics really works for all of his working life, he was nevertheless genuine in wanting to help his members.

Jones and a Wilson aide, Joe Haines, came up with the idea of having a voluntary flat-rate policy of a £5-a-week annual pay rise. This would help the poorest as naturally £5 a week represented the biggest percentage increase to them. The government leaped on the idea and were helped in their promotion of it by yet another sterling crisis. After much argument, the TUC general council approved a flat-rate £6-a-week policy, with zero increases for those earning more than £8,500 a year (approximately £65,000 in 2007 terms).

It is now widely accepted by both main political parties in Britain, as it is across the world, that a free-market economy and fiscal control of the money supply is the best way to grow a 'real' economy. Artificial control such as pay freezes can only work for a time because, when the control is removed, no lessons have been learned and all the old problems return. And so it was in this case. In the short term it worked. Inflation fell from 24.4 per cent in 1975 to 8.3 per cent in 1978. However, anomalies and grievances were being built up that exploded in the 1978 Winter of Discontent. As the Labour MP Philip Whitehead said in his book *The Writing on the Wall*, 'Caught between its rhetoric in opposition on the one hand and the frustrations of its supporters on the other, Labour could not expect an ad hoc incomes policy to be credible for the course of a parliament. Wilson did not solve his problems. He bought time. And time, in July 1975, seemed a very scarce commodity.'

As Wilson and Heath battled against each other, and in so doing ensured that Britain was now clearly the sick man of the western world, both economically and morally, so the young Prince continued to be groomed in his ambassadorial role. Soon after noting his grandmother's guests' delight at the presence of the new prime minister, he was off on an official visit to Canada and the United States.

The crowds in Ottawa were not as enthusiastic as they had been in Australia. However, he was most impressed with the reception he was given at the White House, where he and Princess Anne stayed as guests of the president. The Prince had requested an audience with President Nixon, which had been granted, and although the initial conversation had been a little awkward, once the Prince had steered the conversation away from polo and baseball and on to Russia and China, Nixon came to life and explained his preference for the latter. He spoke with genuine feeling about the threat to the free world of an 'aggressive

The King and Di

Russian communism dedicated to assisting revolution anywhere in the world'.

And yet, when the Prince sounded the president out about the Queen visiting Russia, he was surprised by Nixon's enthusiasm. They went on to discuss China, Cambodia, southeast Asia and the American dream. The Prince had expected the meeting to last half an hour; he was surprised but pleased that Nixon was so taken with him that he forgot the time as he counselled Charles about his own role on the world's stage, advising that he should be a 'presence' while not avoiding all controversy. 'I pointed out that one must not become controversial too often otherwise people don't take you seriously. To be just a presence would be fatal. I know lots of Americans think one's main job is to go around saying meaningless niceties, but a presence alone can be swept away so easily, I feel.' Clearly the Prince intended to be more than a mere presence, and he was not going to heed his own advice regarding controversy in the future.

After ninety minutes, and even though the president seemed happy to continue, Charles felt obliged to withdraw as he felt sure that the Nixon had other business to attend to. However, he was most grateful that the most powerful man on the planet had taken him so seriously. It boosted his confidence so much, in fact, that he now relished this opportunity to play his part in diplomatic affairs and, without being asked, launched into a long letter of report to the then foreign secretary and former prime minister, Sir Alec Douglas-Home: 'The President was extremely hospitable and overflowing with kind remarks. He said that the special relationship between this country and the U.S. was a result of a common language, heritage and traditions. He did genuinely seem very pro-British and anxious to be friendly ...' Of course, Nixon may have been a little bit nicer than normal with one eye on Britain's application to join the European 'club', and could have been excused for worrying that a Britain closer to France could weaken NATO.

A few months later, Prince Charles proposed sharing President Nixon's thoughts on the 'special relationship' in his speech to the guests at the Pilgrims of Great Britain's annual dinner. However, the Foreign Office intervened and had the passage cut from the draft, as Heath's Government was indeed anxious to enter the European Common Market and was therefore keen to suck up to European heads of government. The Prince's secretary informed him that (according to the Foreign Office), 'whereas there was once such a relationship, there no longer is' and that any reference to it would also 'annoy all the Europeans'.

Charles, increasingly displaying a discreet wilfulness, agreed, but talked instead about a 'close relationship': unlike the prime minister he believed that such a relationship did still exist and that the British should keep it alive. Of course history has proved the Prince right and Mr Heath wrong, as the Gulf Wars of 1991 and 2003 display.

In the autumn of 1970, Prince Charles represented his mother at the official independence celebrations for. He was most impressed by the people: 'What was so interesting about this independence was that there were no incidents or demonstrations or anything. Simply peaceful, happy and dignified good behaviour. Personally I found the Fijians some of the most attractive and charming people that I have ever met. They have the most perfect and touching manners and the greatest dignity and good humour I have ever seen. It is a banana skin humour that makes them so marvellous for me, at any rate. Their smiles erase all cobwebs of depression and sourness ...'

This is a gentle prince expressing his admiration for a gentle people. Within a few years he was to embark upon a life's work of providing opportunities for underprivileged children in the belief that it was only by example, love and kindness that could one hope to awaken the self-belief and self-esteem that the Fijians possessed.

He was accompanied on this trip by his newly appointed equerry Nicholas Soames, who was to go on to become a Conservative minister; as a long-standing and very close friend of the Prince, he would in time also become a loud critic of the Princess of Wales. Together they went deep-sea diving and swam among all manner of fish – including sharks, which, the Prince was happy to note in his diary, he did not notice at the time. The Prince was by now taking all manner of sports very seriously indeed. He had decided that any physical challenge wasn't a question of his talent or lack of it, but a test of his character and therefore it had to be overcome. He rode ponies to the limit on the polo field, horses the same way in the hunt. He would also test himself to the edge of his ability on skis and surfboards; soon he was to add flying jet planes and jumping by parachute to his repertoire. The fragile, clumsy and shy little boy had by now easily surpassed the achievements of his father in the world of sporting daring, and had proved that drive, determination and enthusiasm could win through. Perhaps his father's stick and Mountbatten's carrot had played their parts, but it was in the main of his own doing nevertheless.

In November 1970 Prince Charles, representing the Queen at the funeral of French president Charles de Gaulle, flew to Paris accompanied by the Prime Minister Edward Heath and three former prime ministers in the persons of Harold Wilson, Harold Macmillan and Lord Avon. Ever keen to promote the Commonwealth and support its other members, he asked Heath what effect Britain's proposed membership of the Common Market in Europe would have on Commonwealth countries. Heath, quite wrongly as it turned out, assured Charles that the impact on major trading partners like New Zealand and Australia would be minimal.

Keen to use the opportunity to the full, the Prince then pressed Mr Heath to agree that the Commonwealth still had a great deal of value as a multi-racial organisation that covered the four corners of the world. But the prime minister was grudging in his vague agreement, before more truthfully adding that 'there was one thing that he could not stand and that was being told what to do by various African countries'. Membership of the Common Market might have been Heath's greatest achievement, but it was also the biggest splinter in his eye and blinded him to almost anything else.

The delegation stayed at the British Embassy in Paris where the young Prince seemed to have enjoyed the company of the now old but seemingly wise Macmillan and the vain but nonetheless charismatic Lord Avon. Then it was time to attend the funeral service of a man who had much to be grateful to the British for but had never managed to express much gratitude.

From his privileged position, Prince Charles watched as heads of state from all over the world arrived and took their seats. He later recorded, 'Endless African delegations swept down the aisle, rustling like a pile of stationery. Then President Podgormy [of the Soviet Union] appeared surrounded by large numbers of flat-footed henchmen, whose trouser bottoms were about 4 inches above their shoes and hair close-cropped under their ill-fitting hats. Eventually Pompidou and Madame swept past me and settled themselves in separate seats in front.'

This was the last official engagement in a year that taught the Prince much, not least that he would have to push out the limits of his role or he would be stuck with what precedent required and others expected – dressing up in military uniforms in order to travel the world either to open or close things on behalf of his mother. It was a duty that he had been brought up to expect and carry out, but as an intelligent young man with a desire to help right some of the world's wrongs, he was determined to do more than just smile and wave at strangers ...

It had been decided back in 1965 that after university Prince Charles would enter one of the armed services. Some had thought that he should do a stint in all three. Mountbatten was determined that he should only serve in Britain's senior service – the Royal Navy.

Mountbatten was a powerful character within the Royal Family and so his presence was usually sought at family conferences, not so much by Prince Philip, who liked to get his own way, but more by the Queen who wanted to hear all points of view before making her mind up. The Queen Mother also saw the importance of this and so encouraged his presence, especially when discussing matters concerning the Prince of Wales. However, there was to be no conflict here between Mountbatten and Prince Philip: Charles's father had had to pass up a most promising naval career as a result of marrying the then Princess Elizabeth; he was, as usual, keen to see his son follow in his footsteps.

So, following a formal meeting with both of his parents, it was decided that Prince Charles would go into the Royal Navy. Officially this would be for three years, but it was expected he would stay for five: he could not gain command of his own ship for three and a half years, and to reap any real benefit from such a command he would have to hold it for a minimum of eighteen months. Mountbatten was delighted as, now retired from his position of chief of defence staff, he had the time to devote to his beloved great-nephew. Prince Philip was aware of this and did not welcome such close involvement. He wrote a series of memos to his son about his future in the navy, telling him in one that while it was all right to consult 'Uncle Dickie', Mountbatten must not on any account be allowed to use his former influence to intervene in matters concerning Charles's career, as this would create 'a dreadful muddle'. This was a fair and sensible comment, although there is absolutely no evidence that a professional like Mountbatten would have ever contemplated such a thing. It was more likely that the Duke was attempting to put down a marker to remind the former defence chief who the Prince's real father was.

Such memoranda written to Prince Charles at this time shed a great deal of light on the Duke's relationship with his eldest son. In contrast to the fatherly advice and kind encouragement of Mountbatten's letters to Charles, this correspondence, while being concerned and attentive to detail, was remote and businesslike – notes that a man might write to an employee rather than a son. But by now this had become the nature of their relationship: both father and son were busy fulfilling duties around the rest of Britain and the Commonwealth and therefore tended only to meet at official family gatherings at Sandringham, Balmoral or Windsor; when they did, their conversations were stiff and formal. There were no shared intimacies or expressed hopes. Their respective apartments at Buckingham Palace were no more than a short distance from each other and yet, when both men were in residence, neither made the effort to visit the other. In a family where dedication to duty comes first, emotion is positively discouraged, parental criticism comes easily and praise is a rare thing. The Prince had by now become his own man and had done so on his own. Secretly he still craved his father's love and appreciation, but was too proud and had too much of a self-protection system to admit to it. Instead, he was to withdraw from both of his parents into a relationship of pure formality that was often conducted in writing.

Despite all of this, the Prince still loved his father and had come to respect and admire his ability to 'get to the heart of the matter and to analyse things in a practical way'. He also recognised that his father was bound to be frustrated by a son and heir being an 'incurable romantic' and that his father's advice was 'all the more valuable because it came from a perspective so very different from my own'. This point of view was typical of the adult Charles – he was loyal and generous in acknowledging his family's abilities and feelings, but unwilling to cause himself the emotional pain of openly anticipating affection that would not be forthcoming. He loved them, admired them and could appreciate their strengths, but for his own self-protection he would withdraw from them. He was to employ the same tactics years later at the height of his unhappiness during the worst period of his marriage.

It had been decided that Prince Charles would enter the Royal Navy College, Dartmouth in the autumn of 1971. However, before that he would go on a four-month attachment to the Royal Air Force at Cranwell, in order that he might qualify as a jet pilot. He wasn't a complete beginner as during his second year at Cambridge he had taken up flying and had received instruction from RAF Personnel and Training Command. He had done very well – so much so that the captain of the Queen's flight was caused to comment to the Duke of Edinburgh upon 'the wonderful progress he has made'. The duke was impressed enough to make the arrangements for the course at Cranwell, and his son readily assented: this new test of his daring was thrilling, and so the Action Man image was born.

The Prince of Wales flew into Cranwell on 8 March 1971 at the controls of a twin-engine aircraft from the Queen's flight. As usual much attention to the state of security, the briefing of the press and the resolving of protocol issues had to be undertaken before this could happen. Two press briefings were arranged, the second being on the day of his arrival and with access to the Prince in person, in the hope that thereafter the media would let him get on with the course without having to face constant intrusion. It had also been decided that senior officers or those of the same rank as the Prince would refer to him as 'Your Royal Highness' upon greeting him and thereafter as 'Prince Charles', while those of a lower rank would greet him in the same fashion but thereafter would refer to him as 'Sir'.

With the PR and protocol sorted out, attention was turned to the most important issue – security. The Welsh nationalists might have been on the wane, but a new and much more serious threat in the form of the IRA was now apparent. It was of paramount importance that the security surrounding the Prince should be very tight. Two aircraft were assigned to the Prince for his use only. They were separated from the others, kept in a different hanger, maintained only by a specially authorised team and guarded by RAF police at all times. Moreover, while the Prince was allowed to undertake most of the course, anything that involved a higher than usual element of risk was put off limits to him. This caused him much annoyance and he hated seeing young officers of similar age and experience being allowed to undertake operations that he could not.

But despite this, the Prince enjoyed Cranwell from the start: 'I can't tell you how strange it seems to be a serving officer all of a sudden. I am now just beginning to get used to the fact that I have a uniform on and I ought to be calling senior officers "Sir". The latter I find most difficult because I haven't called anyone "Sir" for a long time and I've got so used to meeting senior officers over the past two or three years that the element of fear subsided. They seem more nervous of me than I do of them – but I dare say that element of fear and subservience will soon return to me via the agency of a well-placed boot!'

In addition, his fellow officers were more the kind of chap he had been used to throughout his life than were the students that he had encountered at Cambridge; consequently he immediately felt that he belonged with them. Moreover, as he had proved in Australia as a schoolboy, he had no fear of a Spartan life; it was the uncivilised life he disliked. Here at Cranwell, officers were gentlemen and that made the Prince feel at home: 'the people themselves are really very friendly and the chap who lives on my corridor is charming and likes the Goons – immediate compatibility! ... I have a splendid fussing batman who does very well and uses the Royal "we" all the time, i.e. "What suit shall we put on this evening, Sir?"'

He even wrote to Mountbatten with enthusiasm about the lectures on jet engines while only allowing himself the faintest of whinges about the food: 'To my amazement I find I am beginning to understand some of it and I am convinced that the secret is continuity all day every day. They certainly keep you busy here and I am up early and in bed fairly early as well. The food is pretty revolting, and at unearthly times, but the atmosphere is very like university.'

After just two weeks of ground training he was allowed to take the controls of a Jet Provost and, while he found navigation hard (and was to do so for rest of his naval career), he was soon permitted to make his first solo flight. This was duly noted in his diary entry for 31 March 1971 – only a little over three weeks after arriving at Cranwell: 'the day when I went solo for the first time in the JP. Did it after 8 hours instead of the normal 10. An exciting feeling to be let loose in my own jet. Convinced I flew it far better without Dick Johns in it to criticise my every move ... I did one circuit and managed to bring off a very passable landing ... The feeling of power, smooth unworried power, is incredible.'

Later he was allowed to fly solo aerobatics at 25,000 feet, which he found 'breathtaking'. He was to report to his chum Hugh van Cutsem, 'I can't tell you how rewarding it is when one begins to feel increasingly more professional at some skill. Recently I went on a cross-country solo flight and managed – just – to find my way back here again.' He was 'amazed' by how much he had enjoyed the experience.

But even this paled when compared to his next adventure. He was allowed to fly in the rear seat of a Phantom Jet belonging to 43 Squadron: 'We climbed into the cockpit of the Phantom – on scramble readiness – and when the 2 minute warning was given both engines were started at once and we taxied straight out onto the runway from a shed and took straight off. After a re-heat take-off we climbed to 35,000 feet in 2 minutes at a virtually vertical angle. An attack was then made on a Canberra flying at 48,000 feet and I worked furiously to operate the radar properly.'

Then, and for the Prince of Wales quite wonderfully, they flew over Balmoral Castle. 'Bad weather meant ... dropping down through a hole in the cloud over Ballater. We flew twice over Balmoral at 400 feet, scattering deafening tourists and causing 7 locals to ring up the police in protest. We then roared off at 420 knots past Lochnagar and over Loch Muick ... the whole visit was an unforgettable experience.'

Towards the end of July he made his first parachute jump. Once aboard the plane, feeling like 'a retired tortoise' and extremely nervous, he waited for the plane to arrive at the dropping zone – the beautiful Studland Bay just outside Poole Harbour on the Dorset coastline: 'As I had been clever enough to say I wanted to jump and the press had said I was going to jump I was going to. It was a curious sensation standing in the doorway and just waiting. I was extremely nervous, but since I was longing to experience the sensation of launching myself out of the door ... I kept having morbid reflections on wrapping myself round the tailplane or hitting my head on the side of the aircraft, or even dropping out of the harness before I reached the water.'

When his turn came, and anxious to show no hesitation, Prince Charles jumped almost before the green light and went tumbling over and over. However, as he came out of the slipstream and the parachute opened, he found himself upside down with his feet caught in the rigging: 'I thought how stupid of them not to warn me of this [Prince Charles does have an unfortunate habit of sometimes blaming others rather than himself when things go wrong], but I was extraordinarily calm and in command of the situation and quickly removed my feet ... There was only a short time to admire the view (which is stunning) and enjoy the sensation before my feet touched the water and I was trying to get free of the harness.'

What had occurred is extremely rare, and if the rigging itself had snagged then it could have proved fatal. However, back on the ground, the Prince pushed this near miss out of his mind, now feeling 'exhilarated and happy beyond belief.' Having displayed the sort of courage and presence of mind that even the most sceptical could only admire, he had every justification for his sense of achievement.

Six years later the Prince was appointed colonel-in-chief of the Parachute Regiment. He immediately enlisted on a parachute course. His thinking was, 'I felt I should lead from the front or at least be able to do some of the things that one expects others to do for this country ... I didn't think I could look them in the eye or indeed ever dream of wearing that beret with the Parachute Regiment badge unless I'd done the course ... So they all put their hands up in horror – or rather the RAF did – but somehow it was organised and I did it.'

After five months the Prince was awarded his wings and left the RAF with much sadness. He had made many genuine friends and their expressions of sorrow at his leaving caused him to be 'practically reduced to shamefully sentimental tears'. On his last evening he was called upon to make a speech at a guest evening in the officers' mess. They laughed at all of his jokes and, when he finished, rose as one in a heartfelt standing ovation. Later he retired to bed more than a little the worse for drink – just as his comrades had expected him to be. The next day he was off to Balmoral for the summer.

In September, he returned briefly for the passing-out parade and had to stand to attention for an hour. 'I now know what the poor guardsmen have to go through,' he was to comment. 'However, I avoided fainting and managed to have my wings pinned on my chest without mishap. A marvellous moment.' And it would have been a marvellous moment for most proud parents – but much more was expected of princes in general, and this one in particular.

The prospect of joining the Royal Naval College at Dartmouth filled the Prince with more than a little trepidation. In the long term he saw himself wedded to his ships for at least five years; more immediately, he hated the idea of attending college again. Having enjoyed university and the RAF, now to be cast back into an institution that had been founded early in the twentieth century to train naval officers for the Empire straight from school did not fill him with joy. Having experienced the freedom of undergraduate life and the respect of officer life, he was somewhat indignant at being once again treated like an adolescent.

However, as most of his peers were also graduates, they also found the constraints demeaning and irksome and this was a common cause of annoyance that helped him bond with them. Moreover, the education in seamanship and naval technology was both demanding and intense, so the Prince hadn't too much time for reflection.

Avoiding the easy option as usual, it had been decided to put the Prince on the 'fast-stream' six-week course instead of the more usual twelve-week course. In this time he would be taught about naval tradition, custom and discipline as well as the structure of the service, the art of leadership and, unfortunately for him, navigation, which he hated as his poor grasp of maths meant that this subject was one where he struggled and would continue to do so. Though he could not hope to rival the achievements of his father, who had come top of his class at Dartmouth, the Prince knuckled down and did his best in the time allocated. He became a steady picket-boat pilot on the water, tried his best in the classroom, joined the college sub-aqua club and passed his diving tests.

At first his fellow officers found his presence a little intimidating. However, by sharing with them his feelings of incompetence expressed through a witty self-deprecation, he soon won them over. One of those officers was later to recall, 'If we'd seen him as another officer under training, we'd have thought, what a nice man. What's he going to do for a living? ... He had a sort of endearing vagueness. And yet there was a quality ... a mystique perhaps ... whether that's an innate quality or whether it's part of the royal training ... that's what set him apart from all others.' And his colleagues also admired the 'wonderfully mature, measured, purposeful way' in which he could talk to a senior officer without breaching protocol and etiquette. But perhaps most of all they admired his modesty and kindness.

However, behind the scenes he could sometimes explode in a fit of hot temper, or be irritable and petulant. These moods were usually caused by the anxiety created by the pressure of having to attempt to be the best at everything, while always being polite, smiling and generally behaving in a fashion that showed the monarchy in a good light. The constant strain caused by high expectation on one full of talent and confidence would be enormous, but on one so naturally shy and lacking in confidence it must have been unbelievable, and at times unbearable.

In one such fit of petulance at this time he wrote furiously to his private secretary David Checketts about his future posting. 'What is wrong with everyone? When I asked the CDS [chief of defence staff – Sir Peter Hill-Norton] the other evening at Windsor what ship I was going to, he said ANTRIM – you say NORFOLK. WHICH IS IT?' It never crossed the mind of the young Prince that perhaps the chief of defence staff and admiral of the fleet might just have more important things on his mind than which ship Sub Lieutenant Windsor was going to be resting his weary head at the end of each busy day.

On Friday, 5 November 1971, having passed his exams at Dartmouth, Prince Charles flew from Brize Norton in an RAF Britannia to Gibraltar to join the destroyer HMS *Norfolk*. Once there he met the first captain he was to serve under, and was secretly amused to note his surname was Cook. In the first entry in his naval journal, which like all new recruits he was required to keep for the first six months but was in fact to keep for five years as he recorded his impressions of life at sea, he noted, 'I was to be treated like any other Sub Lieutenant, but there were obvious differences and I suspect no one was sure how I would behave or how pompous I would be.'

One blatant difference between Prince Charles and any other sub lieutenant was the obvious target he posed for the IRA or even the Angry Brigade who had either bombed or machine-gunned several targets in the United Kingdom throughout 1971. Then there was always a chance that an aggrieved or even deranged seaman might attempt to take out his frustration on the heir to the throne. In addition, there was a possibility of someone taking a potentially embarrassing photograph in such confined quarters where men live cheek by jowl, which would fetch a high price on the world market even if the British tabloids could be prevailed upon not to print it. This amounted to a lot of extra responsibility for Captain Cook and his fellow officers. A long and detailed naval memorandum made it clear that the Prince's personal safety was of the uppermost importance. These matters of security were heightened from the navy's point of view when the security services back in the UK yielded to the wish of the Duke of Edinburgh and the Queen that, while at sea, Prince Charles's two personal protection officers be withdrawn from service. To cover their absence, Captain Cook detailed the ship's company to be extra alert.

In addition, for diplomatic as well as security reasons, the ship's programme had to be cleared with the Foreign Office, while the Ministry of Defence had to be informed immediately of any change of plan. Noting that 'Prince Charles keeps himself fit ... is a fresh air fiend and spends as much time in the open air as possible', the memorandum goes on to record that the heir to the throne has a liking for 'slightly dangerous sports' like diving, surfing and water-skiing and that fellow officers should form a discreet presence at all times and a doctor must always be on hand in case of an accident occurring.

Special arrangements were also put in place for handling his correspondence and pay cheque and protecting his personal belongings – including his clothes – from trophy hunters. Add to this the slight chance of the Prince falling overboard in a rough sea, and it is a wonder that Captain Cook had time to worry about anything else aboard his ship.

On his second day aboard, Prince Charles recorded that he was greatly looking forward to 'my first day at sea in one of Her Majesty's finest warships'. He was to have watched her in gunnery practice, but a shell jammed in one of the gun barrels and the exercise had to be cancelled. This caused him to note, 'Not everything in the Navy, as I was to discover, happens like clockwork, and certainly not on time.' Then HMS *Norfolk* set sail for Toulon in order to join a NATO exercise. Once there, the Prince noted with immense pride that 'our ship looked by far the best and most glamorous one in a long line of vessels. No one else I felt could possibly know how to operate at sea as well as we could.' Obviously the frail nature of the Prince's own confidence did not extend to the Royal Navy, his ship or his fellow officers.

In the RAF, Prince Charles had compressed a year's course into five months. At Dartmouth a three-month course had been undertaken in six weeks. Now, on the *Norfolk*, he was expected to gain a Bridge Watchkeeping Certificate in nine months, when a year would be more usual. However, this test had to be passed as it was an important milestone in an officer's career, and without the certificate, promotion would not be possible. He felt the pressure: 'I believe in being well occupied and busy ... but I expect more is learned and accumulated by midshipmen who have longer to explore and investigate ... However I did obtain my wings reasonably fairly ... and I passed the exams at Dartmouth, but I lacked that touch of professionalism which only comes after longer periods.'

After preparing for the NATO exercise, Prince Charles and a group of fellow officers went ashore to have dinner in Toulon. A wonderful meal was enjoyed and washed down with large quantities of champagne, wine and Armagnac. After dinner they staggered into the 'red-light district'. He was to note, 'We went into one bar where a group of our sailors tried, successfully, to force beer down my throat. I had attempted to drink pastiche [sic] but gave up abruptly ... We then moved on to another bar even more crowded with our sailors and Dutch matelots ... A young lady of little attraction grabbed me by the wrist and drew me to the counter muttering "Rum and Coke?" with a heavily disguised French accent. I meekly accepted while the bar reverberated to sound of inebriated voices singing, "There'll always be an England" accompanied by a Dutch sailor playing the accordion.

'At this point I began to think that I was a marked man. Not one but TWO naval patrols appeared outside the bar. Newspaper headlines flashed through my sub-conscious – "Sailor Prince arrested in sleazy French Bar – Admiralty Probe." It all contributed to my general education though.'

It most certainly did, but what the Duke would have made of it all is unknown. On the one hand he would not have appreciated any form of scandal involving his son. On the other, he had always wanted Prince Charles to be more outgoing and it is, of course, a well-know fact that he was quite a womaniser during his days in the Royal Navy. Perhaps he might have taken some comfort that the boy was a chip off the old block.

Once the NATO exercise, with which the Prince hadn't been too impressed as he judged the cooperation between the allies to have been half-hearted, was completed, HMS *Norfolk* made her way back to Toulon. A storm blew up in the Bonifacio Straits and soon she was pounding through walls of white water. He found the spectacle from the ship's bridge to be 'magnificent', but on retiring to his bunk noted, 'the movement of the ship was so violent in the rolling plane that I honestly felt on occasion that the ship was never going to right herself ...'

While on the NATO exercise, he had been allowed to manoeuvre Norfolk to come alongside a French oil tanker in order that she might be refuelled in transit. He had successfully achieved this, but was less confident when ordered, on leaving Toulon Harbour, to set a course for Plymouth, which was over a thousand miles away and required several changes of direction. However, by some 'curious accident', Plymouth appeared where and when it should have done and the Prince's 'relief was ill-concealed'.

But the self-doubt that had plagued him since he had been a small boy was evident again in a letter to Mountbatten: 'I've been made to work extremely hard since I set foot in this mighty vessel. I stumble around the ship, falling down hatches and striking my head against bulkheads in an effort to find my way about. There are so many departments to learn about that the task seems more than any brain can cope with ... I have been "thrown in at the deep end" in the most obvious manner ... I'm afraid that I tend to suffer from bouts of hopeless depression because I feel that I'm never going to cope ... One is surrounded in a ship this size by such scores of hideously professional officers and ratings that I find I appear even more useless than usual. I'm hoping that suddenly all sorts of things will slip into place and I will see the light.'

However, he displayed no such anxieties in public and concealed his real fear of failure behind his usual façade of self-deprecation. As a result, he fitted in with his fellow officers and was well liked by them; and thanks to his kindness and genuine concern for the lower decks, his popularity wasn't just confined to the officers' mess. His journal was to express on many occasions his admiration and concern for the non-commissioned officers and able seamen. This was perhaps not surprising: he had always shown more interest in the palace chauffeurs, gardeners and grooms than his siblings had, and such genuine concern gave him a likeable image in the navy that went some way to making up for his limited technical ability.

Nevertheless, his lack of confidence on the job did not prevent him expressing damning opinions in his journal about government policy regarding the navy. He believed that he had, as future king, the duty to comment on such matters in his private writings, as they would then be recorded for posterity. He was scathing about the decision to scrap the Royal Navy's last two aircraft carriers, as he believed that while the RAF might be a substitute for the Fleet Air Arm in a European theatre of war, it could not hope to be able to do such a job on the other side of the world where it might be denied landing rights, fuel and passage through airspace. Some would oppose such an opinion on the grounds that it was built on the old romantic ideas of empire, without thought being given to current cost and what Britain could really afford. Others might point to the Falklands War of a decade later and declare that Prince Charles's apprehension was totally justified.

While his ship was in dry dock, the Prince was to serve on the frigate HMS *Hermione* and, much to his private displeasure, a nuclear submarine HMS *Churchill*. On the submarine he thought his cabin was particularly tiny; he was shocked to discover that he was sharing it with two other officers. However, he wasn't anti-nuclear or against the submarine in principle. Indeed, on a tour of the vessel he was told that visitors often asked how many hospitals might be built with the £30 million that just one nuclear sub cost. The heir to the throne was to record in his journal with some indignation, 'what they fail to realise is that these nuclears, and the Polaris boats in particular, provide the greatest assurance for peace that the world has ever known. Without such a powerful deterrent (even one Polaris sub. is enough) we could not have the security to build 10 hospitals, let alone 50 for an equivalent sum of money. It is misguided enthusiasm which leads to this unrealistic attitude.'

What he stopped short of saying was that this was part of an idealistic and unrealistic malaise that had become increasingly prevalent in the British way of life since the end of the Second World War, and its effects were serious. You don't, after all, get something for nothing. We would take several years to repair our economy from such thinking, while our social sense of decency and humanity has never recovered: it is now, some thirty years later, poorer than ever and getting worse all the time.

In March 1972 there was a four-week workup for another NATO exercise, which the Prince was to describe rather bleakly in both his journal and his correspondence to his great-uncle. He was taught how to lead a riot squad, but believed that he 'would have been almost more frightened of being shot at by one of the sailors than one of the rioters. The former seem to have no idea whatsoever of how to handle a rifle safely.' He also described how he had managed to throw his simulated CS gas canister, by getting the end caught in his sleeve, at his own men rather than the rioters, and worse how he mistimed an order when lowering a lifeboat, which caused the craft some rather expensive damage – the forward thwart was torn out of its socket as the boat plunged down into the sea.

His recordings evoke the making of a *Carry On* film rather than a serious preparation for action. His commanding officer was later to enter a footnote in his journal that reprimanded him for this account, even though it had been largely self-mocking: 'You paint a fairly black picture of the work-up. It did us all a power of good, and Norfolk is a better tuned weapon as a result.'

Nevertheless, at the end of Prince Charles's nine months aboard, Captain Cook, who was completing his last tour of duty, was more kind when he finally wrote, 'An excellent journal which is fun to read.' And, despite its frank and at times eccentric account, the Admiralty Board in Whitehall seemed to agree. Without reservation, Sir Roderick Macdonald, president of the Fleet Board, observed on behalf of the Admiralty, 'The best journal this Board has seen.'

As it was written by the heir to the throne it was hardly likely to be described as the worst. However, the description 'best' was not a necessary politeness and denotes both a genuine compliment and perhaps an expression of gratitude to the Prince of Wales for sticking up for the senior service against government cuts.

As we now know, the Prince of Wales did not enjoy an immensely affectionate or tactile relationship with either of his parents. This has led many to suspect that Princess Diana's charges that he was a cold and aloof father and husband – damaged by a poor relationship with his own father and the absence of one with his mother – to be true. In fact, as we shall see, there are any number of accounts of Prince Charles being actively involved with his children as they grew up, and enjoying many happy and loving moments with the Princess, as most married couples do.

But for now, let us simply examine the nature of the correspondence that we have read so far. The letters of the Prince of Wales have been full of self-doubt, depression, self-deprecation and at times anxiety and self-pity. They have occasionally shown flashes of petulance and hot temper. But they also highlight a sensitivity for and belief in the importance of art, religion and the soul, as well as a genuine desire to reach out to people. They have always demonstrated a great desire to do his best with what he suspects are very limited talents. They have shown care and concern for all – family, friends, colleagues and their children, employees, the Welsh people, the Australian people, the British people, the ratings in the Royal Navy, and always for those less fortunate than himself.

They have shown resolve in the face of adversity, bravery in the face of danger and kindness, and thoughtfulness when attempting to help others. His letters usually accord a high degree of respect for the 'other man's' opinion. And given any opportunity by a trusted loved one – his grandmother, siblings, an old nanny or increasingly Lord Mountbatten – he is able to demonstrate, and always was from his earliest days, the soft and gentle love that seeps through the pages of his letters time and again. His writing is one of a kind and compassionate individual who is by no means perfect, but nearly always good. Do these letters anywhere demonstrate a coldness or an aloofness? I think not.

These are genuine letters that were written over the first twenty years or so of his life. Other letters to him or about him show him in the same light, and support this impression of him. Together they are much more likely to reflect the true nature of his character than the angry rantings of a woman at a very low point in her life.

In the autumn of 1971, Prince Charles was based ashore at Portsmouth for several weeks. He stayed, at his great uncle's invitation, at Mountbatten's home, Broadlands, in the nearby Hampshire countryside. The Prince delighted in this, as did Mountbatten, who wrote when the time was over that, 'I miss you a lot, for there is no one whose company I enjoy more, as I expect you realise.'

By this time Mountbatten, now in his seventies, was quite prepared to spend as much time as he could moulding his great-nephew into a man who would become a great king. This only served to strengthen their already strong bonds of mutual respect and affection. The Prince took to referring to Mountbatten as 'honorary grandfather', and Mountbatten responded by calling Charles 'honorary grandson'. Soon he was consulting his great-uncle on such matters, and Mountbatten was in a perfect position to teach him. Not only was he gentle and encouraging to the young Prince, he had been a royal insider all his life and had, unlike the rest of the family, wielded real power as both the last viceroy of India and chief of defence staff. This combination was a heady cocktail, and the Prince grew invariably to believe anything that Mountbatten told him.

For his part, Mountbatten was most determined, among other things, to explain how the abdication of Edward VIII came about. This was not only because he was keen to prevent Prince Charles from making the same mistake, but because, unlike the rest of the family, he was very fond of Edward VIII and therefore knew, and would admit to, a much more complex story than the Queen or the Queen Mother would ever concede. Their attitude was that Uncle David was a selfish man who had let everybody down, and as a result should not be mentioned. With this in mind, Mountbatten hoped to recruit Prince Charles to the cause of securing an invitation for the Duke of Windsor and his much disliked wife to return to Britain and finish their lives peacefully having made some kind of reconciliation with other members of the Windsor family. Prince Charles didn't need much persuading: 'I, personally, feel it would be wonderful if Uncle David and his wife could come over and spend a weekend. Now that he is getting old he must long to come back and it would seem pointless to continue the feud ... Apart from anything else it would be fun to see what she was like ... it is worthwhile getting to know the better side of her. I dare say it is much easier for me to speak like this because I knew nothing of what it was like before ...'

The Prince took the case to his grandmother, but he quickly realised that she would find it almost impossible to be reconciled with them, as she still believed that their actions had sent her husband to an early grave. So in the hope of keeping channels open, the Prince of Wales made a private visit to France and arranged via the British ambassador, Sir Christopher Soames, to meet his other great-uncle for the first time. He duly recorded it in his diary thus: 'I drove up with no small degree of anticipation as to what I would find in the Bois de Boulogne and upon entering the house I found footmen and pages wearing identical scarlet and black uniforms to the ones ours wear at home. It was rather pathetic seeing that. The eye then wandered to a table in the hall on which laid a red box with "The King" on it ... The whole house reeked of some particularly strong joss sticks and from out of the walls came the muffled sound of scratchy piped music. The Duchess appeared from among a host of the most dreadful American guests I have ever seen. The look of incredulity on their faces was a study and most of them were thoroughly tight. One man shook hands with me twice, muttering something incomprehensible in French with a strong American accent and promptly collapsed into the arms of a strategically placed black footman ...

'To my relief I managed to escape to into a small sitting room where I was able to have a word with Uncle David by himself. He seemed in very good form, although rather bent and using a stick. One eye was closed most of the time, as a result of his cataract operation, but apart from that he was in very talkative form and used wide, expansive gestures the whole time, while clutching an enormous cigar

The King and Di

…

'We got onto the subject of his relationship with his father and he said he had had a very difficult time with him and that Gan-Gan [Prince Charles's great-grandmother, Queen Mary] was a hard woman and he had been brought up extremely strictly. Hence his feelings against older people and traditions of all sorts. While he was talking the Duchess kept flitting to and fro like a strange bat. She looks incredible for her age and obviously has her face lifted every day. Consequently she can't really speak except by clenching her teeth all the time and not moving her facial muscles. She struck me as a hard woman – totally unsympathetic and somewhat superficial. Very little warmth of the true kind; only that brilliant hostess type of charm but without feeling. All that she talked about was whether she would wear a hat at the Arc de Triomphe the next day.

'Uncle David then talked about how difficult my family had made it for him for the past 33 years … I asked him frankly if he would like to return to England for the last years of his life and he hesitated to ask Wallis if he should give me "the works". It sounded as though he would have liked to return, but he felt as though no one would recognise him. I assured him that would not be the case. On the other hand most of his contemporary friends are dead and there may be very little point in his coming back.

'The whole thing seemed so tragic – the existence, the people and the atmosphere – that I was relieved to escape it after 45 minutes and drive round Paris by night.'

Eight months later, David, Duke of Windsor, formerly Edward VIII, was dead. Prince Charles cut short a visit to Malta to fly home for the funeral, and endured an awkward dinner at Buckingham Palace with the Queen and the duchess. It was the first time the duchess had been to the palace since the abdication and the first time the Queen had shown her any recognition. Both behaved in character, with the duchess nervously babbling on while the Queen was charming but lacking any real compassion. After dinner they were all joined by other members of the Royal Family in order to watch Mountbatten's tribute to the former king on the television, which the Prince was to describe as 'very moving and beautifully done'.

After dinner on the next night, Charles accompanied Mountbatten to St George's Chapel, Windsor, where the Duke was lying in state. They met the duchess in front of her husband's coffin as the Guards

Officers stood vigil – 'their great bearskinned heads bowed as they stood absolutely motionless and silent'. The duchess had not been well that day, and had to be supported by Mountbatten, but at one point she summoned enough strength to move away a little distance on her own – 'a frail, tiny, black figure gazing at the coffin and finally bowing briefly … As we stood she kept saying "he gave up so much for so little" – pointing at herself with a strange grin'.

The Prince was surprised to be deeply moved by the actual funeral. After all, he hardly knew this great-uncle whose name had always been associated with shame during Charles's childhood and who was so disliked by his own beloved grandmother, a lady the Prince no doubt thought to be ten times the woman the duchess was. Nor was he likely to experience the secret feelings of guilt that Granny or her daughter would surely be harbouring following their years of ostracising the tragic couple.

Once inside St George's Chapel for the service, the Prince, walking alone, followed the coffin into the nave. He felt the grief and significance of the moment: 'Somehow I felt deeply moved by the whole experience and felt that it was right that we were honouring Uncle David like this … The service was simple, dignified to perfection, colourful and wonderfully British.' When the state trumpeters of the Household Cavalry blew the last post, he trembled with emotion 'and my eyes filled with tears'. Again, these were not the emotions of a hard and aloof man.

Mountbatten, unopposed as the Prince's most trusted advisor, now also became his confidante in matters of the heart, and Charles began to discuss with him romantic targets to whom he found himself drawn. The idea that he could have had any such conversations with his father is quite unthinkable, but he needed to talk things over man to man with somebody. He could not have his first fumbling sexual experiences in the back of a Mini Cooper or in the back row of the local cinema, and while princes throughout history might have been able to deflower as many young maidens as they wanted, such was their 'divine' power in their day, this sort of freedom was not open to Prince Charles. Getting started in the romantic business can be quite difficult for any shy young man, without the added pressure of living your life in a goldfish bowl. Nor was it very gallant to expect some charming young lady to run the gauntlet of the national press in order that the heir to the throne could satisfy his sexual urges.

All of this presented the Prince with real problems. Luckily for him he had Mountbatten on hand not only to offer sensible advice, but also to provide the perfect private hideaway where Charles and, over a number of years, his potential lovers could meet without the intrusion of a press that was bound to question his intentions and his girlfriends' virtue. That place, of course, was Broadlands. Mountbatten combined a traditional view of love and marriage with a worldly attitude, perhaps as a result of many years in the Royal Navy, to sex. He believed that young men should sow their wild oats before marriage, but then settle down to a life of faithful companionship and affection once the vows of marriage had been taken. This accords with the views of his generation: if the passion of courtship remained in marriage you were very lucky; if it didn't, you got on with an affectionate relationship built on mutual trust, respect, the need to 'keep up appearances' and a family together 'for the sake of the children'.

Naturally, this is in stark contrast to today's perception that if you are not in the first pangs of passion, your marriage is a disaster and should be dissolved in order for you to trawl the aisles of a late-night supermarket to find a new partner, and sod any kids that you might have had along the way. The old route is criticised for being hypocritical, the new for being shallow and selfish. Both criticisms are fair: the question comes down to which route, in general terms, produces a kinder, more responsible and civilised society.

It is clear that without the collusion of Mountbatten when it came to smuggling girls into Broadlands, Prince Charles would have found it very difficult to find the opportunity to give free expression to the normal passions of a young man. Among the young women whom he was to seduce – or would have liked to – at this time, there was just one who was to have an immediate and lasting effect upon him. Since leaving Cambridge he had maintained his friendship with Lucia Santa Cruz: over a year later she had contacted Prince Charles to report that she had found 'just the girl' for him. She went on to make the arrangements for the Prince of Wales to meet Miss Camilla Shand.

Camilla Shand was pretty and had Charles's sense of humour – she loved the Goons. She laughed with her eyes, which lit up with genuine warmth, and wasn't the type to be always doing her make-up and preening herself lovingly in the mirror. Indeed, she didn't care much for fashion and was at her happiest on a horse in the country. She was individual, irreverent and intelligent. She belonged to the unfashionable landed gentry, whom Charles understood and liked, and she was miles away from being one of the fashionable, glamorous and self-obsessed urban socialites, with whom he had little in common and whom he certainly struggled to comprehend. Indeed, Camilla's family background was one that the Prince would have had knowledge of and been comfortable with. It was on the edge of the royal circle: her father, Bruce Shand, was a wealthy wine merchant and her mother, Rosalind, was a member of the extremely rich Cubitt family, which meant that Camilla's grandfather was Baron Ashcombe.

There was also another unofficial family tie between her and the Windsors that she was aware of but he apparently wasn't: she had had the confidence to point out to Prince Charles, at their first meeting, that her great-grandmother Alice Keppel had once been a mistress of his great-great-grandfather Edward VII. The Prince had been both intrigued and amused. She was unassuming, naturally affectionate and he found her to be very sexy. He fell head over heels in love with her almost immediately.

The dashing young sailor prince was, according to the press, having the time of his life. The media put any young lady seen in his company, and there were lots of them, under the closest scrutiny as a potential future queen of England. But they took a more kindly attitude with Charles himself. He, however, was already worrying about how he would ever find the right woman. Who would really want to marry him when she discovered that the rest of her life would be an arduous task, that she would be as much married to the institution of monarchy as to him? His future wife would be committed to life in the goldfish bowl, on constant view and subject to the public's every whim and the media's every lie, a life that would be very hard to retreat from once she had committed to it. Could anybody ever be expected to love him enough to put up with that kind of a life?

In fact, this question had been concerning him since his mid-teens. He had even touched on it in his first television interview back in the late 1960s. Now it was occupying more of his time and causing something of an emotional turmoil. With that self-doubt and gentle vulnerability that has always made him very attractive to women, he was already confiding to those closest to him that any woman he might want to marry would never want to marry him. And then along came Camilla Shand, and he dared to think that here was a woman with all the strengths needed to handle it: she was down to earth, not fazed by him or the institution of monarchy, had the right social credentials, was Church of England and he loved her. He felt at ease with her and felt sure that she could be the friend that he would want to love and spend his life with. Even better, she seemed to have the same feelings for him. In the late autumn of 1972 they became inseparable.

Camilla, while being single and clearly fond of the heir to the throne, had previously been going out with a much sought-after cavalry officer nine years older than her. He was hugely attractive and had a habit of sweeping girls, including Princess Anne, off their feet – and then bedding most of them. His name was Andrew Parker Bowles and Camilla had been going out with him since she was eighteen in the hope that he would marry her. He hadn't yet – sure in the knowledge that she would always have him back.

In the autumn of 1972 Parker Bowles was posted to Germany and it appeared to Camilla that the relationship was finally over for good. She was therefore free to enjoy the kind and gentle relationship the Prince could offer her – a contrast to the swashbuckling, bitter-sweet pain experienced at the hands of her former boyfriend. And so the first of her three love affairs with Prince Charles started because of the army; it was to be finished because of the navy.

In the new year of 1973, the Prince's next posting in the navy was due to separate them for eight months. In early December he had joined his new ship, the frigate HMS *Minerva*, and was to sail on her to the Caribbean in January. This was a commitment to which there would be no escape. There has been much speculation that the Prince wanted to ask Camilla for her hand in marriage before he left, or at the very least tormented himself with the prospect. This is very unlikely: although very strongly attracted to her and hopeful that things would develop, he knew what an enormous step this would be; but as yet he didn't believe he had known her long enough or was certain enough of his own mind to embark on a course from which there could be no honourable retreat for either of them. Furthermore, they were still at a very early stage in the relationship, and it is probable that both would have been far too reserved at this stage ever to think of mentioning the subject.

Prior to sailing, he invited Camilla to make a tour of inspection and then have lunch on board. She returned again the following weekend – 'The last time I shall see her for eight months,' he observed sadly in a letter to Mountbatten. But it was to be much worse than that. There is no doubt that Camilla Shand was very attracted to Prince Charles. Indeed she came to love him unreservedly in the years to come – the way in which she has borne, with quiet dignity, the most unfair and unjust media campaign against her has proved that – but, in the winter of 1973, she didn't know where their short relationship was leading. Perhaps it would develop, perhaps it would not. Andrew Parker Bowles, possibly motivated by Camilla's sudden independence and attraction to the Prince of Wales, returned to claim his woman and they became engaged in March 1973 – just two months after Charles had set sail. She had waited seven years for the man with whom she was infatuated to ask for her hand in marriage, and she jumped at the opportunity, confident that this handsome stud would change his ways in the future.

When the Prince came to hear of her renewed relationship with Parker Bowles he was deeply upset. He wrote to a friend that it seemed so cruel that fate should end 'such a blissful, peaceful and mutually happy relationship … I suppose the feelings of emptiness will pass eventually.' At the time the singer-songwriter Gilbert O'Sullivan was enjoying massive success with a hit song called 'Alone Again (Naturally)'. The lyrics to this song and its haunting melody must have not been lost on Charles as he strove to fight back feelings of loneliness and hopelessness on the other side of the world. However, despite this bitter blow, the Prince remained friends with Camilla and, over the next seven years, as he was to be seen with some of the most glamorous and desirable women in Britain, she became a very close confidante and trusted friend. There was no sexual relationship, but the bond that had formed during that early intimate affair gave rise to a closeness that was very special, even unique.

When the Parker Bowleses' first child Tom was born in 1975, Camilla asked Prince Charles to be a godfather. He happily accepted. Gradually Camilla, without diminishing Charles's love for his grandmother, replaced the Queen Mother as the mother that he had never had. He spent hours on the phone to her and they also met at polo parties and other royal gatherings. The Parker Bowleses were very much in Charles social circle – Andrew was a distant relative of the Queen Mother and his mother was a close friend of the Queen. Camilla and Andrew were thus often invited to stay at Sandringham, Windsor or Balmoral, while Charles often spent weekends with them at their Wiltshire home, enjoying playing with their children, their daughter

The King and Di

Laura having been born in 1979.

Their friendship became physical once more after Laura's birth. By then Camilla had long since realised that Andrew was never going to change his spots: her husband, whom she had chased and forgiven time and again for seven years in order to get him down the aisle, had only continued his philandering ways once he had come up it again. Something of a lothario, and he now lived most of the time in London where he didn't mind being seen out and about with a string of different women on his arm; Camilla was left to spend her time in Wiltshire on her own, attending to the needs of their children and feeding the horses.

Depressed and lonely, she felt drawn to the Prince. She remembered the story of Alice Keppel and Edward VII and enjoyed the idea of history repeating itself. An affair with her best friend would make her feel wanted and needed; an affair with the future king of England would be good for her hurt ego and just what was needed to restore her damaged pride. Moreover, what harm could it do? Prince Charles wasn't married – he wasn't even engaged – and he was seeing many different women, while her husband, given his track record, was hardly in a position to complain.

The Prince willingly agreed to the affair, and both believed it could lead nowhere: she was married, and one day so would he be – but never to a divorcee. So Camilla became mistress to the Prince of Wales, leaving the headlines to those starlets who vied to be seen publicly on his arm. She was not the first married woman to move in royal circles and have an affair, nor was she to be the last.

The Prince of Wales, for his part, was fully aware of his responsibility towards church, queen and country. He knew that they must always come first and that, in time, he must marry a girl who would make a suitable queen and who could bear him a son and heir. This, above all else – including his own personal feelings in the matter – would always be the priority. He was to say at the time, 'I've fallen in love with all sorts of girls and I fully intend to go on doing so, but I've made sure that I haven't married the first person I've fallen in love with. I think one's got to be aware of the fact that falling madly in love with someone is not necessarily the starting point to getting married. Marriage is basically a very strong friendship ... I think you are lucky if you find the person attractive in the physical and the mental sense ... To me marriage seems to be the biggest and most responsible step to be taken in one's life ... Whatever your place in life, when you marry you are forming a partnership which will last for fifty years. So I'd want to marry someone whose interests I could share. A woman not only marries a man; she marries into his way of life – a job. She's got to have some knowledge of it, some sense of it; otherwise she wouldn't have a clue about whether she's going to like it. If I'm deciding on whom I want to live with for fifty years – well, that's the last decision on which I want my head to be ruled by my heart.'

These are not only the sentiments that Mountbatten had taught him, but both the Queen, the Duke of Edinburgh and the vast majority of their generation would have expected no less from a future king. His life held many privileges, but it also had its prices, and this was one. Moreover, these words give a far greater understanding to what was in Prince Charles's mind when he eventually became engaged to Diana Spencer. He was actually putting them into practice: he was lucky enough to find her physically very attractive; she claimed she understood what was expected of her in the arduous task of monarchy and the harsh demands of duty to the people; she expressed her love of Balmoral, the country life and sports and all of his friends. Unfortunately, none of this was true: the Princess lacked the discipline needed for continual duty, only had the stomach for the media when it suited her, hated Balmoral, thought country life was boring, was frightened of riding and was exceedingly jealous of Charles's friends.

Prince Charles was being true to what he had been taught was the best way to select a wife, not only for himself but also for the good of the monarchy in particular and the country in general. He knew his marriage had to last, and he believed that great friendship, common interest and an understanding of what was involved were essential if there was to be any chance of success. Diana convinced him that she was the girl for the job.

Once in the Caribbean, having survived a raging gale while crossing the Atlantic, the Prince had to combine the roles of lowly junior naval officer and heir to the world's most famous throne. As a result he was to attend scores of cocktail parties and, despite the 'alcoholic haze', was happy and touched to note that he was warmly welcomed everywhere by the common people, but he found a number of their leaders to be either aloof, self-important or even sinister. Over the coming months his ship steamed from island to island and state to state, nearly always causing some diplomatic anxiety as the Royal Navy were under instruction that the Prince of Wales was to be treated at all times according to his rank, whereas the governments of the countries where HMS *Minerva* put into port wanted to entertain him as the heir to the British throne.

The Prince handled these very tricky diplomatic mazes with more than a little skill and patience; but the longer he was at sea, the more homesick he became. His only consolation was that it had been arranged for him to spend a week in April on the tiny Caribbean island of Eleuthera, where his godmother Patricia and her husband Lord Brabourne owned a house. Patricia was Mountbatten's daughter, and her father would be there. Charles counted the days until he could board a plane in Bermuda and spend a few days with some of his favourite people.

Then, in March, the plan seemed to have been scuppered by the assassination of Bermuda's governor, Sir Richard Sharples, which led the security services to announce that on no account should the Prince of Wales be allowed to be put ashore there in order to take a plane. Mountbatten regretfully informed the Prince of their ruling and told him that, due to other logistical or security considerations, the trip would have to be aborted. However, Charles was in no mind to have this one ray of hope for the immediate future extinguished and replied, 'I'm afraid I'm taking a leaf out of your book (to a certain extent!) and am putting my foot down and not taking "no" for an answer. I shall use every method at my disposal (including bribery!) to get to Eleuthera and I am determined that I shall succeed.' He did.

He arrived on the island on 13 April, and the next seven days were to surpass his wildest dreams. He swam in the bluest of seas, walked on the whitest of beaches, sailed by the warmest of breezes and found time to sit at an easel and paint it all. At mealtimes he helped prepare the food and at night he enjoyed the conversation before retiring early to bed where he drifted off into a relaxed sleep – soothed by the noise of the surf and the warm wind gently passing through the palm leaves.

As these glorious days passed all too quickly, the Prince found himself increasingly attracted to the Brabournes' daughter Amanda who, at the age of fifteen, was turning from a rather gawky girl into a beautiful young woman. Such was his confidence by now in Mountbatten that later he was able to write to his great-uncle, even though he was her grandfather, 'I must say Amanda really has grown into a very good-looking girl – most disturbing.' In fact it was not at all disturbing for Mountbatten, who secretly hoped that when the young Prince had sowed his wild oats he would settle down and marry Amanda and make her the next Queen of England. His mind loved the idea of a perfect Windsor–Mountbatten alliance, while his heart warmed to the idea of a match made in heaven between the two people he most loved upon this earth. It was so nearly to come about.

At the end of the week Charles flew from the island to join HMS *Fox*, a coastal survey vessel to which he had been temporarily transferred. He was to write to the Brabournes, 'In a cloud [of] deeply despondent homesickness I am back on board this tedious ship. You probably won't believe it … but when I climbed into the aircraft this afternoon and saw you all standing there on the tarmac a terrible lump came rushing up into my throat and the old tears began to trickle out of the corner of my eye. That same ghastly feeling of empty desperation and apparent hopelessness invaded my tummy and I spent a long time gazing rigidly out of the window … It was so utterly similar to going back to school that it frightened me …

'How can I ever convey the pure joy it was for me? Every single moment was savoured to the utmost. Every drop of water, every gamma ray of sunlight, each particle of sand, every glutinous drop of oil was … stored away in the luckiest of brain cells. From now until September I can organise a free film show in my mind to fill me with contented happiness when I am feeling low and desperate.'

These words are instantly recognisable to Prince Charles's close friends as being typical of a man who longed to pass his life surrounded by family and dear friends but knew that despite the pain of it all, duty must come first. Moreover, the Prince knew that other people had to be separated from their families also, not least those on board the ships on which he served. They had to put up with it and therefore so should he. But in great confidence to those whom he really loved and trusted, he could show that he resented that so much of the time he had to endure unhappiness in order to grab the occasional wonderful weekend.

HMS *Fox* moved on to Antigua and the Prince of Wales was to delight in English Harbour, which had originally been Admiral Lord Nelson's dockyard when fighting the French in the late eighteenth century. However, it was here that news reached him of Camilla's engagement Andrew Parker Bowles; he was still reeling from this when in May he received a letter from his father informing him that his sister, Princess Anne, was to marry an army captain called Mark Phillips.

The King and Di

Not only was Charles convinced that Anne was making a dreadful mistake, but it appeared to him that while the Royal Navy held him captive in the Caribbean, everything that was dear to him at home was being taken away from him and there wasn't a thing that he could do about it. Although he didn't enjoy a close relationship with either of his parents, he had come to see his family as something very dear and something to which he had been denied close access for long periods of time since the age of seven. Anne, in particular, had become a close confidante and someone with whom he could play the fool; now he was going to have to face up to the fact that he would no longer have first call on her affection and that her first loyalty would be to someone else. Initially he found this very hard to accept, and it took him several days to be able to contemplate her marriage without a sense of despair.

However, in typical Charles fashion, an inner battle was fought for the sake of the monarchy, and after a few days he recovered his composure; by the time of the public announcement at the end of the month, he was already taking a protective attitude towards Captain Phillips who, apart from being one of the most excellent horsemen in the land, seemed to lack most of the qualities needed to become part of the Royal Family. He was somewhat inept, he stuttered and, in a blind panic, would often say the first thing that came into his head. He was presented in the press as something of an in-bred, upper-class twit ...

As the spring and summer continued, and with the Prince now transferred back on board, HMS *Minerva* cruised through the Caribbean, joining in the occasional Royal Naval exercise but in the main dispensing goodwill in the form of cocktail and dinner parties given in the honour of various local government officials.

In Barbados, Charles went parascending and crash-landed at the first attempt. On the second, he reported, he, 'rose smoothly into the air and cruised happily along at about twenty five feet until a gust of wind caught me and I shot up and down, hit the water, lost one ski, flew violently up into the air again, stalled, regained height again and then did a death-defying dive into the sea at some vast, uncontrollable speed, striking my nose forcibly against an aluminium spar conveniently situated to do just that ... Blood poured out and I decided enough was enough.'

At Nassau he took part in a polo match where both players and ponies had been flown in for the occasion, but the day wasn't entirely successful from the Prince's point of view. He later wrote in his journal, 'I lost my temper completely when the first horse ran away with me and galloped twice through the pony lines, cutting an artery in its shoulder, and second the commentator, Tom Oxley, became so incredibly fastidious and unnecessary in his wet little remarks that I was forced, in a rage, to stump up to the top of the commentary box and ask him to stop making his pathetic remarks. The whole game was an unmitigated disaster.'

However, Prince Charles was in Nassau on official business: he was there to represent the Queen at the island's independence celebrations. He was by now a much stronger personality than in his youth and as a result took charge of the preparations with painstaking attention to detail and a command that left no one in doubt that his will would be done. He even replaced the national anthem at the end of the reception (it had been played at the beginning) with 'God Bless The Prince of Wales' – with the command, 'I am not standing for the latter since it is not a national anthem, and if it is played as I leave I can simply turn and wave.' This meticulous attention to detail was more borne out of a desire to minimise problems so that he could face each ordeal with confidence rather than a wish to dominate his subordinates. He was the one on show and therefore it would all be done in a fashion that he was comfortable with and could be certain of. As a result, there were few hiccups as he delivered five speeches (all written by him), laid several foundation stones, visited schools and hospitals and presided over the independence ceremony itself.

As August arrived, *Minerva* was due to turn for home via the Unites States. She experienced engine trouble and twice had to turn back to port. Prince Charles, thinking that he was destined never to see England again, suffered from a new bout of his all too familiar homesickness, but did his best to remain cheerful. At the third attempt the ship stuttered through a force-ten gale as she finally made her way across the Atlantic. On the last day of August, Charles was able to say goodbye to HMS *Minerva* and escape, at long last, to 'the best place on earth – Balmoral'.

The Prince had not enjoyed his eight months in the Caribbean. It had started with the betrothal of Camilla to Andrew Parker Bowles and had continued with the betrothal of his sister to Captain Mark Phillips. It had also deprived him of one of his greatest delights – an English summer. Nevertheless, the extent to which he was able to conceal his dislike, self-doubt and depression in the name of self-sacrifice for queen and country is best measured by his captain's final report on his progress: 'An honest, loyal and outstandingly cheerful officer whose quick wit and charm have enabled him to integrate most successfully in the ship. He has taken an active part in all the ship's activities and, while there is room for improvement professionally, he has become less critical of his own abilities and has gained in self-confidence as he has become aware of his increasing competence.

'He has an exceptional facility with all grades of society, and on board his division has responded most favourably to his sympathetic handling of their affairs and to his natural concern for their problems and welfare.'

But even this high accolade seemed mild compared to a note that was later added to his West Indian journal: 'In 60 years' experience of Junior Officers' Journals I cannot remember reading any whose accounts were so vivid, humorous and penetrating. I don't suggest that this is the World's Best Journal – all I can testify, I have not seen a better one.' It was signed Mountbatten of Burma.

The Prince's next ship was HMS *Jupiter*. He flew to Singapore to join her. Over the next four months she steamed, rather leisurely, to New Zealand, Suva, Tonga, Western Samoa, Honolulu, San Francisco, Acapulco, Panama, San Juan and Bermuda. It had been decided that the Prince of Wales would have wider duties on board than a dreaded concentration on navigation. Understandably, this somewhat pleased him. Less pleasing was the fact that the wardroom was fairly base and the conversation crude. Moreover his fellow officers, just to remind the Prince that he was only one of them, decided to defy the accepted protocol and referred to him simply as 'Wales'. For a day or so the Prince appeared a little wary and vulnerable, but he bore his new title without reproach and adapted well – even joining in and taking an active part in the mess banter. As a result it was not long before he became a popular member of the ship's command.

Unlike his tour of duty in the Caribbean, the Prince of Wales took much pleasure from this 'incredible Pacific voyage of 1974'. In particular he was pleased to rediscover Australia: 'Every time I come back to this country I find I feel more deeply about it and about the people ... it has engraved itself upon a part of my soul – rather like Balmoral is written deeply on my heart.' He had by now developed a comfortable routine and had found it within his capacity to combine the role of Prince of Wales with the more earthy charge of officer in Her Majesty's Royal Navy. His activities were now familiar – joint exercises at sea, garden parties, barbeques and dinner dances on land, with parachuting, polo and sexual encounters to be enjoyed when off duty.

In Toulon, while serving on HMS *Norfolk*, he had strayed into the red-light district; as an officer on HMS *Minerva* he had managed to see the inside of a Columbian brothel. Moreover, he had succumbed to an officer's daughter in the West Indies, and in Venezuela had let his imagination run riot while running his eyes over the body of the wife of another polo player. He later wrote, 'Never in my life have I encountered such dances as I had with this beautiful lady. She is unbelievable is all that I can say and I danced with every conceivable part of her. I fell madly in love with her and danced wildly and passionately, finally doing a Russian dance at one stage, which cleared the floor because I was wearing my mess boots...'

His self-confidence had now reached new heights and he was able to boast in a letter home, 'You may find when I get back that the Navy and six months out here have made me considerably more extrovert than I was. I am continually amazed at my audacity nowadays.'

As HMS *Jupiter* steamed from island to island across the Pacific Ocean, the Prince increasingly deployed what he called 'the old eye-flashing technique' to great effect. He became a magnet to all unattached women and more than a few married ones as well. The dashing young man in the dress of a Royal Naval Officer, with a flashing smile and a come-on look that twinkled from his eyes, was more than a match for the attempts of any of his fellow officers. Now he was leader of the pack.

Despite these new – and much-enjoyed – adventures, the Prince never got into anything too bad or so deeply as to endanger his reputation or that of the monarchy; he believed that he was only doing what was expected of him. After all, his father had always wanted him to be more outgoing, and Mountbatten's advice had been for him to let his hair down a bit before settling down. But his great-uncle also believed that the girl Charles should have his eye on was none other than his own granddaughter Amanda Knatchbull. He wrote to the Prince accordingly.

Had Charles been more worldly, less reluctant to turn to his own father for an alternative view and less likely to accept the advice of

Mountbatten without question, he might have thought more carefully about what his great-uncle had said. As it was, he accepted Uncle Dickie's views without question. Instead of regarding his honorary grandfather's letter as an intrusion upon his personal life, the Prince opened his heart to Mountbatten and replied, 'Perhaps being away and being able to think about life and about the future (and her) has brought ideas of marriage in to a more serious aspect.' He added that Amanda was indeed 'incredibly affectionate and loyal ... with a glorious sense of fun and humour – and she's a country girl as well which is even more important.' However, the Prince went on to say that he 'couldn't possibly get married yet', but then wrote that the more he thought about it 'the more ideal' the idea of Amanda seemed to him, adding, 'I am sure that she must know that I am very fond of her simply by reading the letters I write to her.'

The reality was that the Prince was dithering: he knew that Amanda Knatchbull fitted the bill; he knew that he liked her a lot; he realised that Camilla could never be his wife, and had long since banished any thoughts of her; and he knew that it would give great pleasure not only to Mountbatten but also to his parents, the government and the country as a whole. On the other hand, he wanted to be certain that this choice was going to be the right one and that he would not meet another woman in a few months' time who bowled him off his feet because he knew that, unlike everyone else in the kingdom, he would not be granted a second chance.

The responsibility for the heir to the throne to marry and produce his own heir was by now beginning to weigh heavily on his mind – along with all the other worries associated with becoming king. It, like all others, would have to be conquered: what was the point of having beaten the rest if he was to allow just one to let him down and by so doing cause him to fail the monarchy and the country? 'Everyone is becoming engaged left, right and centre ...' he wrote. 'I am now becoming convinced that I shall soon be left floundering helplessly on a shelf somewhere, having missed everyone!'

Charles had developed genuine affection for Amanda and he sensed that, given her background and line, she would intuitively be up to the demanding roles of princess of Wales and eventually queen of England. Many observers have commented that he was to become a confirmed bachelor who was bullied into marrying Lady Diana Spencer by his father. This is simply not true. His search for the right girl to take on the almost impossible role of wife, mother and princess had been on his mind since his early twenties; by at the age of twenty-five it was preoccupying him daily. His letters, diaries and journals show how keen he was to marry and become a father. He had always yearned for a female soulmate and had been kindly with children for as long as anyone could remember. But it was his duty to choose a girl who was right for the job.

Reassured by Amanda's 'deep feelings' for the Prince, neither he nor Mountbatten gave much thought at this stage to how Amanda herself might feel about the prospect. For the next five years Mountbatten used his every effort to steer his granddaughter and great-nephew towards marriage, and the intertwining of the House of Windsor and the House of Mountbatten forever.

A reputation for kindness preceded the Prince from ship to ship. Men became keen to serve under this popular officer, and his natural, compassionate manner impressed fellow officers and ratings alike. He upheld all the rules and applied discipline, but was never overbearing and his door was always open to those under his command who needed to discuss the problems they expected to have to face on their return home. An officer who was a good listener has never been common in the navy, but Charles's men were his flock and they responded well to his care.

In Australia, one of his ratings was knocked down and killed while returning to the ship from Surfers' Paradise outside Brisbane. 'I was absolutely shattered,' the Prince recorded. 'Having a division induces an extraordinary feeling of responsibility, I find, and the worst part was not been able to do anything to help. The communications department was shattered by the news and all was very quiet and subdued. Altogether a horrible thing to happen and made worse by the fact that [he] was soon to be engaged when he got home.'

There is a naval tradition, dating back at least to the Napoleonic Wars, that when a seaman is killed his kit is auctioned among his comrades and the proceeds sent to his family. In this case the bidding was slow, as despite the deceased being popular, he left no widow or children to support. Suddenly a voice from the back of the hall bid £400 for a naval-issue suitcase of green cardboard. It was the Prince of Wales. His men followed his lead and they were followed by the whole ship's company. Instead of items going under the hammer for a few pence, the bidding soared and even pairs of socks were fetching £20. In the end £1,500 was raised for the seaman's family. It was a defining moment: a man born to be a leader, but never a born leader, had become one. The men followed Charles the man, not Charles the Prince.

However, this was not as Mountbatten saw it. When news of his great-nephew's success reached him, he attributed it to 'royalty', adding, 'I don't mind betting that when you have done as long at sea you will be a greater legend than your old Great Uncle seems to have been – and for the same reasons.' It was true that the Prince, who saw Mountbatten as the perfect role model, attempted to emulate him in every way. Nevertheless, while lapping up the praise that he so craved, he was quick to reply with genuine modesty, 'I know what you mean about "Royalty" – and it certainly helps to be "known" in the Navy – but in your case there was <u>definitely</u> a great deal extra which transcended any minor considerations of royalty. I shall only be remembered as having <u>been</u> in the Navy from 1971 – whereas you are a legend through indisputably significant and glorious deeds.'

It had become the Prince's opinion that, during peacetime, the Royal Navy's best weapon was the goodwill visit, and he appreciated the positive diplomatic and trading benefits that could be achieved as a result. He understood that the immediate effect was only a warm feeling of friendship, but he realised that such acquaintance led to stronger national ties. With this in mind, he was not always overimpressed with Britain's permanent representatives in the diplomatic corps abroad – especially in America where he believed it was most important to impress. 'I only wish,' he wrote, 'we were represented by higher calibre people in places like San Diego, Los Angeles, Hawaii, etc … it can't do much for our image abroad.'

While in America, he was the guest of Walter Annenberg, the American Ambassador to Britain between 1969 and 1975. He dined at his palatial home along with Annenberg's wife and Ronald and Nancy Regan. Ronald Regan was the Californian governor at the time. The next day he played golf on the Annenbergs' 1,000-acre private course in the middle of the Nevada desert. The Prince, who by now had a pretty good eye from the back of a polo pony, has never been a good golfer; his only consolation on this occasion was that neither Regan nor Annenberg appeared to be any better. At one point Bob Hope appeared from nowhere in a golf buggy. 'I was in swimming trunks and he took one look at me and said "with a physique like that the future of England is certainly assured." I wonder if he was being sarcastic,' the Prince noted that evening in his journal.

Later, Frank Sinatra arrived for drinks and at dinner the august company discussed world politics. Charles was pleased to be included on such occasions, and listened intently, even offering an opinion if his views were canvassed. However, he still waited to be asked, as he as yet did not believe at twenty-five years of age he had the right to interrupt career politicians who had, after all, been elected to office. This view was quite out of step with the rest of his generation who, for at least a decade, had been ripping down anything and everything that stood for the older generation. Charles's ability to listen, always attentive and modest, and then record the arguments in his journals, helped him to fashion a framework upon which he could test and then hang his own views. As a result, he was to become far wiser than the vast majority of the baby boomers of his time.

He slowly recorded his view of life, nature, religion and beyond. For now he felt no great urge to stand on top of a mountain and shout it to the world; but it would not now be too many years before the man who had preached sermons to imaginary congregations as a child would unleash his plan for a meaningful life upon a nation.

By July, HMS *Jupiter* was back in British waters and placed on twelve hours' notice to sail for Cyprus as Turkey was threatening to invade the island. The Prince was at Balmoral for the weekend when the call finally came. For once he was pleased to go. 'I was rather keen to be sent to Cyprus, I had a yearning for some sort of action – some sort of constructive, useful naval operation where perhaps a medal could be won and I could supplement the one I have (for supreme gallantry at the Coronation!) with a proper one.' In the end, however, *Jupiter* was not required to sail to Cyprus after all, and the Prince's journal reflected his disappointment and intense anger at the apparent dithering by the Ministry of Defence. 'Men are not machines and just because they are in the armed services, and therefore expected to do as they are told it is not as simple as that. People are quite prepared to take sensible orders, but patience and willingness wear thin when things are constantly changed, cancelled and then re-instituted. What an extraordinarily good thing it is for me to experience all of this at grass roots level so that I can at least appreciate the things that people have to endure. The trouble is that only a very few of the present government have ever served in the armed forces or in an organisation where other people's decisions directly affect your life and family.'

Instead of going into the Mediterranean, *Jupiter* joined a NATO exercise at Scapa Flow and this proved to be something of a consolation as it aroused Prince Charles's patriotic pride for the force in which he served: 'When I stepped up onto the upper deck it was a most spectacular sight which greeted me. A great line of grey ships stretched out ahead, all creaming along at 20 knots on a glorious Orkney morning with the islands their green and yellow best and the sea positively sparkling. It sent an enormous shiver of excitement down my spine (rather like the Trooping does as well) and conjured up all sorts of images of the old Home Fleet steaming into Scapa led by the battleships, battle cruisers, aircraft carriers and followed by the cruisers and squadrons of destroyers.'

Once anchored in the Orkneys, the Prince used the occasion to take a long walk along the cliffs and later noted in his diary, 'I had forgotten how beautiful the Orkneys were and it was an unexpected and glorious surprise to see them again. The colours were unbelievable – greens, yellows, browns and staggering blues where the sea came in in great sweeping arms.' This is the contradiction of the man: it is not common that one who is drawn to write of the 'shiver of excitement' of speeding warships is also taken to note the glorious colours of nature.

Throughout the Prince's naval career to date, the media coverage had mostly been somewhat muted and generally sympathetic. However, following a series of photographs of the Prince relaxing in Fiji appearing in the *Mail*, *Mirror* and *Sun*, the Queen's press secretary became alarmed that the heir to the throne might be thought by the general public to be living it up in the navy at the nation's expense. Actually, the nation had gained no such impression whatsoever, but the order went out that the media should be manipulated towards taking photos of Charles at work in the navy rather than always being portrayed lapping up the sun with a pretty girl at his side.

This was a mistake by the Palace. While it would be completely irresponsible to have a 'laissez faire' policy towards the press, to attempt to manipulate them costs their respect and sympathy as they can always see it coming and feel insulted. Of course, hindsight is a wonderful thing, and at the time no one questioned the decision. As a result, the press were encouraged to visit Charles when he flew to the edge of the Arctic to go diving beneath the ice in Resolute Bay. He was to record in his journal that, 'There were fascinating ice crystal formations and icicles suspended under the ice and inside the layers of these wafer thin crystal structures were large white shrimp-like creatures. Because of the cold every living creature under the Arctic tends to move slowly and therefore once they have expended their energy in short bursts they are exhausted and you can pick up small fish and tentripods etc in your hand. There were beautiful jelly-like creatures completely transparent which acted like prisms reflecting all the colours of the rainbow inside themselves.'

Eventually he rose to the surface, exhausted but so exhilarated that he was even happy to see the press and couldn't resist the temptation to play the fool. He inflated his suit with air so that 'I looked like some animated form of dirigible balloon. I then stepped outside ... wearing a funny old hat ... and faced an amazed press corps that couldn't believe their eyes. I then had great pleasure in demonstrating the deflating characteristics of the suit which so astonished the press with mirth that they all downed their cameras and all burst into spontaneous applause.'

And yet the Prince seemed even to know that, despite the mutual goodwill created by sharing the discomfort of the Arctic for ten days, he would still have to be on his guard: 'I shall have to make the most of it as it is bound to be the last time!'

In the autumn of 1974, the Prince of Wales was finally allowed to join the Fleet Air Arm and, after a helicopter conversion course in Yeovilton in Somerset, he was assigned to 845 Naval Air Squadron as a pilot on board the commando carrier HMS *Hermes*. There he was to spend the happiest four months of his naval career.

The Prince loved flying and, thanks mainly to Mountbatten, he had great affection for and loyalty to the Royal Navy. Therefore the Fleet Air Arm was bound to hold great attraction. On the other hand, the Ministry of Defence found Palace instruction that the Prince must be treated like all other serving officers while having his life, as heir to the throne, protected to be a complete contradiction and erred on the side of caution. As a result he was not allowed to fly certain aircraft because of their safety record, and had other restrictions placed upon him. Prince Charles found this most embarrassing. Why did the navy employ machines that were too dangerous for him to fly, but were apparently quite all right for his fellow officers to risk their lives in?

He was duly assigned two helicopters that had bright-red nose-and-tail markings to denote that they were for his exclusive use, and they were subsequently maintained to the unique standards of the Queen's Flight. Once the Marines discovered this, Prince Charles became their favourite pilot, which was hardly a great endorsement of their confidence in the rest of the fleet's maintenance.

As it happened, the Prince was a naturally gifted pilot. This was clearly demonstrated one Sunday when a supply ship pulled alongside the *Hermes* port beam. Two helicopters were detailed to collect full crates of beer from the supply ship, deliver them to *Hermes*, then move forward to pick up empty crates and return them to the supply ship. It soon became quite obvious that the helicopter being piloted by the Prince of Wales was considerably outperforming that of the other pilot. 'We were seeing pole-handling of the highest order. He was doing it instinctively, it was terrific stuff,' a fellow officer later commented.

However, that evening Charles arrived in the wardroom looking like thunder. He ordered a drink and explained to his comrades that he had just come from the commander's cabin having been given a severe reprimand for showing off that afternoon. Nevertheless, he soon snapped out of his ill temper when his fellow young officers smiled and said 'join the club'.

Towards the end of his time on HMS *Hermes* he wrote, 'I had more fun flying than I ever had before. The flying was extremely concentrated, but there was masses of variety and interest; troop drills, rocket firing, cross-country manoeuvres (day and night), low-level transits, simulated fighter-evasion sorties, parachuting dropping flights and commando exercises with the Marines. There were no interruptions from any other source and as a result I ended up "Hog of the Month" with about fifty three hours in May!'

Over this period he had logged more than 500 hours at the controls of a Wessex helicopter and had established a reputation as an excellent pilot and a popular officer. All of this only served to enhance his Action Man reputation and the media, now at the high noon of their love affair with the Prince, revelled in his seemingly carefree attitude towards danger. It might have taken two decades, but at last Prince Phillip had the dashing young prince he had sought to create. Ironically, the construction had occurred despite the Duke's actions rather than because of them, and they owed a lot more to Charles's inner will and the encouragement of Mountbatten than anything else.

However, while the nation happily got used to having breakfast with another photograph in their newspaper of Charles getting up to some death-defying stunt, there were those – the ones responsible for his safety – who were not so pleased. In the late autumn of 1975 the Prince, while staying at Broadlands with Mountbatten, had agreed to take a trip in a hot-air balloon. In the event the flight had to be aborted before take-off due to poor weather. When Checketts got to hear of this planned adventure a few days later, he was horrified and wrote to Mountbatten to express his concern at this 'most recent example' of the Prince's apparent desire to dance with danger and potential death. 'Your influence on the Prince of Wales is enormous, and he has immense admiration and respect for your wise advice. I would therefore be everlastingly grateful for your valuable help in avoiding or restraining some of the more adventurous endeavours of this remarkable young man, who is far too important for the United Kingdom and the Commonwealth to hazard unnecessarily.' The flattery worked, as I suspect Checketts knew it might, and consequently Mountbatten replied with both grace and contrition, 'On reflection I agree with everything you have written and the fact that I had an amusing ascent the week before in perfect weather was really no excuse for not thinking about the risks.' He even added a warning that the Prince was planning another attempt at Sandringham.

Despite this letter, however, there is no evidence that Mountbatten made any effort to reign in the Prince's taste for daring adventure: he understood only to well that this apparent 'total lack of concern for his own safety' concealed a fragile self-confidence and pumped up a low self-esteem. He knew only too well that the Duke of Edinburgh, the media and indeed the nation expected this of their prince, which is why he had encouraged his great-nephew to prefer the military sword to the paintbrush, and he was not about to undo all of this good work. Mountbatten, perhaps better than anyone other than Charles himself, understood that the Prince had to go on proving himself to himself and everyone else, day after day, in order to believe that he might just conceal from the nation his own perceived weakness and lack of natural talent to be their future king. He understood that the amazing contradiction of Charles's personality had created a remarkable young man, but that the ties of self-confidence that held it all together under the strongest scrutiny of the Palace, the navy, his parents, the media and the public had to be maintained by constant injections of trial and victory over adversity. Therefore the old man, who had sought to undo much of the damage inadvertently done to the Prince by his father's attitude and the Gordonstoun experience, spent as much time building his fragile ego as he did advising him on his conduct.

The Prince of Wales's next posting in the Royal Navy was no exception. Charles thought it would be catastrophic; Mountbatten assured him it wouldn't be. On 9 February 1976 he took command of his first ship – the coastal mine hunter HMS *Bonnington* at Rosyth in Scotland. He was to record, 'The great and terrifying day had arrived at last. The whole prospect weighed heavily upon me as I drove across the Forth Bridge. There seemed so many things to worry about, particularly as I am not the sort of person who is endowed with supreme self-confidence. Starting off somewhere new is always an effort, not to mention new people and wondering what the officers were going to be like. My head was positively brimming with advice and helpful suggestions from Uncle Dickie and a whole host of naval officers and I could bear the suspense no longer. Above all else was the sensation I simply had to make a success of this particular aspect of my life because so much seemed to be expected of me. No doubt many people were willing everything to go well, but the press will give no quarter if anything goes wrong.'

The navy understood these dangers and had selected the best available set of junior officers to serve him. He set out with great energy, carrying a notebook of questions so that he could check that all was shipshape and Bristol fashion. Sometimes these revealed Mountbatten's influence as they were somewhat out of date, but as the days passed, his officers gained confidence in him and were even impressed by his quiet air of authority.

Two weeks after taking command, the Prince wrote to Mountbatten, 'It really does seem quite extraordinary to be sitting here as captain of this ship! You were absolutely right (as usual) you do feel frightfully grand and not a little confused. Fortunately a considerable proportion of the confusion has worn off since last week and I am now enjoying the whole experience of "being in command."'

Then in his journal he confided, 'There is nothing like being ultimately responsible for everything and therefore kept in the picture all the time, making it easier to make decisions than one imagined.'

A few days later the Duke of Edinburgh arrived to make a tour of inspection, and the prospect of harsh paternal criticism threw the Prince into a mild panic. He was later to record in his journal: 'I was feeling quite nervous, seeing everything from the other side for a change and standing on the fo'c'sle surrounded by clicking cameramen. Papa shook hands with me when he stepped on board, which caused a certain amount of confusion and merriment on my part. I then attempted to introduce him to the officers, but as I forgot their names instantly it was nearly a dismal failure!'

After this nervous start there were thankfully no further hiccups and the Duke does not appear to have been too critical. Neither, though, does it seem that too complimentary – either reaction would have warranted additional journal entries from his son, and there appear to be none.

For the next nine months the Prince sailed his command on the tedious duties that concerned a minesweeper's modest role in the Royal Navy. He remained most mindful that any slip-up would be seized upon by the press and cause not only personal humiliation but also embarrassment for his family and the Crown. He narrowly avoided two calamities – the first when two men were thrown out of a Gemini inflatable but were happily unhurt and therefore an enquiry was avoided, the second when the ship's starboard anchor became snagged on the main GPO cable between Britain and the Irish coast. Having nearly lost two divers in an attempt to free it, the Prince eventually gave the order to slip the anchor. He was rebuked, despite the circumstances, for its loss but interestingly, although in the end both events avoided a naval enquiry and thus public exposure, his two most senior and experienced lieutenants – Clare and Rapp – guilt-ridden for failing their inexperienced commander, were willing to share the blame among themselves in protection of him. This would almost certainly have damaged their own future prospects, but they preferred that to seeing the Prince being torn limb from limb by the sharks of the British press.

As a result of these events remaining under wraps, and with no other disasters to report, the press ploughed on with the Action Man image and, after he had spent five years in the navy, the public's perception of the Prince had by now been completely transformed from that of a painfully shy young man to that of a naval hero. Headlines in the press told the nation 'FEARLESS, FULL OF FUN CHARLIE', 'THE GET-UP-AND-GO PRINCE CHARLES' and 'CHARLES, SCOURGE OF THE SEAS'. This pleased the Palace, the navy, Mountbatten and therefore the Prince. It may also have pleased Prince Phillip, but if it did, it does not appear to have been recorded.

In December 1976, the navy's final report on Prince Charles was written by Commander Elliott. 'In spite of enormous outside pressure,' it states, 'Prince Charles has attained an excellent level of professional competence as a Commanding Officer. He has a natural flair and ability for ship handling and consequently his manoeuvres have been a pleasure to witness. Prince Charles has shown a deep understanding for his sailors, their families and their problems and as a result the morale of his ship has been of an extremely high order.'

Indeed, the Prince's concern for his men's well being was marked by sympathy and compassion, which at times worried the ship's coxswain who was a traditional disciplinarian. On one occasion, a seaman, noted for continually returning late from shore leave, offered on this latest of occasions such an implausible excuse that the coxswain sent him before the skipper for sentence. The man, standing before his captain, explained that after his last offence, he had ordered a second alarm clock to make sure that he awoke on time. Unfortunately, his wife had bought a budgerigar that had escaped from its cage and perched on each clock, suppressing both alarm knobs in the process. As a result neither had gone off and he had overslept once more.

The Prince, hardly able to contain himself, moved quickly to judgement and dismissed the case on the grounds that he accepted the mitigating circumstances. However, the reprieved seaman hadn't even got to the wardroom door before his commanding officer collapsed in uncontrollable laughter and even the disapproving coxswain was forced to see the funny side.

Perhaps he wasn't the sharpest of officers in his generation. There were certainly better navigators and finer sailors, and men like Clare and Rapp were naturally more suited to the sea; but as a captain, Charles Windsor was a natural and the annals of British history have recorded him as such. No editor of any tabloid newspaper will ever be able to take that away from him.

On the day he left the navy, the officers and crew of his ship threw a lavatory seat around his neck and pushed him ashore in a wheelchair. As they proceeded down the quay at Rosyth, crews from every ship joined in the cheering as the Prince waved farewell to a gang, a club, an institution that had embraced him, protected him and loved him. And he had earned it all and deserved every bit of deep respect and affection that was shown to him.

He had come a long way from the bullied and bleak existence of Gordonstoun.

Chapter Five
The Prince Gains a Mission (1977–79)

'Perhaps I'm wrong or have an over-inflated sense of my own importance, but I feel I could be more useful at home than miles away.' These words were written by the Prince of Wales just before he left the Royal Navy, having stuck at it long enough to achieve what Mountbatten, his father and the government wanted from him but by no means achieving the status that one as natural for command as he might have achieved if he had stayed on. To the Prince, climbing to the rank of Admiral of the Fleet while waiting for his mother to die was not an option. Nor would retiring to appear at endless public engagements – dispensing goodwill, smiles, encouragement and compassion – be much better. For while this might endear him to the public and indeed be what a lot of them saw as his function, the Prince yearned for a 'proper job' – one where he might make a difference to the lives of his future subjects.

This was to become an obsession with him. At this time he referred to it in a speech at Cambridge University, saying, 'My great problem in life is that I do not really know what my role in life is. At the moment I do not have one. But somehow I must find one.'

The ever-loyal Checketts searched through royal files in the hope of finding guidance. What should a Prince of Wales do while waiting to become king? The answer from history came back: just wait. Neither Checketts nor the Prince fancied that idea. The Queen might live to be 100, which would mean that Charles would be in his late seventies by the time his life had any real meaning. No wonder so many previous princes of Wales had gone off the rails. Indeed there seemed to be a direct correlation between the longevity of monarchs and the riotous lives of their sons and heirs – George IV, Edward VII and Edward VIII immediately spring to mind as monarchs who perhaps suffered as long-serving princes of Wales with little to do but accept and enjoy the privileges of the position while waiting for their father or mother to die.

Checketts really favoured the idea of the Prince becoming governor general of Australia. The Prince himself, while not being too sure that the job had any real power, was nevertheless interested enough in the absence of anything more fulfilling – not least due to his love of the Australian people. However, wiser powers perceived that such a post could lead the monarchy into controversy by forcing it into political conflict with Australia's elected government at some future date. Indeed, in 1975 a minor constitutional crisis occurred involving the then governor general, one Sir John Kerr, and the Australian government, and the idea was dropped forever.

However, this did not prevent other similar schemes being hatched, and in 1979 Mrs Thatcher's government toyed with the idea that Prince Charles might become British ambassador to France. They thought that he would be better suited than most to the task and that the snooty French would be immensely flattered by his presence. Nevertheless, it was eventually realised that with Mrs Thatcher determined to take on the French in order for Britain to secure European Economic Community budget repayments, the Prince would be placed in an impossible position. The Palace quickly agreed that the idea was a non-starter and it was consequently also dropped.

Perhaps because some in the palaces of Westminster and Buckingham remembered the fate of previous princes with time on their hands, the 'proper job' issue became a general topic of concern. Prior to Mrs Thatcher's election, the then Prime Minister James Callaghan, the Queen's private secretary Sir Philip Moore and others debated what the Prince might do to make proper use of his time. Checketts, acutely aware that the Prince of Wales couldn't just be dropped into some government department for clear political reasons, and indignant that some may feel that he was wasting his time doing nothing, wrote to Sir Philip, 'I find it most revealing that the question "What is Prince Charles going to do now that he is out of the Navy?" is still being raised, when even a brief investigation of the problem would reveal that the true question is "How is Prince Charles going to be able to do all there is for him to do?"' He then listed all of the Prince's current involvements which included the Duchy of Cornwall, the newly formed Prince's Trust, the Prince of Wales Environment Committee for Wales, the United World Colleges, the Joint Jubilee Trusts, the chancellorship of the University of Wales, his role as colonel-in-chief of five regiments and his patronage of the British Sub Aqua Club and the Royal Anthropological Institute.'

In addition, and just for good measure, the ever-loyal Checketts also listed the Prince's formal engagements and foreign tours, some of which were to be undertaken on behalf of Her Majesty. Such a list was hard to argue against, as was Checketts' logic that the position of the Prince as the heir to the throne made it very difficult indeed for him to take any 'proper job' outside the armed forces. And so, in time, Palace officials and government ministers alike had to accept the fact that there were more down sides to him taking on a formal role than positives.

Those wishing to engage the undoubted talents of the Prince of Wales reluctantly accepted this. However, it was never really accepted by Charles himself, who would suffer bouts of depression and low self-esteem as a result of his inner confusion over wanting to be a good Prince of Wales but also wanting to use his talents to do a proper job. He has always found it hard to understand that the two things are not compatible and that his good works through organisations like the Prince's Trust have been a most valuable use of his time. He was not the only one with this problem. While Checketts seems to have understood the problem perfectly and could see a real benefit for the country in not 'limiting His Royal Highness to a specific profession [that] would do nothing but frustrate the growing awareness of this remarkable young man in his responsibility to the people of the United Kingdom and the Commonwealth ...', there were others who failed to realise that the Prince couldn't be both a prince for and among the people, and have a full-time career doing something else. As a result, and with little constructive PR designed to demonstrate clearly how hard the Prince was working on ideas such as those that would benefit deprived youngsters, the Palace remained as sensitive as the Prince did about the proper-job issue. Consequently, it was horrified when, in February 1978, the celebrated gossip columnist Nigel Dempster began an article on his page in the *Daily Mail*

, 'Situation sought: Prince, 29, degree, ex-Army, Navy, RAF, seeks employment. Will go anywhere, try anything once.'

This prompted the Queen's press secretary to write to her private secretary explaining that the public had expectations of the Prince that were not being fulfilled and they were left with the impression that he spent most of his time hunting, shooting or skiing. He copied Checketts in. For his pains he was immediately rebuked by the Prince's secretary who replied, 'As His Royal Highness's relations with the public and general popularity have never been higher, and this is borne out at every public appearance and by the vast amount of correspondence received daily, I do not believe it is the public which hold such expectations, as much as the media ... Perhaps what should be considered is some means of revealing to the media more of the immense amount of important work carried out by the Prince of Wales when not in the public eye, and which seems to be totally unnoticed.'

The Prince, who seemed to understand the dangers of becoming embroiled in something too close to politics, was nevertheless determined to make a difference and didn't see how he would be able to do that through and endless round of public engagements. He wrote, 'I want to consider ways in which I can escape from the ceaseless round of official engagements and meet people in less artificial circumstances. In other words, I want to look at the possibility of spending, say; 1. three days in one factory to find out what happens; 2. three days perhaps, in a trawler (instead of one rapid visit); 3. three or four days on a farm. I would also like you to consider 4. more visits to immigrant areas in order to help these people to feel that they are not ignored or neglected and that we are concerned about them as individuals.'

Not all of these initiatives were arranged, but some were, and they helped give him the information that formed his views that were so often to come to the support of farmers, small businesses, fishermen and especially the ethnic youth in the years to come. It is certainly no exaggeration to claim that Prince Charles has done more than any politician in this country's history to promote the lot of young Afro-Caribbeans and Asians. The work started in the late 1970s when people like Nigel Dempster were writing comical little articles about the Prince getting a 'proper job'.

However, it was not the press who sought to limit his desire to help the most deprived or disadvantaged communities, but courtiers, who thought it was dangerous for the heir to the throne to become too closely identified with such political issues and politicians who either thought it was none of his business or believed that he should only flag up the initiatives and not the obvious failures. Those trying to divert him from these issues were to be disappointed, as their reluctance to allow him to become more closely identified with inner-city problems only served to irritate him and inflamed his passion even more with a fire that, despite all that was to happen to him in the years ahead, has shown no sign of being extinguished.

The media might not have understood that a prince who works towards his own financial gain would have been accused of neglecting his subjects for selfish reasons; that one who took a job in a government might be accused of being politically biased and so damage the monarchy's impartiality. However, they weren't slow to judge the mood of the people – who were increasingly delighted with their Action Man prince and were much more concerned with whom he was going to marry than with a boring discussion about career prospects. After all, in their minds he was 'on the bench', waiting to be called on as a substitute for Her Majesty. That was what he had been born to, and that was his lot in life, for better or worse. As a result, criticism of the Prince in the press remained very minor as republican, socialist or just envious pressmen kept their views to themselves for fear of offending their editors who, in turn, feared their newspapers offending the public.

The proof of the pudding is in the eating, and there was a real test of the monarchy's popularity in 1977 as the Queen celebrated her Silver Jubilee. Socialist and republican commentators had been predicting that the crowds that turned out to celebrate would mainly consist of pensioners and middle-class spinsters. But when 7 June arrived it was greeted by a nationwide rejoicing that demonstrated no discernible difference to the scenes of celebration twenty-four years earlier at the time of the coronation. In London the crowds packed the Mall, many having slept out in order to get a good position. It was an overwhelming demonstration of royalist support. And these royalists were not just English middle-class ladies: they were West Indians and Asians, normal working people, young and old, rich and poor and their children – lots and lots of happy, singing children. The young were actually in the majority and carrying the royalist message forward as the nation erupted into a rash of street parties, bunting, fancy-dress parades and singsongs. The whole country appeared to be wrapped in a Union Jack of unity.

As the golden coach carrying the Queen and Prince Philip made its way from Buckingham Palace to the service at St Paul's Cathedral, there was no space from the Mall to the City as the crowds packed the route. The Prince of Wales rode a large black steed behind the coach and the crowd delighted in the intimacy of his presence. They called out to him, they applauded him and he responded. The much admired author Philip Ziegler observed, 'The nod from the Commendatore's statue could hardly have caused a greater sensation. The Prince of Wales and the crowd had suddenly been transformed into "Charlie and Me"'.

However, despite his newfound self-confidence and public popularity, the Prince still had serious concerns on his mind. What was he going to do while waiting to become king, and who was he going to marry in order to produce a son and heir to replace him one day? The first concern was a self-motivated pressure more than a national requirement, whereas every man jack who wasn't a republican saw the Prince's second concern as his duty to get right and almost took the same interest in it that some distant relative might.

As we now know, Charles took Mountbatten's advice about the marriage question and followed the old man's plan almost to the letter. And to a certain extent he followed Checketts' advice regarding his career. He seemed to understand the pitfalls of working outside the armed forces, but didn't want to work in them any longer; nor did he want to parade around every day just opening new hospital blocks. As a result, he understood that to follow his own instincts and desire to do good works for the under-privileged, especially the ethnic minorities, was perhaps the only avenue open to him as it had purpose and didn't stop him carrying out his duties as either the Prince of Wales or heir to the throne.

Checketts had been quite right to understand that these roles, along with the time needed to manage the Duchy of Cornwall, would involve long and arduous hours week after week, and that the Prince must not neglect his princely duties if he wished to remain popular. But to the Prince, who has always been unafraid of hard work, it didn't seem enough. And although he could understand the logic of what Checketts was saying and could come up with no alternative suggestion himself, he continued to fall into depression from time to time about the fact that he didn't have a 'proper job'.

Of course this is nonsense. Running the Duchy of Cornwall, a multi-million-pound business, is a proper job. Building one of the country's largest and most successful charities is a proper job. Comforting the sick and bringing pleasure to the lives of ordinary people is a proper job. And representing Great Britain at home and abroad is a proper job. So there are four proper jobs for a start. Sir Max Hastings, an ex-newspaper editor and now part-time columnist for the *Daily Mail*, wrote in 2002 that he had no time for the Prince of Wales, whom he considered to be a man full of self-pity who was always complaining. I rather think that Hastings wouldn't last a fortnight as Prince of Wales and if, against the odds, he did, then the monarchy, with him as the heir to the throne, would perish inside the month.

In any event, if, against all sensible advice, the Prince had taken a 'proper job' like Sir Max, then perhaps the Prince's Trust would never have existed and literally hundreds of thousands of disadvantaged children's lives would have not benefited as a result. For if the Prince of Wales had never achieved anything in his life other than the creation of this charity, he would still have achieved more than the vast majority of post-war politicians. Harold Wilson, never slow in coming forward, listed the building of the National Exhibition Centre and the opening of the Open University as his major achievements, and indeed they are both deeds to be proud of, but they are certainly not greater than the setting-up of the Prince's Trust.

In 1972, the Conservative government had brought in a penal reform known as Community Service by Offenders. The idea was that first-time offenders of minor crime would be ordered to work on community projects during their leisure time as a way of paying back society rather than being sent to prison. It was a modest proposal and seemed most logical. Nevertheless, its arrival unleashed a hysterical outburst from the press who believed that Heath and his colleagues had gone soft on crime. One George Pratt, the deputy chief probation officer for Inner London who had been a member of the Home Office working party, came in for some fairly ferocious criticism.

In the midst of the furore he received a call from Checketts. The Prince wanted to know if he could help. A few days later he was received in the Chinese drawing room at Buckingham Palace, and the concept of the Prince's Trust was born. The Prince explained how concerned he was about the effects of alienation on young people. He spoke with enthusiasm about the ideas of Kurt Hahn and even fondly about the bracing environment of Gordonstoun, from which he believed, in the main, he had benefited. He told Pratt that he wanted to help those who hadn't been born with the advantages that he had enjoyed. He wanted to devise schemes that would give the disadvantaged 'a hand up' and not 'a handout'.

Pratt was most impressed by 'this young, enthusiastic and idealistic person' who had scribbled his ideas down on the back of an envelope. The thoughts were sincere, if only half thought-through, and not always very realistic; however, once guided by the experienced Pratt, the Prince gained wisdom without losing passion and against much opposition the Trust was born. It was officially launched in 1976, shortly after he had left the Navy. It was initially funded by his £7,400 naval severance pay, a £4,000 fee from an American television company for an interview regarding his favourite predecessor George III and a handful of donations from friendly celebrities such as Sir Harry Secombe of Goons fame.

Opposition came from the Callaghan Labour government and certain elements of the royal household itself. Their concerns were that the Prince's Trust's very existence would take away from the already established George V and Queen Jubilee trusts, which existed to fund worthy projects for young people. More seriously, they argued, the Prince was insisting that the money was handed out directly to the young people themselves without adequate procedures and checks being applied. Some ridiculed the fact that initial funds had been given to a carver of didgeridoos, a fishing club and young offenders for lifeguard training. Others even questioned his motives: detractors said he only identified with the disaffected as he saw himself as a misunderstood outsider.

But as we now know, the Prince of Wales can be a very stubborn man when the mood takes him, and he was not for being deflected from his goal. He was adamant that anything associated with him should be focused directly on deprived communities; that it should be designed to release talent, which he believed lay within everyone, even the most recalcitrant characters; and it should stimulate a sense of adventure and public service.

After long and at times heated debate, a number of pilot schemes were established under Pratt's guidance, and with a minimum of red tape small grants of up to £300 to individuals and £500 to groups were dispensed. Then, in the 1980s, with the country in full recession and the Conservatives back in power, the Trust really started to find its feet.

Unemployment had soared and there was rioting in the streets – especially in the Afro-Caribbean inner-city areas like St Paul's in Bristol, Handsworth in Birmingham and Toxteth in Liverpool. There, in the ghettos, the young black saw him or herself at the back of every queue for jobs, housing and anything else: not only did they see themselves as outsiders, many were full of resentment and believed that violence and the drug market were the only other routes to take. Against such a background, the Trust was needed as a healing balm and a genuine go-between. Somehow the alienated trusted it in general, and the Prince in particular, in a way they would never have trusted Mrs

Thatcher or her ministers. I first met Prince Charles very briefly on a visit to a youth centre in Handsworth in 1981 and was amazed by his genuine ease with these 'wild' Rastas, and by their delight at his presence.

In June 1977, he had surrounded himself with controversy by becoming directly involved in a bitter dispute between the police and a group of protesters outside a club in Deptford in London. Charles, while visiting the area, had taken it upon himself to walk over to the barricades and ask the demonstrators what their issue was. They replied that they were protesting against what they saw as police harassment of the local black community. The Prince listened and, to everyone's astonishment, they were invited, along with the police, to Buckingham Palace eight days later in an attempt to calm the position and see if reconciliation was possible. Prince Charles promised to do what he could to help. It was the start of the Afro-Caribbean appreciation of what a friend their future king could be. However, this behaviour was seen as unhelpful interfering by many politicians in the ruling Labour Party and this wasn't eased when, in 1978, he went even further.

In November of that year, now most concerned that there was a growing hostility between the Metropolitan Police and young blacks, the Prince organised a meeting between the chief administrator of the Prince's Trust, George Pratt, and the Met's commissioner, Sir David McNee. The latter appreciated the Prince's concerns and explained that it wasn't police policy that was at fault, but the disparity between that and the attitude of some of the bobbies on the beat. In other words, the Met wasn't racist but some of its officers were.

This issue wasn't tackled effectively enough and was to become the subject of much anguish and controversy for another twenty-five years. Over this period, police racism in the capital not only led to riots, deaths on both sides and much unhappiness, it also provided an excuse for much drug-related crime to be committed in the 'no go' black areas where the police were to become impotent to help anyone as they had lost the trust of law-abiding black people because of their attitude towards them.

It was agreed at Charles's express wish that the Prince's Trust would work closely with the police and the ethnic groups in troublesome areas where the Trust was established, and later it was decided that the nineteen chief constables would attend a private seminar at his invitation to see what might be done to arrest the apparent worsening of community relations.

The Prince clearly understood that there was a significant difference between the disaffected Afro-Caribbean youth and those of ethnic Asian decent. Whether he understood that much of the reason for this was down to two clear points is not so obvious from his recorded comments of the time. The Asian communities were then, as they are largely today, held together by strong religious and family ties. This meant that the youth was more disciplined by parental control and less influenced by western inner-city ghetto culture. Many families were entrepreneurial and as soon as they could, they started small businesses, often in either manufacturing or retailing. The children, under their parents' control and guidance, were encouraged to help build up these little enterprises from the 1960s onwards: some of the greatest business success stories in Great Britain today have emanated from these communities, and the vast majority of the nation's small corner shops are now Asian-owned.

Therefore stability was created by parental example and financial security as old established values were passed from one generation to another: the result was that the children of the ethnic Asian population were well policed by their own parents.

However, the position with the Afro-Caribbean youth was quite different. When their parents had arrived in Britain the 1950s they were mainly God-fearing Christian folk who spoke the English language and therefore were more inclined to be influenced by British and American society. They were, in the main, not very businesslike and, with a laid-back attitude, tended to get the worst paid jobs in the community that had been traditionally done by the Irish – those jobs that the British themselves certainly didn't wish to do in the growing post-war economy. This did not help the West Indian status and, as a result, their children were to grow up seeing themselves at the back of every queue in an increasingly materialist world where they were discriminated against because their colour seemed to say that society saw them as inferior.

As a result, and with little financial security at home, the first Afro-Caribbean generation born in the United Kingdom grew up to rebel and reject its parents, their values and British society. Compared to the Asian immigrants, they more frequently had children outside wedlock; such children were never to know a strongly cohesive family unit and were to grow up without the example or steadying influence of a father, and so things continued to get worse as absent ethnic West Indian fathers became a major reason for an ongoing problem with Afro-Caribbean youth.

The Prince of Wales was at the vanguard of concern regarding such issues and it is a great pity that those whose job it was to dampen down a potentially disastrous situation did not heed his warnings more seriously and make a more determined effort to tackle the racial minority problem.

By 1981, lack of any progress on these issues, along with the general economic gloom that accompanied the early Thatcher years of austerity, gave the impression that Britain was becoming an 'every man for himself' society where decency, respect for others and the law were being replaced by greed, selfishness and low moral fibre. It was, and was to continue ever further in that direction for the next twenty-five years.

Over that period, the Prince of Wales attempted to ease the injustice of racism in British society on the grounds of it being morally wrong, socially evil and economically wasteful. His work was to be characterised by the now famous cartoon of him in a crater, sleeves rolled up, on his hands and knees and attempting to defuse a bomb with the words 'inner cities' written on the side. Looking down into the crater and next to a sign exclaiming 'Danger'. Unexploded bomb' is the prime minister and her cabinet. The Prince is saying, 'Come on, give us a hand!'

The employment minister of the time, David Young, later to become Lord Young, became a fan of the Prince's Trust. In particular, the Trust's start-up scheme for small businesses, which would never have even been considered by the risk-averse high-street banks, resonated with Thatcherite ideas and won Young over as he battled to get unemployment down from a frightening three million. Young offered to match voluntary contributions to the scheme pound for pound from government coffers: the Trust had moved up a gear, and with that began the journey to high-gloss professionalism. Now hosts of celebrities queued up to lend a hand, and by the mid-1980s, rock concerts starring Mick Jagger, Paul Young, Rod Stuart, Elton John, George Michael, Phil Collins, Mark Knopfler, Tina Turner, Brian Adams, Status Quo and the mercurial Paul McCartney were being sold out in seconds.

By 1988 Tom Shebbeare had been recruited to run the Prince's

Trust and he, along with his staff, must take a great deal of credit for how things have turned out. In Shebbeare's case this was recognised by his knighthood in the New Year's Honours of 2003. A former Council of Europe official, Shebbeare is today the Prince's director of charities – there is a ragbag of nineteen in total, and it is his new job to attempt to give more strategic direction to them. He is trusted by the Prince not only because of the unqualified success that he has overseen at the Trust, but because the two men share an equal dislike of bureaucracy. Moreover, those in the know say that Shebbeare, while being occasionally outspoken, is very astute in knowing when to be so, and so has an able manner when it comes to handling the heir to the throne. The two men developed a mutual respect from the beginning, and although Shebbeare can moan, with more than a little justification, about the Prince's mood swings or outrageous impatience at times, he, like others close to the Prince, has formed a deep affection for the future king.

The Prince, for his part, while keeping this relationship very much on business terms, has found Shebbeare easy to confide in. In January 1993 he was to write to him, 'For the past 15 years I have been entirely motivated by a desperate desire to put the "Great" back into Great Britain. Everything I have tried to do – all the projects, speeches, schemes etc – have been with this end in mind. And none of it has worked, as you can see too obviously! In order to put the "Great" back I have always felt it was VITAL to bring people together, and I began to realise that the ONE advantage my position has over anyone else's is that I can act as a catalyst to help produce a better and more balanced response to various problems. I have no "political" agenda – only a desire to see people achieve their potential; to be decently housed in a decent, civilised environment that respects the cultural and vernacular character of the nation; to see this country's real talents (especially inventiveness and engineering skills) put to the best use in the BEST interests of the country and the world (at present they are being disgracefully wasted through lack of co-ordination and strategic thinking); to retain and value the infrastructure and cultural integrity of rural communities (where they still exist) because of the vital role they play in the FRAMEWORK of the nation and the care and management of the countryside; to value and nurture the highest standards of military integrity and professionalism, as displayed by our armed forces, because of the role they play as an insurance scheme in case of disaster; and to value and retain our uniquely special broadcasting standards which are renowned throughout the world.

'The final point is that I have always wanted to roll back some of the more ludicrous frontiers of the 60s in terms of education, architecture, art, music, and literature, not to mention agriculture!

'Having read this through, no wonder they want to destroy me, or get rid of me …!'

By the start of 2004 the Trust had helped nearly half a million young people. It now spends more than £30 million a year doing so. It continues to help the kids that everyone else has written off. By providing mentors who make it possible for these youngsters to achieve something tangible and real, be it being taught to play the guitar, learning how to rock climb or starting a business, the Prince's Trust is offering a chance of genuine change for the better.

Over the last thirty years, more than 50,000 businesses have been started. Over sixty per cent were still trading three years after being set up. The top hundred now have an annual turnover in excess of £80 million and employ some 2,000 people. This work has been – and continues to be – a major contribution towards the welfare of this country's most at-risk young. Moreover, in terms of money raised and support given, this work totally and utterly dwarfs the high profile but otherwise quite limited work undertaken by the Princess of Wales, however good such work was. All too often, this supposedly self-pitying prince has not been accorded the credit he, or anyone else doing similar work, richly deserves.

However well things may have turned out for the Prince's Trust, it is easy to forget that such a success, especially given the obstacles that the Prince faced from both Westminster and the royal household, was not guaranteed. Things only really got going thanks to his grim determination. Moreover, as this hard slog was going on behind closed doors, the nation was completely unaware of his objective. These two factors meant that the Prince's view of his own lack of worth was to surface time and again.

Checketts, in his quest to find meaningful work that might cure his young restless master, urged the Prince to take on the role of executive chairman of the Duchy of Cornwall. It was Checketts' opinion not only that the running of the estate that provided the Prince with his income was an entirely reasonable thing for him to be doing, it would also enable him to acquire management and administration skills that would otherwise be denied him. Moreover, this way he could be seen to be working for a living while not neglecting his princely duties.

The duchy was created over 650 years ago by Edward III for his son, the Black Prince. It was added to over the years by land being bought, seized or even stolen. In 1760, when the Crown lands were made over to the state in exchange for the granting of the Civil List, the duchies of Cornwall and Lancaster were excluded. People complaining about the present Civil List should be aware that not only is this money granted by Parliament to meet the expenses of running the royal household (and is not for personal use) but that the Crown gave the state hundreds of thousands of acres of land in order to be granted an income so that it might carry out its job. Those who would like to stop the Civil List should be asked if they would not therefore mind returning this land to the rightful owners. There are always two sides to every contract and in order to break one side then one must be prepared to pay the price to the other.

As a result of the Civil List being granted, the duchy's independence was guaranteed by statute. By the nineteenth century it was being administered by a council on behalf of Prince George. Later, under the skilful direction of Prince Albert, who managed the estate on behalf of his wayward son Bertie, later to become Edward VII, the duchy's affairs were seriously smartened up and, over a twenty-five-year period, income nearly doubled from £25,000 to £46,000 a year, despite heavy investment in beautifying the natural landscape.

By the time Prince Charles began to draw an income from the duchy in 1966, it was much diminished in size from that enjoyed by the Black Prince. Nevertheless, he still had 128,000 acres spread over nine counties, and this made it one of the greatest private estates in England. It had been agreed when the Queen ascended to the throne that she would be allowed to take one ninth of the annual duchy surplus to provide for an income for her eldest son. At eighteen, therefore, Prince Charles was allowed to draw £21,000 per annum. The balance was withheld by the Treasury and offset against the cost of the Civil List. When he became twenty-one, the entire income of the duchy – in 1969 some £248,000 – became his, though by arrangement with the Treasury he elected wisely to waive fifty per cent in lieu of income tax. Top-rate income tax was a staggering ninety per cent at the time.

In 1969 the estate consisted of 70,000 acres of farmland, including

The King and Di

240 farms, 50,000 acres of forest and moorland on Dartmoor, 3,000 acres of woodland, 1,500 dwellings in London and elsewhere, 230 miles of foreshore and 14,000 acres of riverbed. This was no smallholding, and by 1976, when the Prince had left the navy, there was much to be done. The duchy had been poorly managed and was now lagging behind the times in both investment in modern technology and the charging of higher rents: it even needed to sell land in order to balance its books as it faced spiralling costs without the spiralling income needed to meet them. As a result it was contracting instead of expanding. Action was needed, and the ever-sensible Checketts saw this as a chance for the Prince to demonstrate his capabilities and secure his own financial future and that of his heir at the same time.

However, for the time being the Prince was not to find the inspiration to attempt to emulate the success of Prince Albert, and began by being content to chair the Prince's Council meetings while leaving the hands-on management to others. Happily, as we shall see, this was to change – greatly and for the better. It might have been quite disappointing to Checketts that initially the Prince, in his quest for a 'proper job', made a fairly tentative start to this enormous challenge; but if he was, he was far too loyal to let it be known.

It is likely that Prince Charles was as unsure as ever of anything new; unlike Gordonstoun and the armed forces, he now had a choice in the matter and therefore wasn't going to be forced or rushed into anything. But there are two further compelling reasons why his initial performance in the management of the duchy was fairly low-key. Firstly, business would have appeared to the young Prince to be about figures, and the Prince of Wales has the attention span of a child when it comes to accounts. This started with his dread of maths at school and is still with him as he attends meetings concerning the Prince's Trust today: he is famous for looking at his watch within two minutes of being presented with any figures, and aides are forced to explain them faster and faster before he makes his mind up that it is time that the meeting was finished. Secondly, the Prince was only just forming his ideas on agriculture, the environment and architecture at this time, and was yet to realise how the duchy could become a powerful moneymaking machine to fund some of his projects and even act as a guinea pig or example for them. When this occurred to him, and his confidence grew with a determination that the duchy could be more to him than just a source of income, his interest and activity levels grew accordingly.

Charles's involvement in the Trust and the duchy were gradual. Before they became serious interests, he had no clear focus for his energy, and with a growing wilfulness that alarmed Mountbatten; he now began to worry his friends by his obvious anxiety and discontent. To him, the years of discipline and genuine hardship in dreadful places like Gordonstoun, which had made him so unhappy, now all seemed to have been in vain as his life failed to carry the purpose that he had idealistically supposed it would when dreaming of being Mummy's 'liegeman of life and limb'. Although he continued to carry out all of his public duties with discipline and great charm, he sometimes allowed an irritability to invade his relationships with his staff; normally thoughtful and even humorous memos could be ruined by rude and brusque comments.

It was his closest aides like Checketts and Michael Colborne who bore the brunt of this bad temper. Colborne, who had served with Prince Charles on HMS *Norfolk*, had given up his career in the Royal Navy to join the Prince's staff in 1975 as his private secretary. As such he not only organised the Prince's private life, he also became a close confidant. Like Checketts, he became devoted to the Prince and there grew a great bond of genuine affection between them. However, this did not on occasion stop the heir to the throne venting uncontrolled anger over the most minor of lapses and this must have sorely tested Colborne's loyalty.

After one particularly fierce tantrum, Mountbatten, having been told about it by the Prince himself, took Colborne to one side and explained that Charles, in his lonely eminence, had no one else to vent his frustrations on and it was evidence of his regard for Colborne that the Prince of Wales felt able to do so. Colborne was calmed, knowing that as he had not raised the matter with anyone, the Prince, who had not been able to bring himself to apologise directly, had at least felt guilty enough to mention the outburst to the man whom he perhaps admired most in all the world.

This was now becoming a time of trial for Prince Charles. He had been raised to be king. Every major decision about his life since birth had been taken for him, usually by his father, Mountbatten or a committee of them and others. Now, as the heir apparent – a particularly difficult job in the modern world – he felt that he was now trapped in a role that had a veneer of purpose but an inner vacuum. Nor was he able to think of an alternative route – and for once neither could the great and the good. Perhaps there wasn't one.

The Prince had always had a strong sense of faith, and religion had played a major role in the dark hours of his unhappiest days at school. He was not only dedicated to his destiny of becoming head of the Church of England; he had shown a sensitive interest in other religions while remaining a devout Christian himself. Faced with such unexpected inner turmoil, he embarked upon a private voyage of spiritual inquiry. His natural aversion to the laws of scientific materialism pushed him towards mysticism where, like many film stars and others in the goldfish bowl before and since, he found an explanation of the human soul that gave him a life raft to cling on to. This was to provide him with a lasting inspiration and allowed him to build an inner reality, which in itself gave coherence to his feelings and attitudes. It was thus not only a source of inner comfort and stability but allowed him to construct a mental and spiritual foundation upon which his coordinated views on architecture, farming, the environment and social behaviour could be built as an alternative to the perceived wisdom of the time. This fascination of mysticism was not totally dissimilar to the attraction that Princess Diana was to demonstrate, much later, towards mediums and fringe psychotherapists. Obviously the degree of intellectual capacity required for such inquiry is completely different, but the basic instinct to move in such a direction was probably similarly motivated by the same exhaustion of more conventional means of help.

It was this route, as well as a tolerance that had always been there but had blossomed from this period, that eventually led Charles to declare in public that, as sovereign, he would like to be 'Defender of Faith' rather than 'Defender of the Faith'. Given what had happened to a number of his ancestors who had dared to fall out with the Church of England, this was indeed a significantly brave thing to say, and predictably was met by a fierce attack of bigotry.

It was also at this time, during this search for his inner self, that the Prince of Wales fell under the spell of the South African writer, explorer and mystic Laurens van der Post. From very early on, van der Post had formed the view that the Action Man persona that had been built up around the Prince's natural personality, mainly to fit in with the designs of his father, failed to display another dimension to him. This opinion seemed to be further confirmed when van der Post light-heartedly commented, 'I think one should be outward bound the inward way,' and was surprised by the Prince's serious recognition of what he had said.

By 1975 the two men had formed a close relationship, and while Mountbatten remained the Prince's mentor for all things worldly, van der Post had become his main counsel regarding spiritual matters. Van der Post arrived in the Prince's life at a most opportune moment. Charles became captivated by the mystic's book *The Lost World of the Kalahari*. The book described how the African bushmen in the Kalahari Desert had been much more than merely hunters: they had been immersed in the natural world and understood it better than anyone has since due to their mystic qualities. Naturally, this brought about calls of 'charlatan', and much derision from rationalists. But Prince Charles believed he had already experienced this very thing throughout his childhood at Balmoral and felt that van der Post was merely expressing something that had applied to him but which he had never been able to explain to anyone.

In another van der Post book, *The Heart of the Hunter*, he wrote, 'We suffer from hubris of the mind. We have abolished superstition of the heart only to install a superstition of the intellect in its place.' The Prince, unlike most others, seemed to know precisely what this meant.

Then, in the autumn of 1975, van der Post came up with the idea of taking the Prince for a long trip into the interior of the Kalahari Desert with a camera so that together they could record such an adventure for the benefit of the BBC's television viewers. Much to the despair of some at Buckingham Palace, the Prince agreed to make the trip, which would last some seven weeks in 1977. Van der Post was so delighted by this news that he immediately wrote to Charles congratulating him on transforming the monarchy into 'a dynamic and as yet unimagined role to suit the future shape of a fundamentally reappraised and renewed modern society.' Now that was music to the Prince's ears. He needed a purpose; in addition, he wanted to discover who he really was: perhaps with van der Post in the Kalahari Desert he could find both.

In the event, the expedition had to be cancelled because of the troubles in neighbouring Rhodesia, and did not take place until 1987. It was planned as a three-week trip, but in the end got cut back to just four days due to the Prince's busy schedule. Nevertheless, van der Post thought that this was better than nothing. The two men, along with a small party, travelled into the desert by Land Rover, ate around a camp fire miles away from the questionable civilisation of journalists and, even on the last night, ignored their tents in favour of sleeping under the stars. This was considered to be most dangerous as their camp was on the edge of a lions' route to water: silence was imperative if they were not to court disaster.

Perhaps because he had become more jaundiced and less idealistic with age, the mystical truths that van der Post had prophesised failed to reveal themselves to the Prince, and this is reflected in his diary entry of the time: 'On first contact the desert is pretty harsh and unforgiving and I wondered what on earth I had let myself in for! But after 4 days, which was similar to an S.A.S. selection test, it began to grow on you! So did the dirt, dust and hair and I have never been so filthy before. I hardly ate anything and only felt like liquid. It was just the place to be during lent, but the sunsets were out of this world. It was worth going for these alone and there was something very special about lying under the stars in the last night in the bush.' The physicality of it all is there – painted vividly in just a few words; but the mystical qualities are noticeable by their very absence.

The original trip, once cancelled, was substituted by a hurriedly organised excursion to the relative isolation of the Aberdare Mountains in Kenya where they spent five days walking, lost in deep conversation. Van der Post by now was completely devoted to the Prince and saw in him a spiritual vehicle that could be prevailed upon to save the nation if he could help him discover the strength of his inner self. To this end, and at the instigation of van der Post, the Prince began to record his dreams and give them to the older man for interpretation.

In addition, van der Post introduced Charles to the teachings of Carl Jung. Jung was fascinated by the occult, by the mysteries of religion and was, as a result, most interested in the search for the real meaning of life beyond the bounds of accepted natural science. To some he was either a raving madman or charlatan; others, van der Post among them, saw Jung as a man with a brain powerful enough to imagine past the proven rules of life in order to find a world beyond.

The Prince, by now ever keen to continue on a journey towards self-discovery and unlock the creative mind that had always had to play second fiddle to Action Man and duty, was attracted to 'a consciousness detached from the world'. In time he would become so drawn to it that neither others' scepticism nor the mockery that he was to receive at the hands of the tabloid press would deter him. To the outside world, he was still the dashing military man, but there is no doubt that it was then, as a result of the murmuring of concerned officials at Buckingham Palace, that the rumours started that were to give eventual rise to the 'Loony Prince' tag.

In the late 1970s, when the Prince's search for 'an inner world of truth' was strongest, van der Post became obsessed with the idea that Charles, if unable to visit the Kalahari Desert, should withdraw from society and public commitments for a time in order to 'contemplate the inner life of the soul'. The Prince, who might have been tempted, resisted such a suggestion on the grounds that his sense of duty was far too great. Prince Charles may have been searching for an inner peace, but he knew that he would never find it if he was to let the nation and his family down. This dedication was borne out of a pure and genuine sense of duty, a knowledge that to fail in it would cause him more heartache and pain than anything else and the terrible thought that all of the hardship that he had had to endure to get this far would have been in vain.

Nevertheless, his search for this inner world went on, and he shared van der Post's view that Jung's aim to 'restore western man to his soul and recover his religious meaning' was a fine one. As a result he became increasingly at odds with churchmen of his own denomination, whom he saw as at best having no spiritual thirst for new knowledge, and at worst as having hijacked their religion for their own mortal benefit: he didn't like their unthinking pomposity. He took to searching beyond the confines of the Church of England and even Christianity. This was to raise eyebrows in the royal household: alarm bells rang out that the future head of the church in his rather 'loopy' search for a higher meaning to life and religion was exploring the ancient religions of the East. The Prince of Wales sensed that such religions had retained some of the mystical elements that he had seen in Christianity in Fiji but not in England. He learned about Buddhism, Hinduism and Islam. He read up on reincarnation and became drawn to that idea, safe in the comfort that some theologians saw no incompatibility between it and Christianity.

Sir Laurens van der Post gradually began to replace Mountbatten as the heir to the throne's guiding hand in spiritual matters, but the direction in which he encouraged him to travel was hardly the same. The values of Victorian military might and monarchic Christian goodness were now replaced by an almost Beatle-esque search for the mystical. After his death, a biography claimed that Sir Laurens himself had feet of clay and would have hardly been the kind of man of whom Mountbatten would have approved. He was, apparently, something of a fantasist who invented some of his earlier life; worse still, he had even seduced a fourteen-year-old girl who was in his charge and this resulted in the girl becoming pregnant.

Obviously none of this was known to the Prince at the time, who eagerly got to grips with anything to which van der Post introduced him. As his marriage to the Princess slipped into total unhappiness, the old man suggested that Prince Charles might find comfort in reading the work of the British poet and philosopher Kathleen Raine. The Prince did so, and as a result began a mountain of correspondence that was to last some twenty years until Dr Raine's death in 2004. He gave the eulogy at her funeral and praised her friendship and the courage she displayed in supporting his denunciation of the shallow and evil society that had sprung up around the liberal and greedy attitudes that were so readily dreamed up by the nation's opinion-formers and so easily devoured by its people. 'You can perhaps imagine how re-moralising it was to receive such missives when, all around, the world seemed to become periodically madder and the powers of darkness – as Kathleen described them – closed in. She did her utmost to reawaken an Albion sunk in deadly sleep.'

Naturally, when such a comment was made, the liberal voices of a new Britain, who, in a most alarmingly undemocratic fashion, seldom respect an opinion that differs from theirs, launched into a savage character assassination against both the Prince and the poet for daring to disagree with the direction of modern Britain. Writing in the *Daily Mail* on Saturday, 27 November 2004, under the headlines 'IN SCORES OF UNCTUOUS LETTERS, THE POET KATHLEEN RAINE INDULGED CHARLES'S MONUMENTAL SELF-PITY. WAS THEIR RELATIONSHIP, REVEALED THIS WEEK, AT THE ROOT OF THE PRINCE'S WEAKNESS AND SNOBBERY?' Writer Christopher Wilson warms to his editor's commission. He attacks every aspect of Raine's personal life, describing her as a woman, 'who became his mentor but who, in her own life, had abandoned children and ruthlessly discarded husbands in the pursuit of success …' It was something that Raine herself had often admitted to, but according to Wilson this wicked woman had beaten a path to the Prince's door in order to exploit his biggest weakness – his self-pity. While it can certainly be said that the Prince can be most self-pitying, he isn't weak – weak men don't endure the monumental battles with opinion-formers and politicians that he has, especially in the knowledge that the tabloid editors will mock their every word.

Mr Wilson, like so many of his kind, would do well to look in the mirror and think what achievement, however modest, he could place against the workings of the Prince's Trust or whether he would have the Prince's courage to speak out for what he thought was right – however unfashionable such an opinion might be – or whether living in the royal goldfish bowl is really just one lovely life of privilege as he seems to think it is.

Despite years of mockery from intellectual pigmies, the Prince's thirst for spiritual knowledge remains today. It has helped him become a more complete person and thus allowed him in turn to assist in the attempted re-civilisation of his kingdom along the lines of the views expressed to Tom Shebbeare in his 1993 letter to him. It should be said, however, that as an older and more cynical man, hardened by the events of the last twenty-five years, he doubts if too many are prepared to listen. But such is the strange cocktail of negative expectation and steel determination to keep going that this will not prevent him from trying.

As the 1970s drew to a close, none of the constraints or problems of Charles's life were too apparent: he seemed to be having such a good time that he was probably the most envied man in the kingdom. The public image of him was one of a dashing young man who jumped off a hunter in order to leap on to a polo pony; a guy who landed a jet plane before getting into his Aston Martin in order to roar away to a candlelit dinner in some exclusive restaurant with a beautiful woman and then on to a private-members-only nightclub. This image was not too far from the truth: despite his inner traumas, Charles was doing precisely that a lot of the time, and this presented many photo opportunities for the press.

In London, his devil-may-care attitude to girls around town combined with his Action Man image not only made him all the more attractive, it totally disguised his inner turmoil and feelings of worthlessness. Beautiful and eligible young women – including, among others, Davina Sheffield, Sabrina Guinness, Lady Jane Wellesley, Anna Wallace, Lady Cecily Kerr and Lady Sarah Spencer – were paraded on his arm. All in all the nation got the impression, especially as he was often seen in a dinner jacket getting out of his Aston Martin, that the Prince of Wales might make a damn good James Bond when Roger Moore gave up the role.

Flattered by the attention of so many gorgeous women, and capable of using his greater freedom to enjoy them, he determined not only to sow his wild oats, as commanded by Mountbatten, but also to do so with gusto in an act of defiance against his harsh upbringing and as a distraction from his inner insecurity. He was literally spoiled for choice and his closest friends began to worry about how he was getting through all the best candidates for marriage at an alarming rate – often discarding them on a whim without really giving them a chance. This had the effect of frightening the more suitable type of girl away while attracting the wrong ones all the more.

The Prince was to get annoyed by the press taking much more interest in his private life than in the good works that he did or attempted to promote. This was extremely unrealistic of him and just as naive as Diana was to be when complaining about the press, having courted them in the first place. It was not that Prince Charles courted the media in the same way, but to take a girl to watch you play polo when you are approaching thirty, having let it be known that that you consider that to be a good age to get married, and then expecting people to be more interested in your work when your girlfriend may become the next queen of England, is every bit as naïve. He was surprised to hear a Canadian radio announcer describe him as the world's most eligible bachelor rather than discuss his visit to Pearson College in Victoria as the new president of the United World Colleges, a role that he took very seriously. He displayed a similar naivety in Australia, when he announced to Checketts that he would be spending a private weekend with two former girlfriends. Checketts protested that if the media got hold of this then not only would both girls' reputations be in tatters, the image of the monarchy would be damaged as well. Charles refused to listen and insisted petulantly that he had a right to a private life at least every now and then. Checketts refused to be intimidated and made the ultimate threat to refer the matter to Buckingham Palace in order that the Queen may decide. Faced with this prospect, the Prince finally yielded.

So the romantic elements of his life weren't quite as wonderful as the carefree images that the tabloids painted. Moreover, things were often worse for the girls themselves who often not only got a public mauling by the tabloids while Action Man got away scot-free, but the royal household, which was totally inept at dealing with this kind of media attention, sometimes blamed the girls for courting the attention in the first place and exploiting their liaisons with the Prince to their advantage. This was usually not the case and therefore did nothing towards the development of any relationship that might have flowered into genuine affection if given a chance.

It was against this background that Charles, contrary to much public speculation that he was becoming a confirmed bachelor, began to panic that he may never find the right woman. He became most concerned that the combination of the prerequisite credentials, the pressure from the press and the abnormal workings of his family business would conspire to deprive him of a bride at all. The only prospect in sight was Amanda Knatchbull, who, as he had surmised in his letter to Mountbatten, had grown to be very fond of Prince Charles. She was equally impressed with his energy, enthusiasm, sense of fun, kindness and modest self-deprecation. Moreover, she admired his intellect, his wisdom and his love of the natural world. He was in so many ways exactly like his great-uncle and her grandfather. She adored Mountbatten, and she adored Charles for being like him and in love with him. That was a very special bond to her – just to see them together gave her a special feeling.

Nor was she jealous of the fact that the old man paid far more attention to Charles than his real grandchildren. She had also noticed how the Prince had coloured with a warm glow of pleasure when her own mother had called him 'darling' as she always did her own children – an expression that had clearly been missing from his own childhood and for which he had longed. She understood how he held his parents in awe and yet dearly loved them, even though he was clearly perplexed and hurt by their failure to show him the affection that he craved. She was strongly attracted by his tenderness and vulnerability in this regard and considered it to be a counterpoint to his bravery in the field of dangerous sports. As a result she was able to reflect that Prince Charles would be, when the time came, an excellent father.

Between 1974 and 1979 Charles and Amanda saw more and more of each other quite free from the pressure of tabloid gossip. It was one of the best-kept royal secrets in modern times and still the tabloids try to ignore this relationship thirty years on as result of their embarrassment. So how did they fail to spot it? The Windsors and the Mountbattens were two great houses already united by marriage. They were family and hence the couple could go to family gatherings or even visit each other's homes without any of the conjecture or innuendo that was to be associated with other girls.

Therefore, when Mountbatten suggested to Charles that Amanda join them on what might be the seventy-nine-year-old's last trip to India, he readily agreed. But the Duke of Edinburgh objected to Mountbatten going at all on the grounds that his presence, as the last viceroy of India, would overshadow the Prince of Wales and therefore the purpose of the visit. John Brabourne, Amanda's father, was also opposed. His reasoning was that while he felt that Amanda and the Prince were moving towards marriage, if she were to go to India, the press was bound to hound them and make Amanda's life, which to date hadn't been wrecked by them, quite impossible. Mountbatten's daughter Patricia agreed with her husband and said that if Amanda was to join the Prince's entourage, even with her grandfather present, 'action would be needed either to announce an engagement immediately before Charles and she were ready for this or a denial would have to be issued in circumstances which Amanda would find wounding'.

This clearly demonstrates the power the media has over the lives of the Royal Family. As a result of these worries, the old viceroy and his granddaughter were not to make the trip. Mountbatten was to write lovingly to Charles, 'From a purely selfish point of view I must confess that I will be very, very sad to have to forego the great happiness of being able to be with the two young people I love so much and showing them the country which means so much to me. But if my selfishness were to spoil the future happiness of you both then that would be a price that I would not even contemplate.'

Amanda and Charles were not in the first throes of a passionate affair. They didn't have to be. Both knew that love actually has to have a lot more about it than just infatuation and sexual passion. Such feelings usually burn out, and if there is no genuine affection and mutual respect then the relationship will either be miserable or end up in a divorce court. Unlike Diana, Amanda understood all of this. She was indeed a very sensible and loving girl, who genuinely did share all the same interests as the heir to the throne and knew him, his family and what was entailed well. And there was the problem.

When the Prince did eventually ask her to marry him, she had already anticipated the awful prospect of being consort to the heir apparent: the loss of independence, the loss of self-control to an appointments secretary, the invasion of privacy by a prying press ever anxious to discover scandal, or even invent it. The real Amanda would, in reality, cease to exist: she would have to become a puppet of the system, no doubt often caught in the crossfire between the Windsors and their tabloid tormentors. She was a strong-minded girl and not without her own ambition. She had seen it all at close quarters and knew that, while she loved Prince Charles, her feelings weren't strong enough to warrant taking on what she imagined to be one of the worst jobs in the world, even if she was likely to be one of the best qualified to make a success of it. Her immediate response was both gracious and certain. It did not surprise the Prince, who was fast coming to the opinion that however many unsuitable young women might dream of marrying him, no sensible, suitable woman would ever consider the sacrifice worthwhile. Nevertheless, Amanda's refusal was another disappointment in what appeared to be a long line of frustrations.

As a result, instead of being the carefree Action Man portrayed in the press, he was in fact increasingly depressed and irritable. This was to show itself in feats of physical courage bordering on the insane as he pushed himself to every possible limit to get his adrenalin pumping. It was clearly a gesture that gave an indication of his own private unhappiness that neither Mountbatten nor van der Post could help him with and which he would have to resolve for himself now that the shackles of his former institutionalised life had been removed. It was as if he was telling himself that while he might have to be a perfect puppet at the call of the Church, the government and the people for the vast majority of his life, he could at least go wild on the sports field. He even began to ride his own racehorses at steeplechases, and on one occasion came off – he beat the ground with undiluted anger as television viewers watched in amazement. Needless to say, Palace officials were most concerned about the safety of the heir to the throne and some even prevailed upon the Queen at least to consider banning him from some of his more dangerous pursuits on the grounds that he was endangering his own life.

Perhaps because of this frustration and the power that came with the freedom of his position once he was away from the disciplines of the Royal Navy, the Prince, whose behaviour had been described throughout his childhood and adolescence as kind, virtuous and even saintly, was now to show a selfishness that both surprised and alarmed his friends. His closest friends – not the flatterers and hangers-on – were less worried by his unconventional enthusiasms and sporting recklessness, but rather by the lack of focus they appeared to expose in his new life. Some even worried that, if left to his own devices without the disciplines of the navy to keep him in check, he might even start to follow in the footsteps of his great-uncle Edward VIII. Mountbatten was quick to act and in 1978 wrote to the Prince to warn him against 'beginning on the downward slope which wrecked your Uncle David's life and led to his disgraceful abdication and his futile life ever after'. This was hitting Charles hard and perhaps below the belt. He responded with shock that Mountbatten could even think to make such a comparison. Not only had he thought this, he was to repeat the dose a year later when the two men were on holiday in Eleuthera with the Brabournes. This time he rebuked the heir to the throne for showing 'no signs of pulling yourself together'.

It was not that the Prince was being lazy or failing to carry out his duties. On the contrary, they were executed with both charm and great professionalism. The justifiable complaint that Mountbatten was making concerned the Prince's failure to put the interests of others before his own. Even before the holiday had begun, Mountbatten had been alarmed by the Prince who, having accepted the invitation to Eleuthera on certain dates, then asked for them to be changed in order that he might fit in a few games of polo in Palm Springs. The Brabournes hadn't complained to Mountbatten about this, but nevertheless the old man was horrified by such selfish behaviour. He immediately wrote to Charles and advised him to get the Americans to change their dates or give up his polo in favour of honouring the original dates.

The Prince duly took the advice, but almost as soon as he arrived he managed to incur the old man's displeasure. After two days in the sun, walking, water-skiing and painting without proper protection, the Prince had become badly sunburned. In addition, he was suffering from the effects of a very nasty ear infection that had rendered him almost deaf. Worse still Amanda had stayed behind in England to revise for her finals. As a result he became so disgruntled that he even considered cutting his time there short and returning home. Such a discourtesy to his hosts filled Mountbatten with horror and he wrote Charles a note saying as much and once again comparing him to his Uncle David. He even mentioned that the Prince's behaviour had kept him awake at night, as he was 'worrying whether you would continue on your Uncle David's sad course or take a fall'.

Prince Charles flared in red-hot temper as this wretched comparison with his wayward great-uncle was made yet again. However, he soon calmed down, acknowledged his error and stayed. Much relieved, Mountbatten wrote another note: 'What impressed me most was your desire to be generous, kind-hearted, and to think of others before your own interests.'

Charles was later to confide, in a letter to a close friend, 'my conscience got the better of me ... I must say I am becoming rather worried by all this talk about being self-centred and getting worse every year. I'm told that marriage is the only cure for me – and maybe it is!' He does seem to have taken his great-uncle's words to heart and applied more self-discipline to the curbing of his desires. This gave the impression to his closest friends that he had turned the corner and that, as a result, the future didn't appear to be so bad after all. Certainly, normal relations of mutual admiration were restored between the Prince and his mentor after the Eleuthera episode.

It is ironic that the Prince, who was enjoying the height of his popularity with the nation as a result of the positive image that he was given by the tabloid press, had at the same time been alarming his closest friends by behaving in a manner previously unknown to them. This tells us a lot about the effects of celebrity upon human nature when imposed discipline is removed, even when the most trained mind is involved.

It is abundantly clear to all who have ever taken an interest in the life and times of our future king that Mountbatten was a figure of supreme importance, the rock of reliability and the fount of wisdom upon which Charles had come to rely. It was Mountbatten who had seen the Prince's potential and then kept faith with it, Mountbatten who had provided the essential compassion, encouragement and affection that preserved the heir to the throne's fragile self-esteem, while his parents stayed aloof and others fawned over him. His contribution to the development of the Prince of Wales was unique and Charles knew it.

The Prince now resolved that, however troubled he might be in his inner conflicts between who he had been born to be and who he actually was, he would nevertheless never allow himself to drift into the self-centredness of the Duke of Windsor and thus run the risk of letting himself down, wasting the years of effort expended in getting this far and, perhaps worst of all, disappointing his most treasured honorary grandfather. He was to write to Mountbatten after one of their meaningful discussions, 'I have no idea what we shall do without you if you finally decide to depart. It doesn't bear thinking about, but I only hope that I shall have learnt something from you to carry it on in some way or other.'

In August of 1979 the Prince, who had been joined on the Royal Yacht *Britannia* by Amanda, wrote to Mountbatten explaining how she had described to him the beauty of her grandfather's summer home at Classiebawn Castle on the west coast of Ireland. 'I do wish I could come and see it ... I know I would be captivated by it ... I do hope that you are having a rest in Ireland and aren't working unnecessarily hard.'

A few days later, a group of IRA terrorists detonated a bomb on board Mountbatten's small fishing boat as it left the harbour at Mullaghmore. Mountbatten, his fourteen-year-old grandson Nicholas and a young Irish boatman were killed outright. Mountbatten's daughter Patricia Brabourne, her husband John and their son Timothy, who was Nicholas's twin brother, were severely injured. Lady Brabourne, John Brabourne's mother, died the next day. In a flash, and as a result of cold-blooded and wholly inexcusable murder, not only had the heart been ripped out of a very decent family but its head, Lord Louis Mountbatten of Burma, war hero on both sea and land, last viceroy of India, former commander of the Mediterranean Fleet and head of the joint chiefs of staff, was no more. He was to be mourned by a nation and missed by many, but none more than an inconsolable Prince Charles.

The Prince of Wales was in Iceland when he heard the news. He was to record in his journal, 'When I was told some very bad news was about to be recounted to me my heart literally "sank" and I felt quite sick in the pit of my tummy. All sorts of hideous possibilities raced through my mind before the awful truth emerged ... I still can't believe what has taken place and continue, vainly, to imagine that he will somehow revive and prove to everyone that he has yet again survived ... A mixture of desperate emotions swept over me – agony, disbelief, a kind of wretched numbness, closely followed by fierce and violent determination to see that something was done about the IRA …

'All these thoughts raced through my confused mind as I walked back along the river to the house in order to telephone Mummy to find out what exactly had happened and hoping that it was a nightmare … I had always dreaded the day when he would die, but somehow I had always thought it would be several more years – at least until he felt "ready" and no longer felt there was anything to go on living for. Life has to go on, I suppose, but this afternoon I must confess I wanted it to stop. I felt supremely useless and powerless …

'I have lost someone infinitely special in my life; someone who showed enormous affection, who told me unpleasant things I didn't particularly want to hear, who gave praise where it was due as well as criticism; someone to whom I knew I could confide anything and from whom I would receive the wisest of counsel and advice. In some extraordinary way he combined grandfather, great-uncle, father, brother and friend and I shall always be eternally grateful that I was lucky enough to have known him as long as I did. Life will NEVER be the same now that he has gone and I fear it will take me a very long time to forgive those people who today have achieved something that two world wars and THOUSANDS of German and Japanese failed to achieve. I only hope I can live up to the expectations he had of me and be able to do SOMETHING to honour the name of Mountbatten.'

These words would have delighted the old man and made him very proud. They were not written for dewy-eyed public consumption, but as the innermost private thoughts of a grieving man to himself. There is no theatre or dramatic gesture – just naked pain and total truth – and as such they are a magnificent tribute to an outstanding man from one who loved him dearly and owed him much. The very contents prove that Mountbatten had not misplaced his hopes in this young man.

Part Two
The Courtship and Marriage

Chapter Six
The Preparation of a Princess (1977–81)

Having failed her second attempt to pass her O-level examinations, Diana was whisked away to the Institut Alpin Videmanette near the fashionable skiing resort of Gstaad in Switzerland. Her father, while being slightly embarrassed by his daughter's academic ineptitude, was by no means as worried as one might be today in a world of sexual equality. He naturally thought that she would marry into her 'class' anyway: as she would undoubtedly turn into a good-looking woman, and given his family line, this would not pose a problem.

Therefore, being groomed to be an excellent wife for a man of land, or title, or both, who perhaps had a good number in the City while waiting to inherit, was to be the lot in life for this quite unexceptional girl. She had been born, like her future husband, into position and wealth; happily for her, however, she had inherited none of the responsibility that usually accompanies both, and thus she avoided his trials and tribulations.

Diana's younger brother Charles had always been far brighter at school. He would taunt her by shouting 'Brian! Brian!' in her face (Brian was the rather slow snail on children's television programme *The Magic Roundabout*.) Her new school majored on cookery and domestic social graces. It was indeed a classic, old-fashioned finishing school that was much favoured by the British moneyed classes during the first half of the twentieth century. Of course this was humiliating within the family circle, but it was hardly serious – even in the 1970s, girls of rich fathers weren't expected to head up public companies or even map out a meaningful career elsewhere.

The finishing school conducted its education entirely in French. This was normal, and as a result young ladies who were educated this way had always been able to show off an impressive, if unused, command of the language. However, Diana arrived at the school with a very poor command of French and understandably became reticent about speaking out for fear of sounding foolish. The result was that she had difficulty fitting in socially and her class work – which she had always found difficult enough in her native tongue – was now nothing short of pathetic. Her only consolation was that she enjoyed the pleasant, if not too demanding, skiing, but this hardly made up for things and she had a miserable time.

Just as Prince Charles had written to his childhood nanny with dismal tales of Gordonstoun, so Diana now put pen to paper to a former teacher of his, Mary Clarke. However, unlike the Prince of Wales, Diana was also quick to bombard her parents with pleading letters saying how unhappy she was and begging them to take her away without delay. The fact that they acquiesced after just one term is in stark contrast to the years of misery suffered by Charles at Gordonstoun and perhaps offers more than a little explanation as to why, in her later role, she often lacked the discipline that her husband and his family expected of her.

As she was enduring this hell, her sister Sarah arrived in nearby Klosters on the arm of Prince Charles to enjoy a much-publicised skiing holiday. As a result there was some speculation in the British press that the heir to the throne was about to propose marriage. Some friends say that this was never going to be the case as the relationship was close but mostly platonic – Sarah was healing the wounds of a broken relationship while the Prince was only in the earliest stage of seeing whether or not this girl might make a suitable queen. Certainly Sarah was by no means the only one under consideration.

On their return to Britain, Sarah managed, probably by accident, to rule herself out by having a seemingly harmless conversation with the press. In reply to a question about marriage to the Prince, she answered that she would marry only for love and that could be either to a prince or to a dustman. According to Lady Sarah Spencer-Churchill, Sarah did have grand plans in mind: 'Prince Charles, of course, was supposed to rally to Sarah's side, to show the world that he could conquer this pure-hearted girl whose only interest was love – just in case he was wondering if ambition was responsible for her responsiveness.' But Sarah misjudged the Prince. 'He isn't aggressive or domineering. Faced with a personal challenge, he withdraws. The Spencers all rise to challenges like bulls to red flags. Challenges goad them to unthinkable heights.'

At about this time Diana's second sister Jane was getting married. Perhaps her fiancé was less blue-blooded than Charles, but at least there was a royal connection. Robert Fellowes was the son of the land agent who ran Sandringham, and was now the Queen's assistant private secretary. He would in time be promoted and serve Her Majesty well. However, his little-known coolness towards the Prince of Wales was to be most unhelpful in the Queen's relationship with her eldest son; this and her own distance from Charles meant that relations between Buckingham Palace and St James's Palace were to get steadily worse in the years ahead.

In April, a term of pleading paid off and Diana was allowed to leave her finishing school to live with her mother in Cadogan Place, Knightsbridge. The summer was spent fairly aimlessly as Diana and her family considered her future. She needed to start networking socially in order to meet the right sort of young men who might make suitable husbands, and in the meantime she had to find some form of employment. As she was by now growing into a tall and striking girl, and the Spencer family had great social status, the first point did not appear to present a problem although Diana, while showing some interest in making new friends, apparently showed not too much in romantic attachment, believing even then that her destiny lay with marriage to a royal – preferably her idol Prince Charles. The issue of employment was more difficult. Her lack of academic qualification combined with her status and her desire to be a Sloane Ranger in Chelsea seriously limited her choice of jobs, let alone careers.

It was perhaps somewhat surprising at this point that Diana, who had showed such care and aptitude for the welfare of mentally and physically challenged people while at school, did not look to work in this area – even if on a voluntary basis. Obviously, her lack of academic qualifications would have precluded her from entering upon a career path towards a qualified level, but her mere presence among such people gave much comfort throughout her life and would at this point have given her meaningful purpose. For whatever reason, this avenue of activity was ignored, and instead it was agreed that she should embark upon a ten-week cookery course in September 1978. However, no sooner had she started it than her father was taken dangerously ill. He collapsed and was rushed into Northampton General Hospital near the family home at Althorp having suffered a brain haemorrhage. His wife and four children were summoned by a consultant and informed that they should expect the worst.

Raine immediately took charge of things. At her insistence he was moved to a London hospital where doctors were instructed by her to operate without delay. Then she obtained a new and untested drug from Germany and had it administered. She was also to persuade the vicar of All Saints, Northampton, to exorcise the ghost of his father, whom she believed her husband was still frightened of, and finally, as she sat constantly by his bedside, she ordered him not to die. Her powerful and commanding presence made the children feel excluded, but it did the trick and the earl, against all odds, recovered.

Diana had always adored her father, but she was unable to administer her wonderful healing talent to him during this period and so played no real part in his convalescence. Perhaps it was because of her natural fear of losing a loved one, or the fact that she always found it easier to communicate with strangers whom she would be unlikely to meet again as there was no worry of long-term consistency. Or maybe it was because the presence of her stepmother simply overpowered the teenager and pushed her into the background. Whatever the truth, his survival and recovery are attributed to Raine.

Once she had her weak but nevertheless living husband back home, she decided that this was the moment to refurbish the house and leave her mark upon it. Althorp was to have a major facelift that included the building of en suite bathrooms, the installation of central heating, the carpeting of corridors and the replacement of fading silk wallpaper. To pay for all of this she was, according to her stepson Charles, to sell a fifth of the house's art collection. Most of it went to Bond Street dealers at prices that allowed them to make huge profits on resale. An auction at Christies or Sothebys would have undoubtedly fetched a lot more money. Finally, Raine affronted the strong Spencer pride by replacing the huge portrait of Robert, the first earl, which hung on the great staircase, by an equally large picture of herself in her youth. Worst of all, as far as the children were concerned, their father seemed to approve of it all. Prior to his illness, her force of character and his infatuation had given her the upper hand; following it, his dependence and gratitude meant that he passed control of his life almost exclusively to her. His children, especially Charles and Diana, could only look on in silent rage.

Royal biographers have speculated that the seventeen-year-old Diana probably lost her virginity to fourteen-year-old Daniel Wiggin, son of Sir John Wiggin and a friend of her brother's, in 1978. Wiggin has certainly claimed to friends that he deflowered the future Princess of Wales, despite the fact that Diana insisted right up until the time of her death that it was to Prince Charles that she had surrendered this prize. Nobody other than Wiggin knows whether his story is true, but it is widely known that hers is not: Diana had a number of lovers before she became engaged. Nevertheless, she always remained discreet as 'she didn't want to do anything except get married', as Lady Sarah Spencer-Churchill explained, and didn't want her sexual liaisons to damage her chances of first of all attracting Prince Andrew and then, as she became more ambitious, Prince Charles. It was a frustrating time for the youngest Spencer girl.

However, 1979, while proving to be a year in which Prince Charles experienced one of the most horrific and tragic events of his life – the death of Mountbatten – brought about happier times for Diana. Following her marriage to Robert Fellowes, Diana's sister Jane was able to travel with the court and this gave her the opportunity to invite members of her family to attend. As a result, in January Diana was invited for the weekend to Sandringham, where the Royal Family was still in residence following their traditional Christmas visit to the estate.

Prince Charles at the time was, much to Mountbatten's pleasure, pursuing the sensible prospect of courting Amanda Knatchbull. Despite having only met the Prince once before and thus having no reason to suppose that he would ever notice this pretty but still slightly chubby girl twelve years his junior, Diana found herself to be smitten by him, just as she had in the ploughed field on the first occasion; as a result she was increasingly determined to catch his eye and supply the necessary credentials to get her noticed.

In the same month and with her father on the road to recovery under the careful and dominating control of her stepmother, Diana started out on yet another career option: that of dancing teacher. She wrote to Madame Betty Vacani, who ran a school that had taught the Royal Family to dance; to her surprise and great pleasure she was accepted. Her first task wasn't too technical but for Diana, who loved children and took pleasure in their company, it was most enjoyable. Her job was to supervise the youngest toddlers while accompanying their efforts on the piano. For a moment it seemed that at long last Diana had found a useful vocation, if a somewhat modest one given the expense of her education. But in March she went skiing and never returned to the school, much to the disappointment of the children who had liked 'Miss Diana' and were looking forward to seeing her next term.

Instead, Diana had found a chalet party in Val Claret, near Tignes in the French Alps. She was now able to attempt to perfect the skiing technique that she had picked up on the easy slopes of Gstaad, but the more demanding pistes of Tignes put her sorely to the test and she found the going tough, eventually tearing the ligaments in her left leg.

Despite this, she decided to stay on with another group that she ran into. There were twenty in the party and although Diana knew none of them and was the youngest, she immediately got on with them all and became the life and soul of the party.

One of the guests was Simon Berry, whose family were renowned wine merchants; another was a medical student called James Colthurst, who had a brief and apparently fairly superficial romance with Diana. The environment suited her perfectly: it was new and unexplored; the people were fresh and exciting and she could be interested in them safe in the knowledge that it would end before it all got too serious. As a result, she could shine. She was to amaze people under such circumstances constantly throughout her life. Diana on parade was nearly always, even when she was under terrible pressure, a heady cocktail of charm, elegance, beauty and a simple captivating friendliness. Diana, behind closed doors could be a very different person.

However, in this environment, up a mountain with new acquaintances from her exclusive, sheltered life of British class and privilege without much responsibility, it must have looked to an outsider as if she had at last started on her path to adult destiny. Surely this encounter would be a step towards finding a perfect partner and a life of country houses, London flats and happy family holidays. However, Diana had other ideas. One of those present at the time was to recall years later to Clayton and Craig that she was determined to realise her destiny. 'She was going to get married to the Prince of Wales – not "I want to" or "I'd like to", but "I'm going to" ... She was extremely sure of herself. It was fate: she had a strong sense of her own destiny. Then I said, "Why would you want to do that? What's the attraction?" And she said, "He's the one man on the planet who is not allowed to divorce me."'

Eventually she returned to London, vowing to keep in touch with her new friends, and became a cleaner for her sister Sarah and her friend Lucinda Craig-Harvey at the going, if not impressive, rate of £1 per hour.

On 1 July 1979, Diana finally reached the age of eighteen and received a bequest from her late great-grandmother. As a coming-of-age present, her parents decided to buy her a London apartment. Her sister Sarah, who worked at the time at Savills, the London estate agents, was duly instructed to find one. She came up with a redbrick mansion flat costing £50,000 (a substantial sum in 1979) – 60 Coleherne Court, at the junction of Old Brompton Road and Redcliffe Gardens. It was within easy walking distance of Harrods, Harvey Nichols and all the restaurants in Beauchamp Place.

It was quite natural, given her background, new location and recently acquired skiing friends, that Diana would now became a member of the Sloane Rangers – regarded by some as the well-educated and nicely spoken children of the successful, or as spoiled, rich parasites by others. As a property owner, Diana not only now had a home of her own but was also able to earn cash on the side by becoming landlady to various girlfriends. Nevertheless, the family still remained concerned that she hadn't got a proper job and showed little interest in getting one. The Spencers had not been brought up to be cleaners, even if the main client was a family member. They all thought it very demeaning and not the sort of thing they wished to come out during the course of a dinner-party conversation. Something had to be done. In the end, her other sister Jane found her a job, three afternoons a week, that still allowed for shopping expeditions to Harvey Nichols followed by lunch in Beauchamp Place. It was at the Young England Kindergarten in Pimlico, a private nursery for the children of the rich.

At long last Diana had come across something that enhanced her low self-esteem. She was a success from the moment she started. Almost immediately parents were asking to meet the pretty new teacher about whom their children spoke so often at home. Very soon she was asked to work in the mornings as well: to the surprise of some of her friends she agreed to go full-time three days a week. Her parents were both delighted and relieved, for although the pay was modest and the status not great, Diana was no longer a cleaner and had set about her new job with some purpose.

She had received no teacher training, but her ability to gain the children's love and respect was immediate. Moreover, she liked her job and thought it was worthwhile. She was on parade and all of her undoubted and unique qualities shone through. She showed patience, good humour and wonderful intuition. The owner, Kay Seth-Smith, was impressed. 'She was very good at getting down to the children's level both physically and mentally. She was quite happy to sit on the floor, having children climbing all over her, sit on the low chairs besides them and actually talk to them. That's very important, to be able to talk to them, at their level. And they responded incredibly well to her. She would then go and help clean up in the kitchen. She was happy to put on the Marigolds as she called them [rubber gloves]. She would prepare lunch and generally mucked in.'

Diana was to remain wonderfully able to communicate with children, the mentally ill, the sick, the disadvantaged and the dying all her life. None of them would ever challenge her academic ability, so she would never feel inferior and could give to them safe in the knowledge that her help would be valuable, not rejected and would not have to lead to a close, long-term relationship that she might find hard to sustain.

As a result of her success at the kindergarten, Diana determined to occupy the other two days of her week by also working with children and signed up with several nanny agencies. One of them eventually found her a job with an American businesswoman, Mary Robertson, looking after her small son Patrick. Ms Robertson was most impressed by Diana at the initial interview and decided to engage her, despite having serious reservations about the girl's lack of any sort of academic qualifications – but she accepted Diana's explanation that bad bouts of nerves had caused her to fail every single exam that she had ever taken.

Patrick soon became most attached to his new nanny. When Mary Robertson returned from work, she would find the washing-up done, the flat tidy and Patrick clean and ready for bed, snuggled up to his nanny who would invariably be reading him a story. She was absolutely delighted and years later told Clayton and Craig how levelheaded and committed to Patrick Diana appeared. 'It was a huge step to hand over Patrick to a stranger in a strange city where we had no neighbours, we really didn't know anybody. I really had no concerns about her being flighty or irresponsible.'

Robertson's words would appear, at first glance, to contradict those who have indicated that Diana was an emotional mess before she married. And there is no doubt that Ms Robertson's words ring true. However, to point to this as proof that she was enduring no such emotional trauma indicates a complete misunderstanding of who the real Diana was. Throughout her life, at least from puberty onwards, there were two Dianas: the public Diana and the private Diana, the girl on duty and the girl off duty, the girl on parade and the girl at home. People, in her mind, fell into one of two camps: those whom she should impress and those with whom she could let her real emotions show.

In a remarkable way, this was not dissimilar to the behaviour pattern of Prince Charles, who was always a dutiful prince in public but could be insecure and increasingly selfish during his twenties in private. However, there was a difference. With Charles, the people in the first camp – his parents, Mountbatten, the rest of his family and the outside world in general – would only see the acceptable face of a prince, while people in the second camp – Checketts, others on his staff and in particular the employees of Buckingham Palace – were increasingly destined to feel the lash of his tongue as a safety valve against his obvious frustration of having permanently to strain to be a man that he really wasn't.

With Diana things were different. An individual might start in the first camp if they could be the key to obtaining something she wanted, but could quickly be transferred to the second camp once they had delivered or it was determined by her that they would fail to do so. And then as she fell out with other people, so they might be transferred back again. This was often to confuse her family and friends alike. People could be elevated at high speed to being her closest confidante and best friend but suddenly, and for no apparent reason, be dropped stone dead. It would happen time after time throughout her life.

While working on her two jobs and receiving most deserved praise for her efforts during the day, she was seeing James Gilbey of the London gin dynasty in the evenings. This was probably Diana's most serious relationship to date and one to which she would revert after her marriage. Diana may have been perfect at the kindergarten and with Patrick, but when Gilbey stood her up one evening, the other Diana took over. She mixed a paste of flour and egg and went around to his place in the middle of the night and poured it over his shiny Alfa Romeo in the knowledge that it would set and be extremely difficult to remove without ruining the paintwork – something she knew would seriously distress her car-mad lover. Many people have flagged up this story as a typical early-warning sign of how vengeful Diana could be. 'Diana could be a real bitch. If you crossed her – which didn't necessarily mean doing anything awful, simply not giving her her own way – she turned very, very nasty indeed,' was Lady Sarah Spencer-Churchill's opinion as expressed to Lady Colin Campbell. It was shared by many of Diana's friends. Both Rosa Monckton and the Princess's journalist friend Richard Kay have described her in a similar vein; even Diana herself told Lady Colin Campbell, 'I can't help it. I've got a vengeful streak.' Diana did not yet know the Prince of Wales – it was not his treatment of her that developed into this character trait, as she later would wish to convince the world.

On another occasion, when a friend refused to lend her a car, she glued its locks solid. When someone at a house party slighted her, she got up in the middle of the night, unscrewed his car's petrol tank and poured water inside, which did serious damage to the engine. Another friend of hers looked back on these incidents and said, 'People should think about what Diana was really like. She was no saint and certainly no angel. She could be sweet and generous, but she also had a vicious streak in her nature. She could be tremendously and irresponsibly destructive. Malicious really. What she did to James Gilbey's car constituted criminal damage. It was no joke. People have gone to jail for less.' All of these comments come from people who in the main liked Diana despite these flaws, relations or people who considered themselves to be her friends.

Gilbey took one look at his treasured Alfa Romeo and decided that this young woman on the prowl for the best husband that she could get could look elsewhere. He completely lost interest in her. However, he was pleased to make her acquaintance again in 1989, when she was no longer a chubby girl but the celebrated Princess of Wales. Now the boot was on the other foot and she took her revenge on him with glee.

Other early lovers included the Honourable Harry Herbert, the Honourable George Plumptre, whom she continued to see even after she started dating the Prince of Wales, and Rory Scott. She was described by one of her then boyfriends to Lady Colin Campbell as more of an eager lover than an accomplished one, but nevertheless one who had a strong sexual appetite.

In 1980, Diana appeared happier than she had been since the O-level debacle, and was turning into a beautiful young woman. Indeed, at the Duke of Rutland's annual summer ball, she was noticed by many a young beau. Later that summer her cousin Robert Spencer threw a large house party and again the young men singled her out for admiration. One of them was Prince Andrew who danced with her a great deal on that occasion.

Prince Charles, although absent on that particular evening, was also now on the same social circuit. Since November 1979 he had been seeing the extremely attractive twenty-five-year-old daughter of a rich Scottish landowner. Her name was Anna Wallace, but she was known on the circuit as Whiplash Wallace – not, apparently, because of a dominatrix attitude in bed, but because she rode horses like the wind and had a waspish tongue that could be well directed by her ready wit! It was rumoured, that the Prince of Wales had proposed marriage to her, but that she had turned him down for the same reasons as Amanda Knatchbull. This seems unlikely. It is true that she was very attractive, came from the right background and loved the country life, but her fiery temper would have set alarm bells ringing. Prince Charles wanted a woman with a gentle personality – he had always been wary of loud and ill-disciplined people of either sex. Moreover, as the future king, he needed to marry a woman who could be relied on and who would always put the country first. From this point of view, Anna Wallace was highly unsuitable and Charles's comments on the necessary credentials for a future Queen of England, as voiced publicly for over a decade, would have precluded him from asking her in the first place. Instead it is far more likely that this was a fiery and enjoyable physical relationship. He embarked upon it at about the same time as he was enjoying the start of his second affair with Camilla Parker Bowles, all the while waiting to find Miss Right. Indeed, in the early summer of 1980, the Prince of Wales and Anna had a furious row at Stowell Park, which resulted in Anna borrowing her hostess's car to leave in the middle of the night. Her rage had erupted after he had paid too much attention to another woman at the party: Camilla Parker Bowles.

A few weeks later, in July, Prince Charles came across Diana for a third time during a weekend house party given by Commander Robert de Pass at his home near Petworth on the Sussex/Hampshire border. His son Philip had only invited Diana to the bash at the last minute, and he took her to Cowdray Park to watch polo. Playing for Les Diables Bleus was Prince Charles. Unsurprisingly, the place was packed with journalists and photographers. Harry Arnold, the journalist and one-time royal biographer, was on duty with his cameraman Arthur Edwards. This sort of thing had been their job for the last five years. Arnold was later to remember, 'Every weekend in the summer we would go along to the polo matches where he would always take his current girlfriend. Sometimes the girl would be very close to him, on his arm, talking to him between "chukkas" and that kind of thing. But this particular weekend came where there didn't appear to be a current girlfriend and we went to this particular match and Arthur spotted this particular girl sitting in the crowd with a "D" round her neck and had a vague recollection he'd seen her somewhere before. We talked about it and thought: Well perhaps she's the latest one. So Arthur took just one frame of her, just one snap and that was the very beginning of it.'

After the match, and away from the flashbulbs, Diana saw her opportunity and seized the moment. During the evening barbeque she plonked herself down on a bale of hay next to the Prince, who was momentarily on his own. Dispensing with small talk she bravely, but most astutely, cut straight to one of the most sensitive subjects imaginable – the death of Mountbatten. Having met her hero only twice previously, and knowing that he was the future king of England, it was a huge gamble to launch straight into such a deeply personal conversation. She told him that she had really felt for him during the televised funeral, and asked him in that immediate and direct fashion that had won over strangers, the sick and dying, and was to continue to do so throughout her life, how he had dealt with such terrible unhappiness.

She already believed that she was in love with Prince Charles. Moreover, she had made up her mind, in a most bizarre way, that she wished to marry him despite the fact that she hardly knew him and, even worse, had – unlike most of her rivals – given little or no thought to the consequences of this course of action. However naïve this might have been, it was perhaps understandable. Lady Theresa Manners, one of the most desirable women of her and Diana's generation, backed her judgment, saying, 'I can understand why any girl would fall in love with him. He is the nicest, kindest, most delightful man. He is an artist, a poet, a philosopher, a thinker.'

Diana's action was very brave, and she must have steeled herself with the determination that allows so few people in life to grab that unique moment when it presents itself. And, whether or not she was fully aware of her gift, she banked upon immediate intimacy. It was an electric moment that was forever remembered by both of them. Not only was the Prince not used to being asked such direct questions but also, having been lonely for most of his life, he immediately responded. He at once knew this girl wasn't a shallow royal flatterer. He found her to be sincere, down to earth and surprisingly easy to confide in.

As the evening wore on, their conversation became amazingly intense – especially for two people who had only just met and one of whom was a prince of the realm. This was quite abnormal, but Charles welcomed it – he had always yearned for a companion to whom he could open his soul, and had always believed that such people, few and far between as they had proved to be in his life, should be treasured. Relationships had always moved at a remarkable speed with Diana, and so it was now as she, despite being twelve years younger, grabbed the initiative and told Prince Charles how she sensed his loneliness and his need for someone to care for him. These seeds were cast brilliantly on fertile ground: the boy who had craved his father's attention, hated Gordonstoun, been subjected to dreadful bouts of homesickness and devastated by Mountbatten's death found himself immediately beguiled by this beautiful young woman who seemed to understand so much about him. He was, as he has always freely admitted, moved by her patient listening, as he poured out his heart in a most uncharacteristic way to a mere stranger. He did not want the evening to end, and this was someone he clearly wished to see again.

On the videotapes Diana subsequently recorded for her voice coach, she remembered this first evening together: 'I said to him, "You must be so lonely. It's pathetic watching you walking up the aisle with Lord Mountbatten's coffin in front. It's ghastly. You need someone beside you." Ugh. Wrong word. Whereupon he leaped upon me and started kissing me and everything ... And I thought, Waah ... You know. This isn't what people do. He was all over me for the rest of the evening. Followed me around ... Everything. A puppy. And, um, yeah I was flattered but puzzled.'

Everybody there that night remembers them talking. Nobody can remember them kissing, and no wonder – the idea that the Prince of Wales would start to kiss a girl that he had just met in full view of a crowd largely comprising strangers is ridiculous. It is a perfect example of Diana simply having blotted out the truth by the time the last years of her life were upon her.

Commenting on the Prince of Wales's encounter on the hay bale with the young Lady Diana Spencer, former Buckingham Palace press secretary Ronald Allison said, 'I'm sure that one of the things that appealed to Prince Charles about Lady Diana was just how unsophisticated she was. There was a naivety about her ... she was just so young and beautiful, and great fun to be with – in that sense, I imagine, very different from most of the other young women that he's developed some sort of friendship with.'

This might have been what impressed Allison but it was almost certainly not what had impressed Prince Charles. The Prince has often been portrayed as a confirmed bachelor who, unable to marry the woman he really wanted, half decided and was half pushed by his father into marriage with an unsophisticated virgin whom he didn't really love in order to do his duty to the nation and supply a son and heir.

In reality things were very different. We now know that, from the 1960s onwards, Charles had become very conscious of the need to choose the right girl to become the future queen of England. We also know from his letters how desperate he was to find a soulmate. And we know, from their correspondence, that Mountbatten had devised a game plan to help him achieve all of this. Given that the girl must not have a track record, be an Anglican and love Charles enough to sacrifice her life to the ghastly British press, this might not be the easiest of tasks in an increasingly shallow British society. But the plan was the best that Mountbatten could muster and, in the absence of another, it seemed fine. Indeed, it is difficult to imagine that any other course of action would have guaranteed a better result. The plan had been for the Prince to enjoy his bachelor years, play the field, sow his wild oats and then, at thirty or thereabouts, settle down with an aristocratic girl of impeccable character and Anglican stock who could have children and, like the Queen Mother, would be an excellent consort and source of inspiration to her husband. Such a relationship must be built on deep affection, admiration and mutual respect. Any marriage decision must not become clouded by the pangs of infatuation or the power of physical attraction.

Although Diana was completely infatuated with Charles, and he was physically aroused by her, this is not why their relationship was destined to become so very different from the others that had preceded it. Mountbatten may have intended that the special girl be his granddaughter Amanda Knatchbull; she may have said no and Mountbatten may now be dead; but when Diana sat before him and talked of his great-uncle and her feelings for the Prince's pain, it is without doubt that Charles saw immediately that here was another ideal example of a Mountbatten bride – one who might become the soulmate that he had so far been denied.

Diana might have thrust the baton into Charles's hand, but it was now he who made the running. Almost immediately he invited her to a performance of Verdi's 'Requiem' at the Royal Albert Hall, followed by supper at Buckingham Palace. Diana's grandmother, Lady Fermoy, who was also well known to Prince Charles, came along as her chaperone. Diana was then invited to Balmoral in order to stay with her sister Jane and see her new baby. At the time, Prince Charles was a guest at Birkhall, the Queen Mother's house on the estate, and immediately invited Diana to join him on several of his favourite walks. At once he enjoyed her enthusiasm for Balmoral and the surrounding countryside. It was, after all, his favourite place on earth. As they walked, he explained how he felt about life, his love of the countryside, country sports, literature, music and the arts. She didn't profess to know much about any of it, but seemed most keen to learn. He also told her about the rigours and discipline of life as a royal, and she sympathised. And he told her of his loneliness and how he had walked these hills before going back to Gordonstoun with his stomach tied in knots, already homesick in anticipation of another dreadful autumn term.

Their conversations were as intense as they had been on that hay bale, but now it was Charles taking the lead as he enthusiastically poured out his life story and innermost thoughts – something he had found himself able to do with so few people. Suddenly, on the Balmoral estate, it all seemed to fall into place. He was now just over thirty and had played the field; she was aristocratic and beautiful, an Anglican who was twelve years his junior and, although obviously uneducated, she understood him, she was sensitive and she apparently thought enough of him to risk the dangers of royal life.

On the hay bale, Diana had seized her moment; on the Scottish walks, he seized his: it was here that he tentatively made up his mind that Lady Diana Spencer might just become the Princess of Wales – if she would have him.

Was he in love with her at this time? Probably not – he had always said that the choosing of the future queen of England must not be left to the heart for the sake of the nation, the monarchy and the girl herself. He believed, as he had been taught, that it was imperative that passion didn't cloud the issue. On the other hand, he was beguiled by her – not long afterwards he confided to a friend that, while he was not yet in love, he thought that he could be in time. No doubt he had in mind the love built on common interest, mutual respect and deep affection that Mountbatten had told him was the only basis for a successful marriage. Following these walks across the Balmoral estate, the Prince started to tell friends that he thought that he had met the girl he might marry.

The following month, August, saw Diana aboard the Royal Yacht *Britannia* for the week of the Cowes Regatta. By now the word was spreading among the court, and those who hadn't met her were keen to do so. Diana would later recall that they were 'all over me like a bad rash'. In early September, Charles asked Diana to return to Balmoral for the weekend of the Braemar Games as a guest of his house party. Diana remembered that, 'Mr and Mrs Parker Bowles were there. I was the youngest there by a long way. Charles used to ring me up and say, "Would you like to come for a walk, come for a barbeque?" So I said, "Yes, please." I thought this was all wonderful.'

She did, and for the record it was quite natural for the Parker Bowleses to be there. They were part of the social set, as were Charles Palmer-Tomkinson and his beautiful wife Patty, who came to play a central and important role in bringing Camilla back into the Prince's life in the future. Diana found Charles's entourage to be very friendly, but she was nevertheless greatly intimidated by their superior education, experience of life and senior years. It was the natural reaction of a young girl who was coming into a well-established circle of friends who were not just older and wiser but were also well versed in the habits and traditions of court life. She was later to infer that her intimidation was as a result of a concerted plan of negative vetting by Prince Charles's friends, probably orchestrated by Camilla Parker Bowles. This is absolute nonsense, and was probably not even imagined by her at the time. It became the figment of a fertile imagination many years later when she sought to rewrite history.

In time there were those who came to have their reservations about Diana. They were in a minority and really included only two people of any significance: Penny Romsey, wife of Mountbatten's grandson, and Charles's long-standing friend Nicholas Soames. Camilla Parker Bowles was not among their number. She had a sham of a marriage and had enjoyed her second and, on this occasion, mutually convenient affair with the Prince of Wales. However, she was under no illusion whatsoever that what Charles wanted was a wife and that he fully intended to conduct his life according to Mountbatten's plan. It had always been agreed that he would, when the right girl was found, get rid of any other physical attachments. That meant that all mistresses – for she was not the only one – would have to go.

Diana's potential detractors had no problem with her background, religion or apparent devotion to Prince Charles. However, they were concerned by her lack of education, academic skill or worldliness and, as a result, doubted that the couple would be well suited for a life together. It is probable that Soames also imagined that she might not be the wisest choice for a queen. Moreover, they were also sceptical that a girl, who clearly loved racy, urban and fashionable London, was a Sloane Ranger and was known to be frightened of horses, could seriously be genuine about loving Balmoral, country life, riding and all the other things that meant so much to the Prince, never mind being able to stand the strain of royal life and the tedium of duty when faced with that prospect.

Penny Romsey was the most critical. She believed that Diana was devious and that the nineteen-year-old was more in love with the idea of being queen of England than with Charles himself. Soames, on the other hand, believed that Diana thought she loved Charles but, as she would clearly be unable to sustain any interest in his activities, would attempt to change everything about him – including his lifestyle and friends – once she had married him. As she was not his intellectual equal, she would be unable to share in his social and political interests either.

They made their points to the Prince as tactfully as possible. Charles, who believed that he knew Diana much better than them – after all it was he and not they who had had such deep conversations with her – was not disposed to listen. He didn't want to be rushed into a marriage that would be wrong for him or the crown, but equally he didn't want to let Diana go, as she was only the second woman, after Amanda Knatchbull, that he had considered marrying.

Eventually Penny Romsey, concerned that Prince Charles wasn't taking the hint and was about to embark upon a disaster, got her husband to raise the issue more forcefully during a hack at Broadlands. This time the Prince exploded in rage as he defended Diana's honour. News of the incident spread round the rest of his friends like wildfire and as a result anything that could be construed as criticism of Diana was avoided. The 'D' word had to be used very carefully in Prince Charles's presence from then onwards, and this was not to change even after he had married her and discovered 'the other Diana'.

Despite her latter-day views of the Prince's friends, Diana showed no sign of anything but enjoyment during this early period of her romance. She appeared to be delighted by their friendliness and thought the whole Balmoral experience wonderful – or so she said at the time.

Lady Colin Campbell reports that Diana later told her how she tentatively made her way through the early stages of the relationship. 'I knew from Sarah's example, I couldn't put a foot wrong. I didn't either. I was agreeable as could be. Even said I loved Balmoral and couldn't think of anywhere I adored more.' At that point Diana burst out into hysterical laughter as both of them knew how she had always hated the place and had lied in order to 'get the job'.

According to Prince George of Denmark, 'What he found so appealing about Diana was how harmonious they were together. She was sympathetic. He loves fishing. When they were at Balmoral together, she was happy to spend hours together by the riverbank with him in companionable, undemanding silence. He was in real need to be in touch with the elements, with nature, and he seemed to think that she was in the same way. Of course we now know differently. Diana's idea of a nightmare was to be torn away from London for more than a day. But like many women who are trying to hook a man, she was careful to keep her distaste for his interests to herself.'

Charles was fooled, and the more enthusiastic she became, the more he warmed to her. He taught her to fly-fish in the streams and pools; they walked the hills, took picnics to distant cottages on the estate and did all the things that he had longed to share, not with crowds of people, but with a soul mate. Add to this the fact that they had now embarked upon a sexual relationship and it becomes clear that Diana had really awoken the Prince's ardour: as long as she made no mistakes, the prize she so desperately wanted might become hers.

At six they would have drinks with the Queen, before dressing for dinner at eight. Diana was very careful to behave well in front of Her Majesty and had immediately noticed how Prince Charles deferred to his mother. Once at dinner, Princes Andrew and Edward would attempt to ease their elder brother out and get a seat either side of Diana. The Prince of Wales was flattered that his brothers found his new girlfriend to be so desirable. It is said that Prince Andrew, who was much closer to Diana in age, was particularly keen on her. But it soon became clear to him, as it did all the other members of the Windsor family, that she only had eyes for one man, and that was the future king.

The Prince was by now telling his most trusted friends that he found Diana warm, enthusiastic and gentle. In particular, he appreciated her willingness to enjoy all the things he loved and the fact that everyone he introduced her to was impressed by her immediate friendliness. Most of Charles's friends agreed and like Patty Palmer-Tomkinson in particular, came to share the Prince's view that he was extremely lucky to find one so young and beautiful and yet so compatible with his tastes and friends.

It was a glad time and many of his friends still remember it and have since repeated to me that Charles was very happy. Since leaving the Royal Navy he had become increasingly selfish as he began to gain in confidence and occasionally reminded himself and others who he was. He was never vindictive or unkind, but he could have black days, and when he did his temper was foul and it was not always an easy thing to console him or make him smile. Suddenly, Diana had come into his life and had made a difference. His mood was improved and remained good.

As a result of what was to happen in the coming months and years, this early period of their romance gets raked over and over in search of negatives – usually by people who want to find evidence to support Diana's version of events and are looking for the terrible treatment of a nineteen-year-old by a cold and quirky family. There is no evidence of this. The royals were just doing what they had always done on holiday for generations. Indeed, it is remembered by guests and staff alike that they might have been that bit happier that year because Diana, as she had in that chalet full of strangers, had made them so.

For her part, she was happy too. She was understandably perhaps a little nervous at the grandeur of her surroundings and the fact that she was with mainly older and more worldly people than herself; but she was also clearly fascinated by being on the inside track of the personal life of the Prince of Wales and, despite still being in awe of an older man born to be king, she loved the adventure. Did she dare hope for more? She told her closest friends that she doubted if one so handsome, mature and famous, who could have his pick of anyone, would ever choose a teenager like her for a bride but equally she took massive comfort from their universal reply that she shouldn't be so sure of that. She had set her heart at becoming the fairy-tale princess to her perfect prince, and secretly she hoped that it would happen if she played her cards right.

Was it all a confidence trick in order to become the future queen of England? It seems unlikely: Diana was clearly infatuated with the Prince himself as much as with the prospect of becoming a princess – probably even more so. On the other hand, she was less than honest about what really interested her in life, and she clearly had no intention of sticking with these new interests once she had achieved what she wanted. So to that extent she did pull the wool over everyone's eyes – including those of her future husband, who was to agonise over asking her to marry him and would no doubt have come to an entirely different decision if she had revealed the other Diana and her real interests.

Diana probably did not have the intelligence or the maturity to look beyond her immediate goal. Her focus and determination were so strong that she never stopped to think of future Septembers in Balmoral when it might rain, or a life away from her friends and London. As to her mental frailty, like others who are the same, she didn't believe that she *was* frail and so gave no thought to the gruelling royal programme or her ability to cope with it. And somewhere at the back of her mind she probably believed that if she was ever to become the next princess of Wales, she would be able to change what she didn't like – she wouldn't have been the first woman to think that marriage was about 'aisle, alter, hymn'.

Diana's own family were aware of her frailties, but believed that marriage to the Prince, the one thing she had constantly craved, would make her so content that she would become a different person. In addition, not many parents or grandparents are going to speak out against a marriage that their daughter had set her heart on and would mean that the girl would end up as queen of England.

The old guard at Buckingham Palace was more concerned with the virtue of Diana's past than her mental suitability for the role. As a result no questions were raised, and within weeks of their eventual engagement, when the first strains began to show, they were as surprised as anyone and blamed the dreadful amount of media attention that she had been subjected to.

But as yet, none of this had reared its ugly head and Diana seemed to be thoroughly enjoying life. The man she was mad about appeared to be warming to her, and weekends were just one house party after another on the beautiful estates that were home to the van Cutsems, the Parker Bowleses, the Romseys, the Palmer-Tomkinsons and others. Life was rich, relaxed and very grown-up. There were picnics, rides through woods and along river banks (which Diana avoided because of her fear of riding caused by a childhood fall) and early evening drinks before dressing for a candlelit dinner that could have been set in the nineteenth century. And best of all, her man was the star attraction.

The King and Di

This life was also an essential and pleasant distraction for the dutiful Prince who had thrown himself into public duty and social and charitable schemes since leaving the Royal Navy. As a result he was now almost constantly on public display, spied on by journalists and too often in the company of pompous local dignitaries. He had always expected his weeks to be much like this, but he needed these weekends to get away from it all. These estates allowed him to do precisely that.

And when he got there, he expected it all to be done his way. Before his death, Mountbatten had noticed an increased selfishness in his honorary grandson and had, on more than one occasion, warned him of the dangers of becoming 'like great-uncle David'. A courtier of the late 1970s was to comment that while 'he had a lot of charisma ... he was a very selfish and old-fashioned man. Everything rotated around him.'

The flamboyant journalist James Whitaker and his photographer Ken Lennox, both representing the *Daily Star*, were travelling with Arthur Edwards of the *Sun* to the Braemar Games. As they drove alongside the River Dee, they suddenly came across the Prince's car parked by the side of the road. They stopped and, to their amazement, saw the Prince fishing; next to him was a boyish-looking girl who, on seeing them, got up and hid behind a tree. Lennox and Edwards decided to separate and work a pincer movement. As they approached, they realised that the girl was using her vanity mirror to spy on them while still remaining hidden behind her tree.

They were impressed by her cunning, but nevertheless edged forward from their different angles in order to capture her on film. Before they were ready, however, the girl made a dash for the car and they only managed an unprintable fuzzy shot of an unrecognisable face and one of an unidentifiable girl's bottom. Who was this girl, and why was Charlie Windsor so keen to hide her away? These questions went through their minds as the Prince, obviously livid, put his gear away and sped off.

James Whitaker shrugged his shoulders and looked forward to dinner and a few snifters. Arthur Edwards was more determined. He made a number of enquiries that evening and managed to establish that the boyish girl was actually Lady Diana Spencer. Immediately he remembered the single shot that he had taken at Cowdray Park. He and he alone had a photo of her.

He phoned his office and got them to get it out of the files. Then he phoned his journalist partner who was back in Kent, and from there Harry Arnold filed the story. On 8 September, the *Sun* introduced Diana Spencer to the world. The headline read 'HE'S IN LOVE AGAIN! LADY DI IS THE NEW GIRL IN CHARLES' LIFE'. Diana's photograph was on the front page for the first of what was to become thousands of times, and the British love affair that was then to ignite around the world, just as it had for the Beatles seventeen years previously, had begun. Nothing was ever going to be quite the same again.

The following week back in London, Harry Arnold and Arthur Edwards, having got out in front thanks to the Edwards photograph, were determined to stay there and went in search of Diana's kindergarten. Eventually they tracked her down and asked if they could photograph her. Diana agreed, but wanted to be photographed with some of the children. Four were duly selected and their parents contacted in order that they might give their consent. By now other photographers had arrived en masse. Diana, using the children as props, posed for her first real photo session. To the cameramen's delight, the sun suddenly came out and shone from behind Diana through her rather mumsy skirt making it appear transparent – it was a major stroke of luck for them as suddenly her legs were on show. However, such good fortune for them could have spelled the end of Diana's chances. Both the Prince and the Palace had been quick to distance him from any form of indiscretion by previous girlfriends, and for a moment she and her close friends worried. They needn't have bothered. The Prince was very keen on this girl and the photograph only appears to have made him more so. Like the rest of the nation, he saw in it her naïvety along with a combination of motherly care and an aristocratic sexiness. Instead of reproaching her, he is reported to have said, 'I knew your legs were good but I didn't realise they were that spectacular.' The Prince of Wales was to be aroused by Diana's legs for the rest of her life.

With the publication of this photograph came further press speculation that Charles liked this girl a lot, and as a result she might be the one finally to be asked for her hand in marriage by the world's most eligible bachelor.   As a result, media pressure on the kindergarten became intense. The place was under constant siege during working hours: television companies sent crews there to set up camp both at the front and rear of the building, while tabloid and freelance photographers scaled walls and trees in order to breach the children's privacy by taking shots through the windows. At first it all seemed like an exciting adventure, and nobody was enjoying it more than Diana; but in time the novelty would wear off and so the pressure would begin to show.

In October Diana, with the romance becoming ever more serious, was back on the Balmoral estate for a third time. She stayed with the Queen Mother at Birkhall and, while the men went hunting during the day, she spent a lot of her time with the Prince's grandmother. Diana was impeccably behaved and made an excellent impression on her. The Queen Mother, who had never been slow to draw comparisons between her husband and Charles, might have seen a little of herself in Diana at the same age. After all, Diana, like her, was British and thus would pump more English blood into a family that had been mainly of German descent before her marriage to the Duke of York. Indeed, should Diana marry Charles, she would be the first English woman to marry an heir to the throne since Anne Hyde had wed the future James II some 300 years before.

Moreover, the Queen Mother took comfort in the fact that she counted Diana's grandmother Lady Fermoy as one of her closest friends. Both of Diana's parents had court connections, and now Diana's sister moved in court circles as well. In addition, Diana had convinced her that, like herself, she was ready to sacrifice everything for the sake of the country, its monarchy and the future king, whom she appeared to love absolutely. Thus the Queen Mother was convinced and Clarence House became a powerful supporter of the Diana cause.

As a result, pressure started building on the Prince. When the Queen's private secretary, Sir Philip Moore, let it be known among court circles that the Queen was very keen on the match, this poured fuel on the fire. Ironically, the man who is often blamed most for creating pressure over the engagement, Prince Philip, was keeping his opinions to himself at this time.

The following weekend, Camilla invited Diana to her home – Bolehyde Manor. She was driven there at the Prince's request by Charles's valet, Stephen Barry. On 24 October, Diana and Camilla stood side by side watching Prince Charles ride his horse, Allibar, in the Clun Handicap at Ludlow Races. On the Sunday morning the Prince joined Andrew Parker Bowles for an outing with the Beaufort Hunt, while Camilla and Diana stayed at home and chatted. In the afternoon Charles took Diana on her own to see Highgrove House, which he had just bought, and invited her to make suggestions concerning its refurbishment. At the time this must have really excited her and given her hope that her desire to become his wife might not be just the unachievable dream that she had wanted for as long as she could remember.

However, years later, and in different circumstances, Diana chose to forget that elation and focus on the conversation she had that morning with Camilla. She was to remember how Camilla had advised her and seemed to know so much about the Prince's likes and dislikes as well as his private life. She went on to say how she couldn't understand it. The inference was that they were having an affair, and it was made to support Diana's accusations of a continued affair between Charles and Camilla throughout her marriage to the Prince. However, nothing was said at the time, and the Prince and his new girlfriend visited the Parker Bowleses again the following weekend. It is not clear when Diana was to come to know of their relationship. However, it is clear that she wasn't concerned about it at this time – or if she was she was far too clever to make an issue of it, in case it rocked the boat.

At the time, in their elite social circle it was well known that the Prince counted married women among his closest friends, but the tabloids seemed more interested in whom he would choose for a wife rather than a mistress. After all, the previous princes of Wales had always had mistresses, many of whom were already married and therefore couldn't be chosen to be a future queen. The press were never really interested in them and, in 1980, this was still the case – as it was with the public, who understood that the Prince of Wales could not go down to the local disco to pick up a girl for a one-night stand, but still had hormones like the rest of us. This sort of adult public understanding seems to have largely been replaced today by a hypocrisy that decrees that the Royal Family should set a good example, only for it to be totally ignored by the rest of us.

As a result, gossip about the Prince's mistresses was rare, while the official girlfriends took centre stage. Really only the satirical magazine *Private Eye* seemed interested in them. At the time, and largely due to the attention of the *Eye*, and subsequently rumoured in the *Mirror*, Dale Tyron, wife of Lord Tyron and nicknamed Kanga by Prince Charles, was a much more famous mistress than Camilla. Nevertheless, both women moved in the same circles, as occasionally did actress Susan

George, who was also rumoured to be another mistress of the heir to the throne. Many years later, ironically in Diana's favourite restaurant – San Lorenzo in Knightsbridge – Ms George was to explain to me the depth of her love and affection of the Prince and how his wife had painted an outrageously inaccurate picture of him in Morton's book *Diana: Her True Story*. Interestingly, she did so in the presence of her husband, the actor Simon McCorkindale, who seemed quite relaxed and most supportive of her view, which tends to reflect a court attitude. Indeed, Camilla and Kanga were friendly to each other – they often discussed the Prince's needs, what sort of girl he should marry and how, when the time came, she should be helped. This may sound a strange way of going about things, but it is how it has been done at court for hundreds of years.

Penny Junor has always claimed that she believes Charles finished all his affairs when he realised he was to marry Diana. She cites his sense of honour and his attraction to Diana as reasons. Tim Clayton doubts this on the grounds that this all seems just too clean and simple, and in reality life is not like that. Perhaps Junor's opinion is based on her findings as a biographer of Charles, Clayton's as a biographer of Diana.

So who is right? Personally, having studied the available evidence and talked to a number of courtiers of the period, I believe Junor is. I believe that Clayton has made a fundamental mistake in forgetting that court life is completely different to normal life. Just as you wouldn't normally find two women having an affair with the same man and being friends in everyday life, nor would he necessarily just drop both of them when he got married. But court life is different. Mistresses can be companions, stay friends with the king, be loyal to the new queen and know that the physical part of the relationship is over. That is how it has been for centuries.

Moreover, the man in the street doesn't usually work to a plan. Why should he? A lot less is expected of him than of the Prince of Wales. But Charles was working to the Mountbatten plan. In addition, there was a precedent. When Camilla got engaged to Andrew Parker Bowles, she ceased her relationship with Charles but they remained friends and he became godfather to their first child. There was to be six years of wonderful friendship but no physical relations as both Charles and Camilla respected the fact that she had now married. It was only when Andrew had had scores of extra-marital affairs, many with

Camilla's friends, that the second affair started.

Further strength is undoubtedly added to Junor's opinion, when we discover how inaccurate and less than honest Diana's recollections of this period of her life really are. Even Clayton and Craig concede this point in a biography that attempts to offend its intended readership as little as possible by taking as positive a view of the Princess as they can while still producing something that examined the actual evidence and not just her unreliable version of events.

The truth is that by now we have a young woman whose upbringing has ill prepared her for the one thing that she wants so much. Her life had always lacked discipline. She is selfish, spoiled and can be very vengeful. These are disastrous characteristics for anyone who must selflessly give their life up to duty. She, like many children of rich parents, was very used to getting her own way and had absolutely no intention of being selfless. We now know, having examined Charles's childhood, that the Windsors are not like that: witness the fact that he had to ask Mountbatten for a bicycle as his parents thought that to be too grand a gift for Christmas. Diana had showed absolutely no sticking power at anything – even the most undemanding of jobs, yet it does not seem to have occurred to her that what she wanted was probably one of the most demanding jobs on the planet. Whether it just didn't dawn on her, whether she believed that princesses could do anything they pleased as in a child's fairy tale, or whether she was just totally blinded by her love of the Prince and the idea of becoming his princess is impossible to say. Nobody I have talked to who knew her at this time can give me a convincing answer – she does not appear to have discussed it with anyone.

One thing is certain: she couldn't have been marrying into a worse situation. She might have come from a broken family and wanted to be part of one of the world's most famous families, where divorce appears to be unacceptable, but she doesn't appear to have looked further. The Windsors, due to their strange role in life, are a strange family. There is no heart to it: it is an institution, a discipline where one is in constant training, a 24/7 business where participation, however one might feel on the day, is a requirement and a good performance a duty. It is a family where a good queen and her equally good consort have loved their children but found little time for them; a family where, as a result of all of this, the children have grown up loving their parents at a distance, while always being closer to nannies and private secretaries. It is a family and a situation that Prince Charles learned to survive despite having similarly low self-esteem throughout his childhood as Diana.

Diana was now hoping to be admitted to this family without such years of experience behind her, and little to no willpower or discipline when it came to matters that she found boring or tedious. And just as Charles's discipline and determination to succeed had strengthened his capacity to deal with this life, her lack of either would quickly cause her mental frailties to be exposed when she was eventually thrust into the reality of royal life.

Why didn't anyone see any of this? Well, we have the benefit of hindsight, and quite frankly only a few people saw the danger. Her family understandably couldn't bring themselves to do anything that might ruin her chances, while others were silenced by the Prince of Wales's rage. Most people were simply taken in by this beautiful and charming girl: the reality is that Diana was just doing far too good a job convincing those who mattered that she should become the Princess of Wales.

The truth is that the impression Diana had made, on the court in general and on the Royal Family in particular, was most favourable. She appeared to be a fresh and slightly chubby-faced young girl who was delightfully natural, had a terrible wardrobe and dress sense – so much so that she borrowed from everyone else – asked idiotic questions, was completely innocent, knew nothing about anything, told great jokes, made even the Queen laugh and above all appeared to love Prince Charles unreservedly. They all liked her, the vast majority wanted him to marry her and could see no alternative of her age or older. Moreover, they believed that he must not wait for another generation in the hope of improving on this perfection.

They were starting to push against an open door. The Prince became increasingly besotted with Diana. His excitement at finding this beautiful girl that his family liked and the nation had taken to their hearts so quickly, not least because the press liked her, was touching and he let his feelings be known. He couldn't believe his luck and he said as much.

In the meantime, the media attention was growing to fever pitch – with more than a little encouragement from Diana herself, who had developed a good relationship with many of the journalists and photographers who were by now permanently camped outside her flat or the kindergarten. James Whitaker, who was determined to make up for a slow start, had become quite close to her and would continue to write favourably of her, for years to come. Intense pressure was now building by the day from both within the family and the public who, encouraged by the press, made it quite clear that they wanted him to marry her.

Then, out of the blue, came a decisive factor, an event that was a mystery at the time, has remained unresolved even to this day and for reasons discussed later, probably always will be. In November, the *Sunday Mirror* ran a story under the headline 'LOVE IN THE SIDINGS'. It claimed that a blonde woman with an amazing likeness to Diana had driven down from London and been spotted boarding the royal train at night to spend a few hours with the Prince as the train was parked in a siding in Wiltshire. Apparently the paper rang Diana and asked for her confirmation. She replied that the story was quite untrue. Nevertheless, Bob Edwards, the editor, was so convinced by his source that the story was true that he published anyway. As a result it has always been assumed that the source was a royal policeman whom Edwards really trusted.

However, the royal train is always very heavily guarded by many policemen, with foot patrols walking on both sides, others stationed at vantage points like bridges, and still more on board the train itself. This is done to ensure that nobody can sneak aboard and endanger the life of the heir to the throne. In 1980, following the IRA's murder of Lord Mountbatten the previous year, security was very tight: it is most unlikely that anyone could get aboard without several policemen noticing them. But the police were baffled as they had seen no one – and certainly not a mysterious blonde woman answering to Diana's description.

Edwards was shocked by the Palace's reaction. The Queen did something that she had never done for any of her son's previous girlfriends: she intervened to protect Diana's virtue. The clear implication of the story was that Diana had slept with the Prince, and in 1980 that was still not an acceptable act for a potential future queen. Michael Shea, the Queen's press secretary, was ordered to demand a retraction from the *Sunday Mirror*, which he duly did, calling the story 'a total fabrication'.

The message was clear: the Queen wanted this girl to be the next princess of Wales and wasn't prepared to let the media muck it up for her. The effect was to fuel even more speculation about an engagement

The King and Di

announcement. Diana's mother then wrote to *The Times* complaining of her daughter's harassment at the hands of the media. As a result, sixty MPs tabled a motion in the House of Commons 'deploring the manner in which Lady Diana Spencer is treated by the media' and calling upon 'those responsible to have more concern for individual privacy'. This led to the Press Council meeting the Fleet Street editors to discuss the situation. It was the first time in its twenty-seven year history that it had been forced into calling such a meeting.

However, it resolved nothing and the media feeding frenzy went on as never before. The train story had really brought the matter to a head as the tabloids rallied round Diana and implored Charles to act. They made it quite clear that the people wanted him to marry Diana and if he didn't he would be letting the nation down. Britain, at the time, was in deep recession, unemployment was rising and American-style racial tension was growing in the run-down inner cities. The country wanted a distraction, just as it had when Princess Elizabeth had married Philip after the Second World War and again with the birth of Prince Charles himself.

But this was a very different press to then. It was, by now, far less respectful to the monarchy and was changing fast. Rupert Murdoch, the Australian who thought that Britain should be a republic, had bought the *Sun*, which was previously owned by the Mirror Group, in 1969 and turned it into a brash and garish rival of the *Daily Mirror* itself. In turn the *Mirror* had been bought by Robert Maxwell, and so a massive circulation war ensued. Both papers searched endlessly for sensation and didn't seem to mind inventing it if none could be found. Their 'build a celebrity in order to destroy him' policy seemed to be working, and forced other slightly more genteel tabloids, such as the *Express* and *Mail*, to follow suit.

Murdoch had little respect for the Royal Family, and saw being embroiled in sensation and scandal as not just his political standpoint but also as very good business: royal stories sold newspapers, sensation sold newspapers – put them together and you will sell even more. His success had ensured his competitors were forced to imitate him and a road that had been a bit bumpy since the 'cherry brandy affair' was about to get very rocky indeed. It has shown no sign of letting up ever since.

It was against this fever pitch of media madness, political horror and public anticipation that the Duke of Edinburgh wrote to his son and told him that the time had come to make up his mind about Diana. Charles's father clearly believed that with stories like the train mystery, however untrue it might have been, being printed and the fact that it was common knowledge that Diana had spent time at Balmoral without a chaperone, her reputation was in danger of being damaged. Therefore if it was his son's intention to marry the girl, he should do so without further delay. If not, then he should end the relationship.

It has often been said that the Prince took this letter to be not an ultimatum, which it was, but a direct order to marry, which it wasn't. Prince Philip had not always behaved with much sensitivity towards his eldest son, and had made a number of paternal errors, but ordering him to marry was not one of them. If the Prince of Wales chose to misinterpret the letter, then the fault lay with him and not his father. Perhaps it is the greatest sadness that these two grown men, who genuinely love each other, couldn't have chatted the matter through. But, as we already know, to both of their regret this never happened.

Moreover, irrespective of this letter, the Prince was now faced with a tough choice. Should he ask Diana to marry him before he was really certain that she was the right girl – after all, it had been a whirlwind romance of a few weekends and really no time together – or stand to lose the girl that he was very fond of, who seemed so perfect in so many ways and with whom everything looked so promising? He said at the time, 'It all seems so ridiculous because I do very much want to do the right thing for this country and for my family – but I'm terrified sometimes of making a promise and then perhaps living to regret it.' He admitted to being in a confused and anxious state of mind but added, 'It is just a matter of taking an unusual plunge into some rather unknown circumstances that inevitably disturbs me but I expect it will be the right thing in the end.'

We know that the Prince of Wales has always been a man who is very cautious of anything untried and new. We also know that, having dedicated his life and changed his personality to honour his country and please his parents, he would be very keen to get this decision – one that he considered must be taken with the monarchy and people in mind – right. If he had even had one inkling of how such 'unknown circumstances' might come to affect the monarchy, he would have no doubt come to a very different decision.

What would Mountbatten have advised? Well, Charles had sowed his wild oats as commanded by the old man. Diana was younger than the Prince and appeared to want to share his interests. She was an Anglican, came from a good blood line, was keen to have children, was pretty and sexy and clearly loved him. There can be no doubt that, in the absence of a marriage to his granddaughter, Amanda Knatchbull, Mountbatten would have approved. But we can only speculate: Mountbatten was dead, and Charles would have to look elsewhere for advice.

Under pressure to do his duty and marry, but painfully aware that it was also his duty to succeed and not divorce, Prince Charles now turned to his official advisors, friends and family. All of them, with the exception of the Romseys and Nicholas Soames, were keen to approve – most because they liked Diana, but some because they thought that was what he wanted to hear and feared upsetting him and either losing his friendship or their employment. The Queen, however, given her son's predicament, acted with astonishing selfishness and refused to offer an opinion on anything. To others, such as Prince George of Demark, she expressed her doubts. She had strong reservations about Diana's suitability. She thought that the girl was ill-prepared. She hadn't ever stuck at anything long enough to see it through – she might struggle with the rigours of the job. She also worried on the domestic front whether the couple had enough common interests to sustain a marriage when the initial and obvious passion that they had for each other wore off. Of course she was right on all counts: surely it was her duty at least to bring these points to her son's attention once he had sought her advice. She didn't because she believed that it was not her position to interfere.

It was therefore left, as it had been so many times previously, for Prince Charles to turn to his grandmother. The Queen Mother, by her kindness and affection, had always been a very special person to the Prince of Wales. She had continually been an enormous source of comfort throughout the long absences of his parents as a small boy and the tough years of boarding schools that followed. As a result she was only behind Mountbatten and his parents as an influence. The Queen Mother was strongly in favour of the match. She liked Diana, thought she had all the right attributes and was delighted that the girl was the granddaughter of her good friend and lady-in-waiting Lady Fermoy. Lady Fermoy knew of Diana's emotional problems, but failed to speak up. As a result the Queen Mother was in later years to regret bitterly her advice and Lady Fermoy, riddled with guilt, was to acknowledge before her death that she had made a dreadful mistake, as she had known that Diana was 'a dishonest and difficult girl' and that it had been her duty to say something about it. Lord Spencer was to also admit that he had been most wrong not to make Prince Charles aware of his daughter's problems once he had realised that neither the heir to the throne nor his family had an inkling of them.

So the Prince was propelled towards an engagement and eventual marriage by his family, the country and the press, all of whom were convinced it was right and his duty; a few who suspected it was wrong were ignored and those who knew it was remained silent. As a result he was wholly unaware of the real person he was marrying and totally unprepared for what was to follow.

And the pivotal point, the thing that had turned up the heat to boiling point and pushed things along to breakneck speed of a runaway train was the 'blonde mystery'. So who was the blonde, and why has she remained unidentified for twenty-five years?

Some years after the event, the *Sunday Mirror* editor Bob Edwards received a Christmas card from his friend, the columnist Woodrow Wyatt, that simply said, 'It must have been Camilla.' This was a story that was also being put about at this time by Diana herself, by now consumed with jealousy for the former mistress – pointing out that Camilla was also a blonde and lived in Wiltshire not too far from where the train had stopped for the night. So was it Camilla instead of Diana?

Camilla has always denied that she ever set foot on the royal train. Prince Charles and his staff support this. Moreover, it is highly unlikely that anyone would mistake Camilla for Diana. She was much shorter and an older woman in her thirties – as opposed to the teenage Diana – and her hair was much blonder, longer and curlier. In addition, while Camilla was well known to the press, via *Private Eye* and Nigel Dempster's column in the *Daily Mail*, as a mistress of Charles, the *Sunday Mirror*'s article fails to mention her and implies that the woman was Diana. Moreover, somehow the *Sunday Mirror* also failed to include Diana's denial in their story. And given that she was madly in love with Prince Charles, why didn't she ask him, if it wasn't her, who this mysterious blonde was? Might it be that the blonde never existed?

A friend, who was very close to Diana at the time, recalled when I asked her about the scandal, 'Diana just said that it wasn't her and left it at that. Camilla wasn't mentioned at all. Nor was anyone else. I remember thinking, Well if it was me I would be asking if it wasn't me then who the hell was it? But she never mentioned it and nor did I as she was under enough strain and I didn't want to put bad ideas into her head. But I did think it was strange because it wasn't like her to be so sure of something like that. She was not at all concerned about another woman being in the picture.' Therefore, on the balance of evidence available, I think that it is more likely that Lady Diana Spencer managed directly, or indirectly, to plant the story of the 'mystery blonde' on the train, in full knowledge of its potential power.

On 6 February 1981, Charles, Prince of Wales, future King of England and the most eligible bachelor in the world, returned from a skiing holiday in Klosters in Switzerland and invited Diana to Windsor Castle. Upon her arrival he asked her to marry him. He told her to consider his proposal carefully and to take her time. She accepted immediately.

However, the Prince, ever concerned to ensure that he was not entrapping the girl, advised her again about the horrendous pressures of living one's life in a goldfish bowl always observed by an invading and cruel press. Diana hardly listened before rushing back to the flat to announce her conquest to the girls at Colberne Court. They might have done rather better than her at school, they might not have been forced into such menial tasks as cleaning other people's flats – but now that was behind her, for soon they would all have to acknowledge her as the Princess of Wales.

It was the first time Diana had gone out to achieve something and succeeded, and suddenly this one achievement was to dwarf anything that she or her contemporaries could dream about. Somehow, the spoiled Sloane Ranger with little intellect and apparently no sticking power had achieved what she had set her heart on. Eliza Doolittle had won her Henry Higgins, but unlike *My Fair Lady*, the story didn't end there.

In the spring of 1979, the year that saw Mountbatten's horrific murder, Britain elected a new Conservative Government that had as its leader a prime minister who promised to put into effect nothing less than a revolution in government, business practices and the attitude of the people. Her name was Margaret Thatcher.

In the latter part of the 1970s the government and the economy of the country sank so low that people feared it was about to go into absolute decline. In fact, compared to its major competitors, it had been in decline for nearly thirty years. On the back of the inflationary madness started by the Heath Conservative government and subsequently exploded by the Wilson Labour government, a further and more serious crisis blew up in the autumn of 1976. Sterling went into freefall on the currency markets and forced chancellor Denis Healey to make a humiliating return from Heathrow on his way to an International Monetary Fund (IMF) conference in Manila. Healey went on to the Labour Party conference in Blackpool, where the new prime minister James Callaghan (Harold Wilson had resigned in the spring of 1976) had already made a blunt speech to the delegates stating that Britain had lived 'too long on borrowed money, borrowed ideas ... For too long, perhaps ever since the war, we've postponed facing up to the fundamental changes in our society and our economy ... That is what I mean when I say we have been living on borrowed time. For too long this country, all of us – yes, this conference too – has been ready to settle for borrowing money abroad to maintain our standards of life, instead of grappling with the fundamental problems of British industry.

'We used to think that you could spend your way out of recession and increase employment by cutting taxes and boosting government spending. I tell you in all candour that the option no longer exists, and that, insofar as it ever did exist, it only worked on each occasion since the war by injecting a bigger dose of inflation into the economy, followed by a higher level of unemployment as the next step. Higher inflation followed by higher unemployment – that is the history of the last twenty years.'

Indeed he was quite right – except that he could hardly have been referring to his own party when talking of cutting taxes, as they never had. It was a speech as much for Manila and the IMF as it was for the delegates in Blackpool, and it was necessary as the pound was falling like a stone. The government badly needed an IMF loan, and after a much-publicised but nonetheless furtive visit from IMF officials, such a loan was secured, but only on the basis of substantial public expenditure cuts and an agreement to continue an incomes policy.

Throughout the two Labour administrations from February 1974 to May 1979, the tenor and rhetoric had been about the evils of the rich. One Cabinet member, Anthony Wedgwood Benn, formerly Lord Stansgate, attacked both the rich and the middle classes increasingly and supported every strike, official or unofficial. The TUC and its leading members came and went constantly to and from 10 Downing

Street, and expostulated on television about how the country should be run for the benefit of the workers. Accordingly, a moment of complete farce was reached when one union official stated dogmatically on national television that 'every worker should get at least the average pay rise'. It appeared as if madmen were running the country, drunk with power and not possessing enough common sense to run a small market stall.

The middle classes felt they were living in an alien land under constant attack, and this feeling only got worse when Healey, in his budget, imposed a ninety-five per cent marginal tax rate with these words: 'I believe that this type of redistribution through the tax system makes a major contribution to the health of the community as a whole – and I intend to go a great deal further before I have finished.' However, things got inevitably worse as the national lurch to the left only served to stifle incentive and investment and sent the bright and creative rushing for their passports and a new life abroad, while the rest of the nation faced high inflation and the prospect of drifting towards the poor standards of living that were pressed upon the Soviet states of Eastern Europe. Ironically, as the people of those countries were beginning to gather the courage needed to rid themselves of the failure of state socialism, so the British appeared to be heading in that very direction.

As this was happening, the Conservative Party, now kicking its heels in opposition, decided to oust its leader Edward Heath, who had put in place many of the doctrines so loved by his opponents, such as restrictions on wages, prices and dividends. In his place they had elected a woman who, under the tutelage of Sir Keith Joseph, had grasped certain essentials of the remedy required to restore economic sanity to the country. In time much of her thinking would not only be adopted by the Labour Party but also by the Eastern European nations as they emerged from the dark years of communism and economic failure.

Immediately after the election defeat in 1974, Joseph and his student began to exchange a common analysis of what had gone wrong. It was, as they both were to testify, a shared journey of discovery. Usefully, Sir Keith began performing this in public and without delay. He believed that both Labour and Conservative governments since the war had believed in 'unity'. This had meant in reality that for thirty years the private sector had been forced to fight with one hand tied behind its back by government and unions. At the same time and for the same reasons, both parties, when in power, had allowed state spending to be too high, kept defunct industries artificially alive with taxpayers' money and bought industrial peace at any price, again with taxpayers' cash. Was it really that surprising that we had slipped sadly behind our western European competitors? And where would this total disregard for economics end?

Sir Keith then made an obvious, but nevertheless important, discovery about himself. He had joined the Conservative Party in the 1950s, but it was not until the mid-1970s that he had converted to 'Real Economic Conservatism' and realised that, like his party, he had not been Conservative at all. Sir Keith's comments may just seem like common sense some thirty years on, with a converted Labour Party largely applying his beliefs in Britain and with socialism long-since driven out of Eastern Europe. However, it was a very different world then.

Joseph was not destined to become leader of the Tory Party. He was forced to rule himself out of a leadership election following a speech that he made in Birmingham in early 1975. He had stated that people at the bottom end of the social scale were having too many children and were ill-equipped to bring them up. This smacked of racism and elitism and demonstrated an attitude that Prince Charles, among others, was horrified by and saw as both unfair and unhelpful. When Joseph withdrew, Margaret Thatcher was able to take up his challenge to Heath and duly won the election.

From February 1975 until she came to power in May 1979, Mrs Thatcher and her supporters plotted the ground for a revolution in Britain's economic attitudes. She adopted clarity of thought and purpose in a simple and unshakeable dogma that was to become her trademark, a major reason for the country's return to economic health and, for her personally, the defining reason why people either loved her or hated her with a passion. She believed that tax was too high. High-rate tax collected little revenue, destroyed ambition and was a 'symbol of British socialism – the symbol of envy'. Lower rates of tax were also too high. The people had a right to decide how to spend their money rather than have the government do it for them, and if 'earn more' really meant 'keep more', there would be an incentive for people to work harder and show a lot more enterprise. Unless tax rates were to change across the board, she could see no chance of avoiding perpetual decline.

Having earned more and kept more, the nation – families, businesses, local and central government – needed to be 'good housekeepers', balance their budgets and exercise thrift and prudence. This pleased her supporters and sent her socialist detractors into apoplexy. However, the power of this message to a nation genuinely fearful of its future, especially after decades of Labour and Conservative governments that had miserably failed to balance budgets, should not be underestimated. She told everyone who would listen that the government must set an example. Public expenditure must be controlled and it must not exceed public revenue. The nation must create wealth before it spends it. 'You cannot look after the hard-up people in society unless you are accruing enough wealth to do so,' she told a BBC reporter in 1977, 'good intentions are not enough. You need hard cash.' She explained that no government ever had, or would ever have, a magic wand and therefore the more the nation – or more importantly the nation's families – put into life, the more they would be able to get out. The more we expected of ourselves and the less we expected from the state, the more successful both we individually and the state collectively would become.

This was to be the bitter pill of reality and the nation, demoralised by years of failure and distraught by the prospects of the future, had no hesitation in swallowing it when James Callaghan finally called an election for May 1979. Thatcher swept into power – and history – as Britain's first woman prime minister, destined to become one of its most important, both revered and reviled, but nearly always respected.

The financial climate in Britain during her first two years in office was to be every bit as bad as anything that had been seen since the end of the Second World War, certainly in terms of corporate failures and rising unemployment. Tight monetary policy, allied with another sharp hike in the price of oil following the overthrow of the shah of Iran – which in turn brought a sharp rise in the value of the pound as it was viewed as a petro-currency thanks to the development of North Sea oil – created the most difficult conditions seen in Great Britain since the 1930s. Even the accepted British blue-chip star, ICI, cut its dividend and Sir Terence Becket of the normally pro-Conservative Confederation of British Industry (CBI) promised the government a 'bare-knuckle' fight, telling his conference, 'We've got to have a lower pound – we've got to have lower interest rates.'

The prime minister remained firm and declared on the day that unemployment passed two million, 'I've been trying to say to people for a very long time: if you pay yourself more for producing less, you'll be in trouble.' This was of course true but ignored the fact that a lot of inflation had been fed into the system by her carrying out the Clegg recommendations.

The Clegg Commission had been set up to appease public-sector unions following the Winter of Discontent in 1978 – a series of damaging strikes that had been the unions' answer to the Labour Government's incomes policy and had, in effect, put the final nail in James Callaghan's coffin. Thatcher knew it would be inflationary, but was not for alienating anyone who might vote for her. So she promised to implement the recommendations if elected. The result of the commission's findings meant twenty per cent wage inflation – which could have been a reason for going back on her pledge, but she didn't, believing that she would lose credibility if she was blatantly to break such a promise so early in her premiership.

Thus, heavy wage inflation allied to the near doubling of VAT in the first budget of her new administration, meant that within weeks inflation soared again to an average of 13.13 per cent in 1979, 18.1 per cent in 1980 and 11.9 per cent in 1981, before falling back, aided by an overvalued pound and moderate wage settlements, induced by an unemployment rate not seen since the 1930s. In the end a new fitter, leaner and more confident British economy was born, one that was to provide the foundations for a remarkable transformation. However, in the first two years of Thatcherism, things looked extremely grim, especially for those at the bottom of the heap. With unemployment edging towards three million, the percentage of people out of work in these areas was some three or even four times higher than elsewhere, and mainly affected young black males. Seeing themselves as outsiders and discriminated against, they exploded on to the streets of Bristol, London, Birmingham, Liverpool and, to a lesser extent, other cities in the spring and summer of 1981. The scenes of rioting, looting, firebombing and pitched battles with police horrified a nation who had seen nothing like this in Great Britain in the twentieth century.

It was against this depressing background that the news was announced that the Prince of Wales was to marry a girl whom his family liked, the Church of England accepted, the nation approved of and the tabloid press had been pushing for. Just as his mother's wedding announcement had been, in the difficult years following the war, it was greeted with much enthusiasm as a wonderful distraction from all the immediate problems with which Mrs Thatcher and her new government were struggling.

The announcement was officially made on 24 February 1981. The Prince was thirty-two and his bride would be twenty later in the year. Its release prompted an outpouring of national pleasure. Despite the winter weather a large crowd gathered outside Buckingham Palace, where the band of the Coldstream Guards played an old Cliff Richard hit – 'Congratulations'. Also on hand were Diana's father and stepmother, who chatted freely with the large attendant gang of reporters. According to Earl Spencer, his daughter 'had come through [the media pressure] with flying colours … She is obviously a remarkable girl … She never breaks down because Diana does not break down at all.' Her stepmother added that Diana was not highly strung nor did she suffer from depression and that she was keen never to say or do the wrong thing.

The significance of these quotes, which appeared in the next day's papers, was largely lost on most people at the time. Diana hadn't grown up used to media attention, and had received a concentrated amount over the last few months; as the pressure had built up on her, it had on occasion, shown a little. As a result, the quotes were taken to refer to the way she dealt with the media's obsession with her, which was expected to subside somewhat now that the announcement had been made.

However, upon closer inspection, such statements made by family members giving assurances that this young woman didn't suffer from breakdowns, depression and wasn't highly strung seem to be a little strong: perhaps they referred to the very real fears that the whole family held for Diana's suitability for this demanding role. The Spencers have long been a rich, well-connected and extremely proud family. An opportunity for one of their number to marry the next king of England and thus become the mother to a future heir to the throne was everything that the previous earls would have dreamed of; and no doubt Raine Spencer, who in private had often previously described her stepdaughter as being both highly strung and a depressive, could see all the social possibilities that such a match would bring. Perhaps these are the real reasons for what seem to be unwarranted assurances as to Diana's mental state. What is not in question is that they both lied.

Raine shared Diana's grandmother's view that Diana was both difficult and dishonest, while Earl Spencer was later to admit that he had been aware of Diana's problems and that he should have alerted Prince Charles to them.

Margaret Thatcher, no doubt pleased that some good news might lighten the gloom, offered her congratulations during prime minister's question time. A debate in the Church of England's Synod on the state of marriage was interrupted to report the joyous news. Amid all the excitement, the editor of *Debrett's Peerage* announced that Diana would reintroduce Stuart blood to the royal line as she was descended five times from Charles II, four of which were from the 'wrong side of the blanket'. The Prince then announced that he was 'positively delighted and frankly amazed that Diana is prepared to take me on', and then the girl of the hour declared that she was 'absolutely delighted; thrilled; blissfully happy.'

The *Daily Telegraph*, which at that time remained a solid reporter of news and peddler of intellectual concerns, if from a somewhat right-wing perspective, celebrated the affirmation of monarchy that it believed the forthcoming marriage of the Prince of Wales symbolised: 'For a nation more than ever starved of symbols of hope and goodness in public life, the Royal example, far from fading, becomes more important ... The best private feelings inspire the greatest public acts. In its monarchy, the British nation has at its pinnacle an institution that commands such feelings and a family that embodies them. With so many commoners who hate, it matters more than ever that a prince who loves should one day sit upon the throne of England.'

So, amid winter cold and financial gloom, the joy of living monarchy with its fairy-tale pictures and the pride that the institution gives to the vast majority of British people lifted the nation in a way that no cold, faceless republic could have done. Once again the Royal Family had ordered an event that would offer the nation a chance of escape from its present difficulties and glimpse the values, traditions and regal pride that set it aside from other countries. The world would watch the irresistible pomp and ceremony with a reverence accorded to an institution that had lasted for more than a thousand years. The British people knew it, and many were flushed with pride. The country may have been looking into a financial abyss, unemployment may have been soaring and civil unrest engulfing the inner cities, but it had a monarchy that symbolised its pride in its history.

Reflecting this, and capturing the public mood perfectly, the Archbishop of Canterbury, Robert Runcie, announced that he believed that the royal wedding 'could be a healing element'. However, *The Times* went even further by adding that, 'It is fitting that the Prince of Wales should enter married life when one considers the extent to which the monarchy is now regarded as an exemplar of family life.'

In the intoxication of the moment, no one pointed out the dangers of this view, an opinion that had been growing since the end of the Second World War, that the monarchy's function was twofold in acting as the symbol of the state and also as the custodian of family values. Not only had their ancestors never been put under this sort of pressure – and in the case of some, such as Henry VIII or Charles II, it was just as well – but if the monarchy was to fail in its family-values role, even if the rest of the country was no better, this might tarnish or even endanger the symbol of the state role as well. The national euphoria surrounding the prospect of marriage of Prince Charles to Lady Diana Spencer only served to accelerate this dangerous confusion of these dual roles in the minds of the public.

Upon close inspection it should be clear how ridiculous the concept is. It is no different from inferring that the performance of Parliament is indistinguishable from that of its elected members and that marital breakdowns of the latter would guarantee the ruination of the former – a point well made by Dimbleby.

Unfortunately, the point wasn't argued at the time, so a widening chink in the royal armour started to appear and would be concentrated upon in the coming years by those who wanted to bring the monarchy down – whether republicans, intellectual elitists, communists, left-wing socialists or even those consumed by envy of what they saw as the outrageous material wealth of the Windsors. These people, who believed in bringing in equality by moving everybody to the lowest common denominator, were always blinded by their egalitarian principles to the pride and joy that a real and living symbol can bring the people. And as their convictions gave them a superiority complex, so they believed that the people's opinion should be subjugated in favour of their own.

However, at this moment these people bided their time as the tidal wave of national support for the Prince of Wales and his future bride pushed the monarchy's popularity ratings through the roof and made criticism of the Royal Family almost impossible. Only Labour MP

Willie Hamilton, a celebrated vocal critic of them, dared to speak out against the announcement – suggesting that the monarchy had conspired with the Conservative government to create a distraction from the latest set of miserable unemployment figures. This attack only served to force the Labour Party to distance itself from him, as to be seen attacking the monarchy was rightly considered to be courting electoral suicide – as it probably still would be today.

So now, without the wise counsel of his mentor and surrogate father, but still by following the old man's plan, the Prince of Wales was attempting to fulfil one of the most important duties required of him as a future king of England: the production of an heir. The first essential step in that direction – marriage – was now to be met by betrothal to a girl who seemed to delight everyone.

Chapter Seven
The Waiting, the Wedding Day and the Honeymoon (1981)

In 1992 Andrew Morton published a book called *Diana: Her True Story*. Once the shocking contents were digested, many believed he had spent hours talking with courtiers and close friends of the Princess. In fact we now know that the book's main contributor was Diana herself. At the time Diana claimed that she had never met Morton to discuss the work. Indeed she hadn't: she had dictated her life story into a Dictaphone held by Dr James Colthurst, a friend and general factotum, at Kensington Palace before having it smuggled to Morton. The book ripped down the royal veil and let the world see the state of a very miserable marriage. It caused sensation, became an international bestseller, made Morton a fortune, became a book to launch a thousand others and perverted English history every bit as effectively as Henry VII had done so following the Battle of Bosworth Field.

Whether Morton realised the unreliable nature of his information at the time, and whether he chose not to check it out more thoroughly because he was biased in the Princess's favour or because he knew that to water it down would dilute its scandalous appeal is not clear. What *is* clear is that the book is peppered from beginning to end with one-sided accounts and biased judgements against many more people than just her husband, and is full of self-justification as well as events that no one can remember or those that can have a very different recollection of.

The book blamed her parents for an awful childhood before turning its guns on the Royal Family in general and her husband in particular as the cause of the problems that she had suffered in adult life. When Diana was dictating her memoirs, she was at a very low point in her life. Her mental state, that had been causing her family and friends increasing concern for years, was reaching a nadir. As a result, much of the book's contents are vengeful, spiteful and, however hard one tries, cannot be verified. In addition, the account is just as guilty of omission as it is of invention: many kindnesses by others have been left out, as have numerous acts of meanness and sensational scandal carried out by the Princess herself.

The book was eventually to have an effect not too dissimilar to the pamphlet that portrayed Fletcher Christian a hero and William Bligh a villain. Initially it was ridiculed as being an outrageous tale of self-harm and attempted suicides caused mainly by a cold and faithless husband. It was not believed and politicians and newspaper editors queued up to say as much. However, the Princess managed to give the book's account of her life credence without being seen to be involved personally by being photographed on purpose with certain contributors. It inspired a former lover, James Gilbey, to issue a statement that the Princess had told him similar stories to those that had appeared in the book.

In the absence of any correction, for many years it became 'history': writers of sensational biographies, political or lifestyle zealots, or just tabloid voyeurs took it as such and embarked upon works assuming that the Morton book was an accurate account of Diana's life as the Princess of Wales.

It was not. It led them all down the garden path and ensured that they would be writing from the insecure foundations of hearsay, one-sided selective opinion and out-and-out lies. No doubt opportunists who have sought to make their fortune on the back of the late Princess by rehashing the Morton book are not too worried. The more honest but politically motivated zealots who read the Morton book and took it at face value now look very foolish. They hijacked Diana's story in order to promote their own views by using her as an example. Their arguments now hold no credibility because they are built on factual inaccuracy. *Diana, Princess of Wales* by the acclaimed political writer and feminist Beatrix Campbell is rendered completely impotent, as is the less sophisticated tome written by Julie Burchill: both flounder because an argument built on fiction has no basis. Both books will increasingly come to lack authority the more historical revisionists expose the Morton book as a piece of justification. In the same vein, there are hundreds of tabloid columnists and commentators whose pronounced judgements on Prince Charles, the Queen, Prince Philip and others look every bit as marginalised and irrelevant when the truth is uncovered.

Conversely, biographies of either the Prince or Princess of Wales that predate the Morton book were rendered useless as its contents blew away the image of the fairy-tale marriage that was widely accepted as being correct. Post-Morton, the facts started to emerge, despite certain people, among them the Prince of Wales himself, doing everything possible to keep them out of the public domain. But even as the real private life of the Waleses started to come out, still the vast majority of people refused to accept the hard evidence of what the Princess was really like. She has not only managed to rewrite history with the help of Andrew Morton, she seems to have had it indelibly engraved on the national subconscious – despite the fact that new information started coming from books that were written by members of Diana's personal staff, such as protection officer Ken Wharfe or private secretary Patrick Jephson. They were clearly telling the truth, but they painted a very different picture to Morton. However, pro-Diana papers like the *Daily Mail*, which have to please middle England, would have none of it and denounced such people as traitors who were making money from the Princess's memory. Certainly, as ex-employees who were paid to be in a position of trust, it is most questionable as to whether they had the moral right to put pen to paper. Nevertheless, that is not to say that they were lying. Nor did the tabloids place the same moneymaking accusation at the door of pro-Diana books that were not only raking in cash but were perpetuating the lie in the process.

In time, reasoned publications without any axe to grind also appeared. *Diana: Story of a Princess* by Clayton and Craig is one; *Charles: Victim or Villain?* by Penny Junor is another. The long and highly detailed *The Prince of Wales* by Jonathan Dimbleby is a work sympathetically written about the life of Prince Charles and, as a result of his access to personal journals and letters, really does capture, warts and all, the Prince of Wales. However, Dimbleby, by either skirting round or glossing over rather than confronting many facts and issues raised by Morton, left confusion where there should be none. He apparently did this at the Prince's request and for the protection of his wife's memory and the sake of his sons' feelings. It remains a great irony that today the Prince of Wales, by his own silence and his determined protection of the Princess's memory, has become a major obstruction to a balanced and true view emerging and, as a result, many of the myths and inaccuracies created by Morton live on in people's minds.

In June 2004 Andrew Morton published a new biography about the Princess of Wales, claiming, 'This is not a memoir, it is a biography. People are entitled to write their memoirs but they are subjective, and they've all had a different axe to grind.' This sideswipe was intended to indicate that *Diana: In Pursuit of Love* was more objective than the latest rash of Diana memoirs that had just hit the bookshops. He told *Hello!* magazine in an interview that accompanied the first part of the book's serialisation, 'As far as I'm concerned, my first book is the nearest thing to her official biography because it was written with her approval. The latest book is part of that tradition of trying to understand who she was and why she acted as she did.' It uniquely fails on both accounts.

Morton claims that his motivation to write another biography on Diana was that, 'Since her death, she is largely seen in the public imagination as either a sad, damaged princess or a paranoid drama queen. This book challenges that distorted image.' It does not. Instead it seeks to justify Diana's paranoid behaviour by blaming everybody else from Princess Anne to the BBC for it.

In the book he claims that 'the witty, self-deprecating, courageous, caring and humane woman was becoming lost in the riot of lurid allegations', and that his role as her biographer is to show an individual 'irrepressible, kind, vulnerable yet sophisticated' who 'proved to the world that it was possible to combine glamour with integrity, happiness and compassion'. He then goes on to paint a picture of the Princess that is so deeply unpleasant that only the blindest fan or most moronic fool would not see her as a madwoman who thrived on deception, dishonesty, betrayal and wrecking other women's marriages. Whether this was an attempt to clean up the inaccuracy of his first book, or because he could not see the impression that he has given, is not clear. Either way he makes no apology for the factual inaccuracies of the first book and even shows no remorse when admitting that Diana had been less than honest in her taped interviews to the author concerning it.

Moreover, it continues to rejoice at the portrayal of the first book as a well-researched piece of work when it was dictated by the Princess herself. It completely fails to challenge the very questionable accuracy of most of her statements and amazingly simply repeats many of them along with numerous other jealous fantasies while ignoring the actual evidence, which is in the public domain, to disprove them.

Therefore, it clings to the idea that the Prince of Wales and Camilla Parker Bowles were having an affair throughout his marriage to Diana, when it is now widely known that this is not the case. As a result it continues an unfair and spiteful vilification of Camilla as the source of Diana's troubles, while ignoring or making light of the Princess's own various sexual liaisons, many of which were commenced prior to

Prince Charles starting his third and final affair with Ms Parker Bowles, and which brought much sadness to many people.

Worse, in an act of denial of the facts that is worthy of the Princess herself, Morton also seeks to discredit those who have since corrected his first effort's inaccuracies. He does so not by producing new evidence, but by insult and unattributable quotes. For example, he describes Penny Junor as Prince Charles's 'literary apologist'. He then seeks to diminish her book's credibility by quoting others who are not named. This is quite ironic as the vast majority of Junor's quotes are attributed and verifiable, whereas most of Morton's quotes come from unnamed sources. In addition, when Palace sources are quizzed, not only are they unable to verify his quotes but they nearly always refute the accuracy of them. This leads me to believe that Junor's version of events is a lot more reliable than Morton's.

In short, *Diana: In Pursuit of Love* makes a weak, unconvincing and immoral case of damage limitation for Diana while attempting to justify how Morton got some things so very wrong in the first place. It is not a constructive piece of investigative journalism, but rather a tale of continued fantasy and the need for self-justification on behalf of both author and subject. Not surprisingly, the new book completely ignores Diana's repeated claims towards the end of her life that Morton's first book about her did not meet with her approval and was inaccurate – a point that she was rather unfairly to blame Morton for, given that she had helped him to write it and had editorial control – before adding, 'That bloody man has ruined my life.' Consequently, with his 2004 book Morton missed a massive opportunity to correct history and redeem his reputation. Instead, he has written an account of Diana's life that confirms all of her worst characteristics and, by giving no rational explanation for them, leaves the reader with the impression that she was simply a very nasty person. The Princess deserves better consideration than this; but it takes a big man to admit that he was wrong – especially when he has made a fortune on the back of it.

Prince Charles was totally aware of the burdens marriage would impose upon both him and his wife. Twelve years earlier he had stated in a national television interview that, 'You have got to choose somebody very carefully, I think, who could fulfil this particular role … It has got to be somebody pretty special.' Five years later, he told Kenneth Harris in another television interview that in his case, 'A woman not only marries a man; she marries into a way of life into which she's got a contribution to make. She's got to have some knowledge of it, some sense of it, or she wouldn't have a clue, it would be risky for her, wouldn't it?' And he made it clear in yet another interview that, 'My marriage has to last forever.' This conviction was borne not only of his personal religious faith, but from his sense of constitutional necessity: as a future head of the Church of England, he had to set a good example and avoid at all costs the shambles created by Edward VIII.

As if all of this pressure wasn't enough, he also had to consider that convention and law must control his choice of wife. Under the 1701 Act of Settlement, he was forbidden to marry a Roman Catholic, an amazing contradiction in today's society of religious freedom and political correctness, and one that demonstrates beautifully the hypocrisy of modern Britain. Moreover, under the Royal Marriages Act of 1772, he had to get the formal consent of the Queen, the House of Commons and the House of Lords. And, given that their consent would almost certainly be withheld should he contemplate marriage to a divorcee or even a woman thought to have had prior sexual experience at that time, one can see that the choice of spouse for the Prince of Wales is a public matter and therefore cannot be considered in the same light that a normal betrothal of two common people might be.

Morton does not seem to take account of this and makes no allowances for it. This was probably because, despite Prince Charles and others' attempts to explain the nature of her role to her, the Princess did not understand, or at least didn't wish to accept, this circumstance either.

Charles had always understood the implications and constraints surrounding his future marriage. He was acutely keen to make the right choice for the monarchy and the nation. He was part of a long line of royal families from across Europe who had been intermarried by arrangement for over a thousand years towards this end. He feared that few in a 'modern' Britain would really understand the emotional implications for either his future wife or himself. He shared these concerns amazingly frankly with the public at the time: 'Whatever I say is not going to be understood by the vast majority of people ... A lot of people get the wrong idea of what love is all about ... It's basically a very strong friendship. As often as not you have shared interests and ideas in common and also have a great deal of affection. And I think where you are very lucky is when you find the person attractive in the physical and the mental sense ... To me marriage, which may be for fifty years, seems to be one of the biggest and most responsible steps to be taken in one's life ... Marriage is something you ought to work at. I may easily be proved wrong but I intend to work at it when I get married.'

Mindful of the trouble that the opposite sex had brought into the lives of his great-great-grandfather Edward VII and his great-uncle Edward VIII, and wishing to follow Mountbatten's advice in order to prevent the same happening to him, Charles looked towards the marriage of his grandfather George VI and his grandmother Queen Elizabeth as a good example: she was a perfect contender for queen who had married a shy and dutiful man; by a common sense of purpose for the monarchy and through love of their children and the nation, they grew to love each other devotedly.

If he had been a prince in a former time, Charles might have contemplated a marriage of convenience, as many of his relatives had, and supplemented this with a mistress. But then, provided that discretion was displayed and public dignity maintained, the monarch's family's privacy was respected. In the latter quarter of the twentieth century this all changed. Marriage became more about fairy-tale infatuation and passion than longevity, and so was easily and quickly broken, while the media, hiding behind the slogan of 'the public's right to know', was keen to dig long and deep when any whiff of royal domestic scandal was smelled. So Prince Charles was aware that this was not an option, and never even contemplated as much.

Nor did he want such a marriage. As a child and throughout his teens he had doted on his sister. He had written lovingly to her, as he had to his brothers Andrew and Edward, from his hated and lonely life at boarding school. He had even written the story of 'The Old Man of Lochnagar' for the boys to read before bed when he was twenty. Throughout their childhood he had played with them for hours on end and, despite the awkward relationship with his parents, he looked forward to family gatherings, imagining displays of physical affection that he was unlikely ever to receive from them. When billeted with other families – such as the Checketts and the Brabournes – he fitted in as a loving and kind member. He had always craved close family affection and, once he could get over the hurdle of choosing the right girl for the country as well as himself, couldn't wait to start a family of his own, one that would be run very differently to the way his parents had run theirs.

He was fascinated when married friends started their families. He wrote to one, 'I do hope your baby is very well. Does she have all sorts of things now? It's so wonderful having babies in the house again isn't it?!' To another, while confined to his bunk on HMS *Minerva*, he wrote, 'For some time I entirely forgot that I was meant to be feeling sick and had a headache, and leapt about in my bunk with joy for you both ... By the time you receive this I expect you will be out of hospital and beginning to wonder how on earth you're going to cope with a small screaming thing that requires feeding every four hours!'

He further ventured in a public speech that the marital home was 'a secure family unit in which to bring up children, to give them a happy, secure upbringing – that is what marriage is all about. Essentially one must be good friends, and love I'm sure will grow out of friendship and become deeper and deeper.' It was this consistent belief that had made him hesitate. Until he met Diana Spencer it had only been with Amanda Knatchbull that he had felt confident of the fact that mutual respect, affection and common interest were there in sufficient quantity for him to ask her to marry him. Nevertheless, he had been steadfast on what marriage should mean, although he suspected that his views, given his special circumstances, would not be understood by the vast majority of people and that, following the social revolution of the 1960s, they would be thought of as old-fashioned and even wrong. He was right.

Ever since the idealistic 1960s, people had increasingly felt that love was about lust, passion and even infatuation. This was to be the only acceptable reason for marriage and if that then failed, as it often does in time, then the relationship should be terminated and another sought. As a result, divorce rates soared as one in three marriages failed. This also meant that the public was able to identify with Diana's passion for Prince Charles much more easily than with his concept of what might make a marriage work and his desire to balance this with the needs of the country at the same time. This is an important point: it made the Princess's one-sided account of her marriage in Morton's book years later appear to have a common touch in line with popular modern thinking that immediately attracted sympathy, while Charles's views appeared cold and Victorian. As a result, his real position was totally misrepresented.

It was this view of mutual respect, shared interests and deep affection as another view of love that caused the Prince of Wales to answer a television interviewer's question about his love for Diana with the words, 'Yes, in love, whatever love means.' At the time such a comment raised eyebrows, and it was to be cited by Diana later, in the Morton book, as an example for the world to see how the cold bachelor was taking the marriage route as a necessary evil in order to produce a son and heir.

It was later claimed that Charles had made a five-year commitment to produce 'an heir and a spare' before being allowed to return to his old mistress Camilla Parker Bowles. This deal claims to have been made between the Prince of Wales and the Duke of Edinburgh. There is absolutely no evidence whatsoever to support such a claim. No one has ever stepped forward to verify it. It is thought to be quite laughable in court circles, as it not only ignores the character of both men, but also their own difficult relationship with each other. Moreover, the Princess contradicts herself by claiming that the affair with Ms Parker Bowles never stopped anyway, and that the Prince was most disappointed when his second child also turned out to be a boy.

Still, Charles's 'whatever love means' expression was undeniably thoughtless given that he was standing next to an extremely insecure nineteen-year-old as they faced the cameras together following the announcement of their engagement. And while it might have been a genuine attempt to express an opinion, it was disastrous for not being properly articulated. He would have been better off simply to say that he was in love and found her to be very desirable; but the Prince finds it very hard to be less than honest. Diana claimed that he used the same expression in private at the moment of her acceptance of his offer of marriage: 'I said, "I love you so much, I love you so much." He said: "Whatever love means." He said it then.' Surely this is further evidence that he did not realise that the remark might be misconstrued as insensitive, but is a genuine reflection of his belief that there are many kinds of love – that one love is not the same as another and that it is never the same in different people.

Perhaps this was a man who was just too wrapped up with his own insecurities and fears of doing the wrong thing for the monarchy and the country to have understood how the remark might be interpreted. After all, we have followed his progress from childhood and haven't found him to be cruel or cold, but we have found him to be insecure, suffering from low self-esteem and perpetually fearful of failing either his parents or the nation. Moreover, Diana had not yet shown any of the traits or behaviour that were to cause him, the monarchy and those concerned with preserving it the sleepless nights that would soon follow. Rather, Charles thought he had found the perfect girl. He was to write, 'I do believe that I am very lucky that someone as special as Diana seems to love me so much. I am already discovering how nice it is to have someone around to share things with ... Other people's happiness and enthusiasm at the whole thing is also a most "encouraging" element and it makes me so proud that so many people have much admiration and affection for Diana.' The two friends to whom this letter was addressed had no reason to doubt the sincerity of these sentiments.

It is hard to know when Charles started to realise that perhaps he should doubt the wisdom of his decision: once he had made his mind up that Diana was to become his wife, he steadfastly refused to discuss the position with anyone. He was to defend his fiancée to anyone raising concerns about her increasingly erratic behaviour, dismissing it as understandable nerves that anyone might suffer from if exposed to the same set of circumstances at such a young age. However, he did come to have serious reservations about Diana being able mentally to stand the rigours, hardships and disciplines of royal life before the wedding, but he shied away from calling it off. He feared the potential damage to all concerned, and in particular he feared the vilification he would have to endure from a public who in many respects had already chosen their future queen. He hoped against hope that after the wedding it would all work out and told himself that, as there was no guarantee that another candidate would handle the position any better, he had no alternative but to proceed.

It would have been far better for all concerned, especially the monarchy, if he had had the courage of his convictions and walked away; but of course that would have been easier said than done. It is difficult enough to abandon a normal family wedding, but a royal one involving the government, foreign heads of state, the Commonwealth, the Church and the people is quite a different matter – especially as he would then have had to run the gauntlet of a vicious tabloid press. Even the broadsheet republicans would have had a field day. He felt he had no right to put his mother through that: he had made his bed, so now he had better lie on it. Nevertheless, one relative felt that he should have discussed his concerns, telling Penny Junor, that there was a constitutional side as well as a private side to the matter. 'He had chosen Diana with both sides in mind, but equally he needed to think of the consequences of both, if it was going to go wrong.'

This seems a little harsh, especially as his mother had refused to offer an opinion in the first place and he had been told by all concerned to stop dithering and get on with it. He felt that he was putting the nation first by giving Diana the benefit of any doubt in the hope that her behaviour was down to the extreme pressure she had been put under and the unfamiliar world in which she had suddenly found herself following the engagement announcement.

The night before her engagement was announced, Diana had moved to Clarence House to stay with the Queen Mother; three days later she moved again, this time into her own apartment in Buckingham Palace where she remained until her wedding. This was done primarily to protect Diana from the attentions of the media and to give her a chance to acquaint herself with the royal way of life and all that it entailed.

The thinking may have appeared sound and perhaps there was, in reality, no alternative, but this set-up had serious drawbacks. Diana, trying hard at first to impress and get everything right, threw herself into her new life, but it was a strange environment for a young girl. Charles could not be with her all of the time due to his public duties and, having cut herself off from her Sloane Ranger friends, she became very lonely. With time on her hands, demons began to appear. These got worse once mid-March arrived and she was totally deprived of Charles' company. Initially, it hadn't been too painful as Charles would appear and give her an encouraging kiss or a few words of praise and encouragement. This was all she seemed to need, as courtiers still vividly remember. Then the time came for him to make a long-planned official trip that included Australia, New Zealand, Venezuela, Washington and Williamsburg. The tour had been arranged for months and could not be cancelled. Moreover, it was deemed necessary for Diana to stay in London to play an important role in her wedding arrangements.

The royals and their staff are very used to putting duty first and so saw nothing odd about this. Diana, who was used to putting her own feelings and needs first, couldn't understand why it had been organised this way. Perhaps, in hindsight, she should have been flown out for at least part of the tour. It would have shortened the separation and given her something to look forward to – and the people of Australia and

New Zealand would have been delighted to see her. She could have been chaperoned by her grandmother or another suitable person. But all of this would have taken some arrangement and expense and, as one courtier told me, 'It was felt that the sooner she got used to the way things were likely to be in the future, the better.' As a result, the Palace pushed ahead and it was most unfortunate that Diana was deprived of Charles's support at this difficult time. When the time came, she accompanied him to Heathrow and telephoto-lens shots invaded her privacy enough to reveal, despite her bowed head, a flood of tears streaming down her young face.

She was not, however, left totally alone surrounded by the grey old men of royal administration as has been expressed in many accounts. She became a close friend of Sarah Ferguson, whose father managed the Prince's polo team, and she also saw quite a lot of Princess Margaret's children, Viscount Linley and Sarah Armstrong-Jones. In addition, princes Andrew and Edward were both attentive and friendly. Moreover, and despite the fact that the place was full of snooty old retainers and strange customs, the deterioration in Diana's mental state once she became engaged cannot be laid wholly at the Palace's door or the fact that Prince Charles wasn't there all the time to encourage her. It was bound to occur: the only real question was how long would it take.

One man who knew this better than most was Michael Colborne. Without ever being impertinent, Colborne wasn't frightened to tell the Prince what he really thought. He provided an invaluable insight into life that only a man from his background could have given – he was not from the upper echelons of life, and spoke his mind at the same time. The Prince had told him never to change and he never did, despite the fact that from time to time Charles hadn't always liked what he heard and had become extremely angry on more than one occasion. Nonetheless, they enjoyed a warm relationship of mutual respect.

It was Michael Colborne whom the Prince chose to include in the initial and small number of people that he told about asking Lady Diana to marry him before the engagement was officially announced. That same day Diana had gone off to Australia with her mother and stepfather for a holiday. When she arrived back in London, Prince Charles told Colborne that he wanted the biggest bunch of flowers possible to be delivered to her flat, and handed him a romantically handwritten note to go with them. Colborne duly telephoned Diana to tell her they were on the way as he realised that the flat was under tabloid siege. She promised to look out for them. A Sergeant Ron Lewis was then dispatched to Coleherne Court and delivered both the note and the flowers to Lady Diana, who duly thanked him for them. Sadly, some ten years later Diana's memory was somewhat different. She then claimed, 'I came back from Australia, someone knocks on my door – someone from his office with a bunch of flowers and I knew that they hadn't come from Charles because there was no note. It was just somebody being very tactful in the office.'

Colborne didn't actually meet Diana until shortly after that, when the Prince asked him to look after her one afternoon. She had been out in the early morning to watch Prince Charles exercise his racehorse Allibar along the gallops at Lambourne. They were walking home for breakfast when Allibar suddenly collapsed. The horse had suffered a heart attack, and it died in the Prince's arms. Charles refused to leave him until the vet arrived and pronounced Allibar dead; he was so distraught that his detective had to drive on the way back to Highgrove.

Upon their arrival, and while Charles composed himself, it was left to Diana to take Colborne into the kitchen and explain what had happened. However, the Prince always put duty first and so, at two o'clock as originally scheduled, the helicopter arrived to take him off to an engagement in south Wales.

Colborne and Diana went into the drawing room and had a long chat. She told him about herself, her family, her parents' divorce, her father's illness and her stepmother. The story was apparently much kinder and less critical of everyone, except Raine Spencer, than the one she was to tell Morton a decade later. She continued as they wandered around the garden together. Colborne liked her and, being some twenty-seven years older, became a good and reliable friend to her in a paternal way. They were to share an office together as the wedding was being organised.

Nevertheless, at this first meeting he was shocked by how young and naive she was. She still had puppy fat, ruddy schoolgirl cheeks, no dress sense and appeared to have received a poor education. Worse, he could see that she was remarkably ill-disciplined and hadn't got the vaguest idea of what she was taking on. He determined to do everything within his power to help her, even though he understood that this was not going to be an easy job. The role of princess of Wales was always going to be a truly demanding one for any woman, but for one so young and ignorant it looked to him to be almost impossible. He soon realised that first afternoon that this pretty young girl, who appeared to be so perfect at first glance, was far from an ideal choice. He concluded that Prince Charles must have been smitten by her not to have noticed any of this.

Two days later the official engagement announcement was made and Diana was, quite willingly, taken into royal custody. However, as we know, she was soon to be overwhelmed by the palace and its staff of over 200 people who lived a lifestyle little changed from the reign of Queen Victoria. Much has been made of this, and certainly it must have been somewhat daunting to a rather spoiled nineteen-year-old who was used to doing lunch with giggling girls of her own age. Nevertheless, things were never as bad as Diana was to later tell Morton. Not only did Sarah Ferguson et al keep her company, but there were many in the Queen's household who had known her since she was a child and did their very best to make her feel welcome. For example, Lady Susan Hussey spent hours with her. She adored Diana, as she did Prince Charles, and took her shopping, helped her prepare for the wedding and did anything else she could to make the future princess feel at home. In addition, Diana's sister Jane was at court and her mother came to visit her frequently. Moreover, far from being locked away in a dungeon, she continued to meet friends or even lunch happily with the Palace 'old brigade'. Lieutenant Colonel Blair Stewart-Wilson was one – Diana liked him well enough to kiss him in front of the cameras on her wedding day – and Sir Johnnie Johnston and Sir William Heseltine were others. They were all sincerely fond of her and did their very best to make her feel welcome.

The picture that Diana was to paint to Morton is unfair on these people: their kindness has been erased from her story in order to present Buckingham Palace as an unkind place that was orchestrated by the cold, aloof and insensitive Windsors. Further investigation only highlights this, as Diana's memory of the events as told to Andrew Morton is continually at odds with those of countless others who were there at the time. For example, she explained to Morton that no one was there to welcome her when she arrived for her first night at Clarence House. In fact, she had dinner with the Queen Mother and a delighted Prince of Wales.

She went on to tell Morton that during the first week of her engagement her bulimia started, the implication being that it was as a result of her cruel treatment. In fact, she was treated for a completely different eating disorder known as anorexia nervosa – the same disorder that her sister Sarah had suffered from, as had their mother. Sarah had been suffering from it, following the break-up of a relationship, when she first went out with Prince Charles in 1977. Her family would only allow her to speak to the Prince on the telephone if she ate. In the end she sought professional help in a London nursing home and recovered. Frances Shand Kidd was to suffer from anorexia during her latter years of self-imposed exile on a secluded island off the west coast of Scotland, as she battled against alcoholism.

The two conditions are similar insofar as they are both eating disorders that are usually caused by an upset in childhood that lies dormant until triggered by stress in puberty or adulthood. Both illnesses are almost exclusively suffered by females. Bulimia involves binge eating followed by self-induced vomiting, whereas anorexics avoid food, pretend that they eat normally and are thus in denial. Anorexia nervosa can lead to bulimia via a variant called anorexia bulimia nervosa. Both illnesses can become extremely serious, but a dramatic weight loss is usually only experienced in the case of anorexia nervosa. However, both kinds of disorders can bring about a number of other medical problems and can even be fatal.

In time, as her mental state deteriorated, Diana also became bulimic, probably via the ABN variant, but originally, as her mother later confirmed, she was suffering with the same anorexic disorder from which her sister had previously suffered. Diana, who denied suffering from anorexia nervosa at all, claimed at one point that her bulimia was caused by the cold treatment meted out by the Palace and the absence of Prince Charles. Years later, she told Morton that it had also been caused by a flippant remark made by Charles about her puppy fat. She lied. In reality he never made such a remark. This was Diana at her most resourceful, intent on not only gaining public sympathy but also shifting the responsibility for her behaviour from herself to Prince Charles in the process, so that Morton could pillory him on her behalf.

What had actually happened was that, having seen herself on the television, she had commented on how fat she looked. The Prince then slipped an arm around her waist and told her that everyone looked bigger on television than they really were and that she looked great. In reality, and for obvious reasons, Diana started taking the contraceptive pill shortly before her engagement. She, as many women do, gained weight as a result. Her reaction was understandable alarm, which might or might not have been added to by a harmless and innocent remark made in support of her by the man she adored.

Whatever the reason, she virtually stopped eating and her weight loss was dramatic. The blue suit she wore for the engagement was a size fourteen. By the time she was married she could fit into a size ten. She had lost six inches from around her waist in less than six months and it showed. Medical opinion is certain that such weight loss means that Diana's mother's assertion that her daughter was suffering from anorexia nervosa and not bulimia during the early stages of her engagement are almost certainly correct.

Nevertheless, it is very hard to put a finger on the actual trigger. Diana said that she was unhappy and lonely from the moment she arrived at Buckingham Palace. Friends confirm this but add that, while at times she was tearful, she was on other occasions most excited and appeared to be blissfully happy. They were all surprised by her sudden mood swings but most cannot remember her blaming the Prince for any unhappiness at this time, her only complaint being that she wished his duties didn't separate them so often. Nor can they really remember Diana having too many complaints against the household staff at the palace – some can remember her actually speaking affectionately about the Prince's staff. Most put her mood swings down to the media pressure, which was new to her and which she had had to endure for several months. The media attention, the move to a new and different world and the daunting prospect of a massive wedding followed by a strange life of continual duty, which was only now occurring to her, must have put this rather immature and uneducated nineteen-year-old under enormous strain.

In addition to these problems, and fuelled by her own low self-esteem, Diana also harboured fears about the Prince's former girlfriends. She became fascinated by them and started to quiz Charles about them. He made no secret about who had been his previous lovers, and told her everything. He saw no problem with this. He hadn't even known Diana when he was having such relationships. They had been part of his previous life, and that was now finished. He had been told to sow his wild oats before marriage. He had, and now he was to marry and settle down. Moreover, if he was to enjoy a life of great affection and mutual respect with his chosen partner, there could be no secrets. Charles is not a jealous person in personal relationships. He had never experienced jealousy, not even when Andrew Parker Bowles reclaimed Camilla in 1972; therefore he had no idea of the jealous passions that he was unleashing in his fiancée as a result of his confessions. He had absolutely no understanding of how a young girl might feel knowing that he had slept with and perhaps even loved these women whom she imagined to be more intelligent and sexy than she was and some of whom she now saw regularly. It didn't occur to him that this might become a major problem, and in fairness to her, it should have done.

From her point of view things looked very different. She harboured a deep fear of rejection, possibly one that had been dormant in her subconscious since her mother's departure from the family home; now, as a teenager, her experience of life was somewhat limited, with the exception of the sexual liaisons that she had always sought to control. She had achieved nothing, her education was woefully inappropriate, her sense of style was non-existent and her knowledge of the world away from Sloane Square was minimal. These other women must have seemed to her to be sophisticated, intelligent, attractive and worldly. The thought of them made her feel even more insecure than normal, and her ill-disciplined nature allowed her imagination to run riot.

Moreover, her immaturity, mental insecurity and belief that other people behaved like the Spencers meant that she had completely failed to understand who Prince Charles really was. Princess Margaret of Hesse and the Rhine made the point well: 'I know some men are pathological philanderers, and it doesn't behove a woman to believe a word they say. But the Prince of Wales really isn't like that. Everyone who knows him can confirm that his outstanding quality traits are his sincerity and his inability to dissemble.'

Many ladies-in-waiting, observing her concerns, attempted to dispel them. They told her to remember that the Prince of Wales was thirty-two years of age and was therefore bound to have had girlfriends and sexual encounters before meeting her. It was natural that some of these might have been serious at the time. Of course these women would be older and more sophisticated than she was – but she mustn't forget that he hadn't married any of them. He had chosen her. However, her insecurity wouldn't allow her to believe them, and her jealousy gnawed away at her. It even grew to include the Queen. Prince Charles has always placed the letters from his mother in a safe to prevent their theft and sale to a tabloid newspaper. Diana refused to accept this and became suspicious that the Queen was writing about her and Charles was deliberating locking these notes away in order to prevent her from being able to read them.

Gradually the Prince started to become aware of a very different person to the carefree, happy girl who had amused everyone so much at Balmoral the previous summer. He was perplexed, but thought that it could be put down to the strain and stress of the coming wedding. 'Why don't you just ask me about things that are worrying?' he would ask in a gentle manner, but she never would, and so he went on failing to understand the depth of her jealousy and didn't say or do the right things to help matters.

On the evening that she stayed in Clarence House before moving to Buckingham Palace there was a letter waiting for her. It was dated two days previously and said, 'Such exciting news about the engagement. Do let's have lunch soon when the Prince of Wales goes to Australia and New Zealand. He's going to be away for three weeks. I'd love to see the ring. Lots of love, Camilla.' It was genuinely friendly and the intentions were good. She and Diana had by now got to know each other quite well and Camilla thought they were friends. She wanted to support her because she thought she was fun and made the Prince happy. Camilla was genuinely in the pro-Diana camp.

Diana organised the lunch. She later told Andrew Morton, 'Bearing in mind that I was so immature, I didn't know about jealousy or depression or anything like that …' Camilla asked here whether she was intending to hunt on horseback when at Highgrove. On replying 'No', Camilla said, 'I just wanted to know.' Diana continued, 'I thought as far as she was concerned that was her communication route. Still too immature to understand all the messages coming my way.'

Camilla denies that this was her meaning and maintains she had purely asked if Diana intended to take up hunting. She remembers the lunch being entirely friendly with Diana being on sparkling form. She was excited, showed off her ring with great pride and there were no tricky moments at all.

Camilla had been included on the list of previous girlfriends that Charles had told Diana about. Diana had made the Prince promise that none of them remained part of his love life and that there would never be anyone else but her. On both counts the Prince readily agreed. He was being truthful, and as a man of honour and one who is hopelessly honest, he expected her to believe him. This was a mistake: Diana believed that everybody else thought as she did. She made promises, but once made, there was no guarantee that she would keep them. When Diana asked him whether he still loved any of them, he replied, 'Yes' – because he did, and still does today. To him, as we know, there are several kinds of love. He loved his parents, siblings and friends very much but that didn't mean that he wanted to have a passionate affair with any of them. But to Diana, a young girl who really only understood the two-dimensional love of the romantic novel, this meant that he still fancied women like Camilla.

Charles should no doubt have displayed greater sensitivity. He should have tried harder to put himself in Diana's position and ask himself how a nineteen-year-old might be feeling. It was not that he wasn't concerned about her – he genuinely was – but he should have realised that she was a frailer personality than she purported to be and needed a lot of reassurance. Perhaps, after he was to experience jealousy himself in later years concerning Diana's popularity with the public, when her celebrity eclipsed his more serious projects, he would have understood more easily how she felt and acted accordingly.

So perhaps Prince Charles didn't make enough of an allowance for the fact that his fiancée was only nineteen and not as mature as his previous girlfriends. But this wasn't because he wasn't interested in her as his future companion. In fact, her lack of sophistication and style delighted him: she was a blank canvas and he planned to introduce her to all the things that interested him. He thought of his fiancée as an immature girl who was under an initial strain that was inevitable given that she was now destined to become queen of England. He had no idea that she was a particularly vulnerable girl, with an abnormally pronounced sense of suspicion and insecurity that led her to believe that people were conspiring against her. This had not been at all apparent during their courtship; but once the engagement was announced, things changed. Now she was moody, wilful and displayed a terrible temper. He had never seen any of this before and was quite bewildered. She would suddenly blow up, rant, rave and burst into floods of hysterical tears. She would turn against people that she had previously appeared to like and claim that they were out to get her and bring her down by spying on her. Then the rage would go as quickly as it came. Sometimes the offending folk would be forgiven, but more often than not they would be ignored by Diana as if they did not exist – even if she was in the same room as them.

Prince Charles was not the only one to notice this change in her. A number of his and Diana's friends, as well as palace staff, all noticed the same and were most concerned. But still the Prince continued to play down the situation, insisting to himself that Diana would be fine once the wedding had taken place and she had a chance to settle down. He was inclined to ignore her outbursts in the mistaken belief that this would make them go away more quickly.

At the time of the engagement, the deterioration in Diana's stability wasn't helped by the Prince's considerable work schedule. Diana found it very hard to be separated from him and just couldn't understand why he, the future king of England, couldn't just decide to do what he wished – which should be to spend his time with her. She could not grasp that monarchy is a servant to the people, that duty must come first and that his schedule had been decided months, and in some cases years, in advance.

When the Prince was away, Diana was looked after by those members of his staff who weren't accompanying him. By now Checketts had been replaced as private secretary by the Honourable Edward Adeane. The assistant private secretary was Francis Cornish. His predecessor, Oliver Everett, had been invited to return especially to look after Diana before the wedding; afterwards he became her official private secretary.

These were intelligent men – it was a high-powered team. But they were all at least twice her age. They were sympathetic to her, they liked her and they were extremely flattered by her girlish flirting and giggly charm; but they had absolutely no idea how to handle her. She was so young and her experience was so limited that they didn't know where to start. They were not so much troubled by her moods, which were mainly reserved for family, close friends and, increasingly, Prince Charles, but they were astonished by her ignorance when, for example, she asked where Dorset was or what was the capital of Australia. She, in turn, felt threatened by this intellectual gap. No doubt everyone had good intentions, but it wasn't a match made in heaven.

Diana felt more comfortable with former grammar-school boy Michael Colborne. This was not because he was any less intelligent than the others, but because, as he shared an office with her, he could see how lonely she was and would talk to her for hours. The others didn't do this. They were used to dealing with the Prince. His life was very busy; there was no time for idle chit-chat. Everything was run on a businesslike basis – a strictly professional relationship. But Diana was scarcely more than a child, and a disturbed child at that. She had hardly ever been employed herself, let alone employed anyone else. She had never worked in an office and had no understanding of how it worked. She didn't realise what was expected of her. She loved romantic novels, women's magazines and soap operas on television, had no interest in a career and wasn't too fussed about becoming well read – she found anything other than the lightest reading boring. She certainly didn't have a thirst for knowledge like her fiancé. She just wanted to be loved, have babies, be looked after and live happily ever after. Of course, there is nothing wrong with that – provided that you don't also want to become Princess of Wales. So, once she got to the palace, it was a shock: her own frailties and insecurities kicked in and her big dream became disappointing, if not a nightmare.

Many people like Michael Colborne and Susan Hussey spent hours trying to help her, but more often than not she wasn't receptive. She simply refused to be told what to do or when to do it. All her life she had been indulged by divorced parents. She had learned, like so many children in similar circumstances, how to manipulate them. As a result she had grown up never being forced to do anything that she didn't want to. Poor behaviour, bad school reports and failed exams were forgiven without reprimand. This had meant that she had become a charming young lady who expected to get her own way and could be very bad tempered and spiteful when she didn't. Add to this indiscipline her poor education, mental frailties and insecurities, and one is presented with a dangerous cocktail that most families would struggle with, let alone the dutiful but quite dysfunctional House of Windsor. Accordingly, Diana was never to accept the discipline essential to being part of royal life. It seems that she expected that life with the Windsors would be the same as life with the Spencers, only grander.

Diana thought that being royal was entirely different to how the Royal Family saw it. Both they and their courtiers took what they did for granted and assumed that she, as a Spencer, would turn out to be a younger and perhaps not such a bright version of Amanda Knatchbull. They couldn't have been more wrong. However, it was an understandable mistake to make. After all, Diana came from one of the most aristocratic families in Britain; she had been brought up in one of the most traditionally run stately houses in England; the Queen was godmother to her brother and the Duke of Kent was godfather to one of her sisters; her father had been equerry to the Queen; both of her grandmothers had been ladies-in-waiting to the Queen Mother and both the Spencers and the Fermoys had been at court for years and were close friends of the Royal Family. It was not unreasonable for everyone to have assumed that she understood what royal life was about, what to expect and what was expected of her. This was a major reason why the court thought that Diana seemed so perfect for the role now that Amanda Knatchbull had put herself out of the running, and they were pleased to have her.

As things began to dawn on her, she explained to Colborne that she didn't know how she was going to cope with such a life. He replied that she her life would never again be her own. 'In four to five years you're going to be an absolute bitch, not through any fault of your own, but because of the circumstances in which you live. If you want four boiled eggs for breakfast, you'll have them. If you want the car brought round to the front door a minute ago, you'll have it. It's going to change you. Your life is going to be organised. You open your diary now and you can put down the Trooping the Colour, the Cenotaph service, Cowes Week, the Ascots. You can write your diary for five years ahead, ten years, twenty years.' Colborne realised what sort of effect the role would have on the life of a normal young woman who hadn't been trained for the job. What he hadn't realised was that Diana wasn't quite the normal young woman he thought she was. However, it wouldn't be too long before he was to find out.

On learning of the engagement, Lord Palumbo commented, 'I thought that it was a match made in heaven and I think most of us did. I thought that the Prince of Wales would take Princess Diana under his wing and teach her the ways of the Royal Family and the direction that she should follow, and I couldn't think of a better tutor.' He seems to have spoken for the court, according to my research. However, an unnamed senior member of the household told Clayton and Craig, 'Lovely chap though he was, her fiancé gave no indication of thinking through what getting married to this person would be like for her. He carried on with his merry ways, his extracurricular bachelor life, one night in Scotland, one night somewhere else. In her case it was a massively bigger thing.'

This seems slightly unfair as a closer inspection of his schedule over the period of his engagement to Diana indicates a hectic list of official duties rather than bachelor jollies and we already know that he had given a great deal of thought to what marriage to him would be like for any girl who decided to take him on. Moreover, he had Diana worked into as many of his engagements as possible once he returned from his world tour at the beginning of May. These included a visit to Broadlands where Prince Charles opened an exhibition of Mountbatten memorabilia on 9 May. On 14 May they attended a lunch together at Windsor in honour of the President of Ghana. Later in the month they were also together for the state visit of King Khalid of Saudi Arabia. On 22 May the Prince took Diana on a walkabout in Tetbury, a small market town near his Highgrove estate. Jayne Fincher was there with her camera. 'He introduced her to the locals. They did a walkabout and visited the local hospital. And, you know, she was very nervous and he was sort of gently cajoling her round and showing her what to do. She was obviously very new at it, and very shy about it, and he was like a proud peacock showing her off. But he was very gentle and he always had an arm round her showing her what to do, watching her all the time. And obviously was sort of nurturing her into it.'

This quote from a well-respected photographer who saw a lot of the royals at work and play at the time is very interesting as it conjures up the picture of a man whom we have come to know through the course of this book and yet who is wholly unrecognisable as the Prince of Wales described by Andrew Morton. This is a man who was proud of his bride-to-be, happy to show her off and hopeful that her 'other side', as he came to refer to the 'other Diana', would remain at home for the day – if not disappear altogether.

By now Britain had become obsessed by the royal wedding. The *Daily Mirror* reported that there were 971 items of memorabilia on sale, including Charles and Diana mugs, Charles and Diana plates, bookmarks, beach balls, bottle openers, beer glasses and bags. The tabloid press couldn't find enough to write about, no minutiae were too small or too trivial. Even the broadsheets were full of Charles and Diana stories. The nation was building to the explosive excitement of a day that would be watched by the world. The expectation was gripping for the people and profitable for the press, but it only served to put the fragile Diana under even greater pressure.

At a polo match in July, the *Daily Telegraph* reported that she had been 'flustered and tearful when spectators pressed too close'. The Prince rushed to her defence, commenting that it was 'hardly surprising' that the strain of being under such extreme media and public scrutiny would tell eventually.

Indeed, the strain was beginning to show more and more as Diana started to realise the real implications of her future life. Her feelings of inadequacy fuelled her insecurity, which in turn increased her obsession with Charles's previous girlfriends in general, and Camilla Parker Bowles in particular. She was to claim years later that, soon after moving into Buckingham Palace, she discovered that Charles had sent Camilla flowers when she was ill. Diana claimed that with them there was a message that used what she imagined were the couple's former pet names for each other – 'To Gladys from Fred'. It is not clear that any flowers were actually sent. Moreover, no one can be found to verify these pet names.

However, they take on a greater significance when, in mid-July, Diana discovered a bracelet on Michael Colborne's desk with the letters 'G' and 'F' cut into it. It was intended for Camilla. Diana confronted Charles about it and he replied that indeed it was a gift for Camilla. Kanga, Camilla and others would all be receiving presents as expressions of his gratitude for years of constant friendship. He claimed that the initials stood for 'Girl Friday' – a nickname that I have had verified by a friend of his – and that he intended to deliver the gift in person as he would to all his other friends who had invited him to stay and had given him support and advice during his bachelor years. He told Diana that closing this chapter of his life with fond recognition was honourable and shouldn't be seen as a slight towards his new married life. She refused to accept this position, believing that now he was engaged, all contact should be cut with many of these people, especially any former girlfriends.

Diana's account of this incident appears vividly in Andrew Morton's book: Somebody in his office told her that her husband had had a bracelet made for her 'which she wears to this day. It's got "G and F" entwined in it, "Gladys" and "Fred". I was devastated. This was about two weeks before we got married. He said: "Well, he's going to give it to her tonight." So rage, rage, rage! "Why can't you be honest with me?" But, no, he cut me absolutely dead. It's as if he had made his decision, and if it wasn't going to work, it wasn't going to work. He'd found a virgin, the sacrificial lamb, and in a way he was obsessed with me. But it was hot and cold, hot and cold. You never knew what mood it was going to be, up and down, up and down.'

The office was the one she shared with Michael Colborne and he was the man referred to in her account. However, Colborne doesn't remember the story at all the same way. On the day in question a footman brought up a package to his office. He opened it and started to check off a number of items that he had ordered on behalf of the Prince as gifts. According to Colborne, Prince Charles has always used the giving of presents as a way of thanking people. For women it would often take the form of jewellery. There were several pieces: one for Dale, Lady Tyron (Kanga), another for Lady Susan Keswick, another for Lady Cecil Cameron and so on. Among them was a bracelet for Camilla engraved with 'GF', which indeed stood for 'Girl Friday'.

As Colborne was checking off the list he was called into Adeane's office. He left the opened package on his desk and went next door. Diana came in while he was away and had a look at the things on his desk. Colborne had seen no reason to hide the gifts away because, as far as he was concerned, there was no special significance in any of them.

When he had finished his conversation with Adeane he continued on to the main office. A few minutes later he was joined there by Adeane who, having just bumped into an unhappy Diana in the corridor, wanted to know why she was so upset. Colborne then returned to his office. Diana was not there but the individual parcels inside the package had been opened and the lid was off the box that contained the bracelet. He didn't see Diana again until the Monday morning, when she confessed to having gone through what had been on his desk, but said no more about it. Diana's account gives the story a twist that leads the reader to a different interpretation and therefore the conclusion that she wanted them to draw.

But it is true that Diana was upset? She was furious, and an unpleasant row with Prince Charles ensued – this has been verified by several in earshot. Diana begged him not to deliver the gift to Camilla personally. He explained that he felt obliged to give Mrs Parker Bowles the gift in person. A few days later, true to his word, he did, and said goodbye: both of them expected and intended that that would be the last time they would be alone together in each other's company. Indeed from the moment of his engagement in February this was the only occasion upon which he saw Camilla. It was a farewell gift that he truly believed she was owed, and his sense of honour dictated that he should deliver it in person. As he never intended to bed Mrs Parker Bowles again, he just couldn't see the problem, and he wasn't going to be ordered about by a hysterical girl just turned twenty.

There is no doubt that this was Prince Charles' sincere position. However, yet again it shows absolutely no understanding of who Diana really was. He obviously felt that she'd been through the mill during the last few months, but this was no excuse for such unwarranted jealousy and certainly not for having bust-ups in front of the staff. The girl would have to pull herself together.

Not for a minute did he understand that her 'other side' was the real Diana, or that she was completely incapable of pulling herself together – or if he did he just ignored the idea and ploughed on as if she was a perfectly normal young woman who was going through a stressful time. For this reason Diana deserves our sympathy. She was unable to exert any discipline over herself when the black moods fell upon her, but she would show much regret when in a lighter mood. And it seemed impossible for others to help her. Either they didn't understand what was wrong with her or, if they did, she would reject their help (or even them) as she was in denial of what problems she really had.

As the big day approached, Diana's prenuptial tension continued to mount. It seemed to have more to do with the pressure associated with such a great occasion and the future prospect of marriage to duty than worries about Camilla, as her Uncle, Robert Spencer, confirms. 'I am sure that Diana did have reservations about getting married at that stage because her father told me so. But her father and I never discussed the question of Camilla Parker Bowles, her name never came up. We just felt that it was a natural thing to happen because her husband had gone off on a pre-planned trip, she had moved into Buckingham Palace, which was strange and lonely, and there was the tremendous strain of getting ready for the wedding. That was enough to make any girl think, Gosh, I can't go through with this.'

Robert Spencer had reached the same conclusions as Prince Charles, courtiers and household staff. However, Diana, years later, and by then completely consumed by jealousy, places the blame for these prenuptial tensions firmly at Camilla's door. She claimed that she had confessed in tears to her sisters, during a reception given by the Queen two nights before the wedding, that she was not certain that Prince Charles really loved her, and that she wanted to call the wedding off. According to Diana her sister Sarah replied, 'Well bad luck, Dutch, your face is on the tea towels so you're too late to chicken out.'

It was also during this evening that another destructive fantasy of Diana's claims to have happened. About ten years after her marriage to Prince Charles she convinced herself that he had slept with Camilla in Buckingham Palace that night – just forty-eight hours before his wedding. She harboured this imaginary picture in her mind until she finally believed it was true. It was then told to the world and has been repeated in endless books and television documentaries since. It is pure fabrication.

On that Monday evening, the Queen threw an intimate dinner party for Diana's family and other close friends. This was then followed by a huge reception and dance to which hundreds of guests, including most of the crowned heads of Europe, were invited. The Parker Bowleses were not invited to the dinner, but were naturally among the guests attending the ball, which went on into the early hours of Tuesday morning. The Royal Family remained until the end to bid goodnight to all their guests. When the last coach left Buckingham Palace bound for Windsor Castle, where some of the foreign royalty were being housed, as there was insufficient room at the palace, Charles and Diana were the last to go up, exhausted, to their separate suites. There are countless witnesses who saw Camilla leave with her husband much earlier.

However, people sympathetic to Diana's account have since pointed out that Charles and Diana did not sleep under the same roof the next night. Diana had moved into Clarence House for the night, in keeping with the tradition of not seeing the groom from the night before the wedding until meeting him at the altar on the following day. So in theory, they argue, there could have been an opportunity for him to have slept with his ex-mistress then.

Indeed some twelve years later, and possibly motivated by Diana herself, James Whitaker of the *Daily Mirror* was to report that the Prince of Wales's valet, Stephen Barry, had told him some years earlier that Camilla Parker Bowles had spent the wedding eve at Buckingham Palace with Prince Charles. However, as Barry had sadly died some eight years before, he was unable to rebut the charge either against the Prince or his own integrity.

Moreover, it really begs the question why, if Whitaker was correct, did he keep the story under wraps for eight or more years? It would have been a tabloid sensation if he had come out with it when he claims to have been told about it. Whitaker would have been considered to be a hero by his peers, and the *Mirror* would have really got one over on the *Sun* at the same time, as the Waleses' marriage was still considered to be in good shape by the mid-1980s.

This is what really happened. The Prince had spent the evening with the rest of the Royal Family and half a million or so members of the public watching a brilliant fireworks display in Hyde Park. It was an extraordinary outpouring of celebration – the whole country seemed to be partying while millions of people poured into the capital in readiness for the next day's wedding ceremony. Hundreds of people had been camping along the route from Buckingham Palace to St Paul's for days. It was a truly wonderful evening. There were no fights, crime or even drunkenness. Strangers struck up conversations and even friendships; the weather was warm and the atmosphere electrifying. It was a special occasion. The next day was to see the wedding of the century: the heir to the most famous crown in the world was to marry an aristocratic beauty already taken to the hearts of the British public. To witness this, an extraordinary gathering of the world's most noble and powerful people had been assembled. Nearly every king and queen from Europe, Africa, the Middle East and Asia would be there, along with over 160 presidents and prime ministers from the Commonwealth and beyond. The event would not only be watched by the nation but also by one of the world's largest ever television audiences. The Archbishop of Canterbury declared that this was 'the stuff of which fairy-tales are made', and he was right.

The Prince was lucky enough to avoid a ghastly stag night and all the vile pranks that supposed friends get up to, and once the firework display was over he returned to Buckingham Palace. He sat up chatting to Lady Susan Hussey, who was very fond of both him and Diana, and who had an apartment adjacent to the Prince's. Soon after midnight they said goodnight and retired.

About half an hour later there was a knock on her door. The Prince returned, saying that he couldn't sleep. She had been unable to sleep either and so they went into her drawing room and looked down the Mall at all the activity. Both were overcome with emotion as they watched the people's excitement. Some time after 2.00 a.m. the Prince, armed with an aspirin to assist his sleep, returned to his own room. Camilla was nowhere near.

So ended the months of engagement. They hadn't always been unhappy, and were certainly not as black as Diana was later to paint them. However, nor had they been altogether happy months for anyone concerned. There had been difficult times for the palace staff in particular. They had been used to working to a routine and on a strictly professional basis with the Prince of Wales and other members of the Royal Family. They were unsure how to deal with a teenager who would happily take a seat on their desks and chatter for hours one day, then suspiciously interrogate them about Camilla Parker Bowles the next. Diana's behaviour started to alarm them, and they certainly didn't know how to react to it.

Nor had it been a happy time for the Prince of Wales. He just didn't understand her and was thoroughly perplexed. He had never seen behaviour like this before. Until then, the only tempers ever thrown around him were his own. He had never been on the receiving end before and so, like his staff, he just didn't know how to react. His parents' aloof attitude towards family life hadn't taught him too much about the common emotions of relationships, and they certainly hadn't prepared him for Diana's outbursts. His elevated position as heir to the throne, along with his own insecurities and determination to put queen and country first, hadn't helped him understand her either. He probably felt trapped, but knowing that there was no way out he decided to carry on and give it his best shot in the hope that it would all work out the way Mountbatten had promised when the dust settled and they could get on with married life.

And finally it was not a happy time for Diana herself. She had dreamed of marrying Prince Charles. It had indeed been her ambition since puberty. She had met him, made a favourable impression on a bale of hay and grabbed her opportunity with both hands. Then, in the excitement of the chase, she doesn't seem to have given the likely consequences of such a union much thought and had steadfastly refused to listen to advice that she didn't want to hear – just as Charles had with Nicholas Soames and the Romseys. The result was that she was to arrive in a strange and formidable place completely unprepared. She felt lonely, insecure and, I suspect, experienced a feeling of anti-climax.

So where, if anywhere, does the blame lie for the deterioration in the future Princess of Wales health over this period lie? Many fingers have been pointed in many directions – some at the cold and archaic Buckingham Palace staff. It is true that the palace and its customs must have felt very strange to a young, modern girl. But there is absolutely no evidence that anybody was anything other than kind and helpful to her. Diana's criticism of these people is simply not backed up by any evidence, whereas countless stories of their kindness to her can be verified by many people. As a result of the impression created by Diana to the outside world, people like Sir Johnnie Johnston, Blair Stewart-Wilson, Lady Susan Hussey, Michael Colborne, Edward Adeane, Francis Cornish and others have been unfairly portrayed to justify behaviour that came from within and was not caused by them.

What about the Prince of Wales? Charles does seem to have tried to be helpful and encouraging. He seems to have included Diana in official engagements where possible and independent opinions like those expressed by Jayne Fincher would appear to support the view that he was genuinely fond and very proud of her while gently teaching her the ropes. It wasn't his fault that he was away for nearly half of the time during their engagement. And here lies a major problem for anyone marrying into this completely different way of life. Charles however was born to it: he knew nothing else. Amanda Knatchbull had been close enough to it to understand the form. She thought about it but was intelligent enough to understand the price that she was being asked to pay. On the other hand, Diana either failed to heed the warnings from Prince Charles about what marriage to him would be like, or perhaps she thought that in her case she would be able to have a fairy-tale position without the responsibility – the reward without the cost. The fact that the future Princess of Wales apparently became engaged to the Prince without fully understanding the arduous nature of the role of monarch is clearly not his fault. Nor was the fact that she had been less than honest about who she really was and what really interested her in life.

However, Prince Charles was not very skilled at helping his fiancée when tantrums erupted, tears flowed or crazy allegations were made. He had never experienced anything so out of emotional control, and just didn't understand that simple reasoning would not work. Moreover, he is not a man of great self-esteem himself, yet is used to being the centre of attention. This combination rendered him useless to help her. However, to single him out for criticism alone in this might be slightly unfair as nobody – not her parents, her siblings, her friends, her allies, her lovers or her staff – was able to do any better. Therefore it is not a question of whether another man (or woman) could have done a better job, because throughout her life several tried and all failed. In a marriage of commoners Charles might have walked away long before he did.

Nevertheless, Prince Charles must accept one hundred percent the responsibility for asking Diana to marry him. It does not matter that Mountbatten would probably have approved, that the Queen Mother certainly did, that his father had told him to make up his mind or that the nation virtually demanded he asked her, because the decision was his and his alone. It was his call and it turned out to be a bad one. It does him no credit whatsoever not to accept such responsibility.

And so, what about Diana herself? Well there can be no doubt that the whole experience of being propelled from a Sloane Ranger of leisurely lunches, independent means and a complete 'suit yourself' lifestyle to the structure and discipline of Palace life could be described as something very different. But it was surely not so frightening, oppressive or strange as to cause something of a nervous breakdown. After all, she wanted to be engaged, she loved the Prince of Wales and her greatest wish in life was to become his princess. There is no evidence that the palace staff, the Royal Family, Prince Charles or anyone else attempted to ruin her dream or be in any way unkind to her.

The unhappiness of her engagement months stemmed from the moods, tantrums and jealous fantasies. These were of her own making, but they weren't necessarily her fault, as she just couldn't help herself. She was to explain this later to many friends such as Elsa Bowker. ' I was dreadful, really awful, but I just couldn't help myself. It was as if somebody else was controlling me.' Therefore, while Diana might have been mainly responsible for this unhappy period, if one accepts her explanation regarding her inability to control her own mood swings, it would seem inappropriate to castigate her for something beyond her control.

Naturally, this begs the question: should Diana have been about to become a member of the Royal Family and thus an instrument of monarchy? She was already very popular with the public. She was largely worshipped by the tabloid press. She possessed the four great qualities so admired by modern society: youth, beauty, wealth and celebrity. She was to go on to create a mirage of her true self, and in so doing highlight many worthy causes and bring comfort to many poor, ill or dying people.

But these are the qualities of a modern star, a twentieth-century icon. This is about the hero worship of a celebrity image. Monarchy is not about that. Monarchy is about a dedication to the people and not their dedication to you. It has to be a constant, disciplined and selfless force. Duty must always be paramount and no member can ever afford to put themselves first, in the way that Edward VIII did, or above the interests of the nation. In this respect, Diana was quite unsuitable. In addition, she was an emotional accident waiting to happen. Her lack of preparation was almost immaterial because she never possessed the characteristics necessary to continue the long-term promotion of the monarchy. As a result, Diana became the focus that allowed the tabloid press to drag the institution ever more into front-page sensationalism, making it no better than the short-lived sparkle of other mere celebrities. She lifted the royal veil and allowed the public access to a soap opera. The effect was disastrous, as familiarity breeds contempt and overdosing reduces the appetite. The decision of Prince Charles to take this woman as his wife was always going to be an unmitigated disaster and the result was seriously to weaken the relationship between the nation and its monarchy. Diana was in time to become the toast both of most republicans and many socialists as they came to see her as their secret weapon.

Prince Charles made a wrong decision. But in his defence he had tried to make the right one. He had followed Mountbatten's plan and everyone approved of his choice. Moreover, he had been deceived by Diana. Diana's family knew of her problems, but no doubt they hoped, as Prince Charles did, that it would all turn out right in the end. Diana was clearly more responsible for this mismatch than anybody because she had given the impression that she had understood about the life that she was letting herself in for, that she liked the Royal Family, their friends, their homes and their traditions. In reality none of this was true. However, all believed her, welcomed her and tried to help her.

Was she doing all of this on purpose? Or was she really unable at times even to direct her own life? I think that the second option is more likely. Her moods, tantrums, jealous fantasies and general instability caused her as much unhappiness as they did anyone else, and were always far too inconsistent to be a part of a preconceived plan. A former member of her staff told me, 'Diana was really like an expensive computer – lots of exciting features to admire, but the hard drive was broken.'

On the morning of the wedding, Diana awoke in Clarence House to a stunning day. The deep blue sky was a perfect contrast to the odd white cloud and the bright, warm summer sun. She got up and excitedly watched the live coverage of the crowd outside on television. She was on top form. All the moods, tantrums and jealousies were put behind her as she appeared relaxed, calm and to be really enjoying the moment. She was a lot less nervous than most brides, and yet she was about to embark upon the most watched wedding of all time.

Kevin Stanley arrived to do her hair. Barbara Daly did her make-up. David and Liz Emanuel supervised the dressing of the bride and bridesmaids. Diana stood in her ivory dress. Then Stanley placed the Spencer tiara on her head. She looked stunning. The Queen Mother commented, 'My dear, you look simply enchanting,' before leaving for Buckingham Palace.

Then it was time to go herself. The Emanuels packed Diana and her train into the Glass Coach. The train was so long that the last few feet had to be piled on to Earl Spencer's lap. Diana burst into a chorus of 'Just one Cornetto', and everybody laughed. She looked a picture of happiness. She was about to take centre stage, the adrenalin was flowing, doubt was banished and the people's love was a beneficial elixir: this was the fairy-tale day she had dreamed of.

The Prince of Wales, who had had trouble going to sleep, was eventually awoken by the noise of the crowd who were wearing Union Jack pork-pie hats and cheering any sign of activity at the palace where the main balcony was already draped in crimson for the occasion. The Mall was decorated with 150 union flags hanging from flagstaffs crowned in gold. Flowers were hanging from the lamp-posts and every building seemed to be dressed in red, white and blue bunting.

Invited guests were making their way towards St Paul's. Just after ten o' clock, a procession of black limousines transported the world's royalty from the palace to the cathedral in order of seniority. Shortly after 10.20 a.m. the Queen's carriage set out, followed by the Queen Mother along with Princesses Anne and Margaret.

Royalty, politicians and military men on horses were all cheered by a crowd of over a million. The enthusiasm of the people in Trafalgar Square was so loud that Earl Spencer mistook St Martin-in-the-Fields for St Paul's and started to get up; his daughter smiled and held him back. She was wearing a signet ring that the Prince of Wales had sent over to Clarence House the previous evening. It was accompanied by a note that read, 'I am so proud of you and when you come up I'll be there at the altar for you tomorrow. Just look 'em in the eye and knock 'em dead.'

The Prince had been more closely involved with the wedding-service preparations than Lady Diana. With the help of the director of the Royal College of Music, Sir David Willcocks, the Prince had personally chosen much of the music. This included 'Christ is Made the Sure Foundation' and Kiri Te Kanawa singing 'Let the Bright Seraphim'. At his invitation, his fiancée chose 'I Vow to Thee My Country'. In a television interview two days before the wedding, the Prince said, 'I can't wait for the whole thing. I want everybody to come out having had a marvellous musical and emotional experience.'

As Diana entered the cathedral she was being watched by three quarters of a billion people around the world. Anthony Holden, the Prince of Wales's biographer was one of 180 staff supporting Barbara Walters who presented the ABC network's coverage in the US. ABC deployed several hundred cameras, tens of mobile studios, 750 miles of cable, satellites and a balloon floating high in the sky for overhead shots. CBS chose Lady Antonia Fraser, Dan Rather and David Frost to head their team, and the NBC network advertised 'The Wedding of the Century – when England's future king says "I Do" and a shy 20-year-old girl turns into a royal princess. Watch the fairy tale come true.' For all three American networks this was the biggest coast-to-coast, live and open-ended broadcast there had ever been.

In Britain, the BBC backed Angela Rippon with 60 outside broadcast cameras, 12 mobile control rooms and some 300 staff. ITV's coverage was of a similar proportion. The UK audience was the biggest ever – 39 million. It broke the previous record by more than 6 million – when England had played Brazil in a World Cup football match in 1970.

Diana walked gracefully down the aisle, her twenty-five-foot train billowing majestically behind her, held in place by the magnificent Spencer diamond tiara. She was on the arm of her father, who was still a little unsteady following his stroke, but managing fine. This was his family's moment of great glory. Diana was now delivering what the previous seven earls had always dreamed of. Together they negotiated the 650 feet of carpet, with the notes of Jeremiah Clark's 'Trumpet Voluntary' ringing in their ears.

As the bride walked towards Prince Charles, she later recalled, 'I remember being so in love with my husband. I absolutely thought I was the luckiest girl in the world. He was going to look after me.' She then claims to have scanned the congregation for family and friends. She noticed Margaret Thatcher off to the right, and off to the left and some rows back, 'Camilla, pale grey pillbox hat. Saw it all. Her son Tom standing on a chair. To this day, you know. Vivid memory. "Well, there you are, let's hope that's all over with."'

In both cases her observations were recalled years later when self-justification and the vilification of others were on her mind. Nevertheless, they are interesting for a number of reasons. Firstly, a rerun of the video footage fails to detect her looking to either side and secondly, the first thought of love and serenity, fitting with the occasion, seems at odds with the second, which in any event would have been a lot more than 'let's hope that's all over with' in Diana's mind, given her obsessive jealousy towards Camilla. I cannot be certain, but I believe she felt the first and probably not the second as any thought towards Camilla, whom she knew was going to be there, would have been far worse than that if it had sprung to mind in the first place. But her mind wasn't in that set. At that moment it was neither anxious nor neurotic. On this day, the most important so far in her life, she had thankfully left her 'other side' at home. This was Diana at her best, Diana on parade – and no doubt her focus was totally on herself, and not speculating about what the woman in the pale grey pillbox hat was up to.

Moreover, there is a third interesting point – 'he was going to look after me'. Diana continually makes reference to this hope before her marriage and chastises Charles for failing to do so after it. If you wish to become the Princess of Wales, then it is your job and duty to assist the Prince in looking after the realm and not the other way round. It is one of the most arduous, difficult and demanding jobs in the world, not one that should be taken on if one expects permanent pampering. Diana's continual reference to being looked after is yet another indication that she failed, or even refused, to understand what being the Princess of Wales really involved.

Inside the cathedral there were 2,700 guests. Getting the right mix of important people and cherished friends and retainers had been a major problem. The Prince of Wales insisting on finding places for real friends and dependents, including housemaids from Windsor Castle and Buckingham Palace, at the expense of the traditional list of the great and the good that had been drawn up by household staff, made this even more difficult. On one list of prospective guests, which included 21 sovereigns, 20 heads of state and 26 governors-general, he noted against the figure of 281 of the diplomatic corps, 'Ridiculous.'

In addition the Spencers, always a more openly warring family than the Windsors, decided to complicate matters further with the animosities that divided them. Several of Diana's family threatened to boycott the service altogether if Barbara Cartland, Diana's step-grandmother, was allowed to attend. Edward Adeane had even dared to suggest, in desperation, that someone be sent to prevail upon the novelist to stay away. But happily, before anyone had been selected for this unenviable task, the threat was lifted.

Diana and her father continued on their graceful procession through the cathedral. As they reached the front she was now surrounded by the massed royalty of the world. In front of them and on her right were the Queen, Prince Phillip and the Queen Mother. On her left were her mother and grandmother. Then she finally reached Prince Charles, and the Archbishop of Canterbury, Robert Runcie, proclaimed, 'This is the stuff of which fairy tales are made: the Prince and Princess on their wedding day.'

Years later, Runcie supposedly suggested he had privately concluded that he knew it wasn't a fairy-tale marriage and that the Prince was having an affair. In fairness to Robert Runcie, however, this story cannot be verified; indeed it has since been hotly denied on this behalf. It would appear to be yet another story that has sprung up and nobody seems to know from where it came. But none of this was worrying the congregation inside the cathedral or the nation outside on the streets or in front of their television sets as both Diana and Prince Charles slightly fluffed their lines in what was otherwise a perfect advert for fairy tales that even the largest of Hollywood budgets would have struggled to match.

An even larger crowd cheered the couple on their way back to Buckingham Palace in an open carriage. Andrew Parker Bowles was among the guard that rode behind them. Once they had passed, the barriers were lifted and hundreds of thousands of people streamed down the Mall and raced, like an incoming tide, round either side of the Victoria memorial.

Eventually, the Royal Family and their Spencer in-laws came out on to the balcony to face a sea of happy faces, all packed in like sardines and looking up at them. The people called for the bridegroom to kiss his bride. He duly obliged with a rather chaste effort. Then, apparently goaded by Prince Andrew and overcoming his own diffidence and sense of decorum, he had a second go and kissed his bride fully and lovingly on the lips. The newspapers and television were to use the shot over and over again: it was a lasting image that suggested 'and they all lived happily ever after'. And although they didn't, it was nevertheless an immensely happy day. The country was going through a difficult time and the wedding had provided just the reminder of past glories and future possibilities that it needed. Opinion polls suggested that the monarchy was now every bit as popular as it had ever been.

The Prince of Wales was deeply touched by the popular outpouring of love for his princess and himself. He wrote to one of his friends a few days later, 'What an unbelievable day it was that went far too quickly. I couldn't somehow savour all I wanted to savour and I was totally overwhelmed and overcome by the way in which the whole country seemed to have been a favourite guest at the wedding, right down to the way everyone cheered when we said "I will" etc., and then threw confetti at us when we drove to Waterloo. It was one of the most moving experiences I have ever known ... a revelation to find the real heart and soul of the nation being exposed for a moment in good, old-fashioned, innocent enjoyment ...'

And years later Diana's mother was asked by *Hello!* magazine, 'While Diana was certainly love-struck over the Prince of Wales did you ever have cause to doubt his feelings?'

'No,' she replied, 'and I think that if anybody does doubt how he originally felt then they should look at the pictures or film of their wedding day. I think they really did show genuine happiness and deep affection for each other.'

The planned honeymoon has been described by some as a disaster that could have been avoided if the Prince had swept Diana off to a quiet, sun-drenched island where they could have been as alone as members of the Royal Family ever can be. Others claim that it was right that it reflected how royal life was to be in the future for her and so the sooner that Diana got used to her new position, the better. Either way, it is quite unlikely to have made a significant difference to their future.

The plan was to spend a couple of days at Broadlands. The Romseys moved out in order to give the newlyweds some privacy, but

Diana was aware that Prince Charles had taken a number of former girlfriends to stay there prior to meeting her, and she took the fact that he brought seven van der Post books with him as a personal slight, concluding that he was more interested in reading than in her. Charles looked forward to teaching Diana about books and introducing her to a new world of education. Unlike most of his family, he wasn't a philistine, and he expected to help Diana improve her mind. He liked the idea of the two of them sitting out in the sun silently reading while enjoying each other's company and occasionally stopping to reflect and share a meaningful passage. But Diana didn't really like reading, so as he read, she quickly became bored. To make matters worse, when she finally got his attention he only seemed to talk about what he had read: 'He read them and we had to analyse them over lunch every day,' she was later to complain. Prince Charles even attempted to interest the Princess by reading passages of van der Post aloud to her, but his attempts only triggered her inferiority complex and so she would wander off.

From Broadlands they flew to Gibraltar to join the Royal Yacht for a two-week cruise of the Mediterranean and Aegean seas. Of course, having twenty-one naval officers and a crew of 256 men, a marine band, a valet, a private secretary and an equerry on honeymoon with you can't have been easy; on the other hand, how many couples would turn down the opportunity to spend their honeymoon in such luxury? But it did mean that time alone together was limited. Charles was naturally used to this. It had, after all, been his life for as long as he could remember. Diana, unsurprisingly, found it much harder to accept. It was a rude awakening for her that even at private times like honeymoons, the Royal Family is never really alone. When they weren't receiving dignitaries, such as President Sadat and his wife in Port Said, they shared their candlelit dinners on deck with the ship's officers as a band of Royal Marines serenaded them.

However, it wasn't all bad. They often sailed a dinghy together, swam and sunbathed and expressed their delight in each other's company in lots of genuinely happy letters sent home to thank family, friends and staff for gifts and their efforts towards making the actual wedding such a resounding success. Many eye witnesses recorded seeing lots of touching, happy scenes, and felt that the couple were genuinely besotted with each other. And they were: Diana was infatuated with Charles, while he was delighted by her physical beauty and the prospect of the future love and affection marriage would bring – provided her 'other side' could keep away.

The Prince made allowances for Diana's lack of education and her youthful immaturity. Although not amused, he wasn't that annoyed when she discovered Pimm's, got completely drunk and threw a bucket of water over his head in front of half the ship's company. To her it was just high spirits, but he knew that the future king of England should not be seen with a tipsy wife demeaning him. Nevertheless, he also knew that it would take time for Diana to learn the ropes and not become a threat to protocol. If she would try, as she had assured him that she would, then it would all turn out all right in the end. He was to write while on board that, 'All I can say is that marriage is very jolly and it's extremely nice being together in Britannia. Diana dashes about chatting up all the sailors and the cooks in the galley, while I sit hermit-like on the veranda deck, sunk with pure joy into one of Laurens van der Post's books.'

However, behind the scenes his young wife was less at ease. She didn't like being told what to do by people she didn't want on her honeymoon in the first place and with whom she had to share the Prince. In addition, she found it very hard to understand that if a member of the Royal Family is on board the Royal Yacht, local dignitaries would be offended if they were not invited on board to pay their respects when she docked in their port.

By this time her anorexia seems to have turned into bulimia, and it was appalling – up to four times a day while they were on the yacht. 'Anything I could find I would gobble up and be sick two minutes later – very tired. So of course, that slightly got the mood swings going in the sense that one minute one would be happy, next blubbing one's eyes out.'

During this phase of the honeymoon there were two particular incidents that Diana seems to have remembered very clearly. Both related to Camilla. Firstly, Diana claims a photograph fell out of Charles's diary when they were comparing engagements. It was a picture of Camilla. The Prince's official biographer, Jonathan Dimbleby, does not mention the story and nobody else can remember it occurring at the time. Secondly, when dressed for a white-tie dinner with President Sadat, the Prince wore a pair of cufflinks, engraved with interwoven Cs. 'Got it in one,' Diana said later. 'Knew exactly. "Camilla gave you those, didn't she?" He said: "Yes, so what's wrong?

They're a present from a friend." And, boy, did we have a row. Jealousy, total jealousy …'

Neither of these stories can be verified; although the second may well have happened as the cufflinks in question do exist. They probably did have a huge row, but it would have been very one-sided as this was to become the pattern of their disagreements. Diana screamed and shouted and burst into tears. Prince Charles, while being most capable of displaying hot temper himself, was not used to being shouted at by anyone. He was completely perplexed. Her rages were quite terrifying and he was completely unable to pacify her. He couldn't win. If he tried to argue back or even reason with her, she would refuse to listen and would just shout him down. If he refused to engage in the row, this only served to infuriate her all the more and she would become even more hysterical. If he attempted to walk away and allow her to cool down, she would simply respond by screaming the house down. She could often be heard all over Balmoral Castle, much to her husband's embarrassment and the Queen's displeasure.

From Egypt the bride and groom flew to Lossiemouth in Scotland and drove to Balmoral for the third and longest stage of their honeymoon – a month living on Prince Charles's favourite royal estate. Although Diana was to later complain about all three stages of her honeymoon, she had been consulted when the arrangements were made and had played her part in planning it. Perhaps it just didn't turn out the way that she had imagined it would. It seemed to her to have turned into an obstacle course. First there were the boring books, then the bloody dinners with either the Royal Naval officers or some awful dignitaries, and now she would have to put up with her disciplined in-laws and their constant way of doing things – and no doubt some of Charles's dreadful friends, who made her feel so inferior, would also turn up.

So while the Prince settled down with his books and fishing rod to enjoy his favourite time of the year, Diana was starting to bubble over with pent-up anger. Even small things seemed to infuriate her. She didn't like the fact that at pre-dinner drinks Prince Charles would serve his mother and grandmother ahead of her. This was correct as royal procedure dictated that they were served first as the senior royal ladies present. However, Diana wanted him to serve her first, as she was his wife.

Nevertheless, she turned up at a press conference by the Brig o'Dee looking tanned and relaxed and said that she could 'thoroughly recommend married life'. The Prince by comparison looked very gloomy. The press weren't to know that prior to this meeting he had spent an hour persuading her to keep her promise to attend. The apparently happy girl who had charmed the cameras was by now behaving very differently behind the scenes. The Prince's favourite place in the world wasn't hers. They would go up to a remote hill in Balmoral where Charles would read Laurens van der Post or Jung to Diana. She recalled, 'I hadn't a clue about psychic powers or anything....So anyway we read those and I did my tapestry and he was blissfully happy.'

These are interesting words. They come from a woman who was to claim that her husband had only married her in order to produce a son and heir before returning to his permanent mistress and yet, up a mountain alone with his new wife, he was 'blissfully happy'.

Long before they were due to leave, Diana announced that she wanted to go to London. She explained that Balmoral was wet, cold and boring. The Prince reminded her that she had told him it was her favourite place on earth. She cheekily responded that that had been before they were married. He pointed out that the court was now at Balmoral and that they would have to stay. It was part of their job. When she didn't get her own way, she threw a tantrum and declared that if he really loved her he would put her first and take her to London. Later, she remembered 'crying my eyes out ... At night I dreamt of Camilla the whole time ... Everybody saw I was getting thinner and thinner ... Didn't trust him, thought every five minutes he was ringing her up ... It rained and rained and rained ...'

There was absolutely no evidence that the Prince was having any communication with Mrs Parker Bowles, but nothing he could do or say seemed to reassure the Princess. The Royal Family, who had been so impressed and delighted with the friendly and charmingly funny young girl of the previous summer, were now amazed by the change in her personality. Far from being the carefree girl who seemed to like them all so much, they were now confronted by a moody young woman who seemed to sulk permanently unless she was receiving the total, undivided attention of Prince Charles.

So the girl who had auditioned for the job so successfully the previous summer by joining in everything with great enthusiasm now hated the castle, the countryside and the Royal Family's obsession with horses and dogs. And all the time she was suffering from terrible mood swings and continued to lose weight at an alarming rate. The Prince was kind and constantly defensive about her, but he had absolutely no idea what the problem was. He couldn't understand why she wouldn't eat. He would try and encourage her with a 'Come on, darling, this is delicious,' as he passed her a fork of this or a spoon of that at picnics, but to no avail.

These tales of the Princess not eating while at Balmoral are confusing. They can be verified and they seem to suggest that Diana was suffering from anorexia. Anorexics reject food: the very idea of eating makes them feel ill. Bulimics binge-eat and then vomit. Is it possible for an anorexic to be bulimic as the thought of eating is repulsive to them? Diana has admitted in her own words that while she was on the Royal Yacht she was binge eating and vomiting four times a day. However, her mother has confirmed that she was originally anorexic, claiming that she 'saw it immediately because I'd had previous experience of anorexia with my daughter Sarah. It is a stressful illness and I knew quite a lot about it.' Therefore was it possible that Diana was anorexic, became bulimic and then reverted to anorexia in a space of weeks? Or was there another explanation?

What, if anything, was wrong with Diana and how it occurred is the most crucial element of her story. Were Diana's versions of these and later events reliable? This question must be properly considered if we are to unravel fact from fiction. In order to do this, I contacted the Priory Hospital at Roehampton in England. The Priory is world-famous for treating mental illness often brought on by alcohol and drug addiction, substance abuse or eating disorders. They kindly sent me their latest research note on bulimia nervosa, written by Dr Peter Rowan MBBS, MRCPsych.

The paper reports that, 'Bulimia Nervosa is an illness that is most commonly found in girls of later adolescence and early adulthood. It is rarely found in men.' It goes on to explain that there are three types of bulimia, 'Simple, Anorexic, and Multi-impulsive Bulimia Nervosa. There is quite a lot of overlap between them so there are a number of sufferers who show characteristics that belong midway between these subgroups.' As a result it is possible for a patient to progress from one type to another.

Simple bulimia is the type that Diana readily admitted to. It is the least serious. It is 'an illness that begins most commonly when the girls are about eighteen years of age. They are a fairly normal group before the illness...The illness is frequently triggered by a period of unhappiness and this is often caused by a destructive relationship with a boyfriend. The feeling of self-dislike focuses on appearance and dieting is begun in an attempt to improve self-esteem. In contrast to an anorexic the diet is not very successful with the rigid control needed breaking down into bouts of cheating. Vomiting is used as part of increased efforts to achieve the weight loss and so the cycle of bingeing and vomiting begins. There is further loss of control as the body's normal mechanisms of appetite control are overridden and become confused. The weight will remain close to normal but the eating pattern becomes gradually worse. This form of bulimia is the least severe but the severity varies considerably. It is likely that there are a large number of girls with fairly mild symptoms that never come to medical help but there is a significant risk that it will slowly get worse in time.'

The Princess of Wales could claim, as a sufferer of this type, that she was coming from a 'fairly normal group' and that her illness might have been triggered by 'a destructive relationship with a boyfriend'. This way her illness could be portrayed as almost usual and probably the fault of her husband. However, it is extremely unlikely that the Princess was suffering from this type of bulimia. Firstly, she was anorexic before she was bulimic – this is not a route into simple bulimia; secondly, her weight did not remain close to normal but dropped alarmingly; thirdly, her symptoms, by her own admission, weren't to get worse slowly but accelerated quickly; and fourthly, she displayed other symptoms that are unique to the other two types of bulimia.

'Anorexia Bulimia Nervosa is a variant of the illness that is preceded by a bout of Anorexia Nervosa. Quite often this anorexic episode is a brief one and the sufferer begins to recover without treatment. It is followed typically by a short period of stabilised weight just below that at which the menstruation may restart, around 46 kg. The control of the anorexic is not sustained and bingeing begins usually in a very small way but becomes more severe especially once vomiting begins ... The illness becomes dominated by the bingeing and vomiting behaviour but the weight remains low for a while before gradually rising to near and in time above normal. The personality profile and backgrounds of these girls is similar as for a group with Anorexia Nervosa.' The Princess almost certainly entered bulimia nervosa via anorexia nervosa, and her weight pattern throughout her life seemed to have followed this course. Indeed, just before she died she had put on sufficient weight to encourage questions of whether she might be pregnant. However, there is an absence of many other behavioural patterns and character traits that the Princess had and which can only be associated with the third category.

Multi-impulsive bulimia nervosa is a 'severe variant of Bulimia Nervosa that begins in a similar way to Simple Bulimia and in a similar age group of girls. This group suffer with a range of abnormal behaviours all of which indicate problems of emotional and impulse control. Often some of these other behaviours are already causing difficulty before bulimia begins. In association with the eating disorder will be found a mix of other problems including drug abuse, alcohol abuse, deliberate self-harm (usually cutting the forearms), stealing and promiscuity. They have a range of backgrounds but it is quite common to find that there is a high level of disturbance within the family. In personality they are likely to have shown evidence of poor impulse control from an early age and they often have rather poor records of schooling, academic achievement, or making friends last. They have a difficulty in modifying their behaviour because of predictable consequences of their actions and as a result helping them to change the pattern of their lives often requires prolonged help. The severity of the illness, as with all types of Bulimia, is varied and in this group it seems to depend on [the] severity of the underlying abnormality personality.'

I have no evidence of any serious drug or alcohol abuse by Diana, or any evidence of her stealing. However, the rest of this piece could have been written personally for her as it perfectly describes her characteristics and her background. Moreover, someone with multi-impulsive bulimia nervosa is only likely to seek help when there is no alternative left or when a united front of family and friends combine to force the issue. As in similar circumstances concerning alcoholics or drug addicts, the victims are in denial and the problem, as they see it, is with the rest of the world rather than them. However, they are at risk from attempted suicide or self-harm when inevitable bouts of short but sometimes deep depression arise.

In light of this, it becomes clear that without the selfish and misguided support that various so-called friends and hangers-on gave her in the later part of her life, Diana might have listened to those who really wanted to help her and received the treatment she needed. Those friends enabled her to escape that prolonged help by either supporting or even encouraging her deceit. This was to have the affect of condemning her to a frail and unstable life. These people know who they are and, in my opinion, they must now accept at least some of the responsibility for what happened.

The Princess was definitely suffering from both anorexia nervosa at one point and a variant of bulimia nervosa at another. The variant may have started with anorexic bulimia nervosa, but it overlapped into multi-impulsive bulimia nervosa.

What causes these illnesses? Dr Peter Rowan says that the causes remain mainly unknown, 'although there is probably a small genetic contribution'. This would appear to be supported by the Princess's case, as she wasn't the only member of her family to suffer from the illness. He adds, 'Once established, bulimia influences the way the emotions are felt. It protects the sufferer from experiencing feelings that may be to them unbearable. It is paradoxical that bulimia causes them to become increasingly out of control in a wide variety of ways and yet it is the one thing that enables them to feel in control. Their fear of being without this protection maintains and increases the severity of the illness, which comes to dominate all emotional experience. Once the illness has become established the trigger to binge is often partly or wholly related to feelings. Periods of depression, boredom, and anger are likely to increase the risk ...'

So does this mean that multi-impulsive bulimia is or becomes a symptom of an underlying abnormality of the personality? Apparently so, and the collection of feelings and emotions that can trigger and then sustain multi-impulsive bulimia are grouped under the title of borderline personality disorder. When this condition was first described in the US in 1938, it was considered by some American psychiatrists to be potentially controversial. This is not true today. In 2001 the American Psychiatric Association Board of Trustees in the US approved a new practice guideline for the treatment of patients with borderline personality disorder in response to feedback from members that there was an urgent need for one and that case levels had reached sufficient levels for several years in America to supply the necessary data for it.

In the same year, Psychejam.com created a pneumonic to assist easy symptom recognition:

B = boredom easily felt
O = overdoses common
R = rapid mood shifts
D = deliberate self-harm
E = empty feelings
R = relationship difficulties
L = lack of ability to self-soothe
I = impulsive
N = negative self-image
E = emotionally unstable

The Princess of Wales experienced all but 'overdoses common' – unless you count an overdose of the media – on a regular basis.

Also in 2001, *Psychiatry and Clinical Neurosciences* published a research document by Tatsuo Ohshima, MD, PhD of the Chibaken Sodegaura Welfare Centre, in Japan. Its declared objective was to present a study that demonstrated the traits of the psychopathology of borderline personality disorder with hysterical neurosis. His method was to compare them by 'statistical analysis so as to perform positive research'. He pointed out that while the notion of hysteria originated with the ancient Greeks, borderline had only had a history of just over half a century and therefore he thought the time had come 'to discriminate the psychopathology of BPD from hysterical disease by comparative study in our clinical psychiatry in order to treat these patients exactly.' His conclusion was that BPD had some independent traits when compared to hysterical neurosis, but that there was some difficulty in discriminating the two disorders symptomatically.

People who believe that Diana wasn't mentally unwell usually fall into two camps: those who believe she was just an evil manipulator and a less-than-honest drama queen, and those who think she was perfect and that stories of her being 'mad' have been put about by Prince Charles's friends in order to discredit her. It has long been argued by both that the Princess shouldn't be tarred with this borderline personality disorder brush because the diagnosis of such an illness isn't always accepted, and there is still scepticism in some British medical circles as to whether this illness really exists. If the illness doesn't exist, Diana couldn't have had it and therefore she couldn't have been medically unwell.

In fact, as all the symptoms can be proved to have existed by their endless examples, it simply means that if the Princess wasn't suffering from borderline personality disorder, she was clearly suffering from some strain of hysterical neurosis as yet unnamed. No doubt, now that BPD is accepted in the mainstream of medicine across the world, any remaining doubting Thomases will eventually agree to call such a strain borderline personality disorder.

A very well-known Sloane Street doctor she consulted told me that her condition was of a 'nature that that having to live with her might almost be as bad as having to be her. Her illness was serious and must have been hell to live with for all concerned.'

What did he mean? The society psychiatrist Dr Michael Davies explains that, 'In the early eighties, the doctors were not sure whether she was merely mentally ill or psychotic. There's an important distinction between the two conditions. If you're mentally ill but basically normal – in other words, your everyday, seriously disturbed neurotic – you're treatable as long as you want help. With cooperation, you may well be curable. But if you are psychotic, that means you're insane. That makes you a lot less treatable, and the cure rate is not encouraging.

'She was exhibiting symptoms which could be interpreted either way. There was bulimia, which is a serious mental illness and can lead to death. There was the clinical depression, which is another serious mental illness and led to her uncle's suicide. There was the self-mutilation, which was not severe and struck me as histrionic rather than serious, but which nevertheless had to be classified as a mental illness and had to be taken seriously. More worrying, she was exhibiting symptoms of paranoia and schizophrenia symptoms, incidentally, which she continued exhibiting, in varying degrees of severity, until her death. So the question everyone wanted to know was: is she a bulimic/depressive/self-mutilating neurotic, or is she a paranoid-schizophrenic whose symptoms are manifesting in those terms? Her behaviour certainly indicated that she was, if not a fully-fledged paranoid-schizophrenic, suffering from Borderline Personality Disorder. The question the doctors had to ask was – is this a girl who cannot fit in and cannot take responsibility for her actions, so projects her incapacity onto others, or is she someone who has unwarranted suspicions, who imagines plots and schemes where there are none, who has a fractured personality and wavers between seeming reasonableness and overt irrationality?'

I asked the Sloane Street doctor which one it was. He smiled, put his hands up and said, 'Who knows? But I suspect the second.' What did that mean? He said that it meant that without any doubt she was a very seriously ill young woman, possibly untreatable, and that she had probably been ill in varying degrees from puberty until her death.

As a result Diana, Princess of Wales was in need of special care and even if it had been properly administered she might not have been cured. However, if she'd stuck with one doctor or psychiatrist and cooperated with them, there was perhaps a possibility that those who knew her privately would have seen a lot more of the thoroughly decent woman that was glimpsed by them when occasionally her storm clouds lifted. However, it remains highly unlikely that any doctor could have ever got her into a state where she could have coped with the rigours of being Princess of Wales.

Mainly because she was so publicly hysterical and histrionic in front of the servants and some of them couldn't resist the brown envelopes stuffed with ten-pound notes offered by the tabloid press, stories about how unhappy Diana already was started to appear in the *Sun* and the *News of the World* before the honeymoon was over. By the end of September stories had already been printed concerning rows with Charles, her hatred of Balmoral and her dislike of royal protocol. The Prince, while remaining kind and concerned, refused to alter his habits of a lifetime on what was clearly his favourite month of the year. This did not help Diana feel less lonely or bored as she, having declined to accompany him, waited long hours for his return. To make matters worse, that September was particularly wet.

Charles asked Michael Colborne to travel up from London on the overnight train especially so that he could keep the Princess company at Craigowan Lodge on the estate while he went out deerstalking. From nine in the morning, when the Princess, who had arranged to go for a walk with Penny Romsey but instead led Colborne from the kitchen and the waiting friend – without even acknowledging her – into the drawing room, to four that afternoon, Colborne sat with Diana. Sometimes she was angry and poured out her complaints, amid floods of tears, against her absent husband, his family, the boredom, Balmoral and the weather. Sometimes she was silent and sat brooding. At one point she remained so for over an hour. Then she would explode again and kick the furniture as she paced the room. At four she calmly announced that she was going upstairs and left. Colborne felt exhausted.

The Prince was feeling the strain as well. Later that day, and after they had all witnessed another slanging match, the Prince tossed Diana's wedding ring at Colborne in the dark drive as he prepared to leave for London with the Prince. It was already too big for her finger due to her weight loss and needed to be altered. In the car on the way to the station, the Prince rounded on Colborne with an explosion of hot temper concerning a trivial point about his new Range Rover's carpets. He didn't draw breath for over an hour. Colborne had had a terrible day. First the girl that he liked seemed to be disintegrating into a mental wreck and then the Prince, whom he dearly loved and loyally supported, had turned on him over some minor point that hadn't even been his fault.

However, once on the train, the Prince calmed down and opened up to Colborne. For the next five hours they discussed his marriage. The Prince told him that he was at a loss to know why it was going so wrong or what could be done to put matters right – which, he explained, he earnestly wanted to do for the good of everyone, not least the Princess herself, about whom he was becoming increasingly concerned.

In October, the Prince persuaded Diana that she needed professional help and he took her back to London. Diana then explained to the doctors that her only problem was that she needed time to adapt. She refused to accept that she might be seriously ill. She made no mention of her bulimia. They accepted her diagnosis and merely prescribed Valium, which she rejected on the grounds that they were trying to silence her by sedation. When Prince Charles found out he was also appalled, having always been against drugs of any sort.

Later Diana was to complain that an interminable circus of analysts and psychiatrists paid her a visit. 'Put me on high doses of Valium and everything else. But the Diana that was still very much there had decided it was just time; patience and adapting were all that were needed. They were telling me "pills!" That was going to keep them happy – they could go to bed at night and sleep, knowing that the Princess of Wales wasn't going to stab anyone.'

It had not been the happiest of starts to married life, and it must have seemed a long time since that happy day in late July. It had been just over two months.

Howard Hodgson

Part Three
The Birth of Children, and of an Icon

Howard Hodgson

Chapter Eight
It Wasn't Always Bad (1981–86)

Now back in London and preparing for her first joint venture with her husband, a visit to Wales, Diana attempted to pull herself together. It had not been a happy time, but she was still desperately in love with Charles, and he encouraged her every effort, determined that a poor start to their married life could be put behind them if the Princess grew in confidence and banished the doubts and the imagined intrigues from her mind. She remained ill, and the position was far from easy, but she was determined to make the tour and not let her husband down. He remained totally committed to her, and still believed it would only be a matter of time before everything fell into place.

Moreover, they had a secret: the Princess was pregnant, and this made Charles absolutely thrilled. Diana might be struggling in other departments, but she was already proving to be more successful in this area of royal duty than many of her predecessors. Prince Charles wanted more than anything to have a family; in addition, he, like many others at court, could put her continued sickness, changing moods and bouts of depression down to the pregnancy.

He might have drawn comfort from this thought, but that alone would not get his wife through the rigours of their first trip. What could be done? It was virgin territory: there hadn't been a princess of Wales in living memory, nor had there been a family member as obviously mentally fragile. It was difficult to know where to start, and those who attempted found that Diana had become quickly accustomed to her HRH status and would usually dismiss even the friendliest of advice in the belief that she should be suspicious of such people's motives. This belief that courtiers and the Queen alike were plotting against her made advising her almost impossible, and so many people simply gave up.

This was not made any easier by Prince Charles's own lack of confidence and self-esteem, which prevented him from stepping back and perhaps taking a more measured and detached look at the problem. In addition, he suffered from all the problems that monarchy inevitably dumps on its members. He was used to being treated like a star and being the centre of attention. It would be quite impossible for any normal human being not to be affected by such a life. Members of the Windsor family are used to lapping up compliments from their own personal courtiers, friends and staff while handing out no similar praise themselves. The Windsors are known to be jealous of other family members' popularity with the public – no doubt because of their dedication to the job and the public, otherwise why would it bother them? This has led each member of the family to paddle their own canoe and make their own way inside the family business. There are few joint efforts. As a result it must have seemed very strange for Charles to have one so dependent and yet so undisciplined in his care. It was a new and unique experience for him.

The special conditions in which the Royal Family is bound to operate demand a conditioning of the mind in order to complete the unique task of monarchy. Every successful enterprise in life needs essential rhythms and disciplines. However, their particular cocktail of duty, discipline, reserve, being fawned over, privilege and luxury, all the while being expected to play out their lives in the royal goldfish bowl, requires that they adopt a stiff, repetitive and aloof style in order to make the whole thing sustainable. This is the hallmark of any successful monarchy rather than what the natural characteristics of the Windsor family might otherwise be. It is a common failing of authors like Morton to judge the Windsors as normal people when the demands of the public and the nature of the job mean they are guaranteed to be anything but normal.

Indeed, Prince Charles, having been excluded from this way of life during his youth when he was away at school, at university and in the armed forces, was a lot more natural than he might otherwise have been: a prince of genuine kindness as well as intelligence and virtue had blossomed. Nevertheless, while he hadn't become a bad or unkind man, he had become much more selfish after leaving the navy and being sucked into Buckingham Palace and thus exposed to royal life permanently. Mountbatten had noted it, and had warned the Prince against it.

Moreover, by the time of his marriage he had become set in his ways. He jealously guarded his precious little private time, and expected to give the rest first and foremost to the people who would one day become his subjects. This is the pact between a monarch and his people. They give him a life of luxury provided that he accepts that he has no life other than to be their servant. Frankly, it is a very bad deal for the chosen one and only severe discipline and dedication can see it through. Prince Charles had always understood this and couldn't understand why Diana didn't. This meant that, while he was kind to her and tried to help her, he had no respect for her wish to have his constant and undivided attention. He knew that, given his public commitments, this would never be possible. It is therefore hardly surprising that, if the constant combination of duty and discipline accompanied by privilege and luxury that is royal life had affected even a virtuous prince born to it, it might completely wreck the life of a fragile girl, and at times turn her into a monster.

If he had remembered how lonely he had been as a result of his absent and aloof parents during childhood, he might have understood better and attempted to curb his obsessive work rate a little in order to accommodate her; perhaps he thought that if someone as shy and lacking in confidence as he could make it, so could she.

So while it was wholly unrealistic for Diana to have the sort of married life that she had dreamed up as a result of reading too many cheap romantic novels, the Prince might have found a little thoughtful action would have gone a lot further than thousands of kindly words. However, given the depth of her problems and her unsuitability for the task at hand, it is most doubtful that it would have made a lasting difference.

However, there is perhaps a further explanation for the immediate breakdown experienced by the Princess during her engagement and early months of marriage. In 1916 Freud declared that people achieving great success, especially when perceived by others to have done so, were far more likely to suffer such a breakdown than those who had experienced considerable failure. He put this down to a subconscious desire to deflect envy from others. The Princess, by marrying Prince Charles, had achieved her lifelong ambition and was the envy of millions of young women across the globe. She had not only married the man of her dreams, she had made herself the most famous princess in the world. This was success beyond her imagination and one that others could not hope to emulate. Given her frail mental state and the abnormality of her achievement, she would have been a perfect candidate for Freud's theory.

On 27 October they set out for Wales. Anne Beckwith-Smith was appointed her lady-in-waiting for the trip. The visit brought home the hazards of royal life as, once again, Welsh nationalists threatened to punish the Prince for visiting his principality and their country. An incendiary device was found in Pontypridd and there were the occasional anti-English and anti-royal banners, but the Prince had seen it all before and his calm helped Diana overcome any concerns she might have had. Indeed, she was vastly more frightened of the huge crowds that turned out to express their support for their prince and his beautiful new wife. But she coped – this was Diana on parade. She immediately struck a chord with the people who pressed against the barricades for a glimpse of her. She stooped down to chat to children, she touched the faces of the blind, she kissed the elderly and was altogether much more tactile than other royal women in living memory had appeared. The people reacted by holding out their hands and calling out her name as if a saint had appeared among them. And despite the appalling weather and her obviously shocking loss of weight, her demure smile made its way on to the front page of nearly every newspaper in Britain. Diana was a natural – a sensation, and Dianamania would soon be born.

However, in between these public engagements and once back on the royal train, she would break down in tears and protest to her husband that it was beyond her to confront another big crowd that day. Her energy would evaporate once the adrenalin stopped flowing, and she would be forced to yield to the strain of it all. The Prince remained calm and, with encouragement from him and Beckwith-Smith, Diana would dry her tears and summon up enough resolve to have another go.

This must have taken a lot of courage, as the Princess was genuinely overcome by it all. Diana was at this time a far cry from the woman she would later become, and while Prince Charles was in time to become both depressed and jealous by the way the crowd would groan on his side of the street by comparison to the delight they would express on hers, this was definitely not the case on these first walkabouts. His delight at the way the crowds took to Diana was evident. It was further heightened by the hope that this adoration would encourage her to keep going, and in addition he was just relieved that she was out in the street at all. He was to remark with genuine humour and some relief at the time, 'Well, at least I know my place now – I'm a carrier of flowers for my wife.'

Despite the behind-the-scenes wobbles, they pulled off a most successful tour that only confirmed their popularity and the nation's ever-growing infatuation with her.

Once back in London, the Prince of Wales continued with his heavy work schedule. He was, as ever, dashing all over the country, sometimes with Princess Diana, but more often not. On 5 November Diana's pregnancy was announced, and as a result the Prince cancelled a tour of New Zealand, Australia and Canada, scheduled for 1982, in order that he might remain with his wife. The news of the forthcoming birth was greeted with joy by the media, and there was much celebration around the country. The mayor of Tetbury toasted the royal couple under a large union flag, while the Prince, in a speech to the City of London at the Guildhall, paid tribute to Diana. In thanking his audience for the wedding, he attributed the nation's delight in the occasion 'entirely to the effect my dear wife has on the people'.

His words were genuine, and he still hoped that if he kept up appearances to the outside world, he would buy the time for Diana to sort herself out behind the scenes. But his wife didn't see it that way and rather gave up the struggle. On her return to London, she lapsed back into depression and bulimia, which was made all the worse by bad bouts of morning sickness. As a result, most of her engagements with the Prince had to be cancelled. She was apparently angry that her husband insisted on proceeding without her, and couldn't understand why he couldn't cancel as well and just spend more time with her. On the few occasions when she was able to make public appearances with him, she was showered with soft toys for the expected baby.

In late November, she made her first solo public appearance when she turned on the Christmas lights in Regent Street. By now she was looking awfully thin and the newspapers were starting to say as much. This made her all the more self-conscious and less inclined to be seen in public. She spent some of her time supervising the decoration of their new apartment in Kensington Palace, but this was by no means a full-time job and so there were many days when she did nothing but brood. Then Camilla would come to mind. She remained absolutely convinced that her husband's former mistress remained very much in position. There is no evidence whatsoever that she was, but the Prince, try as he might, was unable to reassure his wife.

Life was by now getting to be even more difficult. Diana was both ill and pregnant and nobody – not her husband, his family, her family or even the best doctors in the land – seemed to be able to assist her. Charles really did want to help her and was desperately worried about both her and their baby, but he just couldn't get through and didn't know what else to try. Moreover, he was still putting on a brave face even with members of his own family and was loath to have open discussions about his wife's problems with them. Not only was this clearly not the Windsor way, but also he considered talking about Diana in such terms as being completely disloyal to her. A friend of theirs told me that that, 'Charles was living in a private hell. The world thought she was fine, some in the household knew there was a problem, but only he and a very few knew to what extent. And because he was unable to discuss the problem with anyone he could only keep up a brave face and hope she would snap out of it.'

For her part the Princess just couldn't see things from his point of view. She really wasn't the slightest bit inclined, either due to illness or character, to try. She simply wasn't interested in his needs or duties. She just wanted him to give her one hundred percent of his time. She couldn't grasp why a future king should want to work so hard. Even if he spent time with her he would very likely cause an argument if he were to pick up a book. Those who were close to all of this, people like Michael Colborne, can confirm that the Camilla obsession was a symptom rather than a cause of this behaviour.

Her friends, who were not there at the time, have always attempted to draw attention to Camilla and imply, without any evidence, that her ongoing affair with Prince Charles was the cause of Diana's tantrums and depressions. This is because, later in her life, they were encouraged by Diana herself to believe this. As a result, they claim her behaviour was due to the fact that she felt rejected and worthless. She obviously did, but was Ms Parker Bowles the sole cause of this? Her friends have always refused to accept that she was suffering from an illness, as if to admit to a mental frailty would be to destroy her memory and class her as some insane woman who needed to be locked away. So, in denial, they are forced to find scapegoats – just as Diana had done originally.

Charles's friends, on the other hand, have always claimed that, however affectionate and attentive he was, it was never enough – a view totally supported by Diana's other lovers. A courtier of the period, who was there at the time, came much closer to the truth when he cited the Princess's bulimia, of which very little was known, in telling Clayton and Craig, 'Prince Charles is someone who is very caring, but to have a wife around who was constantly throwing wobblies when he couldn't understand why drove him almost demented.'

Despite these setbacks with the Princess's health, royal officials pushed ahead with ideas about how to define a future role for her. However, progress was slow: certain courtiers, who had originally found Diana to be a delightful young girl, were by now not so certain, and some had to even be reassured by Prince Charles himself that she didn't mean to be insulting. As a result, enthusiasm for this project waned somewhat, and this was accelerated by the Prince's own reluctance to heed the advice of Edward Adeane and his assistants. Adeane was by now alarmed by what he saw as the Prince's wild ideas and unconventional advisors. He did not approve of Charles's continued concentration on the young jobless, and was horrified that the Prince had insisted on visiting a summer camp for teenagers who were on probation. Curbing what he considered to be Charles's 'political ideas' that might bring about a constitutional 'punch-up' with Mrs Thatcher was his priority, so he felt that he couldn't spare much time on Diana's new career – especially as she didn't appear to have any serious interests on which to build.

On top of all this, Diana's education was a real concern to the Prince and members of their staff. Something would have to be done – once conversation went away from emotional issues or chit-chat, her lack of even the most basic general knowledge was a major problem that, if exposed, would soon have her labelled as a dimwit by the press. At first she appeared to want to learn and improve. However, she reacted badly to instruction and thought she was being patronised. She believed that her husband thought she was completely stupid, as he seemed to have Everett spend his day educating her. Those around at the time remember the Prince taking a kind line by continually telling her that she was a natural and that she was doing just fine, but that the media mustn't be allowed to trip her up. She took such comments to be critical and would respond that the press and the nation clearly thought she was 'bloody marvellous' already.

In despair, and for the first time believing that more than just a little time was needed for adjustment, Charles started to spend less time with her. He couldn't stand the tantrums or the outbursts in front of staff. This, to his mind unforgivable, habit of hers of wanting either to embarrass or even humiliate him in front of the household members only served to drive him away when what she wanted was to see more of him. She would wait all day genuinely wanting to see him, and then would often ruin the evening by exploding over nothing within seconds of him arriving.

This in turn put pressure on her staff. The Princess, who often wanted to do nothing but scour every edition of the tabloid press looking for photographs of herself, would often have her mood defined by whether or not the photographs and accompanying copy pleased her. If they didn't, depression would set in and she would seek out a member of staff and engage them in conversations that were far too personal for the nature of such a relationship. She would bare her soul, tell them how unhappy she was, how stuffy the Royal Family was and how heartless her husband was. They would attempt to reassure her, but would inevitably be drawn, as if totally mesmerised by her, further and further into her confidence, only to find themselves then rejected by her for reasons that they could not understand. The reason was probably that when Diana's mood was to swing in another direction, the conversations that she had had with them would have appeared to her to be both disloyal and embarrassing and she didn't wish to be reminded of them. Someone would need to be blamed for this, and her condition prevented her from ever blaming herself. Therefore it must have been the other person's fault and in disgust she would ignore their very existence – sometimes for months.

As the bouts of depression became more frequent, the Princess would sit hunched in a chair, her head on her knees, and be totally inconsolable. Once other staff members failed to lift the gloom, they concluded that it was going to take Diana longer to adjust to royal life than either she or they had expected. However, it was evident to all that something would have to be done.

Matters came to a head in December 1981. The Princess of Wales left Highgrove to buy some sweets in Tetbury. She was spotted and then cornered by some photographers, and her distress was witnessed by millions in the next day's newspapers. As a result, the Queen's press secretary Michael Shea invited all news editors to Buckingham Palace. This was the first time that this had happened since, some twenty-six years earlier, the Queen had felt obliged to do so when Prince Charles had first gone to Cheam School. They all turned up, except the editor of the *Sun*, who claimed that he had a more important meeting to attend with Rupert Murdoch. The newspaper's proprietor had no intention of taking what the Palace said about future rules very seriously, and was not going to be reined in by them.

Once at the palace, the other editors were met by Michael Shea and asked if they could give the couple a little space. He then invited them into the next room for a drink and there they were joined unexpectedly by the Queen and the Duke of Edinburgh, who mingled among them and chatted. The Queen explained to one group that Diana had not grown up used to the sort of press attention that she and her family had to endure. It must be difficult for her to discover suddenly that she was unable to go out and buy a bag of sweets without being followed by reporters and photographers. An editor from a Sunday tabloid remarked that she could always send a footman out to buy the sweets. The Queen looked him right in the eye and said, 'Do you know, I think that's the most pompous remark I've ever heard in my life.'

The battle lines had been drawn. Murdoch was going to show no respect or mercy to the Royal Family, and Diana's apparent instability was their Achilles heel. As his tactic would sell newspapers, it would mean that his competitors were bound to follow suit.

Despite everything, the marriage was not always so bleak. There were, even then, and for a sustained time later, periods of happiness. Times were occasionally like those early days of the courtship – they would roar with laughter and their evident pleasure in each other's company was a pleasure to see. These times, when she was feeling happy, he was there and nothing happened to change her mood, could result in passionate sex. Despite their other problems, both had a high libido and each found the other extremely physically attractive.

Friends can remember riotously funny lunches at Kensington Palace. The key was her mood – if it was good, Charles was usually quick to forgive her past tantrums and hope that they could now build on this current happy moment. The Christmas of 1981 was spent at Windsor Castle and was an extremely happy time. All the usual family rituals were followed as the Prince and Princess spent their first Christmas together with other members of the Royal Family. There were stockings hanging over the hearth, the exchange of inexpensive presents on Christmas Eve, carols at matins and turkey at lunch. On Boxing Day the Prince wrote a thank-you letter to a friend. In it he reported, 'We've had such a lovely Christmas – the two of us. It has been extremely happy and cosy being able to share it together … Next year will, I feel sure, be even nicer with a small one to join in as well.'

However, in early January, once the court had moved to Sandringham, as is tradition for the New Year, this new marital calm was shattered. By this time the Princess's mood had swung back under a black cloud. There was a huge argument and as usual Diana didn't seem to care who heard it. Then, as the Prince was preparing to go riding, the Princess fell down the stairs. A royal servant took the *Sun*'s shilling in exchange for this exclusive tip-off and so the paper was able to report the incident, adding that a doctor had been called and that he was happily able to announce that no harm had befallen either mother or baby.

Years later this episode took on a much greater significance when Diana told Andrew Morton that she was at the end of her tether due to the Prince's indifference towards her. She explained that she was so desperate that she threatened suicide. He apparently called her bluff, said she was melodramatic and refused to listen, and left to go riding. In her desperation she threw herself down the main staircase and landed at the feet of the Queen, who appeared white with shock and shaking with fear. None of this, apparently, had influenced the Prince not to go riding, and when he returned he was as dismissive of her as ever. This recollection, made years later, is confirmed by her friends who recall being told more or less the same story in the early 1990s. They weren't there at the time and so believed Diana's account that a cold and indifferent husband drove her to such extreme behaviour.

Diana even expanded on this version of events just after the Morton book was published by telling certain friends, who included Elsa Bowker, that the reason for her attempted suicide was that she had broken into her husband's desk and had found love letters from Camilla to him; as a result she had concluded that it wasn't worth either living or having a baby. There is no evidence whatsoever that such letters existed. Indeed, I rather think that if they had, Diana would have made dramatic use of them at some later date.

Jonathan Dimbleby's biography of Prince Charles in 1994 repeated much of Morton's story and explains that the Prince had probably reached the end of his own tether by her refusal to be pacified by him, and had decided that from now on he would ignore her rages. Dimbleby also pointed out that this was only the first in a number of 'messages of complete desperation' – feigned suicide attempts or self-harm attacks.

But the story doesn't end there. In 1995 Diana changed her version of events altogether. In an interview with Lady Colin Campbell, probably given as part of a plan to get the writer back on side and thus prevent her from writing a sequel to her critical *Diana in Private*, she denied that any of this had happened at all, and blamed Morton for distorting what he had been told by his sources, referring to him as a creep. She claimed that Morton had invented the 'cry for help' and said that only a man would think like that as it was obvious that no woman would ever harm her unborn baby. She pointed out that the story made her look like 'a mad woman from a third-rate opera'. Of course she was right, but in an act of spectacular denial she apparently forgot that it was her who had made the story up in the first place.

Morton waited until after Diana's death to clear his name. He then published the transcripts of the tapes. This is what she had actually said: 'I threw myself down the stairs. Charles said I was crying wolf and I said that I felt so desperate and I was crying my eyes out and he said: "I'm not going to listen. You're always doing this to me. I'm going riding now." So I threw myself down the stairs. The Queen comes out absolutely horrified, shaking – she was so frightened. I knew I wasn't going to lose the baby: quite bruised about the stomach. Charles went out riding and when he came back, you know, it was just dismissal, total dismissal. He just carried on out of the door.'

So what actually happened? There was a bitter argument. It was detailed in the story given to the *Sun*. The newspaper wasn't quite as brave at that time as they would now have us believe, as they decided not to use it. The informant, who was a royal servant, had seen the argument and then saw Diana trip and stumble down no more than three steps before successfully grabbing hold of the banister. The servant had then added that the Prince of Wales had not 'just carried on out of the door' but had stayed with his wife until the doctor had arrived and pronounced that no harm had been done.

The *Sun*'s photographer, Arthur Edwards, knew the royal servant well and believed his account. He was to tell Clayton and Craig that Diana did not fall down the entire flight of stairs, only three. 'In any marriage there are rows. Of course, they were royal and they were not supposed to row, and certainly not in public and certainly not where the servants can hear. But you see, Diana was very volatile, she just let it rip when she felt she should. And of course Prince Charles was very concerned and called the doctor because she was pregnant to see if the baby was fine and it was fine. But that was interpreted later as Diana trying to commit suicide. Well, of course it wasn't that, she just fell down three stairs.'

Close inspection of the evidence would suggest that a lot of what Edwards said is correct, although it should not be forgotten that Diana did feign other suicide attempts and the notion that it was a suicide attempt at all comes initially from her. As a result, it is quite likely that what really happened was that they rowed. Charles realised that his pleading for calm was falling as usual on deaf ears; fed up with looking like a wimp, he decided that he would change tactic, ignore her and go riding. Diana, in an attempt to keep his attention and regain the upper hand, faked an attempt to throw herself down the stairs. In other words it was deliberate, but it was only ever intended to be three steps. This would have the desired effect but caused neither her nor her baby any real harm.

Can I be certain of this? No, I can't – but the facts are most compelling. Diana had discovered that her outbursts in front of the staff or the threatening of the smooth running of his public duty were an acute embarrassment to her husband. This gave her a sense of power over him. She could threaten such behaviour in order to get her own way. This form of blackmail hadn't always achieved what she had wanted but it had always put Charles on the back foot during a row. Suddenly, on the morning in question, Charles decided to stand up for himself, not by arguing back or striking her, which she would have loved as it would have symbolised attention, made her a victim and put him in the wrong, but by ignoring her – the one thing she could not abide.

As he left the room she followed him out of it and, in a flash, decided that urgent measures were called for in order to prevent him from leaving. The fall may have appeared to be a stumble rather than a deliberate lunge, but I believe it was deliberate as she thought it was the only way she could prevent him from leaving her at that moment; if he did, it might destroy her upper hand by beating one of her best tactics against him. In other words, if he wouldn't bow to her ranting, she would have to go up a gear and force him to pay attention to her. This explanation is logical and the only one that ties Morton, Dimbleby and the royal servant's accounts together. While she hadn't intended to hurt either herself or her baby, it was a cry for attention – if not for help.

Despite this latest scene Prince Charles continued to hope that such explosive behaviour, which he had never seen in anyone else before, was just the consequence of a young girl finding her feet in a very testing position, while also being pregnant. He sought to protect her from the consequences of what would become of her image – and the embarrassment it would cause the monarchy – if her current behaviour became widely known. To this end he trusted that he could rely upon the discretion of his staff, which he could, and he implored all his friends who had seen her difficulties to try and understand them and above all remain silent about what they had witnessed.

It was a strange combination. Diana on parade was more popular than ever. The love affair between her and the British people, which had started before her marriage, was now stronger than ever. Interest in her was both constant and intense. The newspapers were full of photographs and articles every day as they attempted to meet their readers' apparently insatiable appetite. On the other hand, the other Diana, while retaining much sympathy from some of the household staff and friends, was increasingly viewed as a spoiled and unreliable girl by others who saw her at close quarters.

One member of the staff told me, 'The marriage wasn't all bad days, but there were a lot. She seemed only to be happy if he was there, and then not always. It was as if she believed that she could only relax if she felt that he loved her more than she loved him. She needed to know that she was emotionally in control. But she didn't believe she was. Camilla didn't come up too often, and I always thought that she used Camilla as an excuse to blow up at him. It was as if Camilla was one of the excuses she needed to justify her tantrums. She somehow thought that exploding at him would force him to be nice to her and give her what she wanted. Actually, it drove him away little by little.'

On the other hand another staff member from the 1980s told Clayton and Craig of a tempestuous marriage at the beginning, 'Loving at times and confused at times. But two things screwed up the relationship. The Queen and his family were constantly siding with him … and the Camilla relationship. Diana was extremely interested, always asking about it.'

A third commented, 'It was spelled out to Diana. She was told that a lot of the time she would be on her own, that she was expected to be on her own, that she was expected to be his consort, but everyone was telling her, "You're the future of the Royal Family." A young girl like that, it turned her head.'

Interestingly, these are all very different views and yet there is perhaps an element of truth in all of them as they all describe certain elements of the relationship. But as we have already seen, there is no evidence that Camilla was continuing a relationship with Charles at this time. Moreover, it is not true to say that the Queen was continually siding with her son. She was siding with duty and had considerably less patience with Diana as a result than either the Duke of Edinburgh or the

Prince of Wales. She did not express this to Diana's face, but would reserve her comments for senior courtiers. As early on as the couple's honeymoon, the Queen is reported to have told a guest at the Balmoral dinner table, 'I don't know what we can do. Look at her sitting at the table glowering at us! The only time she bucks up is when Charles talks to her.'

By now some of their friends started to believe that the Princess had become obsessed by the concept of possessing the Prince in order to reject him. Like the household staff, they saw her behaviour as either an unacceptable side of her personality or sought to find another reason for it. At this point none of them thought that she might have been suffering from a mental illness. Nevertheless their bewilderment as to how the happy young girl had altered in the space of a year was evident, as was their despair if things didn't improve. One of them told Dimbleby of the sense of joy at the time of the wedding, a 'feeling of a safe future for our country ... this wonderful feeling of them uniting us as one country, one people and this being because one person was marrying the heir to the throne.' The thought that this dream might be shattered because the beautiful princess that the country loved so much was not up to the job was just too awful to contemplate.

Given her pregnancy it was decided that a skiing holiday would be inappropriate for the royal couple, so it was arranged for them to go on holiday to the island of Eleuthera in the Bahamas in February 1982. Prince Charles had enjoyed many happy times there as a young man and genuinely hoped that Diana would enjoy it and find some peace of mind there. As a result of the Queen's hospitality at Buckingham Palace, most newspaper editors decided that it was only fair to give the Princess the break that had been requested. However, the *Sun* was not going to respect that. It hadn't attended the drinks party and didn't intend to comply with the request. The *Daily Star*, which had attended the drinks party at the palace but was nevertheless determined not to be left any further behind in the circulation war, also decided to try and get an exclusive photograph of a five-months-pregnant Princess Diana in a bikini. Harry Arnold and Arthur Edwards of the *Sun* and James Whitaker and Ken Lennox from the *Daily Star* were despatched to the Bahamas on a mission.

The Prince and Princess of Wales stayed in the Brabournes' house as guests of Norton and Penny Romsey. It took some wading through the undergrowth, but the photographers got their pictures and the pregnant Princess was duly exposed semi-naked on the front pages of their newspapers. The rest of Fleet Street condemned the intrusion: the *Daily Mirror*, who in those days still had a little moral fortitude that would later be jettisoned in an attempt to keep up with the *Sun*, denounced the venture as 'squalid in conception, furtive in execution and grubby in publication'. Fine words that they might have also applied to themselves a decade later when they were to publish secretly taken photographs of the Princess working out in a London gym.

The following day, the *Sun* claimed that it deeply regretted any distress that it might have caused the Prince and Princess, but nevertheless reprinted the offending photographs alongside its apology. The Press Council condemned the 'gross intrusion' into the royal couple's privacy, but to little effect, and so another royal veil had been torn down, this time through no fault of Diana's – although one of the offending photographers, Ken Lennox, who had achieved the best shots of the couple, was to claim that years later the Princess had told him she thought the episode had been 'a great giggle' and had 'no hang-ups about being photographed in a bikini'.

Nonetheless, this holiday was a success. The couple swam, waterskied, walked on the beach and the Prince even attempted to teach his wife how to windsurf. In the evenings, each couple would take it in turn to prepare dinner for the other – and it was generally agreed that the royal chefs were better.

Afterwards, the Prince wrote to the Brabournes to thank them for allowing him to experience yet another wonderful time at their house, describing the ten-day break as 'a second honeymoon' that had allowed Diana to 'forget about her pregnancy for a few days and totally relax …' Indeed, Ken Lennox had captured a lot of happiness on film. The couple kissing in the sea, the Prince carrying her out of the water, Diana throwing a towel over his head, them racing across the sand as a very tactile and happy young couple. Years later, when the media seemed to echo her claim that he had never loved her, Lennox thought of these reels of unpublished photographs and asked himself, 'Did my camera lie?'

Of course it hadn't. The Morton book on Diana's behalf, and Dimbleby's rather polite effort to correct some of Morton's inaccuracy, gave the impression that every day was terrible. The truth is that there *were* terrible days, but there were also some that were truly happy. Even so, signs of distress and lack of common interest were ever present, just lurking beneath the surface. If the Prince was swimming just with the Princess, or giving her his undivided attention, things went well. On the other hand, the Romseys noted that the Princess soon became bored by her husband's conversations with them and would be easily irritated if he wished to read or paint.

Back in England, as her pregnancy advanced, the Princess's black moods showed no signs of abating. Indeed, her bouts of misery seemed to become more frequent. Only the closest of their friends knew of the extent of her problems; one or two of them now urged that Charles should take a tougher line with her and tell her to 'pull herself together'. This was also becoming very much the Queen's position. A growing number of the inner circle believed that if he continued to indulge her bouts of depression by offering kind words and understanding, she would never pull herself out of the terrible state that she now found herself in.

Charles would still have none of it. According to him, he and the circumstances were to blame. If she had not married him and been dropped into the royal goldfish bowl, she would not be in such a state. He had always feared that this would happen to whoever he married. It was simply too much to expect anyone to be the wife of the heir to the throne. The demands were too much, the pressures too constant and the loss of freedom too enormous.

As her state worsened, so Diana seemed to become more self-absorbed, until it appeared to some that she could only find comfort in her superstar status. She would have all the newspapers sent to her daily and would read the pieces about her and look at the photographs for hours on end. This obsession was to last for the rest of her life. Later on there would be stories of her laying out the daily tabloids on the carpet in Kensington Palace and admiring photos of herself while crawling over them on her hands and knees. By now she had developed a double-edged attitude towards the press. She loved being in the newspapers and just couldn't get enough of the adulation they heaped upon her; but equally she detested the uninvited intrusion. Moreover, as she had not by this stage learned how to manipulate or control the media, she remained occasionally genuinely frightened of them.

In April 1982, the Falklands campaign was fought in the south Atlantic. The Prince of Wales was, like the rest of the nation, most concerned. He was the heir to the British throne; his country was at war; he was the colonel-in-chief of two regiments fighting on the other side of the world. His brother, Prince Andrew, was a helicopter pilot seeing active service. And he cursed his luck that as the Prince of Wales he would not be allowed to do the same. None of Charles's self-doubt had ever dimmed his undeniable physical courage, nor had his lack of self-esteem damaged his sense of duty.

However, the war did not mean that the Princess was to be distracted from her own concerns, and some who witnessed her disconcerting lack of interest in it were even more astonished that she seemed to resent the fact that the war was keeping her off the front pages of the newspapers. This started alarm bells ringing with those who had sought to give her the benefit of any doubt regarding her suitability for the role of consort to the heir to the throne. Some have seriously questioned since whether or not this really was her attitude at the time, claiming that the story may have been exaggerated later when the marriage had collapsed. It is impossible to be certain if you were not present at the time. Those who were there have no doubt that the facts are correct; nor were most of them particularly biased in the Prince's favour.

Staff members were becoming disillusioned with what they saw as Diana's undisciplined behaviour and mood swings, but they were also increasingly concerned by the Prince of Wales's obsession with unemployment and the ethnic communities. It was not that the old guard did not think these issues were important; they simply didn't believe it was his business to interfere in such political matters. For nearly fifty years George VI and his daughter Elizabeth had played the role of constitutional monarch perfectly by opening conferences, hospitals and bridges. Controversy had been banished following the turbulent abdication crisis. The Royal Family was the symbol of the nation and this was, according to the old guard, their sole job. Political issues should be left to the politicians. Now, along had come a young prince of Wales who wanted to speak up for the jobless, just like his Great Uncle David had, and worse still who wanted to get involved with them and take on projects to help them.

Adeane was overheard on one occasion to say, 'If I hear the word "caring" again I am going to be sick.' Another insider was to comment as the Prince approached, 'What toys are coming out of the box today.' To many such people who had only known the discipline and order of Her Majesty's court, the Prince was playing a dangerous game that could bring the monarchy into conflict with the Thatcher government.

On top of all that, he had shown more poor judgment by marrying a spoiled child, and had made their jobs all the worse as a result. Diana's behaviour concerning the Falklands was clearly unacceptable to these people, and this is generally accepted by all who were close to her on the household staff at the time.

On 21 June 1982, one day after the Falklands War concluded in a resounding victory that lifted the nation as well as resurrecting the political career of Margaret Thatcher, the Princess gave Prince Charles and the nation the son and heir that everybody wanted. It may have been a long and, at times, fraught pregnancy, but it had ended in complete triumph. A people drunk with national pride as a result of the Falklands success now had their glasses topped up by the news.

Diana gave birth at St Mary's Hospital, Paddington. The baby was born at 9.03 p.m. and weighed a little over seven pounds. Crowds who had gathered for the birth, which was actually witnessed by the Prince – he was the first royal father to do so – exploded into a chorus of 'For He's a Jolly Good Fellow' as Prince Charles appeared.

Despite the black moods and bleak days, and however unhappy she had been or had made others, the Princess now basked in the sunshine of her achievement as her clouds of despair disappeared. This was a very happy moment. She felt liberated from her depression, he forgot about all recriminations. They bonded in the joint explosion of love for their son.

William was to be his first name. It had been chosen by Diana. Charles had favoured Arthur, which was one of his middle names and one that he had allowed girlfriends to call him instead of 'sir'. The full name became William Arthur Philip Louis – his third name in honour of the Duke of Edinburgh and his fourth after Lord Louis Mountbatten. In addition, as part of a compromise over the baby's first name, the Prince chose all the little fellow's godparents.

The Queen visited the hospital the following day and joked that the baby had got ears like his father. A jubilant Margaret Thatcher, basking in her own glory, ordered the nation to rejoice. The Prince wrote to their friends the van Cutsems, 'I got back here just before midnight – utterly elated but quite shattered. I can't tell you how excited and proud I am. He really does look surprisingly appetising and has sausage fingers just like mine.'

Diana joked with her beauty consultant, Janet Filderman, about the birth, saying, 'When Prince Charles came I kept saying, "Charles, come and hold my hand, hold my hand." But he kept wanting to go to the front of the engine instead.' Filderman recalls the Princess being very happy, natural and content.

A few days later, when mother and son were safely returned to Highgrove with the Prince, Charles wrote to his godmother, Patricia Brabourne, to describe his great joy at becoming a father at last: 'The arrival of our small son has been an astonishing experience and one that has meant more to me than I could ever have imagined. As so often happens in this life, you have to experience something before you are in a true position to understand or appreciate the full meaning of the whole thing. I am SO thankful I was beside Diana's bedside the whole time because by the end of the day I really felt as though I'd shared deeply in the process of birth and as a result was rewarded by seeing a small creature which belonged to US even though he seemed to belong to everyone else as well! I have never seen such scenes as there were outside the hospital when I left that night – everyone had gone berserk with excitement ... Since then we've been overwhelmed by people's reactions and thoroughly humbled. It really is quite extraordinary ... I am so pleased that you like the idea of Louis being one of William's names. Oh! How I wished your papa could have lived to see him, but he probably knows anyway ...'

After the birth, Diana disappeared from public gaze for the next two months as she and Charles both focused on their new baby. He cleared his diary to spend more time at home. At last Diana, surrounded by her husband and baby son, began to be much more cheerful. The couple had by now been able to move out of Buckingham Palace and into Kensington Palace as their London residence. There Princess Margaret and the Duke and Duchess of Gloucester also had apartments, and Diana's sister Jane lived with her husband Robert Fellowes in the Old Barracks close by. Now Diana indulged in the sort of family life she had always wanted. Charles and William were at home, and she had an extended family next door so that she could enjoy coffee mornings and a quiet and supportive social life. She breastfed William for a short while, and both parents shared the bathing and nappy changing. When William was a little over two months old, Diana hired an experienced nanny called Barbara Barnes and completed the arrangements for the christening with great excitement. It was easily the most relaxed and happy period that the couple had enjoyed in the year since their marriage.

But it was not to last. By the time of the christening Diana's mood had swung back into one of severe gloom. It was assumed at first that she was suffering from delayed post-natal depression, and her condition appeared to be more serious than ever. Once more she began to look thin, pale and unwell. For the first time, Prince Charles and some of his senior courtiers began to realise that the Princess might be suffering from more than just stress. It occurred to them that it was just too much of a coincidence that she was laid low by every external incident. Perhaps she had a disorder and needed treatment? Slowly the Prince realised that something would have to be done or he, Diana and William faced extremely bleak prospects. Moreover, it might only be a matter of time before Diana broke down in public, and that might damage both her reputation and that of the monarchy.

However, the Prince was not a great fan of traditional medicine. Around this time he spoke out to the British Medical Association in favour of alternative treatments and against the influence of the drugs industry. He was to continue with this campaign over the next year as he also produced attacks on modern farming methods and the agrochemical industry, while speaking out in favour of organic food production. All of this produced fierce debate, as well as indignation by the well-entrenched lobbies of these industries and professions, and he was mocked as the 'loony prince' by the tabloid press. And when the press, by now more in love with Diana than the Prince, suggested that he was backing eccentric causes, in private many in the Palace hierarchy were inclined to agree. Adeane in particular remained unimpressed by the Prince's activities and had some sympathy with the view that he had no right to lecture various professionals on ethics, simply because of an accident of birth. He continued to worry that this might even lead to a constitutional crisis. Ironically, many of the Prince's 'loony' views are now the subject of widespread support.

In the autumn the Prince had gently suggested that Diana seek some form of medical assistance. She initially resisted but in the end agreed to see Dr Alan McGlashan as long as he went with her. McGlashan was a dream analyst who was recommended by Laurens van der Post. Charles continued to see him, but Diana was not receptive and instead transferred to Dr David Mitchell, a cognitive therapist.

There were some among the senior courtiers who believed that, by sending her to such people, the Prince had lost an opportunity of really helping Diana. They believed that her condition would only be helped if the talents of more conventional psychiatrists were sought, people who could prescribe drugs in order to redress the chemical imbalance in the Princess. Borderline personality disorder had been brought to the attention of some of them who then believed that the Princess might be suffering from it. What they failed to realise was that BPD is not caused by chemical imbalance, and therefore cannot be directly treated by drugs. It is a disorder that means the personality traits that go together in order to make up every individual are abnormally balanced. This is quite common and there are hundreds of thousands of people who suffer a mild form of BPD and may never know they have it. Indeed, some critics of BPD have looked at the eight main symptoms and joked that a quarter of the population might have it. Mild sufferers usually just need extra amounts of attention and adoration, and provided that they can keep their mood swings under control there is no real problem – until failure deprives them of their much-needed injections of adoration. Then the breakdowns, drug and alcohol abuse and suicide attempts start.

It is universally acknowledged that BPD in serious sufferers is one of the most difficult conditions to cure. It is treated with anti-depressants, tranquillisers and intensive care and patience. A Canadian study in the 1990s reported that up to ten per cent of serious sufferers would eventually successfully commit suicide. Moreover, it takes its toll on the relatives, friends and psychiatrists who attempt to help the sufferer, not least because the symptoms are only displayed to them while the patient behaves completely differently in front of the wider world. In public, sufferers are usually cheerful, outgoing and pleasant. They are often attractive, successful, funny and charismatic people, who give every indication that they are well balanced. They can be so mesmerising that even their doctors, who are trained against the dangers of getting involved with the patients they treat, can be sucked in and emotionally engulfed. It is only then, when one gets too close and fails to give the sufferer what he or she wants, that one gets to see the other side of his or her personality. Many in the medical profession say that while they realise that the patient is ill, and therefore blameless, it becomes difficult not to think of the sufferer as evil.

When a case is serious it can be almost impossible for doctors or family to help the victim: they need care and attention but at the same time repel and detest the people who are attempting to help them, all the while searching for new people to impress.

Diana's position as the Princess of Wales, allied to her popularity with the public and the media's fascination with her as the new face of modern British monarchy, meant that it was even harder to treat her. As one leading expert in psychiatric disorders commented, 'If all sufferers were royal, there might be no more mental illness, because if you are in control you have the power and can use your fantasies and manipulations.'

Not long before Diana's death, one of her closest friends gave a quite unprompted description of her friend's 'terrible' problems, which were to fit BPD in every detail. She then added that, 'She is like someone who has her nose pressed up to the glass looking at the world outside, but never feeling that she is part of it. She can't emotionally, psychologically cope with it.' Most interesting. BPD sufferers are described in US medical journals as being people who are unable to engage in proper relationships or feel any real emotion. They just copy others from the detachment of being 'on the other side of the glass'. The only genuine emotion to come easily to them is a sense of despair at being unable to sustain the relationships that they see others enjoying and yet can't emulate themselves, however hard they try.

On the other hand, another of her closest friends was Lana Marks. Her husband Neville was a member of the Royal College of Psychiatrists and had met Diana several times. He told Clayton and Craig how he had met and spoken to Princess Diana. He said she coped with the pressures of her job, the travelling around the world, the meeting world leaders, but the more personal, emotional role – being rejected by her husband and not knowing how to deal with that – was less easy to cope with.

'If she had a borderline personality disorder she would not have been able to cope with any area of her life. She would have had difficulties that would have been apparent to the world from the day the world first knew about her right through her life. This is the characteristic of a borderline personality disorder, it's a lifelong condition, it's a serious difficulty with emotions, with thoughts and with controlling one's impulsive behaviour.'

Clayton and Craig point out that Dr Marks is the husband of one of Diana's strongest allies and that he would be the first to stress that his opinion was not formed under clinical conditions. However, he is a psychiatrist and he had met the Princess of Wales.

Nevertheless, his opinion is hotly disputed by many other senior psychiatrists who also point out that borderline personality disorder is not only a question of degree but also dispute vehemently the idea that people suffering from it cannot disguise their symptoms to the outside world and that is why it is their doctors and family who suffer the vast majority of their erratic behaviour. In addition they point out that personal, emotional insecurities caused by her marital problems neither explain her advanced state of paranoia in her later life nor do they explain her persistent falling out with other family members, staff and friends. Furthermore, they believe that it is highly unlikely that the Princess of Wales would have demonstrated consistently the eight major symptoms of borderline personality disorder so consistently throughout her life purely on the grounds of an emotional upset, imagined or otherwise, caused by her failing marriage.

The Prince, despite his anger at her behaviour, nevertheless felt extremely sorry for her. He had changed his mind from believing that the fault lay totally with him, to believing that marriage to him had triggered off some form of disorder that was beyond Diana's ability to control in any way. Therefore she was, in his opinion, no more to blame than if she had been struck down by a horrible cancer. He remained loyal and kind to her, but sought her company less.

Ironically, once the idea that the Princess may have been suffering from a psychiatric disorder took hold with certain people who worked closely with her, they found it easier to work with her. It was as if they knew better what to expect. Moreover, it made some sense of the previous twelve months.

In 1991, the Prince of Wales launched the SANE appeal. During his speech he touched on schizophrenia: 'Physical disability, illness, accidents which break bones or upset the functions of the body are painful, yet they can be overcome by strength of personality, good medical care and willpower. Schizophrenia is different: we are talking about an illness which changes the way people think, understand and perceive the world around them and relate to others – the very essence of their personality – so that they are isolated from all sources of comfort and reason. I believe we have to accept that accidents can happen to the mind as they can to the body, and that the consequences can sometimes be even more devastating.' His words were truly born out of personal experience.

No one has ever doubted that the most stable and loving

relationship that Diana was to enjoy was with her children. It was the nearest she came to having a long-term relationship with close family without disruption and serious rancour. However, not even this relationship was untouched by her condition. She would not be able in time to resist using them as propaganda tools in the media war with her husband. Nor would she be able to see that phoning up a young William at boarding school and emotionally dumping on him could be bad for him and make him as unhappy as her mother had made her.

Clayton and Craig tell us how she flaunted her lover James Hewitt in front of the boys; while we know that Camilla was not introduced to them until some time after their mother's death. We are told by Junor how Prince William told journalist Bell Mooney privately, when a young teenager, that he found his mother embarrassing at times (unlike his father), and we are told by Morton how the Princess continually phoned into a television poll on the monarchy, voting each time for its abolition. William, then a boy and aware that both he and his father were supposed to be future kings, was apparently stretched out on a rug watching the programme with her. As usual, Charles's biographer Dimbleby skirts round these issues, at the Prince's request.

As the Princess's resentment to her husband grew to become a complete obsession, she seemed determined that if she could not possess him then she would destroy him and didn't appear to stop for a moment to consider the effect this might have on her children. If she had, she would not have contemplated secretly recording the ramblings of an ill and discredited footman for her own purposes, nor would she have contemplated the notorious *Panorama* interview. Only a very poor mother or a seriously ill one would do either. It is my opinion that Diana was not an awful person, but a poorly one. She could not have behaved any differently.

While Diana's problems had largely been contained behind closed doors, the British public had been distracted by Mrs Thatcher engaging two enemies: the unions at home and the Argentineans abroad. Since coming to power in 1979 she had determined to release the stranglehold that the British trade-union movement had over the economy. She took an extremely tough attitude towards strikes. This was epitomised by the government's approach to a national strike in the steel industry that they were determined to win whatever the cost. The battle was painful and during its course Mrs Thatcher's popularity fell to new depths. But she pressed on, and although she invited people from the whole spectrum of the party into her Cabinet, she took little notice of what many of them had to say. She was not going to 'waste time having any internal arguments'.

Initially the 'wets', as Thatcher dubbed the centre or left-of-centre members of her party, kept quiet as, although the prime minister was not enjoying a high degree of popularity with the voters, the rank and file of the party and the parliamentary party very much approved of her tough line. However, there was to build up a serious resentment among some of them as time went by. I had dinner in Tetbury one summer's evening in 1991 with Lady Prior, wife of Tory Cabinet minister Jim Prior, after we had both been guests of Prince Charles at Highgrove, and was both amazed and horrified by the naked disloyalty and intense hatred that the woman had for her husband's leader. It was obvious to me that Lady Prior was not mouthing her own opinions but also those that her husband had expressed as he put the light out at night.

At the depths of the recession, and with unemployment still climbing sharply, Mrs Thatcher strongly supported Sir Geoffrey Howe's spring budget, which intensified the squeeze both on companies and the consumer. Initially, Howe had been against any such budget, and even the Treasury felt that some relaxation of monetary policy was possible. However, Mrs Thatcher had two extra-parliamentary advisers, Sir John Hoskyns and Alan Walters. The first had built a most successful IT company and the second was a former professor at Birmingham University and the London School of Economics. They had other ideas and Thatcher backed them. Walters had established his monetarist principles long before the phrase was heard of in political circles. Indeed, he had predicted the inflation of 1974 as early as 1972 by analysing the explosion of credit in the Barber Boom.

Hoskyns and Walters helped stiffen Thatcher's resolve in the early months of 1981. To them it was a matter of credibility: the government had to show everyone once and for all that they were not going to move forward 'with enormous insupportable borrowings'. It had to convince the financial markets that it would get inflation down and that you could only build a successful economy on sound money and sensible business practice. Walters pressed for £4,000 million to come out of the public-sector borrowing requirement. Chancellor Howe resisted long and hard. Thatcher knew that Hoskyns and Walters were right, but she also knew that it was Howe and not them who had to sell the package to the House of Commons. Walters at one point doubted if she could see it through and prepared himself for resignation. However, the Iron Lady, as she was now becoming known, stood her ground and as a result Howe feared for his career and in the end agreed to take out £3,500 million, which Hoskyns and Walters agreed was enough to do the trick. As a result, the most important budget for Britain in the twentieth century was born. It was to become a crucial part of the foundation on which Britain's economic recovery was based and therefore a major reason for the country's economic success over the next twenty-five years.

This budget may have been essential for the nation's future, but it was nevertheless a very brave political gamble for the government. Indeed, no government since the end of the Second World War had been so brave, and none has since. The budget produced forecasts of falling output of a further one per cent, while unemployment would possibly exceed three million. However, Thatcher believed this was the price a realistic and, in the future, prosperous Britain would have to pay. She also feared the sack, as she could see many faint hearts among the Tory wets. But it worked. The financial markets saw that here at last was a prime minister who was capable of sticking to her guns, and they applauded her toughness and resolve. There had been tough-talking governments from both parties since the War, but their actions had never lived up to their words. She went to the Tory party conference in October 1981 and told them, 'You may turn if you want to, the lady's not for turning.' The party roared its approval.

If the party faithful, the financial markets and international bankers were applauding, the British public – which was at worst out of a job, and at best subjected to a severe squeeze on its standard of living – was sitting on its hands. However, matters started to improve for her by the spring of 1982: the unions were defeated and at least a portion of the nation started to understand that the short-term bleakness was a price worth paying for a brighter future – a kind of 'cold turkey' that had to be endured in order to kick the habit of living beyond one's means.

Thatcher started to recover in the opinion polls and drew level with the other two main parties – a fact that is now often overlooked some twenty years later. It is overlooked because of what happened next: the Falklands Crisis. Argentine soldiers landed first on South Georgia, a British island in the south Atlantic and then, more seriously, on the

Falkland Islands. As everyone was reaching for their atlases to discover exactly where these faraway islands were, Mrs Thatcher decided that British sovereignty had been violated and that the Argentineans must be removed, if necessary by force. Strong action was called for and, with the Iron Lady at the helm, was taken. A task force was dispatched, a brilliant campaign was waged a long way from home in the Argentineans' back yard, and the British won a victory that had *Time* magazine in the US declaring, 'Great Britain is back.'

Our leader was courageous, our armed forces professional and, above all, we looked, perhaps for the first time in thirty years, to be winners. It was a turning point for Mrs Thatcher. Her ratings in the polls soared, and as the economy showed signs of genuine revival, built for once on a sound base, she was able to go to the country in 1983 and request a second term in office in order to continue the revolution that she had begun. The nation rewarded her with a landslide victory.

Those friends and staff members who were around during the period following Prince William's birth remember the Prince being rather under her thumb as she strove to get rid of many of his staff, his circle of friends and even his constant companion – a Labrador named Sandringham. In her desire to possess the Prince, the Princess wanted him to concentrate solely on her. She gradually realised that she would be unable to prevent his very heavy work schedule, but she thought it would be possible to eliminate friends, staff and even a pet for which he had great affection.

Although she had pretended to like most of his friends and their wives initially, in fact she didn't at all, and was deeply suspicious of most of them – in some cases not without justification. The Romseys were banned from Highgrove and Kensington Palace when the Prince let it slip during the course of one of the Princess's ornament-throwing tantrums that Norton Romsey had warned him against marrying her in the first place. Then there was the polo set and the Beaufort Hunt. They were not so close as the Prince's intimate circle, but he enjoyed their company. On the other hand, Diana thought they were loud, vulgar and far too horsey. At her insistence he distanced himself from them.

As a result, Diana had managed to dispense with the vast majority of the Prince's friends, including those who had genuinely liked her and sought to support her in the first two years of her marriage. Her policy was to write warm and pleasant letters to everyone, while saying terrible things about them behind their backs before adding totally fabricated statements that certain friends or colleagues were supposed to have made about them. Her ability to lie made all of this sound plausible. She accused friends of disloyalty, staff of dishonesty and consequently caused a lot of harm and confusion as courtiers and employees started to be uncertain about whom they could trust.

There have always been petty jealousies surrounding monarchs and princes, and naturally the Prince of Wales was no exception. Diana manipulated the position expertly and did a great deal of damage. As friends started to realise what was happening, they plucked up courage to drop discreet hints to Prince Charles, but still he did not want to hear them. Then even his parents made it plain to their son that they thought Diana's behaviour was somewhat short of perfect, but the Prince wouldn't even listen to criticism of his wife from the Queen. He was fiercely loyal to Diana. He continued to refuse to discuss her moods or tantrums with anyone. He appeared to be determined to make her happy and well by his own devices.

At one point she got so thin that he thought she was going to die – a death, in his mind, that would have been his fault as obviously she had only become like this since marriage to him. So he determined to do everything she wanted in an attempt to make her well again and restore the girl who had appeared so happy when he first met her. As a result he stopped writing, telephoning or visiting his closest friends one by one. He didn't say why and so, without either contact or explanation, they were left to wonder what they had done. Naturally they were hurt, but they nevertheless remained loyal to a man whose friendship they valued, preferring to wait for his contact rather than telephone him themselves and risk upsetting him further.

Not content with banishing the Prince's friends, Diana then insisted that the Prince get rid of his Labrador Sandringham. Sandringham went everywhere with the Prince. He stayed with him at Kensington Palace during the week, before travelling down to Highgrove with his master at weekends. When Charles went shooting in the winter at Sandringham, the dog went too, as he did to Balmoral in the summer.

Diana, who was never really fond of animals despite having had pets as a child, insisted that the dog reminded her of Charles's life before he met her, in the same way that his friends did; she complained that he messed up her house, which was untrue; and more importantly she complained that the Prince paid too much attention to the thing, so it would have to go. The Prince, keen to please her, didn't even draw the line there and regrettably eventually gave in and sent the dog to live elsewhere.

Princess Margaret of Hesse and Rhine, like many others who knew the couple, realised that this attempt by Diana to control the Prince completely was bound to have, in the end, the opposite effect to the one she intended. She could see that the Princess wanted Charles to have 'no rights in his own palace. She believed that the way to keep him by her side was to subjugate him. He kept on appeasing her because he knew she was ill, and because he is that sort of person who will do anything for a peaceful life. But she wasn't training him up, as she once put it to me. She was alienating him. Making him withdraw from her.'

By 1983, and with the elimination of friends and Sandringham underway, the Princess was also turning her guns on the Prince's staff. First to go was a policeman called Paul Officer. He had saved the Prince's life, so the Prince was very close to him. For that reason alone it seems Diana took a dislike to him. Next to go was Stephen Barry. He had also been close to Charles for several years. For Diana, the fact that they went back a long way meant that he had been too closely associated with her husband's pre-marital sexual liaisons. He had also cared for the Prince almost as a wife might have for a long time and was, in fairness to Diana, nearly as resentful of her as she was of him.

Then there was the multi-talented Oliver Everett, Diana's private secretary, who left at the end of 1983. Everett had served Charles as an assistant private secretary between 1978 and 1980. The Prince had then kept him on, thus preventing a promising career in the Foreign Office from developing in order that he might look after the young princess. At first he could do no wrong; then she completely changed her mind. She claimed he fussed over her too much and she couldn't stand it. Perhaps it was because Everett had been instructed by the Prince to improve the Princess's very limited education – nobody seems too sure – but for whatever reason, Diana suddenly cut him off. She wouldn't speak to him, didn't respond to his memos or phone calls and would even ignore his very presence if they were ever in a room together. The Prince was horrified. Everett had given up his career in order to join his team, and this treatment offended Charles's sense of fair play. He found Everett a job as librarian at Windsor Castle, but knew in his heart that this was a shocking waste of his talents. Nevertheless, he still went against his better judgement in order to please his wife.

However, by now the Princess's moods and rages were leaving him in a state of severe depression. It seemed to him that the harder he tried to please her, the worse her tantrums became. It was as if she could only get relief from her inner turmoil and pain by venting her rage on those around her and especially those who tried to be pleasant and who couldn't answer back. Her dresser Evelyn Dagley found herself at the sharp end of Diana's tongue: 'Look at this fucking shirt, Evelyn, look at it you idiot, it's rubbish, rubbish, rubbish – what is it Evelyn? Rubbish … Get out of my sight.' Staff came to expect this treatment when the Princess 'wasn't quite herself', while she hoped that the Queen and the outside world didn't get to hear about it.

Naturally, living permanently in such an atmosphere began seriously to affect the behaviour of the Prince too. His initial concern about the Princess's stability turned to despair, while his delight at the public's love of her turned to jealousy when he realised that they saw her increasingly as his leading lady rather than consort. Not only was he hurt when crowds groaned as they realised that it would be him and not her on their side of the street, he was furious that the newspapers now appeared to prefer covering her having a mindless lunch at San Lorenzo's rather than a serious speech that he had given. He was angered by the unfairness of it all. In his eyes he was attempting to look after the nation's welfare, whereas she was just besotted by her own, and yet the nation appeared to prefer her glitz to his intellect. Slowly, all the self-doubt and lack of self-esteem that he had fought so hard to beat began to engulf him once more.

Unable or unwilling to take any of this frustration out on his wife, who still occasionally had enough good days to give him hope, he took it out on others around him. Inevitably, these tended to be people who could not answer back. We have seen that the Prince of Wales possesses a hot temper himself and had thrown his fair share of tantrums since leaving the navy and working out of Buckingham Palace, but now they became more frequent and less justified. Michael Colborne, who loved the Prince, started to notice this serious change in his master's personality. The usually charming, kind and thoughtful man was slowly being replaced by a person who was shrinking back into his shell, as his fragile self-confidence appeared to be shattering. The easy charm and amusing wit were seen less and less, while the serious and strained side was ever present. Prince Charles was no longer the person that he had fought so hard to become. The press was increasingly seeing him as a hen-pecked husband at home and the loony prince abroad.

When Everett left it was decided that a replacement would not be sought but his job shared between Anne Beckwith-Smith and Michael Colborne. Beckwith-Smith had helped the Princess through her early trials on her first official visit to Wales, and Colborne was apparently a favourite of Diana's, despite the hard time she had given him early on in their relationship. It appeared that a good solution had been found.

However, on an official visit to Canada aboard the Royal Yacht *Britannia*, things came to a head with Colborne. He had been supposed to be working on a reception for Canada's President Trudeau one evening on board, but during the afternoon was called up to the sun deck in order to see the Princess. The Prince had gone off to visit one of his regiments, expecting everything to be prepared upon his return. But when Colborne arrived on deck it became clear that the Princess only wanted to see him in order to have someone to talk to. The afternoon passed and Colborne found himself under pressure in order to catch up and ensure that things ran smoothly at dinner.

On Charles's return, he took Colborne to the Duke of Edinburgh's cabin for a pre-dinner drink and a final check of the arrangements, but instead of running over these he launched into a stinging attack on Colborne for paying too much attention to the Princess. The Prince hardly drew breath for fifteen minutes. Colborne tried to point out that he thought that by taking care of the Princess, not only was he doing his duty but also that such an action was actually helping the Prince. But Charles would have none of it. He continued going berserk. Then he suddenly decided that both men should change for dinner and flung open the cabin door. The Princess had been listening at the keyhole and was just standing there crying.

Charles wrapped her gently in his arms and after an emotional hug that ignored Colborne's presence, led her back to their cabin so that they might get ready. When they reappeared they would both have to smile their way through an official dinner.

But Colborne had had enough. He was tired of being caught in the Waleses' crossfire, and he recognised that there was some truth in what the Prince had said: so much attention lavished upon the Princess had meant that he was now neglecting the Prince and his other duties. He had become increasingly concerned about her. The moods and tantrums that she reserved for the Prince and their staff would disappear when she attended a reception. She became, at least on the surface, a charming and much more attractive personality. However, Colborne had come to the conclusion that this other side of Diana was just as dangerous and might even become an unguided missile that could be used against the Prince and the Royal Family. He had noticed that she was becoming intoxicated with the extraordinary effect that she was having on men. She was still only twenty-two, yet her mere presence in a room caused men of all ages to flock to her, mesmerised and beguiled. This would be enough to affect the strongest head, let alone a girl who had had serious doubts about her own attractiveness for most of her teenage years.

Colborne worried that she was enjoying it more than she should have done and was starting to flirt. A vengeful and spiteful princess of Wales at home was one problem; one that went out to flirt with men other than her husband was quite another. Put together, they were a disastrous combination – more, perhaps, than he felt he could handle.

That evening Colborne wrote the Prince a note expressing that he had done his very best for Charles over the last ten years. He pointed out that he thought the Prince's criticism hadn't been altogether fair as, by helping the Princess, he had genuinely believed that he was helping the Prince. A few days later Prince Charles had a private word with Colborne saying that he understood the note and apologised for his outburst. But it was too late. It had been one rollicking too many. Colborne tended his resignation and the Prince had lost his longest-serving staff member. So ended a relationship of mutual respect and considerable affection. Moreover, the Prince had lost his only actual link inside the household with the real world, as well as perhaps the only person who really understood what he was trying to achieve when it came to issues like inner-city deprivation.

The Prince was shocked and saddened by the news. He tried repeatedly to get Colborne to change his mind. He even phoned his wife, Shirley, several times at home to try and get her to persuade him. In addition, he got several other people to have a go, but collectively they only managed to get Colborne to stay on until the end of the year.

As a result of Diana's interference, Charles's change of mood and stubbornness and Colborne's departure, Sir Edward Adeane now considered his position. He had long disapproved of the self-besotted and non-dutiful Princess. He had also become increasingly frustrated by the Prince's sorties into political and professional areas of life, which he believed should be left to the politicians. The last straw came when the Prince planned to deliver a damming speech to the Royal Institute of British Architecture, criticising a professional body that had enjoyed nothing but acclaim for over a century. Adeane tried to dissuade the Prince who, with typical stubbornness, refused to listen.

As a result Charles delivered his speech as written and caused much offence to the majority of architects. However, he did delight some in the vanguard of that profession and, despite the uproar at the time, he hit a note with the public and probably did more to correct the hideous architectural trends of the time than anyone else. Consequently, his interception is now looked upon as both sage and timely. At the time it was not, and Adeane despaired. Moreover, the prospect of losing Colborne and having to deal more directly with the unstable Diana as well as her increasingly unpredictable husband filled him with horror. On the day following Colborne's leaving lunch, Adeane went to Windsor to see the Prince and, following a blazing row, also tended his resignation.

In less than three years Diana had managed to separate, either directly or indirectly, the future king from his dog, his friends and most of his best staff. Matters looked very bleak for the heir to the throne – especially as there was no obvious sign that his patience towards or his indulgence of the Princess was ever going to pay a long-term dividend.

However, true to the pattern of this complicated, and for the Prince unfathomable, relationship, periods of blue sky, harmony and hope still came along. In March 1983 the couple went on their first international official visit together. It was to the Prince's beloved Australia and New Zealand. They took William with them. The trip was a huge success as the crowds brought every city and town they visited to a complete standstill. Neither country had seen anything like this since the Beatles had toured Australia nearly twenty years earlier – the Charles and Diana show was a complete sell-out. He was popular, but she was a goddess. He didn't seem to mind, perhaps because they were happy and working well together. He even joked that he needed two wives – one for each side of the street. And he tried very hard to help her cope with the enormous pressure of it all, which couldn't have been easy for either of them.

This would have been the case for any young couple coming under so much scrutiny, but imagine the extra pressure that both would have felt given the frail state of Diana's mind and the uncertainty of her mood swings. What would each day bring? It couldn't have been too far from the Prince's mind at any one time that the Princess had not only thrown herself down stairs, but had slashed her wrists with a razor blade, cut herself with a lemon slicer, slashed her chest and thighs with a penknife and chucked herself towards a glass display cabinet during the last two years. These actions had been interpreted more as cries for attention or help than serious suicide attempts. Nevertheless, they denoted the actions of a very frail and poorly mind.

As a result Diana had been receiving medical help since 1982. Borderline personality disorder wasn't widely accepted by British psychiatrists then and so wasn't considered. Instead, the diagnosis seemed to be that the traumas caused in Diana's childhood by her mother leaving the family home and losing custody of her children had blighted her entire upbringing and it would take time and a lot of gentle care to correct. The Prince had committed himself to precisely that. He confided to one of his closest friends, 'The trouble is one day I think some steps are being made uphill only to find that we've slipped back one and a half steps the following day.' The fact that he uses the word 'we' rather than 'she' underlines both his concern and his desire to stand by her and see it through. Their friends and staff members of the time confirm without exception that while his duties took him away from time to time, the Prince showed both tenderness and pity for his wife when she was stricken by these dark moods.

In 1983 both the Prince and Princess were determined to work hard to enable her to escape from this pattern of behaviour for the sake of their son, their marriage and their country. And by the time they reached Australia things seemed to be improving: perhaps the insubstantial foundations upon which their marriage had been built might survive after all. It was certainly felt by those who were there at the time that if Diana's 'blues' could be banished then it would, and in Australia they seemed to have been.

Arthur Edwards recalled that, 'He was always touching her hand or holding her arm. And they seemed to be very much together. And I remember when they looked at each other they looked like they wanted to rip the clothes off each other, they looked so much in love … And there was all these big gaps in the programme where they would go off for two or three days. Because it was a long tour. And it was obvious that they were looking forward to those wonderful weekends and so they really did seem to be very much in love. I am convinced of it to this day.'

The Prince was happy. This was, given his kind nature, just the encouragement he needed. He was in his treasured Australia, with his family and doing his duty. More importantly, his wife was doing hers and for the first time seemed happy to do so. This was all that he had ever wanted, worked towards and had been told by Mountbatten that he must achieve.

An elated Diana wrote home to a friend and confessed that she was now ashamed of her behaviour in London, proud of the Prince and very grateful for his support and guidance. She had, much to the relief of them both, apparently shaken off her inner demons and was suddenly capable of being every bit as pleasant to those around her as the millions of her admirers from around the world supposed she was anyway. It was a truly wonderful time and led many close to the couple to hope that perhaps things would work out after all.

Nevertheless, the Prince still expressed one major concern: the press. The intensity of their enthusiasm was alarming, because he knew precisely how they worked. He wrote, 'The terrifying part, as always in this kind of thing, is that they construct the pedestal; they put you on top of it, they expect you to balance on the beastly thing without ever losing your footing, and because they have engineered the pedestal along come the demolition experts amongst them who are of the breed that enjoy breaking things down. And it is all done for a sort of vicarious entertainment ... Maybe the wedding, because it was so well done and because it made such a wonderful, almost Hollywood-style film, has distorted people's view of things? Whatever the case it frightens me.'

Of course he was quite right. However, initially it would only be him that they would pick on. After all, he had been around a long time and she hadn't. But he knew that her day would come.

The next year Diana became pregnant with her second son, Henry. Born on 15 September 1984 in the same hospital as his elder brother, the little boy was to be known as Harry. In the months before his birth the Princess was to explain that she and the Prince were closer than they had ever been – or were ever to be. Then, 'suddenly as Harry was born it just went bang, our marriage, the whole thing, just went down the drain.'

This is a strange comment, given that Diana had claimed that her relationship with Charles was in trouble before they were even married thanks to his supposedly continuing relationship with Camilla Parker Bowles. Now she was saying that things were fine until the year of Harry's birth. This point is further underlined when she added, 'By then I knew he had gone back to his lady but somehow we had managed to have Harry.' According to Diana's other public statements he had never left 'his lady' in the first place.

Diana went on to claim that she knew from the scan that the baby was going to be boy, but had declined to tell her husband because she believed that he wanted a girl. 'Harry arrived, Harry had red hair, Harry was a boy. First comment was, "Oh God it's a boy," second comment, "And he's even got red hair," something inside me closed off.'

Diana's comments regarding the birth of Harry have been recorded for history and are widely believed. However, those who were there in a professional capacity, or who were close to the couple at the time, remember things very differently. It is true that prior to the birth she told some people that her husband wanted a girl, but none, including those there at the time, can remember the Prince being anything but delighted by the birth of his second son. Apparently he was totally thrilled to witness the miracle of childbirth again, was immensely happy to have been given a second son and made no comment whatsoever about the colour of his hair, which in any event was more blond than red at the time of birth.

Moreover, it is only natural to have a preference for the gender of your child – but whatever the sex is once the child is born, we love it unreservedly. The Prince of Wales was no different from any of us in this regard. In addition, any of us lucky enough to have witnessed the Prince of Wales with Prince Harry as a young boy know that any suggestion that this father did anything other than dote on his son is preposterous. And, following Diana's death, the world could see this great relationship clearly – once Diana's spin was no longer there to jam the airwaves.

In addition, perhaps it is also reasonable to question the consideration and kindness of a mother who tells the world that her son's father didn't really want him. What must have gone through Prince Harry's mind when he read that? Luckily, his relationship with his father has always been so completely different to the one that Diana wanted the world to believe that I doubt if he gave the matter too much consideration.

The King and Di

So who was telling the truth? Diana in her rancorous account given to Andrew Morton some seven years on at a very low point in her life, or the multiple and independent memories of others. Naturally Morton claims that he has verified her statement with others just as he had on other issues. I do not doubt this, but he seems to have ignored one huge and most significant point. Morton went to Diana's current crop of friends for confirmation. They then confirmed that they had been told by her what she had told him. That is all they could verify – none of them were actually there at the time. When it comes to domestic relationships people always take sides – usually in the honest belief that they are right. One only has to listen to somebody gossiping on a bus, one's own mother or even oneself to know that when we tell a story we are always convinced that we are right; from that point of view we start to vilify the other side. That is just human nature. The truth is that there is only one predominant reference point in Morton's version of Diana's story and that is Diana, and her account is constantly at loggerheads with independent witnesses.

Moreover, her words to Morton are often in serious contrast to either statements made or letters written by her at both earlier and happier times or later during calmer ones. For example, Diana's claim to Morton that she was a victim of Charles's cold indifference during her engagement, honeymoon and early months of marriage are clearly contradicted by her letters quoted by Paul Burrell in his book *A Royal Duty*. She wrote to one friend from the Royal Yacht while on honeymoon, 'I couldn't be happier and would never of [sic] believed how content or wonderful I feel. The cruise on *Britannia* was extremely spoiling and we spent most of the time giggling and mobbing each other up. Marriage suits me enormously and I just adore having someone to look after and spoil. It's the best thing that ever happened to me – besides being the luckiest lady in the world.'

To another she wrote, 'We practically blub every time we watch a video of the wedding, and I can just imagine in ten years time, one of the minor Wales's saying "Why did you call Daddy 'Philip'?" Oh well, something to look forward to.'

To a third she confided in a letter concerning her initial depression at the start of her marriage, 'I overcame those depressions all due to Charles with his patience and kindness. I couldn't get over how tired and miserable I got, which was unfair on him.'

Then there was, as previously quoted, her account to Janet

Filderman of the birth of Prince William not long after it occurred, which is both happy and generous to her husband and which she completely contradicted to Morton some nine years later, when she recounted how, 'We had found a date where Charles could get off his polo pony for me to give birth. That was very nice, felt very grateful about that!'

There are countless further examples – far too many to list – that cast serious doubt on the accuracy and truth of a lot of what she told Morton. As a result we are left to contemplate yet again whether Diana was just a wicked and manipulative woman or whether she was simply a young woman who was genuinely troubled and, as a result of the life that she had chosen, had placed herself in an impossible position where no one could really help her.

After Harry's birth, the marriage deteriorated rapidly and irrevocably. The Prince was still polite and kind to the Princess, but after years of torment, tirades and tantrums he withdrew from her emotionally and stopped trying. 'Something happened in his head,' Diana complained to Lady Colin Campbell, acknowledging that she rubbed him up the wrong way. 'I couldn't help it. I couldn't control myself.'

Princess Margaret of Hesse and the Rhine thought that Prince Charles had finally been pushed too far. 'One day he had enough. It was as simple as that. One day – a day neither he nor she nor anyone else can identify – she pushed him over the invisible line. He didn't realise it at the time, but she goaded him past the point of endurance. After that he retreated into himself.' Lady Sarah Spencer-Churchill agreed and believed that Diana had been lucky that he had stuck at it for four years when most men would have walked out on her after four weeks of such treatment.

Given Diana's state of mental health, it was quite impossible for her to accept any of the responsibility for this breakdown. It had to be someone else's fault. She convinced herself that the Prince had never loved her and had indeed never severed relations with Camilla Parker Bowles. 'He was having an affair with that woman all along. That was the problem. That's what caused my behaviour. Wouldn't you have been disturbed if your husband was having an affair? No wonder he couldn't give me the love I needed. He was giving it all to Camilla fucking Parker Bowles.' This was completely untrue, but Diana wanted to believe it and in time wanted the rest of the world to do so also. And thanks to the Morton book, millions across the world do.

It is largely accepted that by 1986 their marriage had irretrievably broken down. Diana would embark upon at least three affairs in that year and the Prince, aware of his wife's extra-marital sex, returned to 'his' lady. However, there are, as is usual in such nasty domestic situations, quite conflicting opinions as to why this happened.

While those at court were in no doubt whatsoever that the Princess had only herself to blame for this state of affairs, people not so close to the couple could only speculate. *Private Eye*'s 'Grovel' and Nigel Dempster for the *Daily Mail* (and ABC's *Good Morning America* in the US) had got wind of Diana's tantrums and the browbeating of Prince Charles from as early as 1982. To them he had become ruled by a fiend with a shrill voice and a foul mouth, and the *Eye* even hinted that he might be forced eventually to run for the comfort of either Camilla or Kanga sooner or later, reminding readers what these ladies did for the Prince prior to his marriage to Diana, and their subsequent redundancy.

On the other hand, some of the other journalists and photographers who spent their lives following the couple around had a different view. For example, Jayne Fincher, who had spent years photographing Diana, had noticed a change in her. She had gone from being a shy girl to someone who was 'very flirty, would giggle like mad, particularly if she went on visits to the military. She loved all the soldiers, and she'd giggle her head off and flutter her eyelashes and be completely silly.'

However, Patrick Jephson believed that the problem in the marriage was more likely created by Prince Charles. The future private secretary of the Princess, 'learned that, among other feelings he stirred in her, many of them warm and affectionate, the Princess also felt fear … when she felt herself to be on the receiving end of his anger, before her characteristic defiance set in, I often saw a look of trepidation cross her face, as if she were once again a small girl in trouble with the grown-ups.'

The view of a senior Buckingham Palace aid was that Charles was still stuck in his bachelor ways. Diana wanted him to spend more time at home with her and the children, and there were tantrums and hysterics. 'She challenged him – it was the first time he had been challenged. It was the first time he had met his equal – he was surrounded by yes-men. Diana accused Charles's friends of being sycophants, but she was her own worst enemy too.'

Another, less senior but closer to them, told me, 'It was inevitable.

Everything seemed to make her unhappy and nothing he did to help did any good. He couldn't do right for wrong and so everything was his fault and she certainly told him so. He hated rowing in public; it was against everything that he'd been brought up to believe in. She didn't give a damn – just like her mother – and when she realised that he couldn't bear it she did it all the more. She thought that she could break his spirit – but in the end she just drove him away … Much has been made of her being a good mother but a good mother doesn't rant and rave and use the F-word in front of the kids I think … Don't get me wrong, the Prince of Wales can be as selfish as the next man, but he really wanted it [the marriage] to work and having been around them for most of their married life, I quickly came to the conclusion that it was only going to be a matter of time before the whole thing went up in smoke. I never changed my mind on that. No man could have tried harder and most would have dumped her after a year or two … He tried time and again for the boys' sake and of course because he was the Prince of Wales.'

One of Diana's former flatmates ventured her opinion at the time that, 'Diana never had a growing-up period of flirtations that most teenage girls have. Diana is now going through that stage, which is something Charles can't cope with.' As it is extremely unlikely that such a statement would have been passed on without the Princess's permission, one is led to the conclusion that this was the message that Diana wanted to get across at the time – one of a fun-loving girl whose older and jealous husband couldn't cope with her light-hearted flirtations and was holding her back.

Interestingly, nobody put the Prince having an affair with Camilla Parker Bowles down as a reason for such troubles in 1986, and nor do they now when asked to recollect what they remember of those times. The marriage was definitely in trouble, and perhaps the reasons are not only unimportant but also none of our business until we all became involved at the Princess's invitation in 1992. Thereafter, it becomes a duty to expose the real position for sake of those unfairly maligned, and for history and truth itself.

And while the world was slowly waking up to the fact that the fairy-tale marriage may be in trouble, Andrew Morton, billed as 'the man who really knows the royals', wrote an odd piece in the *Daily Star* portraying the couple's relationship as a love affair of two strong characters. He concluded that Diana usually had the upper hand but that

The King and Di

Charles, if pushed too far, was a mouse that roared. This was seized upon by the US publication *Vanity Fair*. Journalist Tina Brown, with the help of Anthony Holden, spelled out what was happening. It was role reversal, pure and simple: the shy little princess had become Alexis Carrington from *Dynasty*; Action Man had turned into a dithering old gardener in the form of the Loony Prince. And now neither could understand what they had seen in the other in the first place.

What was without doubt by this time was that the fairy tale would not have a happy ending. Those around them knew that the marriage that the nation had wanted so much, and had put its faith in, was over. In addition, those who were more astute knew that while this might be the end of the marriage, it would not be the end of the story. The dream might have finished, but the nightmare, from the monarchy's point of view, was only just beginning. They had already realised that, whether inside the 'firm' or out, the girl whose unpredictable moods, vile tongue and ability to cause so much personal misery at home, while strutting the world stage with such beauty and wonderful charm, hadn't finished with the Windsors yet.

Indeed, the Princess of Wales had at this time hardly started her malicious campaign that was designed to portray herself as a victim and her husband as a villain – a campaign to deprive him of the crown and bring down the institution of monarchy itself. Much of the British media was by then under the control of the Australian republican, The Royal Family would not be given a fair hearing for many years, and their popularity would plummet as Diana ripped away one royal veil after another in a propaganda campaign that had little regard for fairness or the truth.

Chapter Nine
Affairs of State (1986–92)

Just as Mrs Thatcher had used the enemy abroad to great effect in 1982/3, she used the enemy at home during her second term in government to ensure a further victory in 1987. If her first term, from May 1979 until June 1983, had purged the country of its bad habits under the so-called consensus governments – both Tory and Labour – in the 1960s and 1970s, the second term, from June 1983 to June 1987, completed the purge and began to give the people some of the rewards they had voted for. Just as the Argentinean General Galtieri had provided a convenient whipping boy for the first administration, the miners' leader Arthur Scargill was the adversary to overcome in the second.

The miners had effectively scuppered Heath's Tory administration, initially in 1972 and then finally in 1974. Now there was to be a rematch, but this time the government had done some proper training. One of the reasons that the miners had been successful in the 1970s was due to their organisation of secondary picketing. They won a famous victory, though some see it as Pyrrhic one, when they forced the police to close the vital Saltley Power Station in Birmingham to incoming lorries because of the danger to human life from the violence of the picket lines. This led the miners, and Scargill in particular, as he had organised the pickets, to believe that they would always win. They had the guts and determination to see a battle through, while the forces of law and order would show restraint.

They were wrong: the law on secondary picketing was changed, and Margaret Thatcher was quite capable of meeting the forces of 'wrong' with her forces of 'right', which she ensured were just as committed, well-armed and violent as the other side. She brought in a tough, American-trained, Scottish businessman, Ian MacGregor, to give the Coal Board some backbone, and mobilised the police forces of the country – having been careful to give them a substantial pay rise first – to counter the miners. She also waited until coal stocks were high, having declined a fight in 1981 when she had been advised that they were not.

It was an epic battle. Mining communities are generally impervious to public opinion, and were especially so then when they believed that most of such opinion was formed by softies in the south who didn't know the meaning of a proper day's work. They also had a great loyalty to their union and believed in the eloquent way Scargill expressed their views for them. And he was right: the Coal Board was planning to close many pits and reduce the number of mineworkers substantially. In those days it was still possible to rally a membership with socialist rhetoric that ignored the reality that such pits needed to be closed as they were not economically viable and would thus endanger those that were if they were to remain open.

The miners, however, or more to the point the National Union of Mineworkers, made two errors of judgement. Firstly, the NUM failed to hold a ballot to authorise strike action, which led a significant minority, the Nottingham miners, refusing to strike on the grounds that the union's leadership had been so keen politically to have a go at a right-wing government that it had denied the membership its democratic right to vote in case it voted against a strike. This meant that coal stocks could be replenished sufficiently to avoid having to repeat Heath's three-day weeks of 1974. In addition, other unions, whose members were not keen to help the miners as they were starting to feel the benefits of Thatcher's policies and were not happy with the idea of being left behind in a booming economy, pointed publicly to the lack of a vote as to why they couldn't help. In reality, they wouldn't have been able to anyway.

Secondly, the NUM in general and Scargill in particular failed to realise that Thatcher played to win, whatever the cost, and the cost in terms of both money and the strain on social cohesion was high. But the public, perhaps having remembered the chaos that resulted from Heath's defeat at the hands of the miners, stood behind her. This was especially true once she moved the handling of the strike away from MacGregor – who was tough, but something of a public-relations liability – to the government minister Peter Walker. Walker had been a successful businessman in his own right and knew what was wanted, but he also had the charm and PR skills to deliver it and bring the nation along with him. Scargill was no match for him. Thatcher and MacGregor had the will to win, and Walker made sure that the case was argued in reasonable language and from a moral high ground. This combination, along with a booming economy that ensured little sympathy from other quarters, was all just too much for the NUM.

The strongest and most politically motivated union in the country surrendered unconditionally after a year, its members, first in trickles, then in droves, walking back to work, leaving their union to count both the financial and prestige cost of such a humiliation. It was the final nail in the coffin of union supremacy over government.

Allied with the union legislation that was so skilfully handled through Parliament by Jim Prior and Norman Tebbit, this victory restored the balance of power in industrial relations. Management had been given back the right to manage, and governments the right to govern. Most people were grateful and relieved and it showed in the opinion polls. In 1987, Mrs Thatcher went to the country for a third term in office and was rewarded with another landslide victory.

In her second term Thatcher had also been aided by a bull market on the London exchange, which was reflected around the world. Her government had set out to create more private house-owners and shareholders, the latter being a sector that had been in decline since the end of the Second World War. During its second administration, having spent most of the first firefighting, it realised that it had the ability to stimulate demand for both, but needed a successful economy in each case in order to create investor confidence.

As real confidence grew in the British economy probably for the first sustainable time since 1945, the government prepared to force the sale of council houses to their tenants at advantageous prices, while it intended to privatise British this or that and as a result get rid of incompetent nationalised industries, which were a burden on the taxpayer, by selling them to the public at knockdown prices. Privatisation, or denationalisation as it was also called, was a radical step and it took even the radical Thatcher some time to grasp it totally to her bosom. When she eventually did and put her resulting policies into place, the economic logic became so irresistible that her status grew even higher in the US, half of Europe copied her and she caused the Labour opposition to move eventually somewhere to the right of the previous Heath Conservative government once it realised that not to do so would mean that it would spend further decades out in the cold.

In 1981 she proclaimed, 'The two great problems of the British economy are the monopoly nationalised industries and the monopoly trade unions.' Having dealt with the second in the early 1980s, she then set about dismantling the first. In the twenty-first century this doesn't seem that extraordinary; then, however, half of Europe was poverty stricken under a socialist yoke and Britain had been as nationalised and socialist as it had ever been less than ten years before. The government believed that the nationalised industries were over-subsidised, uncompetitive, inefficient and nearly always loss-making. They did not represent good value for the taxpayer. Initially, the government just tried to ensure that these state monopolies were run more like PLCs as even they thought denationalisation was a step too far. However, as they grew in confidence, spurred on by an electorate that told them that the destruction of the nationalised industries would create much joy and not much sorrow, they warmed to their work during their second term. And to keep the momentum going, the sale of such public assets made large cuts in direct taxation possible in the budgets of 1985 and 1986.

The whole process – the creation of a share-owning, house-owning democracy paying less tax – helped sustain the bull market that had begun in 1982, and was another factor in Thatcher's huge victory of 1987. Indeed, exasperated union leaders and Labour politicians realised that Thatcher, by making voters home-owners who bought shares and had more cash in their pockets than ever before, had given the people middle-class capitalist aspirations, and that meant that she had moved them permanently into the Tory voting camp.

She was right. An analysis of those who voted Tory in 1987 shows how important the skilled manual worker turned out to be: the Tory share of the manual workers' vote, at thirty-six per cent, was higher than in any election since the war. In 1979 Labour still secured forty-five per cent of this vote, not that much less than in 1974. By 1987 Thatcherism had eroded this to thirty-four per cent, which meant that she had taken more of Labour's heartland vote than they had. And the opinion polls showed that these were the very people who were buying their council homes and snapping up the shares on offer in the latest denationalised industry.

Many people believe that there were three great reforming British prime ministers in the twentieth century: David Lloyd George, Clement Attlee and Margaret Thatcher – one Liberal, one Labour and one Conservative. Ironically, many of Thatcher's reforms were concerned with ridding the nation of Attlee's, and were as applauded at the time as Attlee's had been when he implemented them after the Second World War.

Prince Charles, while applauding much of this political and economic stimulation, remained very concerned about the have-nots – those who inhabited the inner-city ghettos and were clearly being left behind in this whirlwind romance with capitalism. He was right to be so, but the nation was in no mood, not even after the 1981 riots, to listen. As a result of this and his then unfashionable views on farming, the environment, architecture, religion and medicine, he seemed to be singing from a totally different hymn sheet to the rest of the nation.

Indeed, one got the impression that somehow, ever since the 1950s, Charles hadn't quite been in step with fashion. In the 1960s he clearly was unmoved by the Beatles and, perhaps wisely in hindsight, worried about the destructive nature of the social revolution taking place as the baby boomers grabbed power. At university, just when people like John Lennon were pretending to be working class, the Prince wore trousers instead of jeans, spoke with a plum in his mouth and seemed more like a don than a student, which meant that he stood for the Establishment in the eyes of the young. By the mid-1980s, it seemed that he had finally found brown rice and mysticism some fifteen years after John, Paul, George and Ringo and their adoring generation had moved on. The 'must be able to do what we want when we want' baby boomers had by now taken Thatcherism to their hearts: materialism became extremely fashionable, and 'we must have what we want when we want it' was the new slogan. In some areas of society, where material gain wasn't conventionally so easy to come by, their children became the second dysfunctional generation, and the further dehumanising of hundreds of British housing estates was underway.

The country had clearly needed such a meritocracy in order to shake off the economic woes that had made it the laughing stock of Europe for some thirty years. Nevertheless, a nasty side effect was seen as people became obsessed by material gain often at the expense of others' loss or pain, moral values, religious belief or damage to the environment. The regeneration of the British economy and the small-business success upon which it was built was essential, and pointed Britain economically in the right direction for the next thirty years at least. However, it also placed Britain at the vanguard of a western society that seemed to have sold its soul in order to buy life's material pleasures on earth – it didn't believe in religion, or that life would be rewarded in the next world.

Unlike Prince Charles, most people don't form their own opinions and then stick to them whatever the current fashion dictates. Increasingly it was only those who were concerned about society's direction and thus could identify with his opinions, or those who worked with him and understood his dedication, who stood by him. The nation – according to the tabloid press that apparently represented it – increasingly wanted an all-glittering world where celebrity, beauty, youth and wealth were the gods to worship. Not only did Prince Charles no longer represent these images, now he was even damning much of the nation's new way of life in his speeches like some Old Testament prophet. As a result, his opinions were open to ridicule.

On the other hand, Diana had no such problem. Not only was she new – Charles was old hat – she was exactly the image that represented the new fashion. She was extremely young, beautiful and wealthy and as a result a perfect celebrity. And celebrity, in modern society, is an addictive drug: the media is the dealer and the public the user. The greater the user's addiction, the sooner an overdose will occur. Then the dealer discards that drug and moves on before returning to destroy it. Only death saved Diana from this fate.

But in the second half of the 1980s, Diana was in the throes of becoming one of the world's most admired icons of the twentieth century. She was a perfect model in the fashion-obsessed UK, where political correctness and the meritocracy were giving rise to greater respect for the female pound and more column inches given to women in newspapers. Moreover, she was half of the world's most successful double act abroad: however troubled their marriage might have become, they worked in public on foreign tours extremely well together, and attracted the attention of the world and his wife wherever they went. But Diana had become more than just one half of a fairy tale; more than a mere consort. She was extremely beautiful, demure and had developed a common touch with the young, old, sick and dying that any self-respecting politician would have given their right arm for. The combination was intoxicating and, as a result, she appealed to both sexes the world over. Men loved her, and women wanted to be like her.

This certainly put some pressure on the dutiful Prince Charles, who grew not only to be hurt by the crowds' preference for his wife, but was seriously annoyed when issues that were important in his opinion, and which he wished to highlight, went unreported in favour of lengthy descriptions of his wife's latest dress. In addition, he couldn't understand how something that he had thought through and done an amazing amount of hard work on for the good of a deserving cause either got ridiculed or ignored, while Diana, who at this time did not dedicate a serious amount of her time to charity work and showed little genuine personal enthusiasm for it by comparison, had simply to turn up in order for the next day's press to be full of pictures of her as a caring princess with a saint-like quality.

This combination of love for the mirage that Diana created and ridicule of the 'Loony Prince' was very mischievous insofar as it was not only grossly unfair and rewarded image instead of substance, but it also completely undervalued the Prince's achievements over these years. Naturally, he had been well supported in all of his endeavours by highly dedicated professionals without whom success would not necessarily have been achieved; but his own dedication, inspiration, enthusiasm, hard work and political muscle made it all possible, and as a result hundreds of thousands of youngsters, who by virtue of an accident of birth were doomed to a life of little inspiration or hope, have every reason to be grateful to him – and most are.

By 1987, the Prince's Trust and its offspring the Prince's Youth Business Trust (PYBT) were enjoying great success. The former was awarding small grants of cash to assist the unemployed, ex-offenders, the ethnic minorities and the disabled to become more self-sufficient, while the PYBT gave out modest loans or grants to similar folk who believed that they were embryonic entrepreneurs. Soon after Mrs Thatcher's re-election in that year, the Prince felt confident enough to write to her to explain why he had established the PYBT: 'I felt very strongly that there was a great deal of hidden and wasted talent in the less prosperous parts of the U.K. and also that it was important to encourage the formation of new enterprises which could, in due course, become some of the major companies of the future.'

Thatcher, who perhaps understandably had been initially wary of the Prince's efforts in this field, seeing them as a criticism of government policy and suspecting them of being left of centre, could not argue with his logic. His aims smacked of Thatcherism because the idea was not to dish out handouts, but to help youngsters help themselves. As a result, she and the heir to the throne started to develop a mutual respect for each other, while often agreeing to differ. This grew year on year throughout the prime minister's time in office. She grew to admire his genuine dedication to the nation, the enthusiasm he displayed and the intellect that he possessed. Thus she came to appreciate a prince whom she nevertheless always saw as interfering in matters that did not concern him.

It is widely known that Thatcher held the Princess in no such regard as she suspected Diana of being a self-obsessed fashion model who was only concerned about her own media image. A former cabinet colleague of the time told me, 'Margaret was always both a little suspicious of and irritated by Charles. She just didn't see it as his business to be getting involved in matters like unemployment, which had been rising under us and naturally we were all sensitive. She believed that it would all come right in the end but wished that Charles would keep his nose out of it and stick to cutting ribbons. At first she saw his pronouncements as an abuse of his position. In the end she saw that he was genuine and didn't have a left-wing bias and she came to respect his views – although I suspect that she always thought some of his opinions were a little idealistic. On the other hand, Diana was a better bet because she had no interest in such matters. She was clearly poorly educated and only seemed to care about how often her face was in the newspapers each day. I think the PM saw Diana as less of a threat and thought that she was a bit of a bimbo really.'

This is rather ironic: Diana was a huge fan of Mrs Thatcher and a loyal supporter of her right-wing policies. Unlike the Prince, with his sympathetic view of the underprivileged, his wife believed that one's surroundings, lack of good example, or even love, were no excuse for committing crime, and those who did so should have the full weight of the law come down on them. The Princess was very much in the 'bring back flogging' lobby.

So the prime minister, who had based the recovery of the British economy on the creation of economic conditions that helped create new enterprises, came to respect the aims of the PYBT, although it is by no means certain that she was ever to share Charles's faith in those to whom he was handing out the cash.

In addition to providing loans of up to £5,000 and grants to the value of £3,000 to people whom Thatcher half expected to run off with the money and spend it on drugs, the PYBT provided specialist advice to those who successfully applied to one of the thirty-eight regional boards that were established across the country. These boards were managed by successful people seconded from private industry, and gave free advice and support to every new business. The formula was more successful than Thatcher imagined or the Prince had dared to hope. In the second half of the eighties it took off to such an extent that by the end of the decade more than 10,000 businesses had been started, involving more than 15,000 young people, 66 per cent of which were still trading after 3 years in business. This was a tremendous achievement and one can't help but wonder what fabulous praise would have been heaped upon Princess Diana by the media if she had ever masterminded and then seen through such a scheme.

It was as a result of this success that Stephen O'Brien, the CEO of a charitable enterprise called Business in the Community (BITC), raised the possibility of yet another new initiative. At a meeting with Prince Charles, O'Brien spoke of the urgent need to break down the barriers of class and race that divided the captains of industry and the leaders of the ethnic minorities. O'Brien, having impressed the Prince with his own eloquence, was then taken aback by Charles's response. 'I was very surprised how much he already knew about the issue. He was very knowledgeable. At the end of the conversation he said simply, "I'd like to help." I said, "If you are ready to take a risk, I'll organise an event."'

A month later in a discreet Windsor hotel, some of the country's most powerful industrialists sat down to dinner with some of the most radical black leaders in Britain, who had decided in advance who should speak and in what order. Some of the Prince's advisers were horrified that O'Brien had been allowed to expose him to such a potentially explosive situation. However, the Prince skilfully chaired a lively and at times heated discussion and the result was that the meeting surpassed everyone's expectations. It finished with Charles urging them to build on what had just been established. Not long afterwards he became BITC's first president and immediately transformed its prospects.

In November 1985, with his new private secretary John Riddell in tow, the Prince flew to Edinburgh to make his first speech in his new role. He was to appeal for greater investment of both money and time into local communities, declaring that this would be the only way to bring about an enterprise culture. Mrs Thatcher certainly couldn't argue with that as she had made the creation of an enterprise culture a cornerstone of Thatcherism, and its appeal was so irresistible that in time both the other two political parties would be forced to ditch their nanny-state dogma and follow her lead. 'The problem is how to change people's attitudes so they realise that they can make a contribution themselves towards job creation and enterprise,' the Prince declared to his audience as he shared his experiences of his work with the PYBT. So far so good – the prime minister's views precisely – but then the

Prince departed from the notes that Riddell had prepared for him and added, 'What really worries me is that we are going to end up a fourth-rate country. I do not want to see that and I am sure none of you do.' This addition not only startled his private secretary and the audience, but also was immediately pounced upon by the press. The Conservative government had been in power for six years, was two years into its second term following a huge election victory and was thought to be doing a good job by most other than the deposed union leaders and diehard left-wingers. Suddenly, the Prince of Wales was telling the world that actually the nation was not out of the woods. Mrs Thatcher was furious as the *Sun*'s headline screamed out 'FOURTH RATE BRITAIN ALERT', and almost every other newspaper made the same point.

The Prince had pushed his case to the boundaries of his constitutional position, and had seriously annoyed the prime minister in the process. However, he hadn't meant to point the finger at the government of the day. While he did believe that the prime minister should pay greater attention to the inner cities, he also believed in her vision of an enterprise culture and was just as opposed to a nanny state as she was. He was purely pointing out that to ignore inner city deprivation would unleash a cancer upon British society as a whole. Some twenty years on, the wisdom of his words seems undeniable.

However, was his controversial comment a naive mistake? The Prince certainly didn't think so. He was passionate about the point and believed that it was his duty to speak out. Moreover, he knew that the press would twist his words or quote them out of context in order to create a controversy of their own devising anyway, and he preferred to give them something that he could stand by.

Nevertheless, by selecting phrases that would inevitably attract attention, he was bound also to generate both conflict and criticism. The Prince was then, and to a certain extent remains today, slow to realise the impact that his words would have. He also has an understandable suspicion of, and dislike for, the media in general, and the tabloids in particular. As a result he has forever moaned about the press. However, on this occasion he was delighted. His sound bite had worked and he had got his point across. By warning against a 'fourth-rate Britain', he had drawn attention to his own deep and rightly placed anxiety while flagging up the role of BITC. Suddenly everyone knew what BITC was, and an important momentum had begun.

Prince Charles had realised immediately the potential of BITC to harness both financial and professional resources to bring out the talents that he was convinced were buried under inner-city deprivation and waiting to be discovered. He believed he could and should make a difference. Not only was it his duty to do so, but also it gave him purpose and took his mind off the increasingly unhappy marriage that he found himself in. He immersed himself in the challenge of his new presidency. Between 1986 and 1992 he was to undertake more than 200 public engagements on the organisation's behalf. Moreover, throughout this period he bombarded entrepreneurs, industrialists, financiers and ministers, including the prime minister, with letters either promoting new schemes or begging for further assistance or greater efforts. Much of this correspondence was littered with expressions of his anxiety about Britain's loss of manufacturing jobs. This further tested the prime minister's patience. Then he developed a passion for import substitution as a means of combating unemployment, and was infuriated when neither the government nor industry seemed to take his 'buy British' campaign seriously.

Charles is a compassionate man but he is not an economist. As often happens when he is passionate about something, he launched into a campaign without thinking it through. He had no idea if such a campaign was either practical or desirable; he just backed his own intuition. His opinion was completely at odds with both the government and industry, which preferred to leave matters to the marketplace. In particular, Margaret Thatcher believed that it was government's job to create the conditions where a free market could prosper, and not its job to interfere thereafter. The performance of the British economy over the next twenty years suggests that she was right and the Prince wrong. However, undeterred and still convinced that he was right, Charles wrote to O'Brien about the inadequacy of British marketing: 'This is what I find so unbearably exasperating about the attitude in this country. There seems to be a degree of complacency, which is little short of incredible. Having just returned from Texas and several visits to High tech companies etc., I find that I want to speak out about all the opportunities we seem to lose in every direction. The trouble is to find the right occasion on which to speak …'

Mrs Thatcher would have shared the Prince's frustration but was sufficiently economically mature in her thinking to know that making speeches about the problem wasn't the answer. The British economy had been in relative decline since the turn of the century and in serious decline since the Second World War. Her advisors had convinced her that if she created the right incentives in an enterprise culture, a phoenix could rise from the ashes, but it would take time to see the effects and at least a decade before these modest beginnings on the newly created business parks that were springing up all over Britain developed into international companies.

With the benefit of hindsight it is possible to see that they were correct and it was the government's policies more than the Prince's speeches that did the trick. Nevertheless, he certainly was sincere, earnest and keen to play his part; this is what he did, and it was not just the deprived ethnic minorities who had reason to be grateful to him. This prince not only stood for David against Goliath when it came to people, he now took small businesses under his wing as well. After a visit to Merseyside, the clearing banks came into in his sights. He deplored their failure to fund small business. He was appalled to learn that two Liverpool firms had been unable to meet export orders to the United States for furniture and engineering due to the fact that their banks wouldn't advance them the cash in order that they might manufacture. When he had asked why, he was advised that there was a certain reluctance to lend money in the Liverpool area. He was livid. How could anyone expect to arrest the erosion of the manufacturing base in the northwest if banks were allowed to behave like this?

This is precisely where the Prince of Wales's views and those of the prime minister went their own ways. Both believed in helping people to help themselves. Both believed in the need to create an enterprise culture. However, the compassionate Charles wanted to rescue the manufacturing base in the northwest of England whereas the practical Margaret believed that if it were worth saving then it would save itself – and if it wasn't then it wouldn't. Economically she might have been right, but that is easy to say when you live in the prosperous south, and many people from all over Great Britain agreed with the Prince and not the prime minister.

On a trip to Boston in the US, the Prince was taken to see an old mill town called Lowell. He was most impressed to learn that there was a 'partnership' working there to revive the community. On his return to London, he proposed that BITC should initiate a similar scheme in Britain. The executive board immediately agreed. Two days later Prince Charles was on the phone wanting to know which town had been chosen. He had wanted an old mill town like Burnley or Halifax.

The board settled on Halifax.

This old mill town was suffering. It had, like so many other industrial towns of the north of England that owed their size and prestige to the Industrial Revolution, come under pressure due to foreign competition. A combination of high productivity and cheap labour costs in the Far East, and poor investment at home, had meant that both the home and export markets for these towns' products were being lost, and as a result mills had closed making unemployment high. Naturally this had affected the whole local community as consumer spending plummeted.

To Mrs Thatcher this was just an unfortunate part of the economic cycle. Tin mining in Cornwall had disappeared hundreds of years before because the tin mines weren't economic. She understood that flogging a dead horse was economic suicide as it poured good money after bad into investments where it would be lost. Prince Charles didn't actually disagree with that, but he argued that whole towns could not just up sticks and descend on London to look for jobs. He didn't want to support dead industries or just dispense cash to the unemployed. Indeed, he understood every bit as well as the prime minister the folly of doing that. But he did want to find ways of regenerating the environment and attracting investment into new business ventures that would stimulate local employment and so help the community recover and once more become self-sufficient.

Halifax became a test bed for a new form of partnership between business and the community. It was soon to be regarded as a model of good practice. It became known as the Halifax Partnership and aroused considerable interest. Prince Charles was keenly involved in the development of the project as a memo written by him to his assistant private secretary demonstrates:

[display text]
1. I am anxious that there should be an input from a good community architect. I strongly recommend he should get in touch with John Thompson, who is the architect involved with the duchy tenants' co-op. scheme ...
2. The point about the community architect is that he/she is badly needed to coordinate the whole project, to encourage the participants, work with local authorities etc. and ABOVE ALL, ensure that the DESIGN of houses is decent. I am worried that they will otherwise just

build hideous little boxes ...

3. I am not entirely convinced that it is a good idea to concentrate this scheme entirely on the unemployed. I would have thought a mixture of people was a better idea. I don't believe, for instance, that the self-help scheme I saw in Macclesfield 2 years ago was exclusively involved with unemployed people. The important thing is to try and recreate, or rejuvenate, COMMUNITIES as a whole ...

4. I re-emphasise this question of DESIGN. If it is at all possible people should be able to express their own feelings about the design of their houses, the layout of the scheme, gardens, front doors and windows. A community architect understands all this and knows how to work WITH people who have never had any experience of this sort of thing. They have to convince the local politicians to let them coordinate such projects and to be flexible about the interpretation of building regulations etc.

Please make sure I am kept fully informed about progress. C
[end display text]

Soon Charles felt confident enough to write to Margaret Thatcher in order to promote the scheme: 'I felt that we had much to learn in this field from the United States and as a result we decided, as a pilot project, to concentrate on one town in the north of England and to encourage a partnership approach towards regenerating the local economy, rehabilitating old buildings, restoring confidence ...'

Suddenly Thatcher saw what the Prince was up to. What he was talking about could work and, as it did not involve government subsidy dressed up as artificial investment, it wasn't against the ideals of Thatcherism after all. By championing the idea of partnership so vigorously, the Prince managed to change government thinking and set it on course that both John Major's governments and those of Tony Blair were to follow. Indeed, Mr Blair became so impressed by the concept that to hear him talk about partnerships two decades later one might be forgiven for thinking that the whole concept was his brainchild in the first place. Mrs Thatcher and her ministers might have reached the same conclusions as the Prince in the fullness of time anyway, but it is unlikely that the rapid momentum would have been acquired without the success of BITC's brave initial pioneering scheme. Thanks to its success it was not long before this approach became an established feature of government policy, and it remains so today some twenty years later.

Mrs Thatcher had once famously said of herself, 'The lady's not for turning,' but on this issue she had, and as a result government not only embarked on a more humane policy but one that greatly assisted the regeneration of local wealth without wasting any of the Exchequer's valuable cash. By now she and the Prince were not only getting to understand each other but there was a mutual, if at times somewhat grudging, respect developing. She probably now saw him as a Tory wet, but at least that meant he wasn't a socialist. He still wasn't convinced that she gave these matters enough attention, but was nevertheless extremely grateful that she was listening and had now even acted positively.

In reality, their beliefs were more similar and complementary than either had at first realised. Charles's compassion had dictated that help reached the deprived areas of British life; Thatcher's general economic regeneration of the British economy – based on sound money and economic principles – produced, in time, a wealth that could sustain enough investment in the enterprise culture to keep it moving forward with a momentum that eventually recaptured Britain's position as the world's fourth biggest economy, able to afford the long-term investment in programmes that were so enthusiastically supported by the heir to the throne

By 1989, BITC had established nineteen partnerships led by British leadership teams. The success of these encouraged the government to set up the first Training Enterprise Councils (TECs), which were actually modelled on the BITC schemes. Ministers in general, and the prime minister in particular, were slightly reluctant to give too much of the credit for this to the Prince in public – as one might expect from politicians who needed every piece of useful propaganda to get themselves re-elected. Nevertheless, most were happy to concede in private that Charles's own involvement had played a very significant part in establishing what, in the nineties and beyond, came to occupy an important place in Britain's economic and social life. This was not just because he was the Prince of Wales, but because he had made himself an expert on the subject of social regeneration and had found solutions to difficult problems. This meant that Mrs Thatcher could present herself and her government as caring, as well as bringing economic realism to a country that had been living beyond its means for most of the twentieth century.

The King and Di

It was also at the Prince's instigation that BITC started more than sixty inner city 'compacts' between local schools and local employers. Once again Boston had been the place where the Prince was introduced to the idea. There he discovered that in a run-down area of the city, employers, schools, parents and children had made a formal 'deal': any child who agreed to meet a set of social and academic targets would be rewarded by going straight to the top of the job queue in those companies that were involved in the scheme. The idea was to promote social responsibility by all, reward those who were attempting to help themselves and become good citizens, and offer hope to the most deprived children in the city by involving local business in a partnership of training and education. Prince Charles was once again most impressed. He felt that the scheme was working because the people of the community were actually solving their own problems. Once again he urged the executive board of BITC to promote similar schemes in Britain. He believed that with a little encouragement and explanation, schools could go on to run the scheme themselves.

As usual, Charles pulled out his pen and started lobbying heads of industry and government; he followed this up with a series of dinner parties at Kensington Palace where the guests, once captured around the dining table, were subjected to lengthy and enthusiastic explanations of how such a scheme could transform employment prospects in the deprived areas.

Norman Fowler, the employment secretary of the day, was duly dispatched to take a look at the Boston Compact. He returned equally enthused and became a staunch ally of the Prince. In 1996 Norman and I spent time together as we were involved in a two-venue debate against the likeable Denis Healey and Chris Haskins of Northern Foods, sponsored by a leading insurance broker for the benefit of their corporate clients. Fowler, who is both genial and a gentleman of principle, told me over dinner on the first evening that throughout the 1980s Prince Charles had blazed a trail through the problems of inner-city deprivation with such passion and energy that Mrs Thatcher had been forced to follow. At first this had been almost against her will, but she had later become converted when she understood that the Prince was offering solutions of self-help and not opposing Thatcherism by advocating the ruinous cash handouts favoured by the Labour Party.

Not long after Fowler's return from Boston, BITC's compacts were turned into government-sponsored 'education and business partnerships', and once again the Prince had had a direct hand in defining the course that the government was following, and thousands of less well-off children would be the beneficiaries.

O'Brien was delighted and even amazed by the speed at which results had been achieved. He put this down to the indefatigable energy and enthusiasm of the Prince. To celebrate the Prince's first year of presidency he wrote to Charles, 'I wanted you to know just how much your Presidency has meant to Business in the Community ... The development has been enormous ...' He went on to cite a rapid growth in membership, a surge in funds, a renewed sense of motivation and cooperation that 'has come about directly as a result of your injunction to everyone in this area to "work together" ... Your visits to depressed areas have lifted spirits and made a real difference. Your visits to Skelmersdale, Brixton, Deptford and Handsworth live in our minds in this connection. The comment by the Chief Constable in Birmingham that your visit in the summer contributed substantially to easing tension was, I am sure, absolutely accurate. We repeatedly hear comments from the black community to the effect that "at least the Prince of Wales cares about us."'

Just another sucking-up letter? Not quite. In September 1985, an outbreak of ethnic violence in Handsworth had left two people dead; several injured and had caused an estimated £16 million of damage. The following summer the chief constable of West Midlands Police, the respected Geoffrey Dear, warned that once again tension had risen to breaking point. The Prince of Wales then made a visit to Handsworth that coincided with the anniversary of the previous year's riot. Afterwards Dear was able to tell the press that Charles's visit had 'quite dramatically' eased the tension. I consider myself one of the few white men who know the West Indian Community in Handsworth well. I was their personal funeral director for nearly twenty years, and there were many fewer family homes that I hadn't been inside than those that I had. I lived and worked with them cheek by jowl and I know how much love and respect they have for Charles Windsor and how hard he has had to work to earn it.

The Prince responded to O'Brien's praise enthusiastically. He endorsed his proposal that for the next annual general meeting the members of the BITC board should be invited to a 'field day' in Hackney and Tower Hamlets. He replied, 'I think it would be a very good idea. This is just what is needed – less sitting round a table and more persuasion "on the ground"!'

This idea of O'Brien's was immediately seized upon by the Prince. He quickly realised that the best way to get the decision-makers in society to help him was to force them to confront the problems and challenges facing BITC. This led directly to the establishment of the Prince's now famous 'Seeing is Believing' campaign. The idea came to him as a result of O'Brien's suggestion for the location of the AGM and the slogan was thought up by him to express neatly the belief that business leaders and politicians would only understand the sense of urgency about the needs of our inner cities if they saw the deprivation at first hand. He hoped to make them realise the potential of young people to restore both pride and hope into these ghettos through the self-respect gained by helping to regenerate the area, rather than expecting government to correct everything by pouring in good cash after bad.

The Prince was most astute in this. The reason why so many of his projects have been successful over the last twenty years, whereas so many of New Labour's have failed in recent times, is precisely because Charles understood that a community can only help itself. New Labour mistakenly believed that by pouring cash into deprived areas for better housing and community facilities, people would be grateful and respond accordingly. They didn't, and within a very short space of time things were as bad as or even worse than before. A child will only be inclined to keep his room tidy if he has tidied it himself – he understands the effort that went into doing it and experiences the reward of achievement. This is only basic human nature, but the heir to the throne, despite his privileged life, understood it.

Now the Prince added to his avalanche of personal letters and persuasive vegetarian dinner parties forays into deprived areas. He would lead his guests into an uncharted world of decline and despair. Quickly he realised that this was much more powerful than any picture that he might paint with his pen or at a dinner party. By the end of the 1980s, 'Seeing is Believing' had already galvanised several hundred business leaders into direct support for a range of BITC projects by providing training and work in some of the most run-down areas of the country. By now the Prince had really got the bit between his teeth. He was not a figurehead but a man on a mission. He wrote to O'Brien, 'I can't tell you what a difference it makes to me to have someone like you who actually takes up some of my suggestions and puts them into practice.'

It is quite easy to get the impression from Andrew Morton that the Prince of Wales spent the 1980s on a polo pony, hunting, bedding Mrs Parker Bowles or depressed about his own insecurities. This is not only a distortion; it is clearly a deliberate perversion of the truth. In addition to his involvement with the Prince's Trust, PYBT and BITC, the Prince was still chairman of the Royal Jubilee Trusts, the management of which was finally merged with the Prince's Trust in 1988 after what had been a long and hard-fought battle with the old guard at Buckingham Palace. In addition, he was also the driving force behind another organisation, the Prince of Wales Community Venture, which was set up in 1985. He informed Margaret Thatcher by letter that, 'The aim of this venture was to try and find a way by which young people from ALL walks of life – those from state schools and private schools – could be brought together for a short period in their lives in order to live and work as a team, making a contribution to their communities in various ways. The important element of this project is that it involves several voluntary organisations agreeing to co-operate, together with the active participation of the Fire Service, the Ambulance Service and the Police, to whom the young people are attached …'

The Prince, despite having hated his time at Gordonstoun, had retained the influence of Kurt Hahn and therefore had a vision that the nation would regain some of its former discipline if it engaged in a compulsory community-service programme for teenagers. He hoped that he would in time be able to persuade the prime minister to introduce such a scheme. She had some sympathy with the idea, but believed that such a plan was far too close to the idea of returning to compulsory national service and that it would be, as a result, unacceptable to the electorate and therefore a vote-loser.

As a surrogate initiative, Community Venture provided a year-long programme of 'service and training'. The first pilot scheme took place in Sunderland and was followed by others in Llanelli, Blackburn, Bradford and Strathclyde. The Community Venture ran for six years before being phased out in 1991. Only a thousand young people had participated over that period, which meant that while it was by no means a failure, it wasn't the roaring success that his other projects had been. Perhaps this was because the benefits were less personally directed at the participants than in some of his other schemes.

However, this setback did not deter him, and he continued to argue the case for compulsory community service to any government minister or high-ranking civil servant that he came across. He even made a passionate speech about it to Tom Shebbeare at the latter's final interview for the post of director of the Prince's Trust. In the end he finished with the question, 'Don't you agree?' Shebbeare said he didn't, and even had the guts to tell the Prince why. He still got the job. Thereafter, he spent quite a bit of his time ensuring that the Prince didn't waste any of his valuable media coverage banging on about these sincerely held but nonetheless unfashionable views.

The Community Venture was eventually replaced by the Prince's Trust Volunteers programme, which was based on the principles to which Prince Charles was so committed, but which had also been modified enough by Shebbeare to be acceptable to the public. By 1993 the new scheme had seen 4,500 youngsters go through the six-day intensive programme, and this was projected to expand rapidly towards 25,000. By 1994, after much personal lobbying of ministers by the Prince, the government committed itself to providing matching funds for the scheme. A Whitehall working party involving twelve departments was also set up to find ways in which government employees might participate. Then the Labour Party's Commission on Social Justice also adopted key aspects of the scheme. Indeed its proposals for Citizens Service seem to have been virtually lifted from the Prince's Trust Volunteers programme. Unfortunately, New Labour was even less keen than the Tories had been to give credit to the imagination and enthusiasm of the heir to the throne, but at least the Prince had the satisfaction of knowing that his thinking on many areas of social concern had now been adopted by both of Britain's main political parties. How many political, church or social leaders can say that?

By the end of the 1980s, the Prince of Wales was carrying the BITC message to the rest of the world. He wanted the multinational companies to share his perspective. He and his team held a two-day seminar in Charleston, South Carolina. More than 100 senior executives attended it from the United States, Britain, Japan, Europe and Australia. The Prince talked about the responsibilities of big business to the environment and to each local community. Then, after the Prince had led them all on a tour of the traditional town, the delegates broke up into small groups in order to debate the issues raised by Prince Charles. The event was a tremendous success and within months the Business Leaders Forum (BLF) was in operation. Over the next few years, seventeen similar international meetings were organised and as a result over 4,000 business leaders from North America, Europe, Latin America and Asia came to debate the best ways that business could defend the environment and look after employees and the local communities where they lived.

Some critics saw this as little more than an elitist talking shop for jet-setting VIPs who liked the idea of meeting the Prince of Wales. Undeterred, the BLF was to form nearly 100 partnerships with businesses from Russia, Poland, the Czech Republic and Slovakia, setting up a range of essential training and environmental programmes as these countries struggled to convert their societies and economies from the yoke of communism to the bitter realities of a free-market economy. A task force was formed to regenerate the cultural life of St Petersburg. The old Red Army barracks near Budapest were converted into units for the use of new small-business ventures. As other similar projects sprang up around what had once been the old Soviet Union, whatever the critics were saying, it was clear that Prince Charles's message about what business could do to help and stimulate prosperous communities was by now reaching an international audience and people were benefiting around the world as a result.

All of these initiatives, both at home and abroad, were born out of concern by a compassionate and caring man who wanted to improve the lot of the worst off in life and believed that by helping them to help themselves he was going to benefit everybody else as well. He also believed that the converse was true: if nothing were done, a cancer would develop in these areas that would in time create a way of life that would be detrimental to all. Of course, he understood how important good press was in order to promote his projects; but while he appreciated how positive media coverage was a huge help, he wasn't obsessed by it in the way that his wife had become. While it might have frustrated him from time to time, he realised that the media would think of a lot of what he was doing as worthy but too complex and dull to fire up the tabloid press. Although the trusts had made a real difference to the increasingly ugly inner-city misery in Britain, and both major political parties had been forced by him to sit up and take notice, 'THE CARING PRINCE SAVES THE POOR' is hardly the sort of headline they wanted.

The King and Di

In Britain, information and good news are continually buried under shallow scandal and the trivial opinions of self-important columnists. However, editors can always find column inches for bad news. And so it was in October 1987 when a blunder by Kensington Palace had meant that two of the Prince's causes launched appeals on the same day. 'FURY AS BLUNDER WRECKS CHARLES' CHARITY' is how the *Daily Mail* headlined the story. Its competitors blazed out a similar message.

The previous year, an architect called Rod Hackney had had the idea of setting up a charity called Inner City Aid, and persuaded not only important men like Lord Scarman to become trustees, but also the Prince of Wales to become its patron. The Prince saw the aims of Inner City Aid as being completely in line with his thinking and so was happy to accept. Inner City Aid was then launched at a conference set up by Hackney and devoted to community architecture. Unfortunately, the date was the same as that of the launch of a competing campaign also involving Charles for the Prince's Youth Business Trust.

Hackney was suspected by sceptical developers and hostile architects of doing all of this in order to promote himself and ensure his election as president of the Royal Institute of British Architects the following year. Once the Prince had declared the conference open, Hackney took to his feet and made an appeal for funds. He told the audience, 'This is about regenerating Britain's inner cities,' and went on to explain that he hoped to receive £10 million for 'the renaissance of the United Kingdom from the inner cities outward'.

This exaggerated rhetoric had the effect of grabbing the attention and completely overshadowed the PYBT launch, which the Prince attended later in the day. Hackney was delighted, but the Prince was furious at what Riddell was to describe as a 'cock-up'.

Within days, Charles Knevitt, the director of Inner City Aid, was summoned to see Riddell and told to stop fund-raising. He was also told in no uncertain terms that the PYBT had been horrified to discover that Hackney had set a target of £10 million, which was bound to affect the PYBT appeal – something that not only carried the Prince's name but also enjoyed matching funds from the government. As a result, every pound not raised cost two in reality. Naturally, Knevitt was bemused: if he wasn't allowed to raise funds then how was Inner City Aid going to operate? However, when he reported back to Hackney, the ICA chairman seemed undeterred.

Then, in February, the Prince summoned Hackney to Kensington

Palace where he was forced to listen to the complaints of the disgruntled trustees of the PYBT. There was a fierce argument at the end of which the Prince instructed Hackney to postpone his fundraising for two years. He proclaimed that by comparison to PYBT, Inner City Aid lacked both clear objectives and the strategy to achieve them. As a result, PYBT should be given a clear run while Inner City Aid withdrew to identify a role for itself and find a suitable project for development.

Fine logic, but perhaps Charles should have thought about all of this before he lent his name to Hackney's idea in the first place. In his haste to promote anything that he genuinely believed would help those in need of support in the inner cities, he seems to have completely missed the potential for a conflict of interest between the two organisations. Moreover, the double booking speaks volumes about the administrative ability of the Prince, his advisers and the complicated politics of his overlapping network of charitable interests.

The Prince was to come to repent his rather ill-conceived support for Inner City Aid. Hackney's burning ambition and expansive rhetoric seemed to drag the Prince ever closer to a public showdown with Mrs Thatcher, who by now had won her hat-trick of election victories. Despite having been converted to the Prince's brand of inner-city assistance, she was still extremely sensitive to the charge that her government didn't really care about a raft of people who had been left behind in the inner-city ghettos as the rest of the country enjoyed the fruits of a share-holding and home-owning democracy. Those close to the Prince became concerned that unless Hackney's wings were clipped, he risked exposing the Prince to the charge of interfering in party politics as anti-Thatcher. This had to be avoided at all costs as it was not part of the heir to the throne's job and could bring about a constitutional crisis. In addition, Charles wasn't personally anti-Thatcher: he thought that her governments could help more in the inner cities than they had, but he was sympathetic to her ideals.

On the first anniversary of the ill-fated launch, Hackney held a press conference at which he declared, 'For the sake of the country, this venture will not be allowed to fail … The other charity [PYBT], which does a fine job, has had a chance to raise money. Now perhaps it is our turn.' Not only did this outburst expose to the media the tension between the two charities, it also inferred that ICA was saving the country from the government and was an open act of defiance against the Prince's two year ban on fund-raising. Not surprisingly, Prince Charles was embarrassed by the headlines. Something would have to be done.

Originally, Hackney had been seen as a kindred spirit, but now Charles was reluctantly persuaded by the likes of Shebbeare, O'Brien and Riddell that he would have to be eased out of the royal circle. At a meeting in June, Jim Gardener, the chairman of the Prince's Trust, persuaded the Prince of Wales that he should tell Hackney that he was no longer prepared to be the patron of ICA unless it was to become an advisory body only.

A meeting was duly fixed for the Prince to meet Hackney in July. However, Charles found it an uncomfortable affair and failed to be as forthright as he intended to be. As a result Riddell then wrote to Hackney and was quite explicit. Nevertheless, Hackney still failed to take the hint and insisted that Prince Charles had not resigned as patron and that Inner City Aid had no intention of becoming an advisory operation. The Prince's advisers continued to make the point. One commented that Hackney 'is resolutely resisting attempts to shove him back in the bottle'.

He was right. Hackney managed, despite the best endeavours of Charles's aids, to keep Inner City Aid going into the 1990s. Happily it became only a shell and therefore failed to cause the Prince the embarrassment that his advisers feared, but it continued to use the name of Prince Charles as its patron right up to the bitter end. Charles had got away fairly lightly, but the episode clearly demonstrates how much fine work can be undone by one loose canon, poor planning and a lack of caution when people flatter to deceive.

Immediately after her third election victory, Mrs Thatcher had made a public commitment that in this term her government would tackle the inner-city problem. Prince Charles seized on this and, at his next meeting with her, urged her to visit the inner cities personally and meet the local leaders who were heading up BITC's plans for regeneration. He followed up his suggestion by proposing a lunch at Kensington Palace where she could meet some of the people involved in his various schemes.

After some prevarication, his suggestion was rejected. But Charles is a stubborn man and didn't intend to take no as an answer. He continued to lobby senior ministers to establish better coordination between ministerial departments, business and local communities and, a year after the election, he tackled Mrs Thatcher again. This time she agreed to host a lunch at Number Ten to meet the inner city 'enablers'. The Prince insisted on compiling the guest list and then sent everyone involved a memo: 'The important thing is for the PM to meet the REAL people at the grass roots level who have struggled to get their housing co-ops, or whatever, off the ground. Inevitably, by the nature of their situation, they will probably not be Conservative voters and will have "radical" views. But then so does the PM! If she is going to have an impact on the situation in these inner urban areas etc., then she must hear at first hand from such people what it is like and what their problems are. I only hope that she won't allow herself to be put off by people who may tell her that she shouldn't be seeing "left wing" characters ...'

However, Thatcher then withdrew the invitation on the grounds that news of the lunch was bound to leak and the press would then exploit matters by flagging up once more the reported antipathy between the prime minister and the heir to the throne. She believed that this would obviously provide her opponents with the valuable point that the Prince of Wales, although supposed to be politically neutral, was in fact opposed to Thatcher and her uncaring policies. She thought that this was in neither of their interests. Perhaps she had a point. Publications such as the *Guardian* or the *Observer*, who love to ridicule the Prince of Wales, are only too happy to use his name to support their position against a person or a policy that they don't agree with.

Nevertheless, the Prince refused to be put off and at their next meeting persuaded the prime minister to attend a reception organised by BITC. Charles's persistence had paid off and the prime minister, after all, was to have a meeting with the community entrepreneurs whom she had hitherto rejected. Thatcher had had no need to be so fearful. The meeting was a great success and caused O'Brien to write enthusiastically to Prince Charles, 'The atmosphere was extremely light ... She said that she had learned a great deal, was enormously impressed by the scope and scale of activity and felt that leaders, like those in the room, were the starting point for local regeneration ... I think much will flow from this and everyone present was deeply grateful to you ...'

The Prince replied, '"Hooray" is all I can say – and I do HOPE that this first encounter will bear fruit ultimately. Please keep me in touch with what transpires ... I have written a note to the Prime Minister to thank her for seeing these characters and to say how important it is to encourage them.'

However, Thatcher still felt that the Prince had used both his position and the moral high ground to push her into a corner. She told one of his staff, 'I really think that after all we have done we could expect a little more support from you.' Without waiting for a response, she turned and walked away. The prime minister had become accustomed to calling all the shots and wasn't pleased that the Prince seemed to be exploiting this Achilles heel in her portfolio of policies. Nevertheless, she later requested a list of inner-city 'enablers' that she might meet on a visit to Liverpool, and she subsequently agreed to host the long-postponed lunch. Charles was delighted, but warned those who had been invited, 'If you are going to do this you must not make political points, you must not ruin the whole thing by getting at her and scoring points.'

At the three-hour lunch in the Cabinet Room at Number Ten, Margaret Thatcher listened politely to an endless litany of proposals for action and investment. Afterwards, nothing seemed to happen, and the Prince concluded that all of his efforts had been in vain. However, his perseverance with the prime minister, which perhaps only either he or the Queen could have attempted, was not quite as unproductive as he had imagined. A number of inner-city programmes were expanded and the government agreed to match the amount raised by BITC for a series of community-based projects.

Meanwhile, the Prince persisted with a range of parallel initiatives at the BITC's behest, which by the end of the decade was growing towards a membership of over 400 companies, 75 per cent of which were large household names. As a result, BITC became the most influential organisation linking business to the community, not only in Britain but also perhaps in the world. By 2004 it could boast 750 corporate members with another 2,000 companies participating in their programmes and campaigns. As a result, member companies employed one in five in the UK private-sector workforce. Seventy-two of the FTSE 100 were members, and BITC had a further sixty global partners.

According to men like O'Brien and Shebbeare, who know their own value, the Prince's role has been absolutely crucial in all of this. They know him well. They know that he is far from perfect and that he can be bad-tempered and self-pitying, but they also know that his qualities far outweigh any failings. However, the prime minister wasn't always quite so sure of these qualities. They clashed over issues other than inner-city deprivation when Charles, in Thatcher's opinion, overstepped the constitutional line and involved himself in what she saw as matters that should be left to the democratically elected politicians.

One such occasion was when, following a successful official visit to the Middle East in 1986 by the Prince and Princess of Wales, it was decided by the Foreign Office that relations with the region could be furthered by the Prince. The desert rulers presumed a special affinity with the British Royal Family in general, were clearly impressed with the Prince's knowledge and were flattered by his interest in their customs and religious beliefs. Plans advanced to the point where it was agreed to set up a special unit in St James's Palace. Then someone remembered that it would be in order to tell the prime minister what was going on. Thatcher was not amused. One Foreign Office official remarked that the sound of breaking furniture could be heard all over Whitehall once she learned what was being planned. To her it seemed as if the Prince, who had an annoying habit of getting involved in domestic policy, was now planning to set up a miniature Foreign Office of his own. She explained politely but firmly that this was not part of his constitutional role. Prince Charles replied that she had got 'the wrong end of the stick', pointing out that the idea had not been his but had come from her administration. As a result the position was resolved amicably.

Then there was the position concerning President Ceausescu of Romania. The Prince became infuriated by government policy to treat him as a friend and a valuable ally when in Charles's opinion he was no better than Hitler. The government's position was dictated by the Cold War – Ceausescu was anti-Moscow and was therefore a friend to be cultivated. Prince Charles saw him as 'a monster and a tyrant' who had destroyed both the environment and local communities by his dictatorial and corrupt policies. In 1978, the previous Labour Government had awarded the Romanian dictator the honour of becoming a Knight Grand Cross, the highest Order of the Bath. The Prince was seriously unimpressed by this political hypocrisy and wanted something done about it.

In August 1988, he asked the Foreign Office, who had originally made the recommendation for the award in the first place, what was the government's attitude to the socially destructive policies of this man.

He was less than impressed by their reply, and kept pressing over the next five months before eventually writing directly to the foreign secretary Geoffrey Howe in February 1989 to tell him that Ceausescu's 'systematisation', a policy that projected blitzkrieg on the environment by dictating the destruction of some 8,000 villages and their replacement by 'agro-industrial' centres was both 'inhuman and diabolical'. 'The point of this letter is really to say that I do believe the situation in Romania should be an URGENT priority for the European nations to address. After all, for WHAT did so many of our courageous countrymen die during the last war? Was it merely to see one system of tyranny and misery exchanged for another? Somehow, we in Western Europe seem so complacent about these matters ... I do so hope it might be possible for there to be a greater public awareness of what is going on ... The press is full of Gorbachev and glasnost but seem to ignore those other parts of Eastern Europe where abominable tyranny still reigns. Are there no members of Parliament exercised about the situation? Why doesn't the Foreign Affairs Committee report on it?'

Howe's soothing response, which seemed to agree with Prince Charles without indicating that anything satisfactory would be undertaken, fell somewhat short of what the Prince wanted to hear. On 30 March he wrote again, this time suggesting that Ceausescu's GCB should be withdrawn. Howe consulted Thatcher, only because the letter had come from the heir to the throne and as such couldn't be ignored. She was livid. Who did this idealistic young man think he was? A Cabinet colleague replied, to the amusement of those present, 'I suppose he thinks that he is the future king of England, Margaret.' The PM was not amused. In her mind it was all very well for the Prince to keep taking these moral stands, but he didn't have to run the country's policies either at home or abroad and therefore did not really appreciate the way either that economics dictated domestic policy, or diplomacy dictated foreign policy.

The Prince suspected that the government would ignore his request on the grounds that a dangerous precedent would be set if they followed his advice and withdrew the award. He was right. Nevertheless, he wasn't going to be silenced and so increased Mrs Thatcher's annoyance further when he decided to make his case public on 27 April 1989. In a speech at the Building a Better Britain Exhibition, he became the first significant person in Europe to condemn unequivocally the tyrant. 'President Ceausescu has embarked on the wholesale destruction of his country's cultural and human heritage ... The object is to reshape the nation's identity, to create a new type of person, utterly subordinate to its dreams ...' The speech was well, and for a change positively, covered by the British press and this alerted it to the rest of Europe, where other political leaders took up the point, having noted that the remarks carried the weight of coming from the heir to the British throne and supposing, quite wrongly, that they met with the government's approval.

Again Mrs Thatcher was furious. It was not that she disagreed with a word that the Prince had uttered, but she doubted his right to involve himself so closely with political matters and thought that such statements were an abuse of his position, which was after all an accident of birth. Thatcher was certainly a royalist and even found the Prince both charming and intelligent, but she was once again dismayed by what she saw as his deliberate interference in government – something that she thought had been more or less resolved when the Prince's distant relative and namesake had lost his head in the seventeenth century.

Initially, the government refused to be moved, citing, as the Prince had suspected, the need not to set a dangerous precedent for depriving the holder of an honorary award in peacetime. However, eight months later, as Ceausescu was in his final days of power, it did a U-turn and was shamed into heeding the Prince's request. Yet again, Charles's unshackled idealism had won over the prime minister's need to be practical – something that she had come to be frustrated by, but which had grudgingly earned her respect. This young man at times seemed to present more of an opposition to her than the Labour Party. This was to become the unconventional, and not always well-received, role of the Prince of Wales. Years later, when Labour were back in power under the leadership of Tony Blair and the once all-conquering Tories were a shadow of their former selves, many who follow political life in Britain noticed that Charles had once again stepped forward as a major political adversary of the government. He was not frightened to expose the immature shallowness of 'Cool Britannia' and the ridiculous political correctness that was being imposed upon the nation.

Charles, given his drive and the willpower that all zealots possess, but remembering his constitutional position, had by now started on a charm offensive to win over hearts and minds in the government in order to influence policy. Some see this ongoing attitude as the actions of a caring man determined to leave behind him a better Britain than the one he saw develop in the 1960s; others think his behaviour is an outrageous abuse of his constitutional position and that he should confine himself to state occasions, waving from the back of a limousine and cutting tape in order to declare a new hospital open. A third section of the public, much smaller but including people in influential positions, hope he will exploit his position to the extent that he will eventually bring about a constitutional crisis that will lead to the abolition of the monarchy.

Despite the distractions of children whom he adored and a wife whose illness and moods meant that a contented married life with a loving companion was all but impossible, the Prince continued on his mission of salvation, as he saw it, or nuisance as Mrs Thatcher perceived it. He not only barraged ministers with letters but he invited them to lunch at either Kensington Palace or Highgrove. None failed to accept his invitation – after all, it was from the heir to the throne – even though they must have realised the dangers of going.

One such victim was Peter Morrison, the minister of state at the Department of Energy in 1989. Trapped at Highgrove he was subjected to an 'HRH grilling'. The Prince can be extremely forceful in private, and sometimes surprises his guests with his aggressive tone as he bangs the table with his palm in order to emphasise his point. Morrison, who had known the Prince of Wales for many years, was not going to be intimidated and did not hold back in response. The matter of dispute between them concerned the fact that Prince Charles did not believe that the Thatcher government was doing enough to conserve energy and thus prevent further damage to the environment. Charles knew his subject well – by all accounts every bit as well as the minister. He held, as he did on many conservation and environmental issues, very strong beliefs.

Having been slightly mauled by opposing the Prince over a subject on which Charles was well read and passionate, Morrison wrote nonetheless to thank his host for lunch but could not refrain from adding, 'I wish that the answers to the questions were quite as easy as Your Royal Highness would like them to be ... You see, everyone without exception wants energy efficiency, unless they are an idiot, but the trick is to teach them how to put the theory into practice.' He went on to lecture the Prince on how the hard-pressed farmers had to burn straw and just couldn't afford to adopt the Prince's conservation ideas.

Charles must have found the tone condescending to the point of impertinence. He wrote back and pointed to several ways that straw might be disposed of without burning it and went on, 'You say that the solution is ultimately having more wealth to be able to afford the necessary costs. But how, then, do you achieve the wealth to afford those costs if by creating that wealth you are compounding the damage that is being done – especially if you assess these costs simply by using the economic theory which has succeeded in bringing us face to face with an environmental crisis in the first place ...'

The minister replied that Prince Charles's letter had pushed him into some constructive work and thought, and concluded by inviting the Prince to open a forthcoming conference on energy efficiency, adding, 'I can assure you that neither I nor the Department will try in any way at all to put any words into your mouth ...'

The Prince of Wales answered dryly, 'I am grateful for your assurance not to try and put any words into my mouth, otherwise I might be tempted to quote from Tony Paterson's recent Bow Group Paper "The Green Conservative". Writing on page 56 about Energy Efficiency, I see he says: "There is probably no more inadequate area of policy in the whole spectrum of the Government's policies on any topic!"'

A year later the government announced the ban on straw burning for which the Prince had fought so strenuously. His persistence, along with others, had paid off and again he had brought about change from behind the scenes and without the public's knowledge.

However, he considered this to be but a small victory in the war against those who seemed to him to be so complacent when it came to protecting the environment. He kept up his pressure on the department by criticising the secretary of state, John Wakeham, for the government's poor response to the Commons Energy Select Committee report on the greenhouse effect, asking what proposals were in hand for developing renewable sources of energy as alternatives to the use of fossil fuels.

Wakeham responded by sending Charles a report that he had recently commissioned on the subject. The Prince was quick to spot an appendix indicating clearly that Britain lagged far behind other countries in expenditure on research and development in this field, and he pointed this out to the secretary of state. Wakeham parried the point by stating that the figures were wrong, as they did not include British Coal's own research and development spending, which was financed by government grants. However, he failed to provide the Prince with what that figure was and so Charles was unable to see if its inclusion made any real difference in closing the enormous gap between Britain and the other developed countries. He suspected that it didn't, and was unimpressed enough to scrawl in the margin, 'Why publish such a misleading table then?'

This sort of exchange was most common between the Prince and ministers of Margaret Thatcher's government as Charles bombarded them with questions and requests for information. They might have been forgiven, as Dimbleby has pointed out, for wondering who would rid them of this turbulent prince. For his part, Charles believed that as a privy councillor, a member of the House of Lords and heir to the throne, it was both his job and his duty to question government on behalf of the people. This paternal view gave him the right to warn, protest and advise. The Prince's interpretation of his role inside the British constitution is obviously open to question, but it cannot be perfectly disputed, as there is no written constitution to prove that such an interpretation is wrong. And at least his intentions were genuine, as was his devotion to the nation and its people.

However annoyed or frustrated ministers became, they still felt obliged to furnish him with a considered response as they were respectful of his unique position. This often – although perhaps not as often as Charles would have liked – led to a frank exchange of views and an answering of questions that either influenced or even on occasion changed government policy.

It was over the course of the 1980s that the Prince, who had long held his views on inner-city deprivation, the environment, architecture and other topics, came to see that his view of a better Britain would only occur if the government supported it both by research and development finance and, where necessary, by legislation. He came to understand more and more that it was only they who in the end could make the real difference. The Prince's Trust might do a lot of good, but it couldn't alter the course of the country's future – hence his intense carrot-and-stick campaign with a government that initially thought warily of him, but came to respect the logic of many of his ideas and suggestions.

Many ministers entered Highgrove or Kensington Palace

convinced, by the picture that had been painted in the tabloid press, that they were about to have lunch with a woolly-minded, utopian vegetarian. They came out two or three hours later shocked by the Prince's grasp of the subject under discussion and the practicality of some of his suggested solutions to difficult problems. As a result, as time passed there were more ministers who came to admire the Prince than there were who would be seriously irritated by him.

Nor should it be forgotten that the Conservative Party is a royalist party – the only one of the three main political parties in Britain that is. This is an important point in understanding the relationship between the Prince, his views, his work and the Thatcher government. As a result of its royalist principles, its leaders were disposed to honour his peculiar status and so were of a mind to be drawn to his seriousness of purpose, his charm, his modest behaviour and his humour. Despite their frequent differences, most ministers looked forward to a meeting with the Prince and usually came away at its end, even if an agreement of views could not be arrived at, encouraged. And because of who he was, they were obliged to hear him out and address his views with a more open mind than they would have done with an opposing politician.

At the peak of Thatcher's economic boom, when developers had never had it so good, Lord Northfield, head of a leading building consortium, accused the Prince of being hijacked by the 'loony green brigade' because he had had the temerity to make a speech suggesting that it would be better if new developments took place on vacant inner-city land rather than the developers constantly pushing the planners to allow more and more invasion of the Green Belt.

At this point in time, the Thatcher government was basking in the glory of winning the Falklands War, while the prime minister toughed it out with the Russians and demolished any EU leader who challenged her; at home she had created a booming economy, while delivering the nation from the strikes and blackmail of tyrannical and power-crazed union leaders. Against this hard-nosed and hard-won success, it was easy for papers like the *Sun* to paint the Prince as a utopian idealist who had found the 1960s twenty years too late.

But in 1987 things started to change. The publication of the Brundtland Report, 'Our Common Future', shifted the environmental debate on to an elevated and wider stage. Suddenly millions of people across the world seemed to get the message that what the Prince, and people who shared his views, had been saying was far from being idealistic rot. In fact it was most sensible, and unless something was done to save the environment, the whole future of the planet might be in jeopardy.

It almost became fashionable to become green overnight, and suddenly world leaders were falling over themselves in a dash to address environmental issues, alarmed in 1989 when people associated with Charles's beliefs – the Green Party – secured fifteen per cent of the vote in the European elections. Even Mrs Thatcher was forced to take notice as her minister for overseas development, Chris Patten, seized on the theme and declared that, 'What is needed is growth that can be sustained ... Growth must be pursued within – and not despite – the limits of ecological resilience.'

The Prince was delighted, took courage and went on the attack in a most controversial way. At the opening of the North Sea Conference in London, he made a stinging attack on the secretary of state for the environment, Nicholas Ridley, without actually naming him, as he sat in the audience. He told the gathering, 'Some argue that we do not have enough proof of danger to justify stricter controls on dumping or to warrant the extra expenditure involved ... If science has taught us anything, it is that the environment is full of uncertainty. It makes no sense to test it to destruction. While we wait for the doctor's diagnosis, the patient may easily die.'

Those associated with the Green movement were delighted. More significantly, so were many in the government and even civil servants inside Ridley's Department of the Environment who had become increasingly frustrated by his indifference to the issue. It is widely believed that much of the information quoted by the Prince in the speech was actually supplied by Sir Martin Holdgate, a senior adviser to Ridley's department at the time.

This open declaration by the Prince for the need to have a 'precautionary principle' not only broke new ground in the public debate, it assisted those like Patten in the government to push the prime minister towards a more positive stance on the subject. Ridley was furious and saw the Prince as having not only attacked government policy but one of Her Majesty's secretaries of state as well. As far as he was concerned, the Prince had gone beyond the unwritten rule that precludes him from involving himself in party politics. He expected Thatcher to come out on his side and rebuke, preferably in public, the

Prince. Ridley was after all one of her oldest allies in government, and she had been annoyed by the Prince's interference on many less serious occasions before.

In fact, Mrs Thatcher stayed silent. She was a clever politician and she realised very quickly that the Prince had struck a cord with the people and it would not be wise to swim against the tide.

The Prince and Patten became close and had a number of private meetings. Charles was impressed by Patten's political intellect, the minister by the Prince's knowledge and conviction. This became an important relationship and helped Patten alert Thatcher to environmental points that would have been considered heresy in earlier years of Thatcherism when no one worried about such issues. To Thatcher's credit, she started to listen.

The following February, as patron of the European Year of the Environment, the Prince, secretly encouraged by Patten, again urged the government to do more. 'Why then are we so slow in this country to respond to what is, I think, a growing public feeling? Why has environmental regulation of one kind or another taken so long to come about here when you find that in West Germany, for instance, or the United States, they have had many more regulations and controls for a long[er] time than we have?' He went on to attack the General Electricity Generating Board for 'doing too little too late' to combat the effects of acid rain. He criticised big business for being out of step with the man in the street and even told the audience that he had banned the use of aerosol sprays at home when referring to the depletion of the ozone layer.

This salvo of shots against government, nationalised industry and big business was bound to capture the headlines. Naturally, as might have been expected, a couple of tabloids chose to major on his autocratic attitude towards the banning of aerosols in Kensington Palace. However, the others joined the broadsheets in treating this speech seriously, as they were to again and again in the latter part of the 1980s. The media, like Mrs Thatcher, knew he had touched a public nerve and wasn't going to risk circulation figures by criticising him.

One journalist reflected, following the transmission in May 1990 of the Prince's environmental film *The Earth in Balance*, 'The loony prince of tabloid fable begins to look like a man in harmony with public opinion, not to say at the cutting edge. We're all friends with the plants now.' Also at that time, the *Sunday Mirror*, which had been more sympathetic than most tabloids to the Prince and was enjoying the *Sun*'s predicament caused by the Prince's newfound popularity and their previous ridiculing of him, observed, 'Prince Charles could be forgiven for adopting an air of quiet self-satisfaction these days. For the years of sneers and cheap jokes are over. The causes and the enthusiasms that earned him taunts like the Potty Prince have suddenly become everyone's concern. Now it's his bandwagon everyone wants to jump on. He's the champion of the Green Revolution. A man admired for his foresight.'

And one person already on his bandwagon was his old adversary – the prime minister. She had been pushed aboard by Patten and colleagues as far back as the end of 1988. She had then astounded environmentalists when she told the Tory Party conference in October, 'No generation has a freehold on the earth. All we have is a life tenancy with a full repairing lease.'

Although the persuasion of people like Chris Patten and Sir Crispin Tickell, Britain's permanent representative at the United Nations, were important in securing her conversion to the 'precautionary principle', there can be no doubt that the greatest influence on Mrs Thatcher was the lead taken by the Prince of Wales and the public's reaction to it. She had been obliged to act as a result, and knew that she must join him rather than oppose him – even if she was secretly furious with his intervention in what she saw was a political matter. But she had to acknowledge that he had, armed with the courage of his convictions, marched into a major political debate, had taken on the government and industry, and for the first time had emerged as the clear winner without even a scratch of damage to himself.

Margaret Thatcher knew that only public opinion could deliver that sort of victory and so, like the *Sun*, believed that discretion was the better part of valour in this instance. However, her rhetoric was more than she was prepared to deliver as the economy stumbled following the stock-market crash of 1987 and the inevitable downturn in world trade. Nevertheless, she was astute enough to realise that the environment, with more than a little help from the Prince of Wales, had found a seat on the top table of politics and could no longer be ignored.

Now it was too late to shut the Prince up. One or two ministers, like Ridley and Norman Tebbit, thought that the prime minister had let him go too far, but others were prepared to play along as they agreed with a lot of what he was saying. Convention demanded that his speeches were sent to the relevant minister for comment before delivery. They sometimes suggested a minor alteration or request a passage be omitted, but in general a good working relationship between the Prince and Thatcher's ministers existed, and he often found their advice helpful. However, the passage that had offended Nicholas Ridley so much had only been added after he had approved the speech, and it was this almost as much as what had been said that had angered the minister. He believed that on that occasion the Prince had fought dirtily and had outrageously ignored convention, and it must be said that he had a point.

It wasn't too long before they were to clash again. When the final draft of a speech he had written about the threat to the ozone layer was sent to the Department of the Environment, he received word that the secretary of state was not entirely happy. The Prince commented, 'I've just heard that Nicholas Ridley has seen the speech and wants to cut out two pieces. I'm afraid that I'm not going to.' Ridley was exasperated, and seriously believed that the Prince had jumped over the constitutional line with both feet. Of course he was right, and at another time and on a different topic Charles might have caused a major constitutional crisis by his actions. However, world opinion that was enthusiastically reflected in the United Kingdom made him pretty much untouchable.

However, it made him enemies within the government who would be slow to forgive. Much later, in the mid 1990s, I was chatting to Norman Tebbit, with whom I was attending some City gathering. We were discussing how Prince Charles had influenced public opinion since the middle of the 1980s. Quickly it became clear that while we both agreed that he had, I was in awe of this achievement and Norman clearly wasn't. Eventually he erupted, as I was reluctant to yield my position, and he declared with a discernible raise in the tone of his voice, 'The achievements of the Thatcher government were not helped by an idealistic wet that had never had to really run anything in his life.' The straight and brutal Norman, so roundly hated by the trade-union movement, was one of those rare Tories who might just put party and principle before queen and country and had been genuinely outraged by the Prince's attacks on chums like Ridley, whom he saw, as Margaret Thatcher did, to be part of an elite club informally known as 'one of us'.

By the time the 1990s were well underway, the Iron Lady and her 'one of us' club had been removed from power as the nation – now feeling less financially threatened than when it had swept her to power nearly twelve years earlier – seemed to want more caring and less brutal policies. Many senior Tories had wanted to react to this movement in its heartland and both keep the boom going, despite the 1987 world stock-market crash, and present a softer face – one more in keeping with the now much-admired Prince of Wales.

As a result of this utopian and economically ignorant view, the British economy had severely overheated in 1988, and by 1989 was beginning to pay the price for it. The Chancellor of the Exchequer, Nigel Lawson, had not appreciated how strongly the economy was growing in 1987 and 1988, and had guessed the effects of the stock market crash wrongly. Mrs Thatcher had guessed more accurately, but she knew she was in a minority and so allowed Lawson, who was backed by most British and American economists, the City, the financial press, the majority of Tory MPs and, according to most opinion polls, the electorate, to ignore her concerns.

After the tax-reducing budget of 1987, Lawson clearly feared some overheating and, as was in his power in those pre-1997 days, raised interest rates in August. This was totally unexpected in the market and the FTSE 100 share index plunged 100 points in a matter of minutes. However, this only proved to be a hiccup and London soon recovered and continued to roar along with New York, Tokyo and other leading markets.

Then came the crash, and Lawson reacted by cutting interest rates sharply. He continued to do so right into the spring of 1988, trying to keep the pound below three deutschmarks, a level necessary to keep British manufacturing competitive and so prevent recession. He continued his tax-cutting budgets, and in March 1988 simplified income tax into two bands – a standard twenty-five per cent and a higher rate of forty per cent, both of which survived many future budget adjustments under different chancellors.

In the real world, away from the stock market, the British consumer – feeling prosperous thanks to generous earnings settlements, relatively low inflation, and a sharp rise in the price of his house fuelled by loose credit – was spending money like never before or ever again until a similar set of circumstances in 2003/4. By the middle of 1988 this expenditure showed itself in a series of balance-of-payments deficits that would have defied belief only a year earlier. In the year to

March 1989, the total deficit in the UK balance-of-trade deficit was £20 billion, or nearly £2 billion a month. Such deficits worried economists and politicians alike – it was widely believed that the one factor that had cost Harold Wilson the 1970 election was the publication three days before the poll of a trade deficit of £57 million. Even allowing for the subsequent inflation of which Wilson was a major cause, this figure was mere petty cash by comparison.

Lawson's reaction was to change direction once more. He raised interest rates again, and sharply. From a low of 7.5 per cent in the spring of 1988, the base rate doubled to 15 per cent in the autumn of 1989, and stayed there as British consumers, still encouraged by the rise in the equity value of their houses – many of which had been bought at bargain prices from local councils – simply refused to stop spending.

To Mrs Thatcher's intense irritation, inflation rose too. The Tories had always told the electorate to judge them on inflation. And despite a bad start in 1979, some of which was of their own making, they had brought it tumbling down to four per cent in time for the 1983 election. Thereafter it had stayed in that region, which was unheard of following the economically foolish years of Harold Wilson and Edward Heath. Moreover, they had rejuvenated both the country's economy and its attitude to work that not only led the British economy to regain its place as the fourth biggest in the world, but also allowed it to sustain a position as the best in Europe for several years.

But late in the day, they had failed to take their own advice and had allowed too much money into the system and that, as Thatcher had always preached, would produce inflation. Furious that she had allowed Lawson to go down this route, even if she had been fairly powerless to stop him, she now blamed him for pumping liquidity into the economy following the crash. He blamed her for not permitting the pound to join the Exchange Rate Mechanism of the European Monetary System – whether he had a point remains unclear, but by that time she wasn't in a powerful enough position within the party or even the Cabinet to push her will through. No wonder she hadn't wanted the added strain of a punch-up that might have even led to a constitutional crisis with the Prince of Wales.

Now she became like a troubled Roman emperor, or even like Princess Diana across town in Kensington Palace – seeing plots against her everywhere. Around this time I had lunch with John Gummer, a minister in her administration, a close ally and a great admirer. He informed me that the prime minister was seriously displeased with me. I replied that I was amazed that she even knew who I was. 'You wrote the lead article in this month's *First* magazine, and she didn't like it,' he countered.

'But it was very positive. It listed all of her achievements at home and abroad,' I answered in complete disbelief.

'Yes, but you had the cheek to criticise the erosion of the manufacturing base in the north-west and seemed to side with Prince Charles on the fact that there weren't enough self-help schemes being established in inner-city areas. When did she tell you how to run Hodgson Holdings plc?' I left the lunch thinking that Margaret Thatcher's days were numbered.

When the end came it was painful and humiliating, as it always is when your own side stabs you in the back. The Iron Lady was bleeding and it showed. At that time, a sensitive letter arrived in her hand from an unlikely source. It congratulated her on her receipt of the Order of Merit. It reminded her of her remarkable contribution to world politics and in particular for her 'extraordinary determination and courage' to which it was attributable that major and fundamental changes in the Soviet Union and Eastern Europe had occurred for the benefit of those people and the safety of the world as a whole. 'That's an astonishing and famous achievement for which your name will go down in history as one of this country's most remarkable Prime Ministers.' The handwritten letter came from Charles, Prince of Wales.

This was to the Prince's credit; perhaps it was less admirable that he couldn't then stop himself from going on to point out, having paid her such a magnificent tribute, that they hadn't always seen eye to eye on domestic issues. He reminded her of his frustration at the reluctance of her government to pay adequate attention to the idea of partnerships 'between the different sectors that make up the life of our nation'. He wrote with genuine passion, but seemed to have forgotten that Mrs Thatcher was no longer in a position to do anything about it – his rebuke served no purpose and only detracted from an otherwise kind and heartfelt letter.

So ended one of the most interesting, yet little commented-on, struggles in modern political times between the government and the monarchy: the caring prince verses the pragmatic prime minister. And yet, in the end, they weren't really that many miles apart. Both believed in helping people to help themselves, and both bled red, white and blue. Mrs Thatcher had always been wary of many of the Prince's ideas, which she saw as unnecessary intervention. It had taken her some time to discover that not all were and that many helped regeneration in a sustainable way. For the Prince's part he had been often frustrated by her closed mind and the charge made against him of meddling in matters that were no concern of his. And although there was considerable movement by the Thatcher government towards his views in time and on many fronts, it was never quite as much as he had hoped for.

On the same day as his letter was dispatched to the deposed Thatcher, the Prince also wrote to the new prime minister, John Major, congratulating him on his appointment, before launching into the need for his government to pay attention to the vital importance of partnerships in the community. He concluded by stating that he very much hoped that they would be able to meet before too long and discuss the issue.

They did, and not only did the new Prime Minister demonstrate a more open mind to such ideas, which blossomed under him and his successor Tony Blair, but the two men became firm friends. They recognised in each other not only many common beliefs and interests, they genuinely liked each other.

So however the shallow tabloid press portrayed Prince Charles during the 1980s, the amount of work he tirelessly undertook on behalf of his causes and beliefs of how a better life might be delivered to the people of Great Britain should not be underestimated, nor its effects belittled. There are very few princes of Wales from any historical period who can lay claim to an equal record with this regard. Nor should it be forgotten that such work was always undertaken in addition to civic ceremonies, royal duties and official foreign tours that any member of the Royal Family has to undertake – and as heir to the throne he has traditionally had the heaviest schedule of any member, something that increased when he married Princess Diana and the world wanted a visit from them above all others.

A typical 1980 year for the Prince of Wales may be exemplified by 1988. As well as his work for BITC, the Prince's Trust, other inner-city concerns and the environment, the Prince also gave his support to a campaign to save the National Fruit Collection in Kent. He launched his book, *A Vision of Britain*, to accompany his television programme of the same name, which was an assault on British architectural trends. He made an impassioned defence of the Book of Common Prayer against the 'crassness' of the Alternative Service Book. He was deeply involved in plans to create a village of his design, which he believed would produce a better environment for people to live in, near Dorchester. In time Poundbury, as it was called, was built, and despite some scoffing from the architecture establishment, was applauded internationally and by the vast majority of British visitors, many of whom appeared to be ready to exchange their bland box on some awful housing estate, as designed by a British Establishment architect, for a new home in Poundbury.

At this time he also got locked into a serious argument over plans of how to best preserve Henry VIII's flagship, the *Mary Rose*; he gave an hour-long lecture at the Botanical Gardens in Kew warning of the serious effects if we continued to allow the rainforests to be destroyed; he warned students at Budapest University about the evils of communism; he made another television film called *The World in Balance*, in which he told of the consequences of human greed and folly upon the planet's future; he planned an international seminar on the Royal Yacht as part of the groundwork for the Earth Summit in Rio; and he made official visits to Indonesia, Hong Kong, Nigeria, Cameroon, Hungary and Spain.

During the same period, he had private meetings with ten government ministers and three from the opposition, one of whom was a young Tony Blair. He wrote more than 1,000 letters to people who included heads of governments as well as ordinary citizens of his mother's realm about such issues as, among others, the disabled, South Africa, the Gulf, Romania, appeals on behalf of a much-needed centre for Islamic Studies, his Architectural Summer School in Italy and a schizophrenia helpline set up by the charity SANE. He also organised a concert to celebrate his grandmother's ninetieth birthday.

This hailstorm of activity was perhaps too much and meant that many of his projects were slowed down by competition for his time from others. It was also a nightmare for his office to plan in advance against such a backdrop of diverse commitments, all of which had to be fitted around the standard pillars of national events such as Remembrance Sunday. Even Mrs Thatcher had offered help and advice in trying to streamline the Prince's diary in order for it to become more focused and therefore effective. This job was made no easier by the fact that John Riddell, although a pleasant man with an agile mind, was no administrator and the Prince's mood could go up and down depending upon the progress on his projects or the state of his disintegrating marriage.

In addition, the Prince's own scattergun approach and desire to throw himself into every worthwhile project that he was presented with only made matters worse. Even Charles could see this, but was either incapable or unwilling to help. He confessed with typical honesty, 'The trouble is, I always feel that unless I rush about doing things and trying to help furiously I will not be seen to be relevant and I will be considered to be a mere playboy!'

This all served to make life in his office a bit of a roller-coaster ride. He would expect officials to be available at all hours to respond to an idea that he had just conceived, which gave his critics the cause to label him both a 'butterfly mind' and a thoughtless employer. The first charge is certainly unfair as most of his 'brilliant new thoughts' were linked to his longstanding concerns. The second is fair. The Prince had enough royal blood running through his veins and inherited Windsor characteristics in his mind sometimes to be the very picture of unacceptable aristocracy. He could throw his papers around the room – he did throw a book at Paul Burrell – and he might easily flare up if challenged, even when a staff member did so in the politest of fashions. These instances usually occurred when he was looking for a release of pent-up frustration and depression as to why his plans weren't taken more seriously by Mrs Thatcher or why, however hard he tried, his marriage only seemed to descend ever more into a lonely dungeon of private despair.

But this was only one side of the Prince as an employer, and it was but a small side compared to his other. He has been generally kind and compassionate with staff throughout his adult life. We have already come across many examples to date and will learn of other most notable ones as the story of the royal couple's life progresses. The Prince has always been ready with help and compassion when any among his staff were ill or found themselves having to confront a personal misfortune. He would not only send flowers or bottles of whiskey, but would handwrite copious notes to them and leave their jobs open until they could return. If former aides fell on hard times, he would make it his business to angle for a job for them, and if that wasn't successful he would often ensure that he provided one instead. Most amazingly, he would find time in his ridiculously busy schedule to visit them. A very good account of what a decent man the Prince is to work for was given by both Mr and Mrs Paul Burrell before Paul realised how much money there was to make out of saying something else. When one of his trusted advisers, the secretary to the duchy John Higgs, was terminally ill with cancer, the Prince wrote, 'John is still determined that no-one should know and thinks that no-one does. He is without doubt the bravest man imaginable but I do wish he could have talked to someone. He won't talk to anyone and it must be agony for him mentally. I really don't know what to do. I am devoted to John ... I really can't bear the thought of losing him.' When Higgs was close to death, the Prince, who had personally gone out of his way to bring pressure to secure a knighthood for him, went to his bedside to confer the honour. Following his death he erected a memorial to him at Highgrove.

These pictures of the Prince at work during the main years of his marriage to the Princess have almost been lost under a barrage of tabloid ridicule from the period, and are never really alluded to by the Princess in her misleading biography as penned by Andrew Morton. Throughout the period, she also took on charitable work, but it demanded fewer hours, and she was more of a figurehead patron. It demanded none of the passion or intellectual input that her husband's did. It was not until the mid-1990s that Diana, on a cut-down and more focused charity programme and fuelled by a new energy and a mission to be seen as 'going good', really started to participate in her projects with anything that might be described as the same intensity that Prince Charles had maintained all his adult life – even this tended to be work in front of the cameras rather than intellectual input behind them.

Diana's ability wasn't to find solutions to the problems that the charities she supported were fighting. Unlike Prince Charles, she lacked both the ability and the inclination for this. Her great ability was to bring such problems into the public awareness and she was uniquely talented, perhaps the very best in the world, in this regard: her work to make people more aware of the suffering caused by both Aids and landmines was of incalculable value. She was a famous and beautiful woman and she used her fame and beauty to very good effect, and thus benefited millions in the 1990s.

This does not mean to say that those charities that recruited Diana earlier in the 1980s did not benefit tremendously from her name being on the letterhead, her attendance at a charity dinner or a well-planned photo opportunity that the press adored so much. In the main it worked very well – maximum reward for minimum effort, and never a cross word with Mrs Thatcher or her ministers. Diana wasn't really interested in politics at this time, had no burning passion to help the deprived in the inner cities and never felt intellectually strong enough or, given the debilitating nature of her illness, had enough interest or energy to think of new initiatives or challenge existing ones. Moreover, if she could muster a criticism of Thatcher then it was simply that she wasn't right-wing enough – a true but unlikely view from a woman years later to be labelled by a new socialist prime minister, Tony Blair, as the People's Princess.

In many ways, although Thatcher did not hold Diana the individual, or the lifestyle that she stood for, in high regard – seeing it privately as an necessary but unattractive side of capitalism, as I have been told by one of her former colleagues – she could see that in many ways she was preferable to Charles when it came to the business of monarchy. After all, Diana didn't challenge or embarrass the government in the way that he did – she just turned up, did her job, looked beautiful and was enormously popular. Surely this was what a constitutional monarchy was all about. Mrs Thatcher appreciated that she never got bombarded by Diana with letters requesting meetings with wretched inner-city leaders, or demands that foreign leaders accused of human-rights violations were stripped of their knighthoods, or barbed accusations, sometimes made in open speech, of doing nothing to save the environment. To Thatcher, Diana seemed at least controllable in the workplace.

Ironically, the Princess was anything but controllable for long periods at home, where she seemed incapable of summoning the strength to pull herself together in the way that she somehow managed when undertaking public duty. There were the occasional breakdowns in the early years, but amazingly few given her state, and the Princess must take enormous credit that she got through as many as she did without further mishap.

It is by no means certain to what extent Mrs Thatcher was any more aware of Diana's mental state or the royal couple's marital problems than the rest of the nation at that time. She was not the sort of woman to pry any more than Prince Charles was the sort of chap to want to talk about it, and although Diana began to give her friends and confidants her rather one-sided and selective version of events after a few years, Mrs Thatcher was not one of that group and was therefore highly unlikely to have had such a conversation with the Princess.

The King and Di

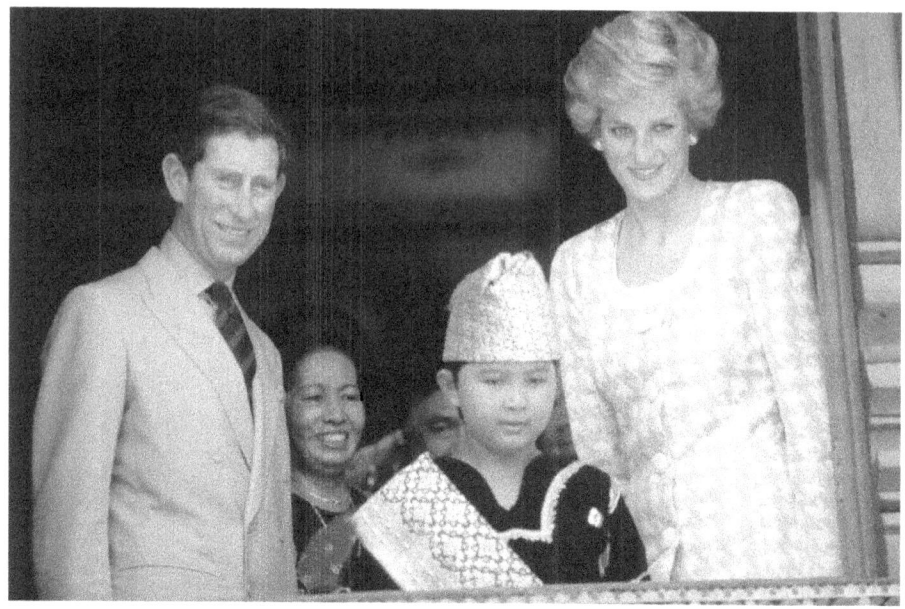

Above : Prince Charles and Princess Dianna working together well on a state visit
Below: 'Charles and Diana at a polo match early on in their relationship

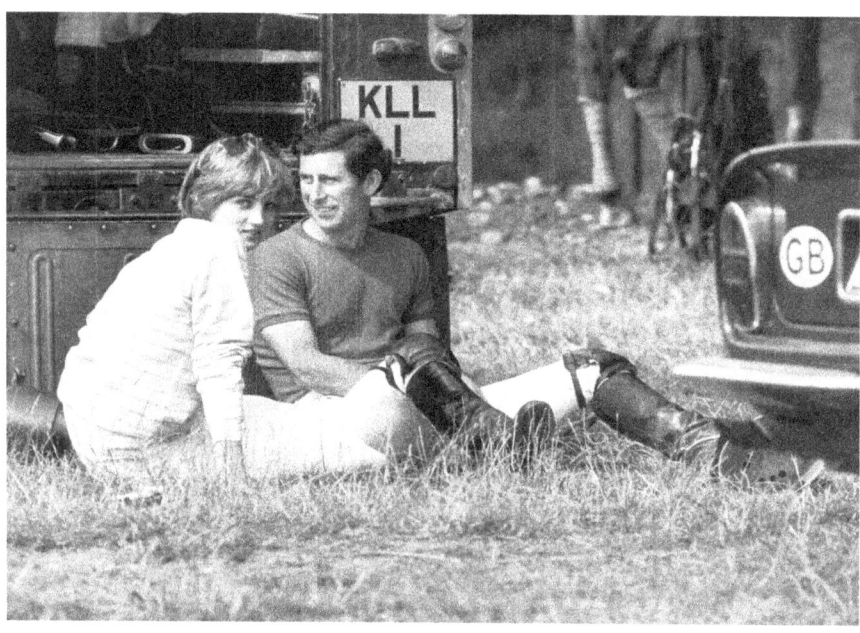

Howard Hodgson

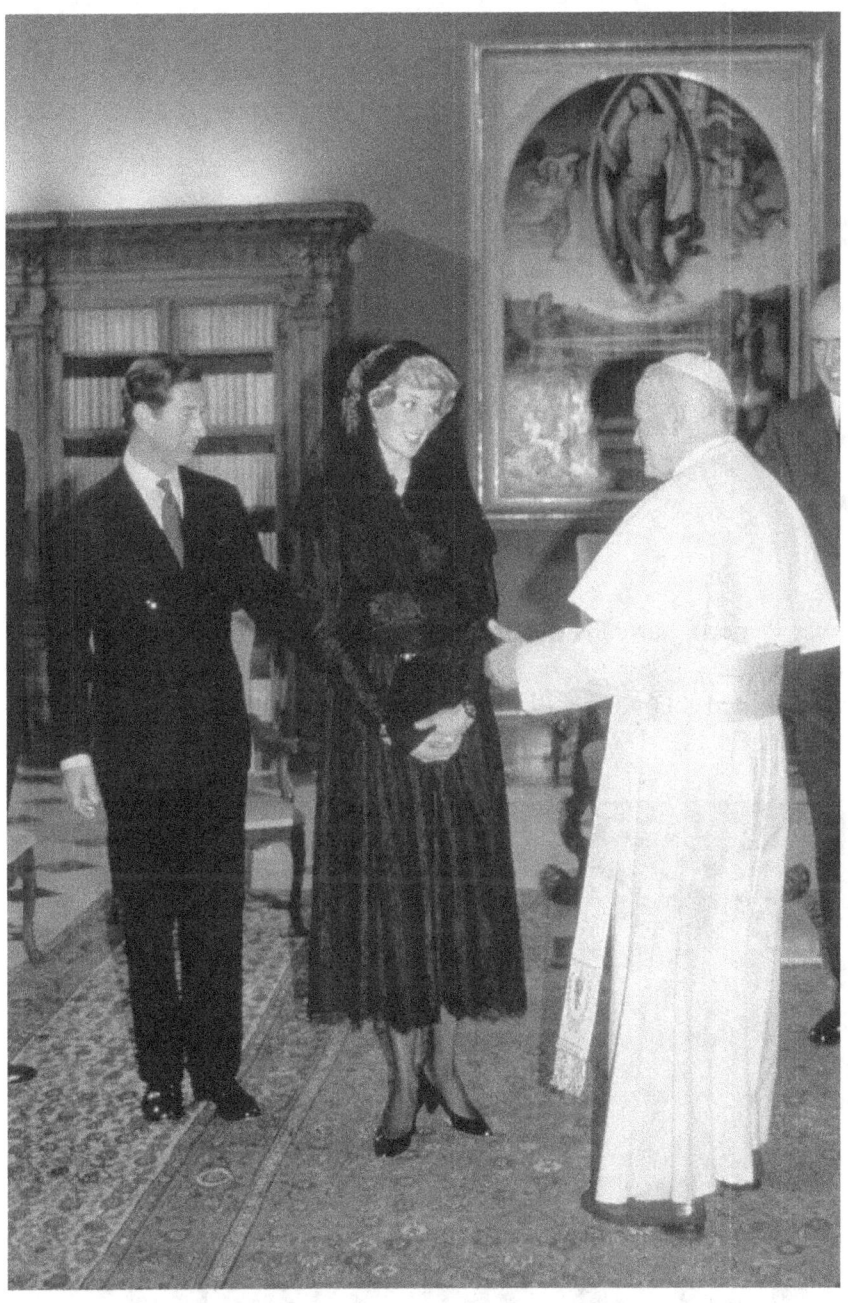

Prince Charles and Princess Dianna with the Pope
© Camera Press

The King and Di

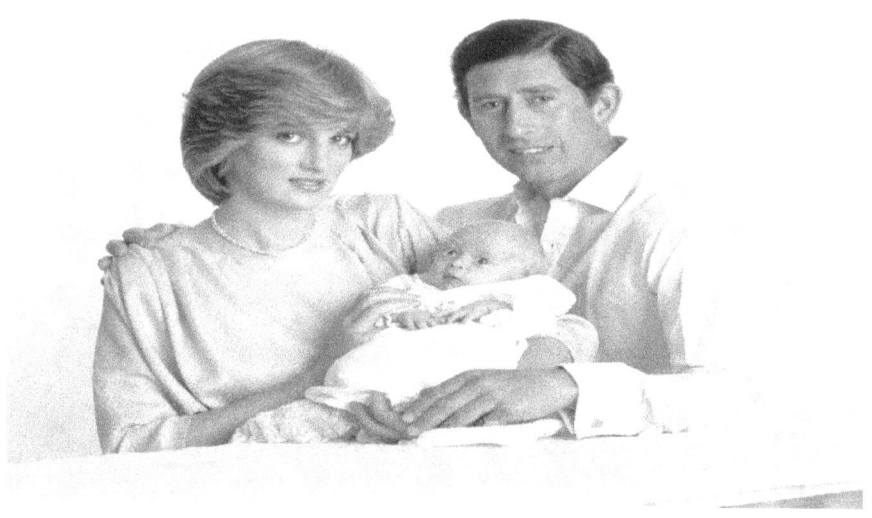

Above: Prince Charles and Princes Dianna with a new born Prince William.
Below: Princess Dianna with Princes William and Harry
© Camera Press

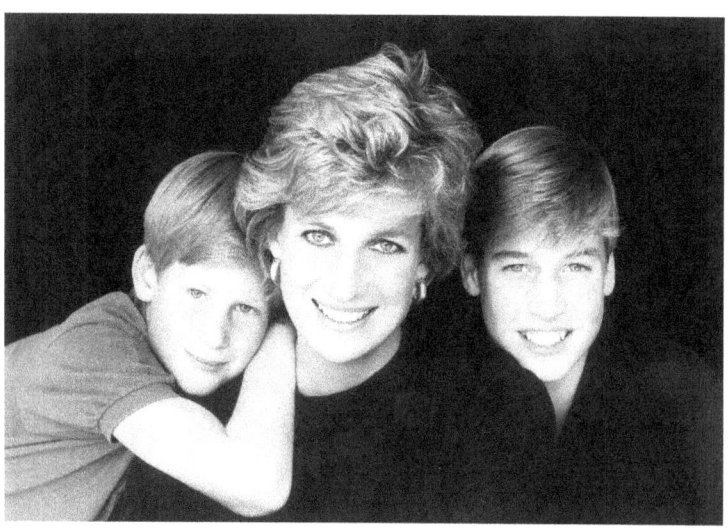

Chapter Ten
Affairs of the Heart (1984–92)

As her marriage to Prince Charles proceeded in an increasingly unhappy fashion, the Princess of Wales tended to confide only in those whom she considered to be part of her own personal circle, people whom she felt were hers and hers alone. She knew that she could fall out with such people, and almost without exception she did; but she also knew that she could return to them later, safe in the knowledge that they wouldn't have 'changed sides', as she saw it, and gone over to the Establishment. In Diana's mind, the other side not only contained all their mutual friends, with the exception of Peter Palumbo, who had known Prince Charles since he was sixteen, but everybody connected to the Palace and the government as well.

Diana always assumed that all these people would side with the Prince, as it is likely that she felt in her heart of hearts that the fault lay with her rather than him in the first place – she would occasionally admit as much to friends like Elsa Bowker. She was also daunted by the Establishment intellectually, and so didn't trust them. In addition, these people worked around the monarchy, knew the form and knew the Queen, her son and their courtiers. As a result it was much more difficult to paint the picture of cold unkindness that she wished to in order to explain away her depressions and moods. Moreover, those known to her would immediately know that she wasn't exactly telling the truth.

This is not to say that all of Diana's friends were unintelligent – far from it. Indeed, men like Lord Puttnam are extremely intelligent and could easily see Diana's failings in both honesty and manipulation when it came to their experience of her. Nevertheless, they swallowed almost everything that they were told about her life at home and at the palace without serious question. This prompted men like James Gilbey, whether a lover at the time or not, to report to the world that Diana believed the Prince to be a poor father. Puttnam himself revealed for common publication that he would have been most upset if his daughter, who was the same age as Diana, had married into a family like the Windsors and had been treated in such a way. And then there were the countless others who lined up to verify how badly Diana had been treated by the Queen and her family and how hurt she had been by the affair between Prince Charles and Camilla Parker Bowles that had never ceased and had continued throughout their marriage.

The problem is that, as none of these people witnessed any of these events, they could only repeat what they assumed was the truth as told to them by the Princess. The facts reveal that Charles was always a loving and besotted father, adored by his children; that his affair restarted with Camilla Parker Bowles only once Diana had been unfaithful to him with several men; and that those who were actually there at some of the events to which she refers in Morton's book remember things very differently from Diana. Worse still, no one can be found to come forward and totally support her version.

The Windsors, like all families, have their faults: they are certainly not perfect and the very nature of the disciplined world that they must endure as the nation's first family sets them apart from the rest of us. However, they are certainly more kind to each other than the Spencers, and there is no real evidence to justify Diana's character assassination of them. Her motives appear to be no more than self-justification and spite on the surface; it is only when you consider her condition that you find a kinder reason for her behaviour. Either way, a false account was given by her.

So what? Is it that important? After all, it is only a domestic affair that we are talking about, and she is now dead; perhaps her sons and her ex-husband should be allowed to remember her in peace. Naturally, there is an argument for this. However, it was Diana herself that made a public issue of these private matters and therefore for the benefit of those unfairly maligned as much as for the benefit of truth and the presentation of an accurate history, we should be presented with the accurate facts – whether we like them or not.

So should Puttnam and Co hang their heads in shame and apologise to the nation for the unintentionally misleading impressions they may have been guilty of giving all of us? Perhaps not, as she was, like many in the ghastly clutches of borderline personality disorder, a seriously accomplished liar and capable of brilliant deception. It should never be forgotten that Diana was able to convince Morton of Prince Charles's continuing affair with Camilla Parker Bowles without ever revealing that she had ever had an affair with anyone. And this was not just mindless deception. It was part of a brilliant plan. If Diana could convince Morton that her husband had been having an affair throughout her marriage to him and that he and his family had treated her harshly, she would be presented as a victim whose life had been wrecked by these old-fashioned, dysfunctional folk. She would be seen as a young, beautiful woman who had only wanted to bring up her children in a modern and decent way but had been prevented from doing so by archaic tradition, a heartless queen and a cold and faithless husband who was obsessed by his mistress, polo and duty to the exclusion of his children.

If this version of the story could hit the streets first and unopposed, not only would it cause such sensation as to seep into public consciousness, but it would also create enormous sympathy that would tend to excuse her own infidelities or other failings if or when they were exposed. Surely across the nation men who loved her or women who admired her would say, 'But you can hardly blame her when you think of what it must have been like being married to him and his dreadful family.'

And she was right. Her plan worked perfectly. Initially, no one would guess that the person behind the book was Diana herself. When it was serialised in the *Sunday Times* in June 1992, it took Prince Charles and his staff completely by surprise. Charles's hurt, embarrassment, humiliation and concern for the effects on his children were complete. Would Prince William be taunted at school by the front-page headline, 'DIANA DRIVEN TO FIVE SUICIDE BIDS BY "UNCARING" CHARLES'? The article went on to detail Diana's bulimia, her husband's indifference towards her, his love of his mistress, his various failings as a father and the complete isolation that she had felt locked inside a loveless marriage and surrounded by hostile courtiers and a cold and disapproving Royal Family. Of course in the absence of any statement from Diana denying that any of this was true, the public was bound to draw the conclusion that it was. They were not to know that she was really the author and that she had either made up or completely twisted most of it.

A book that explained that Charles had had one true love since 1986 while she had been sleeping her way round Kensington would have been a truer story, but it certainly wouldn't have had the effect that the Princess desired; nor would the idea that a mother could willingly allow her children to suffer the hurt of such humiliation of their family by publishing a one-sided account of their parents' lives for her own selfish reasons. Therefore it was absolutely essential that Diana was not seen to have had anything to do with the writing of the book; it was equally essential that it didn't contain anything that she didn't wish to be published. Giving Morton the unique opportunity provided her name was kept out of it assured the first point; dictating it and then editing it secured the second. This beautiful young woman might have been academically dim at school but, as is often the case with borderline personality disorder sufferers, her naked, streetwise, animal cunning was highly tuned.

One former lover, who refused to talk to me directly but did so through a mutual friend provided that I promised not to name him, said, 'She was very convincing. She could be very funny, bubbly and extremely good company. At first it was just like one of those schooldays flirtations we can all remember. She had an ability to make you feel that there was just you and her in a special world and that everyone else was on the outside and that some were enemies. Sometimes she was very sad and appeared to be very vulnerable. It was when she was like this that she might talk of how dreadful her life was with Prince Charles and his family, whom she sometimes referred to as "the fucking Germans". By the time she had finished I would be amazed at how I had been fooled into thinking what a decent chap Charles was when all the time he had been nothing short of a cold-hearted cad, preferring polo and his lover to his wife and children. Then she turned on me and I couldn't understand what I had done wrong. I just put it down to the damage that she received as a result of her horrid life. It never occurred to me that I had become a sort of Windsor to her and that she was probably having lunch with a new man and telling him what a shit I was! But that was Diana – wonderful, beautiful, vulnerable, but extremely selfish and at times perhaps the most spiteful person I have ever met, and then suddenly wonderful again.'

It would appear that Diana had the same initially positive effect on most people who came into contact with her and were flattered by her charm, beauty, position and, in the case of men, her wicked cocktail of vulnerability and flirtation. This apparently affected her protection officer Ken Wharfe, who didn't have an affair with her, almost as much as his predecessor, Barry Mannakee, who did. If you were in a crowd, her look could be piercing and might seem to be directed at only you. If you were sick or dying, the genuine concern and intense interest in you alone would have been wonderful if delivered by an old matron, but when freely given by a truly beautiful and extremely famous princess, it was overwhelming. For a longer relationship than these brief encounters, however, life was trickier.

The Princess, as she progressed through puberty, increasingly became obsessed with particular individuals and demanded devotion back in return. Later in life she would bombard trusted friends with as many as twenty phone calls a day, and a lot more if they also happened to be a lover. It would be necessary for them to drop whatever they were doing and rush to her side if that was what she wanted. Failure to put her every need first was, in her mind, a massive betrayal and a sign that they might be disloyal, were abandoning her or just didn't love her.

Her first love and obsession was Prince Charles. It was controllable initially as she focused on winning him. However, after the announcement that they were to be married, it was inevitable that such obsession would come head to head with Charles's own obsession: he was obsessed that if he wasn't working flat out for the good of the nation, they might find out that he was really as worthless as he believed himself to be. Two such people both lacking self-esteem and balance are highly unlikely to be able to help each other along a stable path. Therefore, the marriage was likely to be an unhappy one even before the couple had ventured down the aisle. Add to this the fact that Prince Charles was completely taken in by Diana's dishonesty and therefore initially thought that they shared common interests in friends, places and lifestyles when in reality they shared none, and it becomes obvious that the marriage was bound to be doomed even before she had thrown her first tantrum or taken her first desperate slash with a penknife.

So the marriage, blighted by her moods and his inability to understand them or help her, was further weakened by their common lack of interest in anything the other liked except their children. Slowly Prince Charles came to see that his wife's moods were more than just a symptom of getting use to royal life. Bit by bit the brighter periods became fewer and fewer as Princess Diana's love turned to hate. She had been almost permanently depressed throughout her marriage. Now he was slowly sinking into such a deep personal despair that some of his friends, many of whom had been banished by the Princess but were now returned to his life as the royal couple drifted apart, feared for his safety.

In November 1986 he wrote, 'Frequently I feel nowadays that I'm in a kind of cage, pacing up and down in it and longing to be free. How awful incompatibility is, and how dreadfully destructive it can be for the players in this extraordinary drama. It has all the ingredients of a

Greek tragedy … I fear I'm going to need a bit of help every now and then for which I feel rather ashamed. All I want to do is to HELP other people …'

By this time the Prince had given up the ghost on his marriage and was about to return to the intimacy and security of a renewed relationship with Camilla Parker Bowles, although she may have had to fend off the competition of Eva O'Neill and Marchesa Bona Frescobaldi in the early months. Both were close to Charles at this time, but both have always denied having anything other than a platonic relationship with the Prince.

However, and while things were never good in his marriage for more than the briefest of periods, this was not the case until then. Prior to 1986 his reserves of compassion and sympathy for the Princess still had to be exhausted. He believed that despite all her moods, tantrums and depressions, she really loved him and therefore it was his duty to be as good a husband as possible in such difficult circumstances. He had always determined that for the sake of his children, the country, the monarchy and the church, he would do everything to make his marriage work. The discovery of his wife's affairs was to change all of that and allowed him, in his mind, to believe that his marriage had by now, as he was later to put it, irretrievably broken down.

When he came to know of her infidelities is not exactly clear, but it would appear to be in 1986, and the knowledge seems to have allowed him to embark on the course that both Prince Philip and Mountbatten had advised him that he should adopt if his marriage didn't work out: they had told him if that happened, divorce was unthinkable and that a façade should be kept up while he found a married woman with whom he might conduct a discreet affair.

The Prince, being rather more idealistic and less practical than either his father or great-uncle, had held on to idea of a faithful marriage. However, once he knew about his wife's affairs, he knew that his guilt would be far less profound: he would, after all, only be doing the same as her, and as they were by now leading almost totally separate lives, he felt his conscience was clear. As long as the façade remained in place for the benefit of the children and the nation, he could organise a private life that might lift him from the morbid gloom that had engulfed him of late.

The Princess's first affair had almost certainly taken place without his knowledge. He was not a jealous husband, didn't spy on his wife, wished her moods would get better and was happy for her to go off and do things if it improved her humour. This meant Diana had a sort of freedom that she had always denied her husband for fear that he would use it to go off and have an affair. So, with her usual approach of 'one rule for me and another for everybody else', that is precisely what she did.

What Diana had in mind was a man whom she didn't really know and therefore with whom she could relive all the flirtatious fun of a new relationship. It would be an escape from her surroundings and herself. She later claimed that the affair happened because Charles was 'dead from the waist down', but this seems to be unfair – she told others such as Sonia Palmer the contrary: 'The Prince is an intensely sexual man. Diana herself told me.' Understandably, the Princess realised, just as she had before her marriage, that discretion was essential. She wanted a fling, not a marriage break-up that would wreck all the hard work she had undertaken in order to become the Princess of Wales.

The year was 1983 and the man was the seventeenth earl of Pembroke, Henry Herbert. He was a dashing, middle-aged man, in the Clint Eastwood mould, who came from a senior aristocratic family and lived in one of the finest houses in Britain – Wilton House near Salisbury. Pembroke wasn't in the army and didn't work in the city or for the Foreign Office like most men Diana knew. He had produced films, such as *Emily*, starring Koo Stark, an erstwhile girlfriend of Prince Andrew who may have lost her chance to become the duchess of York as a result. He was his own man, and that fascinated Diana at a time when the aristocracy rather looked down on celebrities rather than rub shoulders with them as they do today.

He was forty-five; she was only twenty-two. He was the older man that girls of the Princess's age can be easily seduced by. He was different and she wanted him to want her once he had caught her eye. From that point of view, she made the running – as she had with Prince Charles and would go on to do with all her lovers. Very few people in the upper echelons of the aristocratic circle knew about the affair, and that explains why it has never appeared in the tabloid press. One thing that I have learned while writing this book is that the bluer the blood, the less likely they are to talk – and if they do it will be for the sake of truth and conviction.

The Princess's affair was not a long one, and the divorced nobleman was just a confidence-boosting memory by the time she was ready to start thinking about adding a second child to her family. However, either thanks to the positive feelings that she took from it, or perhaps a feeling of guilt, or even because she had confirmed in her mind that the Prince was the better man, she returned to her marriage with a softer and more balanced attitude to her husband. The result was that he responded and they were to enjoy an especially harmonious period during the conception and run-up to Harry's birth.

Because the Pembroke affair had gone unnoticed, rumours of Diana having affairs first started in 1985. Courtiers had long realised that the marriage, which had suffered from her moods and their rows from day one, was getting worse. It became clear that not only was the Princess not keen to undertake joint engagements with the Prince any longer, she was also determined to remain in London when the court moved to places like Sandringham or Balmoral, while the Prince seemed not to mind any longer and put her under no pressure to attend. It was also at this time that the Princess's staff became aware that something was going on between Diana and her personal protection officer, Sergeant Barry Mannakee. Telling conversations were overheard. 'How do you like this dress?'

'Fine. I could fancy you myself!'

'Well you do anyway don't you?'

He started displaying signs of intimacy that she clearly encouraged, but at first there was very little gossip: Kensington Palace is a small place and most were frightened of the Princess getting to hear about it. Diana's reputation for being capable of taking fearful revenge on those who displeased her was well known, and most wished to keep their jobs.

Then, in July, shortly before the marriage of the Duke and Duchess of York, Diana and her personal officer were apparently caught in too much of a personal position. The Princess had apparently returned to her Kensington Palace drawing room after kissing William and Harry goodnight; her protection officer was waiting. She was twenty-five and the future queen of England. He was fourteen years older, not particularly good-looking and could only boast an annual pay packet that perhaps equated to the cost of a couple of dresses a year for the extravagant Princess. It was an unlikely match, so what could the attraction be?

Of course it is possible to become very attached, and even attracted, to people you see at work. It happens all the time: bosses are forever running off with their secretaries or assistants, and there is some sort of attraction when people are thrown together but are supposed to keep a dignified distance. It is forbidden fruit. For Mannakee, a married man reaching middle age, the wife of the future king of England, was the most forbidden fruit in the world: the temptation of being given the 'come on' by the Princess was just too much to resist. But what was the attraction for Diana?

Diana's very condition meant that she needed everyone to love her. She needed her picture to be in the newspapers every day. She needed to be the most popular member of the Royal Family. Even in the early years she never worried about upstaging either the Queen or the Prince of Wales; in latter years she positively delighted in doing so. She became, by her own confession, amazingly jealous of Sarah, Duchess of York when her sister-in-law looked like becoming more popular than her. Having sexual relations is a huge expression of desire, and Diana needed to be desired by some men for a long time, by others for less. The duration depended on how long it took her to tire of them, and that was usually established by how long it took either to control them completely or, in her husband's case, to give up trying.

On the evening in question, the couple were caught in a compromising position by a senior member of Prince Charles's staff who entered the room unexpectedly: what he saw only confirmed what had concerned him for about a year as he, along with other senior staff members, had begun to notice a closeness between the Princess and her detective that went far beyond the proper nature of the relationship. For some time, the Princess had increasingly done things, like go for long car drives on the hills near Balmoral, on her own – which meant in effect on her own with her protection officer. Initially most staff members put this down to the princess's desire not to spend time with Prince Charles, and this didn't surprise them; but as the intimacy of their glances, Diana's giggles and the nature of Mannakee's remarks, which started to go far further than those being made by a mere guard should have done, became almost open, senior members of the Kensington Palace staff became alarmed. When this particular courtier was confronted with exactly what was going on, there could no longer be any doubt.

According to Sue Reid, writing in the *Daily Mail* in September 2004, 'Within hours of the embarrassing Kensington Palace encounter, Prince Charles – who was, at this stage, still faithful to his wife – was informed by his loyal courtier of Diana's alleged dalliance.'

What! Prince Charles had been faithful to his wife and not carrying on an affair with Camilla Parker Bowles throughout the course of his entire marriage as the paper had been screaming out in headlines for the last twelve years? According to Sue Reid, a couple of days after Prince Andrew's wedding in Westminster Abbey, the Queen was also informed of what had happened by Diana's brother-in-law Sir Robert Fellowes, who had by this time progressed to become Her Majesty's deputy private secretary.

This part of the story is disputed by others who claim that the prince was only informed that Mannakee would have to go, and that the Queen was told nothing at all at the time. If their version is correct, it seems curious that Prince Charles just accepted the advice and never questioned why. Penny Junor believes that despite this point, the second version is true and that Mannakee was not the only lover his wife had that the prince knew nothing about until much later. She points out that, unlike Diana, Charles had never been a jealous person when it came to where his wife was or whom she was seeing. If he thought that she had been unfaithful he never confronted her or moaned to others about it. 'Even during the darkest periods of his marriage, when life, as a friend puts it, was "one long whinge, it was not always directed at Diana and even at the worst times he did show understanding and sympathy for her personal position."' In addition, my own research has led me to the conclusion that the Prince, by this time, had realised that he and his wife were both locked into an awful marriage that there would be no getting away from. Therefore, he understood that Diana's position was no different to his and that the best way forward was for them both discreetly to live separate lives. As a result he had no intention of rocking the boat and enquiring what she might have been getting up to.

However, I also believe that Charles either knew about Mannakee at the time, not long afterwards, or of another of her numerous liaisons around this period, otherwise he would never have allowed himself the pleasure of being put back in touch with Camilla Parker Bowles by Patti Palmer-Tomkinson, and this was to happen later in the year.

Unfortunately, for him, the Princess didn't see it this way. For her there was no logic to the notion that as she was being unfaithful, why shouldn't he. Instead, her attitude was exactly the opposite. So while he turned a blind eye to her numerous affairs over the next seven years, she pursued him with espionage and violent rages concerning his renewed relationship with Camilla. When confronted by those who questioned the fairness of this, Diana would simply reply that she was jealous because it was Camilla. Not even the obliging Mr Morton buys into this theory, wisely commenting that whomever the Prince had taken as a mistress, Diana's reaction would have been the same.

Nevertheless, whether the Prince knew what he was up to or not, Mannakee was sent for and told that he was being removed from royal protection duties and would now work for the Diplomatic Protection Group instead. There are those who believe that Diana continued to have Mannakee smuggled into Kensington Palace after his move to the Diplomatic Protection Group. I have not found anyone who actually saw him there, but some are convinced that he was and claim that he and Princess Diana still spoke very regularly on the telephone. Mannakee made no complaint about his fate; indeed he seemed, according to one colleague, 'bloody relieved that that was all that was going to happen to him.'

It wasn't: within a year Mannakee was dead. At 10.15 p.m. on 14 May 1987, his spine was fatally snapped in a horrific motorcycle accident in east London. At the resulting inquest the coroner decided that he had died due to a tragic crash involving the motorbike on which he was riding pillion and a Ford Fiesta driven by a newly qualified driver, seventeen-year-old Nicola Chopp. That appeared to be the end of the matter until the Princess some years later talked openly about her affair with Mannakee and went on to claim that as a result of it he had been brutally murdered by secret-service agents. She described Mannakee as 'the greatest fellow I have ever had'. Asked if Mannakee provided the 'intimacy you weren't getting', she admitted, 'Yeah.' Then she added almost as an afterthought, 'I think he was bumped off, but I will never know.'

On the night in question, the Suzuki motorbike was being driven by Mannakee's friend and fellow policeman, Stephen Peat. He was travelling along Woodford High Road at between thirty-four and thirty-eight miles per hour, with Mannakee on the pillion seat, when the young rookie driver Ms Chopp pulled out of Hermitage Walk in front of him. Peat, an experienced rider, lost control of bike, which skidded sideways before going to ground and sliding past Chopp's Ford Fiesta; as it did, Mannakee fell off and crashed into her car. Peat, who has always claimed that the crash was nothing more than an accident, suffered chest, head and eye injuries but was allowed home after two days. Mannakee wasn't so fortunate.

Nicola Chopp told the inquest that followed his death that a vehicle opposite her had turned left into Woodford High Road just before she had turned right to follow it. She claimed that the vehicle had its headlights on full beam. Police investigators also told the coroner that this vehicle's lights could have temporarily blinded Peat. Nevertheless, Nicola was later found to be at fault. She was fined £85 and found guilty of driving without due care and attention.

How could this have been a murder plot rather than another unfortunate road accident, the like of which are all too common in urban areas like east London? Could the mystery car have masterminded the whole thing and caused the accident deliberately? It must be considered extremely unlikely to the point of being impossible. How could the driver guarantee that his lights would blind Peat to the extent that the bike would crash? How could he guarantee that Nicola would turn out into the main road to provide the barrier needed for Mannakee's body to slam into? And how could he then guarantee that this would have the desired effect of killing Mannakee – especially as Peat didn't die. To ensure all of this happened, one would need the compliance of both Nicola Chopp and Stephen Peat. Chopp, a seventeen-year-old at the time, who had only passed her test six weeks before, doesn't strike me as a natural secret-service stunt driver. What's more, she would have had to agree to drive her vehicle out into the main road at a given signal in the knowledge that Peat would somehow manage to push Mannakee's body from behind him off the bike and into Chopp's path, while ensuring that he and the bike missed her car.

Moreover, both Peat and Chopp risked serious injury themselves and in the case of Peat he received injuries that could have easily been fatal. In addition to this, Stephen Peat and Barry Mannakee were friends. Therefore both Peat and Chopp are the most unlikely of accomplices, and yet without their help the elimination of Mannakee would have been practically impossible. Such a plan would be unwieldy, messy and have a huge chance of failure. No decent novelist would ever dream up such a sloppy plan in a work of fiction. If MI6 wanted Mannakee bumped off, surely all they would have needed to do was to assign him to some Israeli diplomat who was highly unpopular and controversial with the Arabs and then shoot him while he was guarding the diplomat: the world would assume that the assassin's bullet had hit the wrong man and the job would have been neat, tidy, almost guaranteed and no questions would ever have been asked. A decent novelist might write that fiction – it does, after all, make a lot more sense.

But the *Daily Mail* was proud to throw new light on the case and help Sir John Stevens, the Scotland Yard chief heading up the inquiry, solve it and possibly even exonerate Nicola Chopp. In her article, Sue Reid went on to claim that the *Mail* had learned of the existence of a file, copies of which were locked away in three separate bank deposit boxes in different parts of the country. The file was said to contain 'dynamic new evidence supporting the princess's theory that her bodyguard was murdered'.

It continues: 'The file is said to show the results of a secret forensic examination of PC Peat's motorbike which reveals that it was tampered with prior to the crash. Copies of the file were placed in banks in Devon, the South Coast and Norfolk by a friend of Mannakee's, a police officer of 30 years standing with links to the Royal Protection Squad.' So might there be something in this theory after all? How did the expert know when the tampering was done? The article didn't say. And how did MI6, or whoever, know that Mannakee, whose bike it was not, would be on the Suzuki when it would all go wrong? The article didn't say.

But the *Mail* had found out that two men, one the aforementioned police officer and the second a peer of the realm, knew all about it. They had apparently met while serving time in prison together for financial fraud. What? A policeman who had close links with the Royal Protection Squad and yet had done time for financial fraud. There can't be too many of those. Surely it wouldn't be hard to discover who he was, would it? Apparently it was, because the peer wouldn't tell them. So who was the peer, then? The hereditary peer was one Charlie Brocket, whom I happen to know well. Lord Brocket, who starred in the TV series *I'm A Celebrity Get Me Out of Here!*, was jailed in 1996 for his part in a multimillion-pound insurance fraud involving a part of his collection of forty-two Ferraris. The eccentric Lord Brocket refused to name his police-officer friend, and apparently the *Mail* didn't feel the need to check the records and find out who he was, despite the fact that Brocket told them that they were together in Springhill Open Prison when he was first told of the existence of the mysterious Mannakee file. The announcement of the existence of this file might, to the less charitable, appear only just to have been remembered by his Lordship in time to coincide with the launch of a book that he had written.

Lord Brocket explained to the *Mail*, 'I was talking to this former policeman, who was also serving time, about the death of Princess Diana in the Paris underpass. It was March 1998, seven months after she was killed, and five months before I was released.

'The policeman suddenly blurted out that he knew Mannakee. He said that he and another group of detectives, angry at any suggestion that the princess's bodyguard had died in a motorcycle accident after Peat had lost control of the bike, took the remains of the vehicle to their own forensic expert.

'Apparently, the expert – who was not told who owned the bike or who was riding it – wrote a report saying that the machine had been tampered with deliberately. The resulting file is the one that is sealed in the banks.

Brocket, who vaguely knew the Princess socially, and had often hunted with the Prince of Wales, went on to explain that he tried to contact his policeman friend, who was released soon afterwards, once he had secured his own release. He doesn't explain why he intended to do this. We are left to guess what his intentions were. Perhaps he intended to run his own investigation into the matter and sell the results to a grateful daily paper. But, according to Lord Brocket, whatever he said didn't go down very well: 'I rang him at home last December. I spoke to his wife who sounded terrified. She told me: "Leave us alone – we want to stay alive." The implication was that whoever killed Mannakee would be prepared to kill them.'

The *Mail* did, in fairness to them, point out that this revelation by Charlie Brocket might be 'the wild ramblings of two men with dubious records of honesty'. Moreover, I am obliged to point out that it might also be the deliberate lie of a man keen to impress a lord, or even the work of a vivid imagination by a lord wishing to be a self-publicist. As the *Mail* failed to track down the policeman, I cannot say.

Nevertheless, James Hewitt, who was to start a romance with Diana not long after Mannakee was banished from her life, has also stated that not only did the princess tell him that she and Mannakee were lovers, but also that she was certain the secret services had had Mannakee murdered. However, this did not prevent her from having further liaisons with several other men: if she seriously believed that this would lead to their deaths, I like to think she wouldn't have done so.

In a more alarming revelation, Hewitt also claims that during the height of his affair with Diana, he was visited in his London flat by an officer from MI5 who warned him, 'If you do not stop seeing Diana you will suffer the same fate as Barry Mannakee and die in a road accident.' Hewitt may be charming and a bit thick, which went in his favour with the Princess, but there is little evidence that he had the capacity to lie like the Princess of Wales. However, his story cannot be substantiated by anyone and perhaps the greatest indication why it isn't true is that he carried on seeing her. In fact, their relationship became more brazen, but he still lives happily today, making many bucks from his association with her. If MI5 or MI6 had murdered Mannakee and the Princess, I am sure they wouldn't have worried too much about getting rid of Hewitt too. And why were they all so insistent that everybody had to die in a car crash? It simply defies belief.

What is not in doubt is that the Princess took the news of Mannakee's death very badly, and this clearly indicates that she held more feelings for him than just an employee, albeit a close one. The Prince had been tipped off about what had happened moments before he and the Princess were due to leave for RAF Northolt in order to take a plane to the Cannes Film Festival on the day following the fatal accident. A former staff member said that the Prince looked deeply troubled: not only had Mannakee been at one time the children's protection officer, he had also been Charles's as well, and the Prince, who was by now clear about what had been going on, was not looking forward to telling the Princess what had happened. However, he also knew that he must, as it would be quite unfair for her to learn about it from a journalist asking her to comment on the death of her former protection officer.

So as the car made its way towards the airport, the Prince brought up the subject of Mannakee, apparently with some hesitation as he struggled to find the right words. The Princess is said to have frozen with the fear of one about to be confronted about having done something that she shouldn't have. However, when it became clear that her husband was not going to confront her about her affair but was trying to say that Mannakee was dead, she started to cry uncontrollably, became hysterical and tore her clothes.

The Prince and Diana's lady-in-waiting, Anne Beckwith-Smith, both desperately tried to console her. Somehow they managed to get on to the flight, but she remained in complete despair and continued to sob. Then she stopped and went to the toilet. There she slashed herself to such an extent that the dress that she was due to wear for the film festival had to be altered by her dresser to cover up the damage that she had inflicted upon herself.

The Princess has a different memory of this event to others present. She believed that her husband had told her bluntly in order to catch her out and thus prove that she was having an affair. She recalled, 'Charles told me that he was killed in a motorbike accident. And that was the biggest blow of my life, I must say. That was a real killer. Charles thought he knew but he never, never had any proof. And he just jumped it on me like that, and I wasn't able to do anything … I just sat there going through this huge high-profile visit to Cannes … Thousands of press. Just devastated. Just devastated. Of course it wasn't supposed to mean as much as it did.'

Following Mannakee's death, Diana started to have disturbing dreams about him. She consulted a clairvoyant and then decided to visit his grave. It was only then that she discovered that his wife had had him cremated. 'He was just chucked over the ground. That absolutely appalled me, but there we were. I wasn't in a position to do anything about it.' From then on the Princess is supposed to have visited the London crematorium where Mannakee's ashes were scattered on each anniversary of his death. This cannot be verified, but could easily be true. I have not been able to substantiate a story that once, following a row with Prince Charles, she was seen walking alone on a Norfolk beach wearing a headscarf given to her by the bodyguard.

However, the death of Barry Mannakee was obviously a traumatic experience for the Princess and there can be little doubt, especially given her own testimony, that she was involved in an extra-marital affair with him. Whether he was murdered by somebody as a result is completely in doubt as there seems to be no evidence to support the accusation – only, as usual the hearsay of Diana's cronies and the ramblings of a man who in all honesty cannot be considered to be a reliable source of information until he produces the proof to support his claims. What is not in doubt is that Mannakee wasn't the first person that Diana committed adultery with. Moreover, it seems likely that he was a temporary infatuation whose relationship with her was cut short, rather than a man with whom the Princess was truly in love.

Around the time of his transfer – the time when they were discovered and supposedly at the height of their passion – Diana attended a party to celebrate Sarah Ferguson's forthcoming marriage to Prince Andrew. The Princess danced outrageously with a city financier. Like Diana, he was married. Eyebrows were raised by her open flirtation.

John Rendall, who later became the social editor of *Hello!* magazine, was at the party. Around midnight he went outside for a cigarette and heard sounds coming from the bushes. He looked up and nearly swallowed his cigarette when he 'saw the Princess of Wales with this man. They were necking. I moved away, finished my cigarette quietly, and went back inside. They didn't return for ages.'

The following month, August, the Prince, the Princess and their children went to stay as guests of King Juan Carlos of Spain, his wife Queen Sofia and their three children in Majorca. The king was rumoured to have a wandering eye, and when the two families took his yacht around the Balearic islands, stopping off to swim in secluded coves and play on private beaches, Diana could not resist the temptation. A cousin of the king's speculated to Lady Colin Campbell that it was just a fling for him but that Diana was using it as a weapon with which to try and make Charles jealous: 'But it didn't work. He couldn't have cared less. In fact he upped sticks and left them to it, and went to Puerto Andratx, where he stayed with Jose Luis de Villalonga. I don't believe Queen Sofia knew anything then. If she had known she would not have welcomed Diana back.'

The following year the Waleses were to return again, but this time the trip was less successful. The Prince and Princess were still going through the motions of a marriage for the sake of their children, but as the king and Diana attempted to pick up where they had left off the previous summer, they were rumbled by Queen Sofia who now saw through what she had previously thought was Diana's innocent flirtatiousness. She concluded, as did the king's cousin, 'There is no question about it. They were having an affair.' The Prince and his family weren't invited back a third time.

So if the Princess really did love and mourn Mannakee as much as she said she did, she had an odd way of showing it. Moreover, not only was Mannakee not Diana's first act of adultery, she was not even faithful to him while they were having their affair. Indeed, there is some doubt as to whether or not she was actually faithful to any of her lovers thereafter, as their dates appear to cross over. In addition, it is almost certain that there are many that we do not know about – men who have been decent enough not to kiss and tell. Penny Junor reflects that several other men seemed to have a claim on her affections at one time or another, men who would visit Kensington Palace at all hours of the day and night. 'She appeared to enjoy the power she had over them, telephoning and having them arrive at her bidding, and dismissing them when she wanted them gone.'

One quite junior member of one of the Princess's royal neighbours' staff was less delicate, stating, 'Blimey, it was just like a red-light district round there at times. Men coming and going all the time and sometimes only just missing one another. I told the wife that we should tell the *Sun* … She said, "Na, we'll lose our bleedin' jobs if we was found out." Sometimes she used to smuggle them into the Palace in the boot of her car in broad daylight. She thought no one could see, but I could and at first I thought that I must have been seeing things. Imagine – the Princess drives up and opens up her boot and some bloke gets out.'

The Princess was summoning men to worship at her feet, and if she were attracted to them, sex would follow. It was simply part of a need she had almost to devour men that she wanted to the point of overdose when she would either tire of them or imagine that they had badly let her down and reject them – in the way she had her husband. The relationship with Charles had been long and painful. Now things speeded up and most of her romances were short, although one with James Hewitt, perhaps because of his forced absences, and another with Oliver Hoare, because she never felt that she had quite captured him, were longer.

All men summoned could not resist going, and most would have certainly been only too happy to be seduced by this enchanting and apparently vulnerable woman who was not only extremely beautiful but seen as such by the whole world. However, while many were invited into the bedroom, not everybody was.

Having worked hard to recover her figure from the birth of Prince Harry, the Princess, with her relations at home deteriorating, looked around for the kind of social life that her early marriage to Prince Charles had precluded. So during 1985 while her affection for her protection officer grew before blossoming into a physical relationship, she also became closer to Sarah Ferguson in the hope of dropping back into an exciting and youthful social circle that might enable her to enjoy the discreet flirtations that she felt she needed in order to drive her blues away. She no longer enjoyed the garden at Highgrove, never visited the farm there and would use any excuse to cut short weekends and return to London early, where she would increasingly delight Fergie's set of friends, doing the drinks and dinner parties energetically while also revamping some of her own old friendships.

But then Sarah Ferguson was elevated up the social ladder and into the inner sanctum of the royal circle by becoming engaged to Prince Charles's younger brother Andrew. The press happily depicted them as good friends, which indeed they were, and rejoiced that at last Diana had another woman in the family who was closer to her own age and therefore could be a confidante and ally.

Princess Diana saw matters somewhat differently. How could a woman sleeping with her husband's brother be a trusted confidante? Moreover, with another royal wedding looming, her playmate was bound to turn from a friend into a rival. The Princess was right. She had been around for more than five years, had had two children and of late had been spending time, quite rightly, bringing them up, which meant that she had been less in the public eye. Then suddenly along comes Fergie – a fresh-faced, unsophisticated 'girl next door' whom the press adored. She was clearly relaxed, irreverent and determined to have a good time. She appeared to be a breath of fresh air that was blowing Diana off the front pages. Suddenly the Princess, who had never been confident throughout her life, now became even more insecure as it appeared that her comfort blanket of being the favourite of the national press was going to be snatched away by her friend who was going to marry into the Windsors and would no doubt be soon siding with them against her. As she later admitted, 'I got terribly jealous.'

Her behaviour became ever more erratic. She would swing from not being able to do enough for a charity to cutting it dead and completely refusing to do anything. Her friends also began to feel the effects of her violent mood swings, hitherto only seen by a few. She blew hot and cold with them and caused them much anguish. One minute she couldn't see or speak enough to a friend, perhaps having lunch several times in one week or phoning them up to twenty times a day, sometimes for hours at a time, telling them the most intimate details of her life and buying them expensive and thoughtful gifts. The next minute, and for no apparent reason, she would cut them out of her life completely and refuse even to receive their calls. Then, a week or a month or even a year later she may return to them as if nothing had ever happened.

Vivienne Parry, a very good and loyal friend who worked for her and became a trustee of the Diana Memorial Fund following her death was later to say, 'At some time all of her friends were frozen out.' And if Diana's behaviour was erratic with her friends, it was certainly no less so with her staff. One day she could be kind, thoughtful and very informal, the next she might cut them dead and might not speak to them again for a month. Oliver Everett, Richard Aylard, Anne Beckwith-Smith – who is supposed to have survived as long as she did because Diana didn't think she was as good-looking as she was and therefore wasn't a threat – and others all received what was known in the KP office as 'the treatment' at one time or another. One reported to Penny Junor, 'I would have given up all the flowers, all the niceness if only we could have avoided the sheer bloody-minded sarcasm, the silences, and the sending to Coventry that went with it.' By all accounts it was not uncommon for the Princess to scream and use obscene language at the staff either in KP or Highgrove when a sudden and uncontrollable anger overtook her. The only good thing about these outbursts was their duration was a lot shorter than the sullen moods and the extended silences.

This kind of behaviour towards those immediately around her only got worse as time went by and she increasingly came to see conspiracies against her at every turn. She started to leave disturbing messages on people's pagers or answering machines. She never signed them off with her name, but everyone knew that it was her leaving the message. Patrick Jephson would receive them regularly. A typical message would tell him, 'We know where you are and so does your wife. I know you are being disloyal to me.'

In the late 1980s Camilla Parker Bowles would receive late-night phone calls telling her things like, 'I've sent someone to kill you. They're outside in the garden. Look out of the window: can you see them?' Mrs Parker Bowles was well aware that it was Diana, although the Princess would never admit as much. Nevertheless, as a woman in a large house on her own in the middle of the country, it must have been very upsetting.

But the most poisonous messages were reserved for Ms Alexandra

Legge-Bourke, known as Tiggy. She became the children's nanny and friend when they stayed with Prince Charles once the royal couple had separated. The Princess was to wage a completely unwarranted campaign against Ms Legge-Bourke as she wrongly became convinced that the Prince had adopted the nanny as a second mistress. This was made all the worse, in her mind, by the fact that the boys appeared to be very fond of Tiggy, which made her insanely jealous.

No one dared confront the Princess about these messages, as they knew the tantrums she was capable of and the revenge she may wish to inflict. In Camilla or Tiggy's case that might mean a horrible public scene; others would just be sacked.

Diana's sackings were well known inside the royal circle of employees, and they cost the Prince a small fortune over the years. In the United Kingdom it was no longer possible to dismiss staff without a warning procedure being followed and good reason given. The Princess had no intention of following the law with this regard, and most people she took against had done nothing wrong in the first place. Diana would simply decide, usually quite arbitrarily, that she no longer wanted them around. As a result, the Prince's office would have to calculate what an industrial tribunal would award and add on an extra twenty per cent in the hope that the ousted member would honour their contract and not squeal to the press about 'the mad cow', as one put it, they had been working for. In those days the maximum settlement was £11,000, and therefore the Prince paid off a succession of usually perfectly reasonable cooks, housemaids, dressers, secretaries and, until Burrell, butlers at a rate of around £13,000 a time to disappear and not work for him. He would then have to find and pay replacements.

One person sacked for apparently no good reason was a chauffeur called Steve Davies. He had been having an affair with one of the Princess's pretty young dressers named Helen Walsh, who lived in a grace and favour cottage at the back of Kensington Palace. For some reason, perhaps because Davies really had eyes only for his girlfriend, the Princess decided irrationally that she didn't like the relationship and that they were taking advantage of their position. She had the chauffeur paid off and told Helen that her boyfriend was barred from the cottage. Infuriated by the unfairness of it all, she consulted the Royal Personnel Department. They advised her that she was free to have any guest she wanted, provided that the police on the gate knew who they were. When she heard about this, the Princess was livid with what she saw as the girl's complete impertinence and got one of her staff to check over the rules. When they reported back that, technically, all guests had to be off the premises by midnight, she was delighted. The next night she was round at the cottage by ten past midnight and banging on the front door while shaking with rage and ranting, 'I know he's in there, I want him out now!'

I asked my source the obvious question: 'Why didn't she just sack her as well as the boyfriend?'

'Fairly obvious, isn't it? If Helen had been sacked as well, they would have been able to live together and Diana would no longer have any control over their lives.'

The way she treated Victoria Mendham is perhaps the most chilling reminder of how awful the Princess could be to staff, especially those who loved her and only wanted to do their very best for her. Mendham, who is mentioned by Morton but surprisingly not in this context, was a junior secretary at Kensington Palace for seven years and much admired the Princess. She even began to imitate Diana in the way she dressed. Diana rewarded such heroine worship by making the girl a close confidante, indeed a perfect one – one who would be happy to listen to her for hours and never disagree with a word. So things proceeded very well, and Victoria was invited to go on holiday with the Princess to America and the Caribbean, and she paid for her on both occasions. Then at Easter in 1996, Diana invited Victoria to go a second time to the Caribbean; Mendham, having loved the previous two holidays, readily accepted. Halfway through the holiday, Diana announced that she had instructed that the bill be split in two and that Victoria's share would be about £5,000. The secretary stammered both in fear and absolute shock that she had been invited to come. 'Yes,' replied Princess Diana, 'but you always knew you would have to pay your way.'

Mendham phoned KP the next day in floods of tears and explained that she didn't have anything like £5,000. She was told not to panic and that a senior courtier would approach the Prince of Wales on her behalf. Charles duly paid the bill quietly. When the Princess returned home she asked if the bill had been settled and was told that it had, but not by whom. Initially she assumed that it had been by Victoria. However, she did find out and was clearly furious that everybody had conspired behind her back to help Mendham out. Nine months later she invited her confidante again on holiday but, now understandably wary, Victoria informed the Princess that she would love to go but that she could only afford the economy-class airfare to the Caribbean. The secretary thought that the Princess had agreed to this, so she went, but on her return was presented with half the hotel cost, which at £1,700 a night before meals and extras was huge. Mendham couldn't pay and the Princess chased her relentlessly for the money, having appeared to have forgotten about their agreement. Now Victoria was frozen out as others had been before her.

When Diana went to Angola on her anti-landmines campaign she took Burrell instead of Victoria, who was heartbroken as a result. While there, and in between some of the shooting of the now-famous film footage that recorded her brave and thoroughly good work, Diana was either on the phone to the accounts department back in London to see if they had collected the money from Victoria, or actually pursuing Mendham herself. Prince Charles again came to the rescue and settled the unpaid bill.

However, this was not the result that the Princess wanted. On Diana's return there was a showdown and Victoria Mendham, somebody who wanted no more than to serve loyally a woman whom she had loved for years, was axed and told to clear her desk and leave at once. In tears she did precisely that, and was cast out forever.

Notwithstanding this treatment, and to prove that Diana could exercise a hold over women as well as men, Victoria Mendham phoned in following the news of the Princess's death and offered to return to her old desk in order to help arrange the funeral. Somebody who can treat another person so shabbily and still receive that sort of love from them must have some very strong redeeming qualities. Therefore there can be no doubt in my mind that notwithstanding these dreadful acts of tyrannical cruelty there has to have been a very special side to the Princess of Wales that allowed people like Victoria to forgive her.

Nevertheless, these terrible stories of staff abuse and manic messages illustrate what life with the Princess could be like for other people, not just her husband. Nor can they be dismissed as smears put about by the Prince's friends or staff. The Prince gave his staff clear and definite orders not to spin against the Princess, not only for the sake of their children and the monarchy and even the Princess herself, but because, like others, he was fearful of what pouring oil on to the fire could bring.

Happily for the Princess, the 'Fergie problem' wasn't to last forever. Soon after Sarah's marriage to Prince Andrew, Diana asked her office to arrange additional work for her and gave them three dates when she would be available. This was most uncharacteristic, but was nevertheless achieved. When it had all been fixed up, a policeman from the Royal Protection Squad commented that the dates happened to coincide with the first three official public engagements of the Duchess of York.

Diana had come out of her corner fighting and had upstaged her rival to perfection. There were to be few occasions in the future when Sarah would come close to challenging Diana's position again.

With Mannakee now unable to satisfy Diana's unquenchable desire for sex and adoration, the Princess cast her eye around for a new conquest: it fell on Philip Dunne, the brother-in-law of Rupert Soames, Nicholas's younger brother. Dunne was a Clark Kent look-alike and worked in the City for the banking firm Warburgs. The papers would report a whirlwind romance that got so careless that diners at a top London Restaurant, the Ménage à Trois, even noticed them playing footsie under the table.

However, the Prince was aware of these reports and, as long as they remained discreet and caused neither his children nor the monarchy any embarrassment, he would tolerate them as a way of keeping a woman happy with whom he had to share a public life but had by now totally given up any idea of sharing his private life with. Given this semi-official seal of approval from her husband, the Princess lurched from careless obsession for her new toy to using him as a weapon in order to tempt her husband back to her. She enjoyed many public and private dinners with the banker, and even a weekend at his parents' home, Gatley Park in Herefordshire, while they were away skiing. The following summer the Prince included Dunne on his invitation list to Royal Ascot, much to the Princess's delight. However, this approval and freedom was blown away by Diana's inability to be as discreet as she had once been, and the reason for that was probably that she wanted to make her husband jealous.

The wedding of the Marquis of Worcester to the actress Tracey Ward was a very big affair. Not only were the top members of many aristocratic families present, but more dangerously there were many less discreet individuals there as well. The Princess first took the floor with Dunne and danced in a highly provocative way: she started to comb his hair with her fingers before cuddling up to him and burying her tongue in his ear. It was either done to cause the Prince extreme embarrassment or to make him jealous, but it didn't work because he remained in deep conversation with his ex-girlfriend Anna Wallace and never looked his wife's way. At two in the morning he left without her, leaving her to continue with a floor show that would end her relationship with Dunne.

Needless to say the gossip columnists began to speculate widely, and pieces about the Princess and Dunne started to appear in the press. When they didn't stop, the Princess became alarmed and wanted out. She had no intention of being blamed for the marriage break-up – she would be seen as the villain and her position and reputation would be ruined. She feared that the Queen might even restrict her access to the children, and she hadn't given up hope of winning back her husband – even if she was absolutely clueless about how to go about it.

She didn't have to tell Dunne herself: the Palace was only too willing to do this for her as they were equally alarmed by where the press speculation was leading. The papers were by now full of stories concerning the fact that the royal couple hardly ever saw each other. For once, the 'grey men' and Diana agreed: Dunne was telephoned by them and warned off.

The Princess was pleased when the Dunne stories stopped, but then alarmed again when she heard rumours that Mannakee was planning to sell his story. Who told her this is not clear – it might have just been a story invented by her later in order to make her tale of an MI5 murder sound more plausible. We shall never know.

By the time Mannakee died in May 1987, Diana had formed yet another attachment, this time was to Major Waterhouse, whom she had met while skiing with Prince Charles, Dunne and the Yorks. Waterhouse was a distant cousin of Diana's. He was the grandson of the previous Duke of Marlborough, who is the true head of the Spencer family; his mother, Lady Caroline Spencer-Churchill, was a well-connected lady.

David Waterhouse was a tall, dark, army type to whom Diana found herself drawn. Soon he was enjoying evenings at Kensington Palace, intimate dinners at the Princess's favourite restaurants, trips to the cinema and even, it was claimed, bridge games with the Princess at his apartment. Her detective would sit downstairs in her car smiling to himself that Diana must think him an idiot: he knew perfectly well that bridge requires four players, and there were only two people up there alone. These supposed bridge games would go on for hours.

Lady Colin Campbell writes that the Palace saw Waterhouse as a safe pair of hands. He had been brought up to be an English gentleman and was the model of discretion. No attempt was made by them to break up their friendship, which ran for some time – certainly long enough for another of her long-term lovers, James Hewitt, to become jealous of him. However, despite Waterhouse's caution, the gossip columnists were starting to receive little titbits from other punters of the posh eating houses frequented by Diana, and the press began to speculate that the marriage was by now in real trouble. Then one night, as the Princess was emerging in the early hours of the morning from her friend Kate Menzies' mews house, a waiting photographer captured her and Waterhouse on film apparently indulging in the kind of horseplay that would have been explosive if it had been splashed over the front page of a tabloid newspaper.

Diana knew that she was in trouble and did what any beautiful girl does when her back is to the wall: she cried and appeared very distressed, which she almost certainly genuinely was. While Waterhouse lurked in the background, the Princess and her new protection officer pleaded with the photographer to hand over his film and say nothing of what he had seen. At first he resisted, knowing that such a picture could be worth something and it would certainly do his career no harm either, but whether it was Diana's distress or the officer's bullying, or a combination of the two, eventually the film was recovered. However, the photographer obviously had second thoughts: he went straight back to his newspaper and told his editor what he had seen. Naturally it became headline news, but it was somewhat less damaging than it would have been if the story had been accompanied by a sensational photograph. A photograph would have screamed out that this was a true story; without one it was passed off by most people as having been exaggerated or even made up – such is the reputation of the British tabloid press. As a result, Diana had managed another close escape.

Nobody that I interviewed when researching this book, even those sympathetic to the Princess, denied that there was a physical relationship between her and Waterhouse. No one was positive that there *wasn't* a relationship of that nature. Furthermore, everyone I have interviewed speculate that Philip Dunne was more than a passing phase: he was seen entering Kensington Palace alone on more than one occasion, and not always at the usually polite social hours court etiquette required, despite her rendezvous with Waterhouse and Hewitt. And at the same time, it is believed that Mannakee was still being smuggled into the Palace for secret meetings. One advisor of that time has stated, 'For certain she drove more than one car at a time, and I know that she applied the same rule to her men.' It was around the time of the discovery her affair with Barry Mannakee that Diana also became interested in James Hewitt.

The relationship with Hewitt would last some years, but was not one that Diana appears to have been faithful to despite her claim to have been very much in love with him. Indeed, after her flirtation with Waterhouse, he was briefly replaced by James Gilbey, the car salesman who had known the Princess since she was seventeen. Many other male friends were constant visitors to Kensington Palace and it was always presumed by her staff, given the Princess's desire to spirit them in and out again secretly – sometimes in the boot of her car – that at least some were lovers. The arrival of Hewitt in the Princess's bed might have slowed the flow of other male guests to the Palace, but it certainly did not entirely stop it.

James Hewitt came into the Princess's life in the summer of 1986 when he was invited to a drinks party at Buckingham Palace. Hewitt was cornered by Diana and happily spent most of the evening talking to her, which he found easy and natural. He later recalled, 'I think that she wanted to find out more about me and what I did and she learned that I was a riding instructor, and that's really how we started. She said that she would like to learn to ride again. She had hurt herself as a young child falling off, and lost her nerve, and wanted to get her nerve back again. So I said I would be able to help, and so it was arranged.'

Diana had spotted her prey and, even though she was deeply involved with Mannakee at the time, she knew how important the conversation was in order to build an opportunity that would eventually lead to what she wanted. I suspect that if Hewitt had been teaching her how to pass her hated O-level exams, the Princess would have volunteered for lessons all the same, such was her determination to create a platform upon which she might develop a relationship with this army officer: because she was already in at least one extra-marital relationship, she understood that she needn't rush but could bide her time and establish a believable cover – that of ensuring that she learned to ride so that she could participate more with the horse-mad Windsors. Weekly encounters would give her both something to look forward to and the opportunity to capture Hewitt's heart without undue or undignified haste. It was one of many separate plans to relieve her misery and give her lots of different little fantasy worlds that she might dream about without ever really having any intention of going there. She would usually tire of the man long before there ever came a need to confront such issues, but as long as she felt that she controlled everything around her, she felt better in control of herself.

James Hewitt, who knew Prince Charles vaguely through polo, got permission from the colonel at Hyde Park Barracks and soon the lessons, which also included a lady-in-waiting called Hazel West and occasionally others like Sir Christopher Airy and the Duke of Luxemburg, took place two or even three times a week. The group would be followed by a few police cars and there would be various bodyguards along the route. The Princess, who was quite genuinely frightened of horses, wasn't very good. She was never very fond of animals, despite having been surrounded by dogs as a child, and her nervousness told the horse that he was in charge. But she was determined to persist with the lessons and everyone, especially Diana and her instructor, seemed to enjoy them.

Soon she was asking James what she should wear at various forthcoming engagements. She had done this with Mannakee and would do it with most of the men she wished to attract. Naturally it wasn't a serious question: while Diana knew that she needed fashion advice, she also knew to seek it from men like Bruce Oldfield, who had more fashion sense in his little finger than men like Mannakee, Waterhouse or Hewitt would ever have in their entire bodies. She asked because it kept the conversation focused on her and gave the man plenty of opportunity to flatter her by remarking upon her various attributes. This in itself might lead the conversation on to a more flirtatious or even intimate nature. The man would think that it was him making the running, but actually it was her.

When she rang him to arrange for a lesson, they would talk on the phone for an hour or more. The relationship was developing nicely in her opinion, and she would say as much to one or two very close female confidantes. Then disaster struck: Hewitt was promoted to acting major, and took charge of Headquarters Squadron at the Combermere Barracks in Windsor. Hewitt thought that would be the end of that. However, Diana, who was never one to be thwarted in her desires and who never for a second forgot that she was the Princess of Wales or how to get her own way, decided that it wasn't. Hewitt was delighted, but also surprised to discover that Diana would travel to Windsor, at some personal inconvenience, in order to be taught by him.

It suddenly dawned on him that the growing attraction he felt for the Princess was reciprocated: 'It's something that I wasn't expecting or wanted to happen. I mean, sometimes when you don't expect something you don't see it until it hits you in the face.' Hewitt might have been hit in the face, but the Princess had hoped for this outcome as she had crossed the room in Buckingham Palace.

Such measured and wonderfully executed flirtation – an amazing cocktail of happiness followed by sadness, vulnerability, loneliness, sensitivity and the ability to make any man feel that she really needed his help – would not just be employed in order to entrap lovers. She would use the very same technique to flatter all men who might be able to deliver a particular favour that she wanted.

Sir Michael Peat, now the Prince of Wales's private secretary but for many years the Queen's accountant, would loathe it if he was requested to attend upon the Princess. On his arrival she would tap the settee where she was sitting and invite him to sit down next to her. He would do so, and the flirtation would begin – only to end, if he was unable to grant what she wanted, by his being dismissed coldly or with a hail of bad language. A few months later the scene would be repeated as if any previous one had never taken place.

On another occasion one very senior courtier, who remains in an extremely important position at court today, was propositioned by the Princess. He explained that while he was most flattered, he was nevertheless happily married and that his religious beliefs inclined him to stick to his marriage vows. At this the Princess became uncontrollable with rage: she cried and attempted to punch many of the priceless paintings in the room. It took much diplomatic effort to calm her down. Understandably the courtier, who happily for him didn't work at KP, kept out of the Princess's way for several weeks, worried that she would deliver a fearful reprisal for his rejection. However, it would appear that the Princess realised how important this gentleman was to the royal household and, with too many other rumours circulating Buckingham Palace concerning her behaviour, she obviously decided to bide her time.

Riding in Windsor Great Park there was a lot more space and a lot fewer police in attendance. As James Hewitt commented, 'You can get lost in there. She said, "I wish we could be alone."' And so he arranged for a radio telephone to be given to him so that he could ride alone with her while still being in touch with the police. 'I enjoyed her company, we enjoyed each other's company, and the more time we could spend together, the more we'd enjoy our week.'

Then one day they were sitting in the anteroom of the officers' mess at Windsor. They had been riding and were warming up with coffee and biscuits as it was a cold day. Diana poured out her problems to Hewitt. He was amazed, as he hadn't realised until then that she was unhappy in her life. 'She explained that underneath the veneer of calmness meeting big crowds of people would really make her very nervous. She explained what bulimia was to me, which is the first time I'd ever heard of it. She said she wasn't as appreciated as much as she should be by those who were asking her to go and meet the crowds and go and be a public figure and go and work for the firm, the firm being the Royal Family.'

Not unreasonably, Hewitt, like Charles had been before him and clever men like Puttnam would be after him, was totally convinced that she was telling the truth. Why would she make these things up. Hewitt was not to know that many back at the 'firm' might not 'appreciate' her sarcasm, tantrums, silent moods, sackings or violent rages because he had never seen them, and she was never going to admit freely to an intended lover that those kind of problems existed. It was only occasionally that she would admit as much to herself, and as time went by such occasions became fewer. Unfortunately, it never occurred to Hewitt that if someone was finding the time to come by car from Kensington to Windsor three times a week just to ride round the Great Park, their workload was hardly paralysing – the vast majority of mums, working or otherwise, would love that sort of free time. Neither did he wonder why, if she craved tranquillity, she was so very fond of being in the newspapers every day.

'She was in a tearful state – she apologised for that afterwards – and I remember she was sitting on the back of one of those leather chesterfield sofas with her boots on the cushion and I was sitting in the middle, sort of looking up. She was very tearful at that stage, so she came and sat next to me and we hugged each other.'

Diana had decided that this was the moment: she could make an advance for physical contact by needing a cuddle and see where that led. She always realised that she would have to lead her suitors on as none would be brazen enough to make the first move with the future queen of England. Hewitt, who was not to know that Diana could turn on the tears at the drop of a hat, made enough of a positive response to give her the courage to phone him that evening and invite him for dinner alone at Kensington Palace. He accepted, and ended up staying the night.

Some have unfairly accused Hewitt of being irresponsible and not keeping his distance when he must have known that their relationship was impossible. Many stronger and brighter men than James Hewitt have fallen under the magic of Diana's initial spell, however, and very few had the willpower to turn her down.

After that first night, they continued to ride together in Windsor Great Park, but Hewitt would also visit Kensington Palace about twice a week and usually leave in the small hours. Occasionally they would entertain Diana's closest friends like ex-lover Harry Herbert, Kate Menzies or Carolyn Bartholomew there. Sometimes they would go out to dinner, usually at San Lorenzo, where the owners Mara and Lorenzo Berni were friends of hers and where the tables had a celebrity ranking and therefore she would be seen to be the most important of important people. When eating in public places, Diana would use the company of friends like Carolyn Bartholomew to throw other diners or waiting photographers off the scent of either Waterhouse, Dunne or Hewitt. Men like Mannakee didn't get to go to places like San Lorenzo for obvious reasons. Diana and Hewitt also managed the odd trip to the opera, where they could hold hands in the dark. This must have been the attraction to the Princess as she never managed to develop a genuine liking for any form of classical music and much preferred the pop music of her generation.

She initially appeared happy with Hewitt – so much so that apparently Bartholomew told him that he was good for Diana, 'the one light in her life'. She did appear to be getting what she wanted out of the relationship, even if she was running it parallel to others. She felt desired, received love poems and gifts and shared secret moments and confidences. Other men might desire her and be as besotted as Hewitt, but he was more than infatuated with her – he really did love her: 'It's a great thing to be in love with someone. And if they're in love with you, I mean, you know, it makes you want to sing and walk with a bounce in your step. And all the things that you can do, you can achieve, if you've got those feelings. I mean, she told me time and time again how much she loved me, and what our relationship meant to her.'

Anyone who has been in love and believed that such love is being returned can recognise the genuine emotion in James Hewitt's words. However, either because love is blind or because the man is as stupid as the Princess was later to describe him, he clearly did not get to know the real Diana. He continued to believe blindly what he was told by her: 'She would say, "The Queen doesn't appreciate what I'm doing. I try to do my job. She's not helping me." … She would much have preferred to be involved and supported and seen to be supporting the Royal Family – very much so … she wasn't a rebel, you know. It was her choice to get married to Prince Charles. She knew what she was getting into – the wider implications – she knew the importance of the monarchy. And let's face it, her son was going to be king one day. There is no doubt in my mind that she would have loved to have been supporting, and would have loved the outcome to have been completely different … When she told me, "I think they're jealous because I seem to be more popular," this complete expression of disbelief must have come across my face because, you know, I just didn't think that people could be so petty about that.'

Now if there was ever a case of more the fool rather than the knave, this is it. Hewitt, who was later ridiculed by the media as a 'cad' for writing a book about his love affair, was more accurately described by the Princess herself as a man who 'couldn't be trusted to open his mouth and come out with joined-up sentences'. If she could fool intelligent men, foxing a gullible person like Hewitt was effortless.

He couldn't have got the Princess more wrong. She had clearly no idea of what she was getting into when she married Prince Charles. She had refused hundreds of kind offers of help and support from the palace staff for years, often preferring to terrorise them instead. She had refused to be told what to do or when. She rejected all advice. She hated the constraints and disciplines that went with the job and mostly hated every aspect of serving the people. In short, she adored the privilege and position of being royal, but hated of the hard work and self-sacrifice that went with it. She had no idea what modern monarchy was really about and seemed to think that it certainly wasn't a team game but a sort of beauty parade or celebrity contest where her job was to win by becoming the most popular. To this end she would utilise not only her charm and beauty, but also the sick, the dying and even her children if necessary.

In October 2004, Patrick Jephson published his second book, *Travels with Diana*. His first, *Shadows of a Princess*, had not only reportedly earned him a fortune, but also a rebuke from the Prince of Wales when his appeal to the ex-secretary not to publish fell on deaf ears. The former naval officer's second book goes even further than the first, portraying the Princess as a cruel and paranoid figure who would tip off journalists ahead of visits to hospices, hostels for the homeless and hospitals. He claims that she was particularly likely to do this if any member of the Royal Family was enjoying media attention – especially the Duchess of York.

In a synopsis of the new book, Jephson claimed, 'It would be nice to say that all the compassion I saw was genuine but sadly I can't. Her visits had more to do with manipulation of the media than compassion.' He then added that so-called private and caring visits to families hit by personal tragedies not only drummed up support for the Diana camp, 'But we all knew an equally desired outcome was for the discomfort of the rest of the [Royal] family.' The synopsis also claimed that the Princess, who was to develop a fondness for exercising in public gyms in the late 1980s and early 1990s, was not an 'innocent victim' when photographs appeared in the press. He claims that it was all part of a conscious effort that produced 'flattering images and comments about her well-toned physique'. My research confirms this, and I would further add that the only time the Princess really hit the roof about such photographs was when some purported to show that she had cellulite on the back of her legs. She called in a few favours to get the claim that the marks had been created only temporarily by her car seat published in the next day's tabloid press.

When the actual book was published, Mr Jephson confirmed as correct the salient points of my assessment of Diana's personality. His comments help to correct the gross deception created by the Princess, with the innocent help, or otherwise, of Andrew Morton. Nevertheless, I can't help thinking that it is wrong of former aids, who were paid for their position of trust, to betray that trust for easy profit. Nor do I think that such books, whether or not they agree with my interpretation of events, give a complete picture: all too often they portray both the Prince and the Princess as two-dimensional cardboard cut-outs the way the tabloid press does, as opposed to the complex people that he is and she was. Nor do I believe that many of these books take the trouble to let the reader understand either of their childhoods or the crazy cocktail of discipline and spoiled celebrity that royalty really is and which would drive most people mad and in Diana's case was just too much for her. In addition, I feel obliged to add that *Travels with Diana* is a singularly unimpressive piece of work and in the end just another example of someone cashing in on their association with Princess Diana.

The mid eighties were not just proving to be a hard time for Diana; they were a testing time for her husband. He found that Adearne was missed, but not as much as Michael Colborne – a departure that he found particularly tough to deal with, not least because he was well aware that his own foolish and selfish behaviour had caused it. His home life with the Princess was dismal; Mrs Thatcher and her government weren't as receptive to his ideas as he would have liked; his courtiers were always cautioning him against upsetting her; the press ridiculed him; his father was unsympathetic; he had no close relationship with his mother; he still missed the guiding hand of Mountbatten; Anne had drifted out of his life; and his wife had banished most of his friends – and even his dog.

He knew by his work in the inner cities that it was wrong to feel sorry for himself, but he couldn't help it as his fragile self-confidence ebbed away, leaving his self-esteem at an all-time low as he sank deeper into depression than at any time in his life. Even the miserable years at Gordonstoun had not been so bad because he had always known that while they had to be survived, they would nevertheless eventually pass. Now there was no light at the end of the tunnel. He didn't have, in his mind, a proper job and although he adored his children every bit as much as they loved him, he couldn't relax at home as Diana's moods and tantrums remained with her and were all the more distressing to him as first William and then Harry were to witness them, as were many of his staff. He increasingly found it hard to accept in her a behaviour that was so upsetting for the children and undignified and embarrassing in front of employees.

Moreover, he feared that it would only be a matter of time before the sort of tension created by her moods found its way into the press. He readily understood that tales of screaming and the smashing of ornaments, not to mention self-harm, would not only be highly embarrassing for the Queen but would somewhat dent the nation's fairy-tale picture of the monarchy, which it still held despite rumours that all was not well with the marriage – a marriage in which the monarchy had invested so much faith only four years earlier.

Given her own problems and the fact that she was a major reason for his, Diana was the last person to be able to help him and, as he was now cut off from most of his old trusted confidants, he felt completely isolated. Nevertheless, his depression at least helped him appreciate how miserable life must be for her, as he had by now completely come to understand that there was more to her state of mind than just the necessary adjustment she needed to make in order to deal with to royal life. As a result he still maintained some sympathy for her, even if he now found it hard to be left alone in her company.

As his mood worsened he became increasingly temperamental and hard for his staff to please. He cut back on his engagements, and found solace either by digging the Highgrove garden for hours on end, riding like a man possessed and jumping walls and fences that invited the devil to 'bite his arse', as a friend put it, or playing polo as if he wished to cause or receive serious injury. The Prince may lack self-esteem, but his courage has never been in doubt and he has always tested it to the limit as a method of punishing himself in the hope that this would make him snap out of his depression. His theory was that if he nearly died, it might make him happy to be alive, and thus the depression would disappear. Perhaps a crude idea, but it neatly depicts that he was by now hardly in a better state of mind than his wife. The great difference was that he would hide it away and still attempt, by the discipline ingrained in him since birth, to do his duty, whereas she would, as the American expression of the time so succinctly put it, let it all hang out.

The press began to pick up on his falling number of personal engagements and compared them to his mother's, his father's and even his sister's. He was well down on them, and it seemed to the media that he was never off the polo field. They let him, and the nation, know what they thought about that. The criticism, for a man who believed that he must fill every hour doing good or the nation would reject him, was exceptionally stinging. However, he was honest enough to admit that it wasn't altogether unfair. At the time he said, 'If I can get a game of polo I feel five hundred times better in my mental outlook. But without some form of exercise I'm afraid to say I get terribly jaded and, well, not depressed, but below par.'

His friends thought this was a brave but ridiculously understated comment. By 1985 he was much further down than 'below par': he was chronically depressed as he blamed himself for what had happened. At the time he wrote, 'I never thought it would end up like this ... How COULD I have got it all so wrong.' Some of his friends thought that the heir to the throne might even be suicidal and decided that something needed to be done about it.

They knew that he had always got on well with Camilla Parker Bowles before he met Diana; indeed they believed he might have developed a lifetime commitment to her if she hadn't married Andrew Parker Bowles. Naturally, they also knew all about his affair with her prior to his own marriage. And they knew that she was now sitting at home in Wiltshire as her charming husband bounced his way from one woman's bed to another and that many of those beds belonged, humiliatingly, to her friends. They suggested to both of them that they should contact each other.

Camilla understandably believed that it was not her position to contact the Prince of Wales. Initially Charles, in a morose mood and full of self-pity, didn't see how it would help if he got in touch with her. Moreover, he had had virtually no contact with Camilla in the last four years: they had been at the same social gatherings very occasionally, but had never met privately since their meeting when he gave her the 'farewell' bracelet. He had only spoken to her once on the telephone since then, and that was when he was telling friends that Diana was expecting William.

He didn't really see what good having a chat with Camilla would do, but friends like Patty Palmer-Tomkinson persisted and eventually he and Camilla exchanged notes, which soon became long letters. Then they started to speak on the telephone. This took months, but eventually Patty got them to meet at her house in Hampshire. Camilla had a good effect on the Prince as he started to tell her about the difficulties of his life with Diana. He had never spoken to anyone about this for fear that to do so would be disloyal. It may be supposed that his previous close relationship with Camilla made this possible: he was certain that he could talk to her and whatever he said would remain secret.

Slowly the original attraction of a warm and selfless woman, who made him laugh and gave him the confidence that he so desperately lacked if not supported by a loved one, awoke in him once more. He began to fall in love with her all over again. He was to feel very guilty about such feelings, but consoled himself that Princess Diana had commenced several affairs before he and Camilla had even written to each other; it was with some relief that he felt able to commit himself to a physical relationship that he knew would make him feel alive again.

Just as Diana's relationship with Hewitt had helped her, so the Prince pulled back from the edge of his black hole; but many of his friends thought that some of the damage done during those first four years of marriage to Diana had left permanent scars that would never heal. They feared that he would remain more dour, petulant and negative than he once had been, his nerves having been shot to pieces. They were probably right, although his sense of duty to both the Queen and the country were in no way diminished, and he remained as determined as he ever had been to be a great king of England and to continue to serve the nation with his excellent work for the deprived and the less well-off while he waited. It should not be underestimated how much his recovery was assisted by Camilla Parker Bowles. She bolstered his confidence, listened patiently to his whinges, took a serious and genuine interest in his work and above all made him believe that he really did have a contribution to make and that by doing so he would make a real difference to ordinary people's lives.

Now that the Prince had a lover and the Princess had several, a kind of civilised if uneasy peace broke out as they tried to keep out of each other's way except when with the children and working together on foreign trips. They both tried hard to keep up appearances for the children and it would appear that Diana even attempted at times to curb her tantrums and crying in front of them. Instead they confined their war to sarcastic digs across the breakfast table. He reportedly once read out a headline from a newspaper – 'DIFFICULT DI CAUSES MALICE AT THE PALACE' – before adding, 'Sounds about right to me.' On another occasion she was apparently heard to ask, 'Who is getting the benefit of your wisdom today? The sheep or the raspberry bushes?' There appears to be no one who actually heard these barbed comments, which are reported in Clayton and Craig's account, but there are those who can confirm that they depict the atmosphere of the time very well.

Despite this, it was during this period of the mid- to late 1980s that, as their personal standings were high with the nation, they put on some of their most sparkling performances as the world's most formidable double act while representing Britain abroad. The Prince, now encouraged by Camilla, became an increasingly controversial figure and, although the press had initially mocked him, he had struck a chord with the public and was bouncing back, both to the embarrassment of the pro-Diana papers, and at times the annoyance of the government. Meanwhile the Princess, while looking as beautiful as ever, started to make speeches that helped bring attention to serious issues such as Aids, and her skill to communicate, charm and empathise with ordinary people helped create the image that she needed so badly. Put them together and they were dynamite. They seemed able to join up and represent the nation abroad convincingly enough to scotch the rumours that were permanently circulating about the poor state of their marriage. An impressive display by both of them on a visit to the Vatican had the world's media purring.

But their domestic life was in reality miles away from this image. Their peace was very fragile and the civilised aristocratic behaviour was capable of being blown away by Diana at any moment that a fit of jealousy rocked the boat. By 1987 it was a well-known fact among the royal household that the marriage of Charles and Diana was in anything but a happy state. New recruits would be taken on one side and discreetly told that both of them had someone else but that a tacit understanding had been reached that would preserve the marriage for the public good and the sake of their children. As a result, nobody expected the marriage to end in divorce, but everyone seemed extremely nervous of Diana's ability to stick to the deal. One employee was to tell Clayton and Craig years later on, on his arrival at the Palace, he was told that they could occasionally bear to be together in public, but being alone together was a different matter. 'There was an accommodation for a couple of years, Charles and Camilla, Diana and Hewitt. The problem was she couldn't stick to it. This was a girl who has no stability, didn't have the intellectual rigour or concentration, or the sense of duty to stick it out.'

This was typical of Diana: as ever it was one set of rules for her and another for him. When she had the children with her, she would invent last-minute excuses to stop them going to see their father play polo or go shooting or fishing, which was not only unkind to him but acutely unfair on them as they worshipped him and really enjoyed such outings. The Princess was astonishingly jealous of her sons' relationship with their father and, by reducing his time with them, she sought not only to promote herself in their affections but also to exclude him. She appears to have given no thought to his feelings and very little to how this might affect the princes. If Charles had ever pulled these sorts of tricks on her, there would have been tears and perhaps even a public sobbing to attract attention to his unkindness. And while it was quite all right for her to see Mannakee, Waterhouse, Dunne, Hewitt and others, she continued to be obsessed about her husband seeing Camilla.

Diana encouraged Hewitt to strike up a relationship with her sons as early as 1987. He would play with them either in the garden of Highgrove or at Kensington Palace before going into their bedroom to read them bedtime stories. A visit was organised to his regiment, and Hewitt had uniforms made for them. The Princess thought that was a great idea. But would she have been happy for Camilla to have enjoyed the same relationship as Hewitt did with William and Harry? Given her undignified and cruel behaviour towards their nanny, Tiggy Legge-Bourke, some years later, when she worried that the princes were becoming too fond of her, I somehow doubt it.

The Princess was the odd one out. The Prince, the Parker Bowleses and Hewitt played by the rules. Hewitt played regularly either with or sometimes against the Prince on the polo field: 'We saw each other from time to time at polo – weren't, you know, closest buddies but knew each other to say hello and how are you and how's it going,' is how Hewitt later described his relationship with the Prince. The Prince even invited him to his fortieth birthday in November 1988, which Hewitt took as a tacit sign that he approved of him.

Hewitt also saw Andrew Parker Bowles from time to time in his regiment's officers' mess. Parker Bowles was now the Colonel Commanding the Household Cavalry, and therefore Hewitt's commanding officer. They would exchange pleasantries with each other. Perhaps only the British aristocracy could employ such finesse. Hewitt would be standing there, having a drink and a chat with the husband of his lover's husband's mistress. All the parties knew what was going on, as did some others in the mess, but no one ever referred to it. It was an unwritten rule and it gave Hewitt comfort that his relationship with the Princess was approved of at the highest level. He certainly wasn't worried about being bumped off by MI5 at this point in time.

He could take further comfort when, in the summer of 1987,

Princess Diana started spending weekends at Hewitt's mother's home in Cornwall. The royal Jaguar would arrive with a police escort and, after dinner, Hewitt would play poker with Ken Wharfe, the Princess's new protection officer, before Wharfe went to sleep on the couch and Hewitt retired upstairs with Diana. Hewitt naturally assumed that not only would the Prince have been briefed for security reasons about where his wife was, but also that he apparently didn't seem to mind.

The truth is that the Prince was a fair man who believed that he and the Princess should live by the same rules. He knew that he and his wife, for whatever reason, had endured, by that time, six years of hell. There had been years when her ranting, violence, self-abuse, moods and cruelties had clearly expressed her unhappiness and in the end nearly driven him to the same state of mind. He had remained extremely loyal to her throughout and, until he discovered one or more of her affairs, he had also remained faithful. But now that she was enjoying other men and he had rediscovered Camilla, this seemed to be the best solution. She could have Hewitt and whomever else she wanted, provided there was discretion and neither the crown nor the children were embarrassed or hurt, and he could have Camilla.

The Prince believed that this was the best that either of them could hope for given the desperate state that they found themselves in. Furthermore, while he continued to be kind to her and would remain so for the rest of her life, it was now his opinion that they were better off looking forward and making the best of the future rather than looking back. Slowly Diana came to understand that she had finally really burned her bridges with Charles, and even though there were days when she would tell friends that she hated him, the thought of him rejecting her made her want him back. The one man whom she had always wanted to possess had finally turned his back on her, given up trying to make his marriage work and no one could help her get him back again.

But she hadn't given up trying. When the tantrums and suicide bids didn't work, she attempted seduction. One night, as she told Lady Colin Campbell, 'I went into his dressing room. I am wearing this fabulous eau-de-Nil silk nightdress, low-cut and slinky. I sat down on the bed beside him. He was reading one of those deadweight books by Laurens van der Post. I said something nice and touched his fingers. He winced when my fingers brushed past his. I've never been so hurt in my life. The idea that my own husband can't stand me touching him ...'

Of course, it is not impossible that the Princess, as she had done in the past and would continue to do until her death, had just made up the story. But if it is true, it shows the completely different nature of their characters. He, having tried everything possible to make his marriage work for four years, had now mentally left home. She, who couldn't begin to understand this, thought that a quick flash of her forbidden fruit would bring him to heel once more. Lady Sarah Spencer-Churchill later explained, 'She turned off the Prince of Wales completely. He's basically a compassionate guy and he wanted her to be happy. But he was not going to have her browbeat or blackmail him into loving her when he no longer did. She'd killed his love with her antics and she should have been counting her blessings that it took four years instead of four weeks. She was lucky he's a decent guy and the monarchy did not want a divorce. Most men would have walked out on her after a month.' Strong words – especially from a woman related to the Princess and not in Prince Charles's circle of close friends.

Curiously, she didn't start a massive charm offensive. Perhaps she knew it wouldn't work. Perhaps, after so many years of fighting him, she had forgotten how to charm him. Instead she made a special visit to the Queen to ask her to order her son to stop seeing Mrs Parker Bowles. A courtier at Buckingham Palace at the time told me that Diana waited calmly for the Queen, who had a very busy day of engagements and had agreed to squeeze the Princess in between two of these provided she was prepared to wait. The Princess appeared to be quite relaxed and happy reading an edition of *Country Life* until the Queen entered, upon which she sprang to her feet and ran over to the Queen in floods of tears before being led away by Her Majesty. 'It was an Oscar-winning performance that appeared to catch the Queen completely off guard,' is how he recalled the scene.

Unfortunately for Princess Diana, it did not have the desired effect as the Queen refused to get involved. Over the next few years she would try again and again, but would never get the result that she wanted. When this failed, she appealed to the Duke of Edinburgh instead. She wrote to him and their resulting private letters came into Paul Burrell's care and used by him, as was much of her private correspondence that had fallen into his hands. Philip was blunt with his daughter-in-law: 'Can you honestly look into your heart and say that Charles's relationship with Camilla had nothing to do with your behaviour towards him in your marriage? ... Being the wife of Prince

Charles involves much more than simply being a hero with the British people.... We do not approve of either of you having lovers. Charles was silly to risk everything with Camilla for a man in his position. ... I cannot imagine anyone in their right mind leaving you for Camilla. Such a prospect never entered our heads.' He also told her that any fair-minded person would recognise that she had been a poor wife, and while she wasn't a bad mother, she was nonetheless far too possessive with her sons.

The Princess, according to Burrell, was absolutely delighted with the Duke's comments about her rival, and 'leaped around the room with unbridled joy'. However, it is extremely unlikely that she would have been able to square up to his criticism of her as a wife or mother. By this time her ability to see that her behaviour would make it impossible for any man to live with her permanently had diminished to virtually zero. There were now no more letters or confessions to friends that she was ashamed of the way she had behaved; instead there were constant angry, late-night phone calls to people complaining about Camilla, her husband, the Duchess of York, the Queen, Stavros (as she called Prince Philip) and their 'fucking German family'. Diana was no longer able to see the reality of any of it. It couldn't be her fault as, in her own mind, she hadn't done anything wrong. Sometimes she would claim that Prince Charles and Camilla Parker Bowles had been having an affair throughout her marriage to the Prince; on other occasions she claimed he went back to Camilla before the birth of Harry. But then she came up with a third version in the late 1980s when she wanted to stop him seeing Camilla.

She had been seeing Hewitt, Waterhouse, Mannakee, Dunne, Gilbey and others for years. For nearly a decade her tantrums, moods, sulks, rages and scenes had made life at one time or another miserable not only for the Prince, but their children, the Royal Family, their staff and most of the couple's friends. The Prince had almost succumbed to a nervous breakdown as a result and most people close to her divided clearly into two camps: one, which included Prince Charles, felt extremely sorry for her, believing that she needed help but knew that she wouldn't hear of it; the other believed that she was a very spoiled and spiteful girl who had let the people's worship of her go to her head. But the Princess didn't see any of this. In her mind her marriage had broken down because of her third theory on the Camilla affair. She convinced herself, and then set about convincing her friends, that

Prince Philip had struck a deal with Prince Charles that if he produced 'an heir and a spare' in the first five years of his marriage, he could return to Camilla. Where did this story come from? Diana's head. Why did she invent it? Because there had to be a reason for Charles going back to Camilla and the truth was something in her increasingly neurotic and paranoid state that she just couldn't face.

Should anyone take it seriously? Of course not. For a start the Princess peddled three different versions of the same story. No one can be found to verify any of them. Secondly, scores of people can be found to verify the Patti Palmer-Tomkinson version. Thirdly, Diana's lie about the Prince's reaction to the birth of Prince Harry contradicts this third version, as the birth of the 'spare' would have pleased him. Fourthly, the Duke and the Prince have never enjoyed a relationship that would have allowed such a deal to be struck. And fifthly, the Duke had made his feelings on the Camilla issue plain to Diana herself.

Did anyone take it seriously? James Whitaker, writing in the *Daily Mirror* in May 2004 as the newspaper serialised the paperback version of Paul Burrell's *A Royal Duty*, wrote, 'All over again, but in rather more detail, we here that dear Diana was told by Charles that he no longer loved her, and worse never did. We are told that the Princess felt she was a "sale or return" bride because, according to her, Prince Philip apparently told his son that if the marriage didn't work out he could return to Camilla's arms. And even more tragically, we learn that Diana came to believe that she only got to marry Prince Charles because she was a suitable brood mare and would produce the two requisite children – an heir and the necessary spare. Can there be anything more brutal for a young bride to take in?'

His article raises an interesting point that demands an answer. As a journalist of many years' standing, how did he come to write such rubbish?

The *Mirror* had not only spent a lot of money serialising the Burrell book, it had previously spent a fortune tying Burrell to them. In a typically silly celebrity-style move, the former editor, Piers Morgan, had made Burrell the 'royal correspondent' for the paper as part of a deal to ensure that they, and not the *Daily Mail*, got to buy his story exclusively following the collapse of his trial at the Old Bailey in 2002. This must have pushed Whitaker's nose out a little as the current holder of the 'royal correspondent' title at the time had been Whitaker himself. However, with Burrell in such favour with his bosses, it might not be very clever to start questioning the quality of the information that his readers were lapping up. Apparently, a tabloid journalist has got to write what a tabloid journalist's got to write. Add to this a discernible bias against the Prince that Whitaker, along with other royal journalists flattered by Diana, has displayed for years, and you have the answer.

James Hewitt was easily Diana's most important lover during this period, and would not be rivalled until Oliver Hoare arrived in her life in the 1990s. However, he is not the father of Prince Harry as has been continually rumoured. This whisper has circulated for years and owes its origin to the fact that Harry has red hair and does not have the Windsor nose. As a result, and because his features and colouring are similar to Hewitt's, many people have jumped to the wrong conclusion. In fact, Harry has features and colouring that are common to many Spencers: Diana's siblings, Charles and Sarah, are good examples. In addition, the Princess didn't even meet Hewitt until Harry was nearly two years of age.

It is clear that Diana found Hewitt's simple, easy-going style and obvious devotion to her a comfort. Moreover, Hewitt seemed to take in his stride her obsession with stopping her husband seeing his mistress, although it must have been hurtful that on occasion she only wanted to talk about Charles and Camilla and not them and how they might work out a future together. There were times when Diana would visualise that dream with him, but it would never go any further than that as in her heart of hearts the Princess knew that being the wife of an ex-major was not nearly as iconic as being the future Queen of England. She was addicted to such hero worship and this, along with her inability to let Charles go and her other sexual liaisons, meant that a future life with Hewitt was never more than a hazy dream after a couple of drinks, a warm feeling that was never actually going to happen.

Nevertheless, Hewitt encouraged her and even advised her to attend a party in February 1989 at the home of Lady Annabel Goldsmith. The Princess had told him that Camilla would be there. Hewitt told her to hold her head up high and act regally. Instead Diana chose confrontation. 'I said: "Camilla, I would just like you to know that I know what is going on between you and Charles, I wasn't born yesterday ... I'm sorry I'm in the way, I obviously am in the way and it must be hell for both of you but I do know what is going on. Don't treat me like an idiot." ... In the car on the way back my husband was over me like a bad rash and I cried like I have never cried before – it was anger, it was seven years' pent up anger coming out.'

After more than two years of a civilised and adult approach, Camilla might have been confused by this outburst as she was well aware by this time that the Princess had enjoyed several lovers herself and had clearly been the first to be unfaithful. But she wasn't taken aback. The royal circle had by now experienced more than eight years of Princess Diana's erratic and neurotic behaviour. Camilla said nothing in reply, limiting herself to a deep and over-elaborate curtsy. This slight act of impertinent defiance doesn't appear to have been noticed by the future queen as she swept out of the room, but it was not lost on the other women present, who smiled to themselves; later one or two complimented the older woman on her restraint.

Although Hewitt was well aware of the Princess's desire to end her husband's relationship with Camilla, he clearly wasn't aware of Diana's other love interests. Nevertheless, he couldn't have failed to notice that by 1988 she had become close to Philip Dunne, as there had been much speculation about this relationship by then in the British press. Some biographers have suggested that this was a clever plan by Diana to lead the press away from Hewitt. This is most unlikely, as Diana didn't want the press to write about any man – be it Hewitt, Waterhouse, Mannakee, Dunne, Gilbey or whoever – as this would tarnish her reputation, and any future possibility of playing the wronged faithful wife who was never loved by a heartless husband would be very difficult. It goes without saying that this image would be totally destroyed if news got out that the future queen of England were sleeping around. Of course, some of her adoring fans may have said good luck to her, but as the mother of the future king of England, an awful lot of people certainly would not have done. Diana may have had many failings, but spinning out her image in the best light was something she could usually manage just fine.

Many people who were genuinely fond of the Princess have commented upon how she was at her best when others were in crisis. They not only point to the love and kindness that she found she could so naturally dispense to the poor, the old, the sick and the dying, but that she could suddenly forget a dispute with a friend if that person was suddenly facing a crisis.

Sir Elton John is a good example. Sir Elton had argued with the

Princess in the 1990s and so an unflattering cartoon of him was placed in the Princess's bathroom, next to one of Camilla, and she ignored his very existence. Then, seeing his complete distress at Versace's funeral, she made a very public display of comforting him. Naturally, there are those who comment that it would have been completely impossible for Diana to have resisted, and thus missed out on such a wonderful PR opportunity in front of the world's press. And of course there is much evidence of this sort of behaviour from the Princess from the 1980 kindergarten press photographs onward to support their claim.

However, people suffering from Princess Diana's condition can apparently respond well to the problems of others as it gives them an opportunity to help them; the combination of this and an immediate feeling of superiority gives their low self-esteem a boost. Another such occasion was in 1988 when the Prince was involved in a skiing accident near the Swiss resort of Klosters. On the afternoon of 10 March, the Prince and his friends Major Hugh Lindsay and Charlie and Patti Palmer-Tomkinson were being led down a difficult off-piste run known as the Wang by an experienced local guide called Bruno Sprecher. Sprecher had been hired to escort Fergie, also an experienced skier, but she had fallen in the morning and hurt herself. She was pregnant and it was thought that it would be better for her to rest for the remainder of the day. Prince Charles invited the guide, one of the best in the resort, to join him for the afternoon. Diana, who could ski but not to the standard of her husband or his party, decided to remain behind in the chalet with Sarah.

The party came to rest at the top of a steep and narrow gully so that Bruno Sprecher could take the lead before descending the most difficult part of the run. They were wedged between a precipice on one side and a sheer rock face on the other. Suddenly there was an almighty roar and the party turned to see giant blocks of snow, ice and rock tumbling down towards them and destroying everything in their path. Sprecher screamed for the party to jump to one side. Charles and Charlie Palmer-Tomkinson reacted quickly and made it to the rock-face side of the gully, as did the guide himself and an accompanying Swiss policeman. Patti and Major Lindsay were caught under the wall of falling snow and were hurled over the precipice and 400 feet down, before hitting the slope again and then tumbling another 400 feet down the mountain before halting, lost under the snow.

Sprecher, an expert skier since childhood, was first down to the scene. By the time the Prince arrived he had already found Patti Palmer-Tomkinson and was giving her mouth-to-mouth resuscitation. He had a spade and together with the Prince they worked her body free. She was in a very bad way. Sprecher then went off in search of Lindsay and eventually discovered his body a few metres away under three feet of snow. He was dead.

In the meantime, Prince Charles worked to bring Patti back to consciousness, talking to her reassuringly all the time. He told her that Charlie was all right and that the helicopter was on the way. Her face was blue and, as he gently rubbed it, it felt very cold and at first there was no reaction from her. Nevertheless, he kept talking as he remembered that Patricia Brabourne had once told him that it was the sound of the doctors' voices that had prevented her from dying following the bomb attack that cost her father and one of her sons their lives. Later Patti was to say that Charles's voice had helped save her life: 'I was hanging on every word, it was like a lifeline. He was so calm, so conversational.'

Eventually, Patti Palmer-Tomkinson was taken to hospital and placed on a ventilator. She was critically ill and there was doubt as to whether she would survive. She had appalling injuries and would have to undergo countless operations over several months before making a miraculous recovery – she was even able eventually to ski again. The Prince visited her in hospital with her husband the next day before he returned to London. He was most troubled – it had been the worst day of his life since the death of Lord Mountbatten. Not only had Lindsay been a good friend, he was his guest and had died while with him and in so doing had made his young wife a pregnant widow. The Prince, forgetting his own courageous behaviour of ignoring the danger and skiing down to Patti, blamed himself. So did the media. The *Sun*'s headline read, 'ACCUSED. OFFICIAL: CHARLES DID CAUSE THE KILLER AVALANCHE'. Others repeated stories that foolhardy Prince Charles, a man known to love dangerous sports, had led his party down a closed run and ignored avalanche-warning signs. This was nonsense: the official enquiry, found him to be in no way culpable. The run was not closed, he did not ignore any warning signs because there weren't any, and his party did not start the avalanche.

The Prince had been most concerned that Bruno Sprecher was not made the scapegoat either, and had to be persuaded not to give an impromptu press conference to say as much. In the end it was Diana who helped his press secretary persuade him that a written statement by him should be read out on his behalf at the airport. It was then typed out by Sarah on the plane home and handed to the media.

Throughout the manic thirty-six hours following the accident, the Princess had been calm, extremely sensible and for the first time in a long while a real support to her husband, which those there readily accept – if not quite to the extent that she was later to claim. She forgot about tantrums, sulks, sniping remarks and even photographs of herself in the press and really did rise to the occasion.

Sarah Lindsay, whose baby Alice was born just two months after the accident, understandably went through some very difficult times. However, she was not forgotten by either the Prince or Princess of Wales. Charles talked to her endlessly, and unlike others was never frightened to speak about Hugh. He understood her need to talk about him and he accommodated that need selflessly. The Princess's support was even more exceptional. For three years she telephoned Sarah once a week on her 'bad' day. When I lost my second son in 1982, my 'bad' day was always a Wednesday. Sarah Lindsay's was a Sunday evening, and every Sunday evening Diana was there for her. This was an act of genuine goodness and not one that she was doing to win brownie points with the press.

In addition, when Alice had her first birthday she was invited round to Kensington Palace to enjoy a birthday cake with the two princes. The Princess told Sarah that she would never go back to Klosters. She was as good as her word. The press considered this very sensitive, and thought Charles was most insensitive for returning every year. However, Patti Palmer-Tomkinson explains, 'We all agreed that we would never go anywhere else ... It would have been like turning our back on him and leaving him there. We can't ski together, the three of us, without remembering Hugh.'

There can be no doubt that, despite acts of selfish, cruel and at times cynically calculated behaviour, the Princess could be both selfless and extremely caring, and this was not always undertaken as part of some cleverly devised plan. Perhaps this is why she has some friends or associates who only see one side of her, others another and just a few both. With Diana, as Morton rightly says, you only got to see what she wanted you to see, and then only when she wanted you to see it.

Howard Hodgson

The 1980s had been an important decade for both Charles and Diana. He had started it as Action Man, married a beautiful bride, been upstaged by her in public and nearly driven mad by her at home. He had survived with a little help from his friends and by the end of the decade had recovered and largely destroyed the 'loony' image given him by an unkind press as his beliefs were endorsed by the people.

She had grown from a shy and slightly chubby girl into a world icon of beauty, fashion and compassion. She had learned how to deal with this most of the time in public, but had steadily slipped into a serious mental state in private that had caused everyone around her unhappiness and pain and would have her brother and others urging her to receive medical help in the coming decade.

Despite these incredible strains, they had become the world's most famous couple, spread a little magic, done tremendous good among the needy and produced two wonderful sons.

Chapter Eleven
Charles and Diana at Close Quarters (1991–96)

In February 1991 my telephone rang at our home in Wilton Place, London. My secretary, Lynn, answered almost wearily as the thing hadn't stopped for days. I had sold my shares in PHKI plc for several million pounds the previous month in order to enjoy a quiet life with my family. I was looking forward, in particular, to watching my two younger children grow up, as my work had prevented me from doing this with the elder two. Since then the phone had never stopped ringing – papers about articles on how to spend millions, a publisher for a book on how to make millions and lots of people who wanted to tell me how to invest millions – which, as you have no doubt already guessed, was with them.

It was the middle of the afternoon and I was in bed – not because I was now living the life of the idle rich, but because two discs in my back were shot to pieces and were in danger of having to be removed if bed rest didn't effect a recovery, as the injury had caused my right leg to become paralysed.

It was the urgency in Lynn's step as she thundered up the never-ending staircase of the typical Belgravian house that made me think that this call might be something a bit different. Eventually she arrived breathless at my door. 'Guess what?' she panted, and then continued before I could. 'Guess what? I've got St James's Palace on the phone and the Prince of Wales wants to have dinner with you at Kensington Palace. What shall I say?'

'What do you mean what shall I say?' I roared. 'Say yes, and be quick about it before they ring off. He might never invite me again.'

'But what about your leg?'

'Sod that. Don't even mention it. Just accept.'

And before she had descended the mountain back to her office, I was already on the phone to my doctor. 'Well, Crockard won't like it one little bit,' Anthony – my doctor – warned. Mr Crockard was the specialist and Anthony was quite right: he would have had a fit if he had known what I had in mind.

'But he won't know. Look, if you shoot some morphine into my bottom, I'll get by. I've got a dinner in the House of Commons the night before so we can have a trial run then.'

Anthony duly obliged. At the House of Commons I just about

managed to get to my table in the main dining room and during the meal I was in no pain whatsoever. But the dose had been a little too strong, and the first glass of claret, which admittedly I'd been advised by Anthony not to have, put me to sleep – embarrassing for me and most boring for my host, the late Anthony Bevan MP, and made all the worse by the fact that he had been a friend of my late father.

So the next night my doctor Anthony arrived and duly administered a smaller dose in order to prevent a reoccurrence of the previous evening, as to fall asleep at dinner with the Prince of Wales might be considered more than just bad form. Then I took off in the car, which had been sent for me, resplendent in my dinner jacket and supported by an antique cane with a beautiful silver top – hardly as practical as the crutches the hospital had provided, but much more elegant and fitting, I felt, for an occasion that I was determined to enjoy even if I suspected that I was only going on the strength of my newfound disposable wealth.

The car sped up the drive and was rather casually waved on past a single police officer, before stopping in a dimly lit yard. The car door was opened and I was welcomed and invited in. I struggled up a fairly unimpressive flight of stairs that opened on to an even less impressive hallway. From there I was shown into the drawing room, where I joined a dozen or so similarly dressed men. This room was comfortable rather than grand and, although tasteful, I remember it as being perhaps slightly faded.

A butler offered me a drink from a tray he was carrying, and I accepted a glass of champagne with some difficulty and more than a little fear that to drink it might put me out before I even made it to the table. The charming and long-serving Tom Shebbeare made his way over to me in time and explained the form. When the Prince arrived he would mingle with his guests before dinner, and we would then proceed to the adjoining dining room, where I would find my place by name card. I should address Prince Charles as 'Your Royal Highness' on the first occasion, and thereafter as 'Sir'. He was sorry to see that I was in a bad way, but reminded me that nobody could sit until the Prince did. I proudly informed him that I had been presented to Her Majesty the Queen and other minor royals in the course of my charity work and that I understood the form. He smiled, as I guess spiders do when inviting a nice juicy fly into their parlour.

This is a well-worked format. The Prince has amazing pulling power: captains of industry the world over are willing to pay a fortune for the privilege of being in his company and basking in the reflected glow of his royalty, perhaps for just a day or, if their shareholders can afford it, for several. They relish the chance to become associated with, if not a friend of, this genial man. He is charming, and he needs to be in order to undo the purse strings of these multimillion-dollar corporations. He wants their money for his projects and uses everything at his disposal to get it.

Tom Shebbeare and his crew work the room as warm-up acts before the main man enters, and when he does you know about it. The crowd parts before him as he moves across the room, trying to look happy with a nervous smile on his face, but an unmistakable kindness twinkling in his warm and friendly eyes. He plays with his right cufflink as he looks knowingly at people he is supposed to recognise and avoids the glance of those that he doesn't for fear of upsetting the planned introductions that will follow. He has obviously done this thousands of times and, like a seasoned cabaret star, he is very good at it, although staff say he is clearly better when his confidence is up and he doesn't feel as if he is being undermined.

I started to wish these introductions would hurry along. They seemed to take forever as guests naturally wished to savour the moment, and while it was Shebbeare and Co who were clearly running the timetable and not the guests, it was important to them that we all felt that we had had our personal moment with the Prince. I had been standing for over fifty minutes and still there was no sign that dinner was to be served in the near future allowing me to sit down. The lower dosage of morphine had prevented me from falling asleep, but at a cost of not killing off the pain. The antique stick was bending under my weight, its silver top was digging into the palm of my hand and I began to feel faint. 'You mustn't pass out in the Prince of Wales's drawing room,' I kept telling myself. Drastic measures were called for, so I threw caution to the wind and knocked back all the contents of the large champagne flute that I had been holding rather than sipping at for the past hour.

Eventually it was my turn. The champagne seemed to have had a good effect and I felt a little better – or maybe the fact that the Prince of Wales was shaking my hand and talking to me made me forget about the pain. He was not as tall as me, but was nevertheless taller than I had expected. He was tanned, and looked very fit for a man of forty-two.

Howard Hodgson

He congratulated me on building up Hodgson Holdings plc (which had become PHKI in 1989), cracked a couple of funereal jokes, which were no worse than anybody else's I'd heard, and then asked why I looked as if I had been in the wars. I explained my problem, and he told me about his back and how he suffered with it. Then he was off, but a couple of paces away, he stopped and half turned and looked back into my eyes before saying, 'We need men like you. You'll not get away from us now, you know.'

Well that was it. I had grown up a royalist, always a cavalier, never a roundhead, and later on had come to share Prince Charles's concerns for the nation and admire his work. Nevertheless, Shebbeare and Co might still find it hard to prevent my hard-earned cash from going to my kids; but after that statement, if Charles Windsor wanted me to go to Moscow in a blizzard and walk there with that bloody awful stick as my only form of support, I was his man. The effect was amazing. I was almost able to march into dinner, enjoyed the meal, despite the appalling nut cutlets that were served as HRH was going through his vegetarian phase, and ended the night by going off to Annabel's nightclub with Tom Shebbeare and some of the other guests. My recovery wasn't enough to allow me to dance, but I chatted to Tom until the small hours before returning home to Wilton Place a very contented man.

The next morning I received a call from a member of the Prince's staff. The Prince hoped I had enjoyed the occasion. I replied that I had. Would I agree to serve on a new steering committee chaired by Richard George, chairman of Weetabix, that was being assembled in order to guide the Prince's Trust's future? I readily agreed. Could Tom Shebbeare and an associate called Manny come round to Wilton Place and explain the form (and, no doubt, attempt to tap me for some cash)? I agreed.

'Er, one last point,' the guy stammered rather nervously. 'When cigars were offered last night, you declined.'

'Yes, I did. I prefer a cigarette after dinner,' I replied, not then the non-smoker that I am today.

'Well, that's the point. The Prince of Wales has asked me to inform you that you are the first person to smoke a cigarette in that room for at least fifteen years and he'd prefer it if you were to be the last for the next fifteen. If you get my meaning.'

Tom and Manny duly came a week later. I offered them shares in a new company that I was investing in. They accepted, knowing that this was better than nothing and if the company floated they would receive a windfall (it didn't). I joined the committee and at the first meeting was pleased to help design the now famous 'Jump' advertising campaign featuring heads of industry jumping off the ground.

Over the next few months I was sent on various assignments. There was a mission to Birmingham with the Earl of Shrewsbury to meet 'Deadly' Doug Ellis, chairman of Aston Villa Football Club. An amusing lunch was had – Shrewsbury was an excellent fellow whose company was most enjoyable, and 'Deadly', for whom I had worked as a youth, regaled us with many amusing stories. Then it was down to business, and after a little cajoling Ellis promised to get Nigel Kennedy and Elton John to head a concert at Villa Park, the profits of which would be donated to the Prince's Trust. Apparently Ellis had entertained Kennedy, who is a fanatical Villa fan, on his yacht in Majorca and had taught John everything that the tantrum-throwing star knew about how to run Watford Football Club.

The earl and I returned to London very pleased, and were more than a little flushed with success when Shebbeare duly praised our efforts. But 'Deadly' did not deliver. Perhaps he couldn't hold the two stars to account to the degree that he had hoped. Perhaps the price of an Empire medal or even a knighthood was simply too high. After all, Aston Villa was still a private company in 1991 and all the financial risks associated with such a concert would have landed at his door if the event had not been a success. Ellis was a man made good from a modest background who liked the association that the Prince's Trust offered with the Prince of Wales. Some twelve years later, at a 2003 visit to the headquarters of the Prince's Trust in Regents Park, a young female graduate informed me that a tension between one's money and one's title was still going on. In the 2005 New Year's Honours, Mr Ellis was rewarded for his services to football and the community in the West Midlands with an OBE, which was described to me jokingly by one of his previous managers as being apt, given that he thought that it so often stood for 'Other Buggers' Efforts'.

Over the next few months, other missions followed, the most awful of which was being sent to Cardiff to hand out various awards to young people who had turned their Prince's Trust grants into successful small businesses. As I entered the room, the first thing I noticed was the glance through and beyond me to see where the Prince was; this was followed by an expression of total disappointment when they realised that he wasn't coming and I was all they were going to get. I know exactly how the Prince of Wales must have felt on a walkabout with Diana when the crowd would groan on his side of the street, realising that she was about to walk down the other side.

In early summer, I was asked to go to Highgrove to attend a cocktail party that was to be held in aid of Macmillan Nurses. As I arrived with my wife, I remember thinking how casual security was – we were hardly checked by anyone before entering the house's hallway where we were introduced to Lord and Lady Zetland, served with champagne and offered delightful little canapés by William and Harry, who were identically dressed in blue and white striped shirts, pale blue trousers and dark brown loafers.

The Prince eventually made his entrance. He looked very smart in a dark grey double-breasted suit, blue shirt and red tie. Like many women before her, my wife was immediately taken by his presence, warmth, kindness and charm. She thought him to be very attractive. We chatted about various things before he remarked on my back. 'You're looking a lot better than the last time I saw you.' He obviously hadn't read my letter to him. Following our last meeting and my carefree trip to Annabel's, I had been rushed into the Wellington Hospital and both discs had been removed in an emergency operation.

'I had them both out, Sir. I wrote to you about it. Mr Crockard did it. I made a series for the BBC travelling all over Europe three weeks later and I'm already playing cricket and riding horses again. You should consider having it done, Sir,' I told him.

'Oh, I don't think so. I've got a room full of suggested cures sent from all over the Commonwealth,' he replied with uncharacteristic pomposity.

'Well, you should be so lucky that your subjects love you so well,' I replied, hurt by his dismissal.

He glared at me. The Zetlands looked down into their drinks. My wife looked at me. I looked at the Prince. And then suddenly, after what my wife was to describe as 'a good minute' but was probably about two seconds, the Prince's glare evaporated into a kindly smile as he said, 'Of course, you are right.'

A couple of weeks later, I was to receive this letter from him.

19th August 1991. Highgrove.

Dear Mr. Hodgson,

I am afraid it has taken me a very long time to find your kind letter, and I heartily apologize, but with so much going on at present I can never get to my letters! I was very touched you should bother to write and I have since seen you at Highgrove when I could see for myself that you were a new man! However, my back is now considerably better, owing to endless exercises recommended by the physiotherapist, and I will do anything to avoid an operation!

Yours sincerely,
Charles.

I believe this shows the real reason for his pompous remark – understandable fear of the knife – and it further shows him to be a man of a good and generous nature. There is no other explanation as to why he sought out my original letter and took the trouble to reply to it.

I don't know if it was the frank exchange concerning back cures, or the fact that, when asked as we walked through the gardens, I was pleased to explain that I thought the various arms of the Prince's Trust seemed to me to be uncoordinated, but he was keen to talk. We walked for nearly an hour with scores of other guests in tow as I, perhaps driven by what I saw as an opportunity of having him to myself, pressed home my points. He listened, questioned, thought a little, questioned again and, at times, became quite excited. Eventually he told me that what I was saying was quite right. Things could be better organised. And yes, we should do something. Moreover, he told me that he understood what I had said about the dangers of raising money for the Trust by granting medals for cash. I had told His Royal Highness that, when I was chief executive of Hodgson Holdings plc, it had been put to me by a very high-profile CEO of another public company that a gift from Hodgson Holdings to the Trust would, as long as I never mentioned it, gain me great recognition. He then showed me a list of PYBT contributors, and how much they were donating. He advised me to look at the next honours list and see who got what. At the bottom of the list was written 'Anonymous – £500,000'. He pointed to this and said, 'Howard, that guy will get a knighthood.'

Having repeated this to the Prince, I went on to explain that there were dangers here. I understood that there was nothing wrong with 'king's patronage' in bygone years when a merchant might support the

Crown financially and in exchange be granted a title – the money was his to give. However, I pointed out that CEOs of publicly owned companies didn't own them and therefore were giving other shareholders' money away in order to buy a title for themselves. I told Prince Charles that this was very dangerous and that if the press were to get to hear of it, a scandal would ensue.

He took my point. He looked concerned and was silent for a few moments. Then he asked me to write to him about it. 'Give us your ideas on how we should organise things.'

I did, and the next time I met Richard George he hardly passed the time of day with me. Some time later someone telephoned me from the Trust. He was not happy. How dare I go down to Highgrove and give the Prince my private advice? Didn't I realise that with Prince Charles the last storyteller always told the best story? Had I no idea of the disruption I had caused? People who had worked on projects for ages had had them endangered thanks to me. It would take a lot of time and effort to get the Prince calmed down.

I replied that I wasn't really sorry and stood completely by what I had told the Prince. At the time, before the Princess Diana and Duchess of York marriage traumas were to hit the press, the monarchy's status was high and, despite the 'Loony Prince' tag, Prince Charles himself was still well respected. I pointed out that a 'somebody else's cash for a title' scandal would alter that. We would have to beg to differ whether I had done the Prince a favour or caused problems for those who worked at the Trust. And I still believe today that a press more concerned with rooting out true stories than inventing titillating ones would have picked up on the fact that a CEO had promised a donation of £300,000 from his company to the Trust. In return he received a CBE. However, the company went into receivership and so in the end the Prince's Trust didn't get their hands on the cash, but the businessman had still got his reward – a fact that Tom Shebbeare was understandably angry about, as he recalled during a 2003 meeting with me.

Anyway, after that and for whatever reason, my phone stopped ringing; as my own marriage was going through difficulties at the time, life just moved on and we drifted apart. However, back on that summer evening I observed many things about the Prince of Wales that were quite at odds with the image promoted by the media. He explained to me, for example, how he had grown a hedge so that Princess Diana could sunbathe on a terrace free from the telescopic lenses of the press who had found a site in a nearby lane and had congregated there on many occasions in the hope of photographing her in a bikini. We now know, and even suspected then, that their marriage wasn't in the best of health. However, he referred to her fondly and with a tone of genuine care and sympathy in his voice.

He asked me about my children and then spoke very warmly about his own. On his way around the walled garden, suddenly a number of lady guests, who were taking up the rear, squealed as a salvo of rotten apples rained down on them and dislodged at least one hat. The culprits were William and Harry. The Prince turned to me and said, 'Little devils,' with a warm smile of amusement at such mischievous exploits. In a wooded area, where the Prince had constructed a tree house for his sons, we watched them clamber up their ladder before descending again to earth by a rope, and he roared with laughter when Prince Harry asked, 'Papa, shall we do it again in case the back people didn't see.'

A little later, Prince Harry was tugging so hard at his father's sleeve that the Prince of Wales's shoulder was bouncing up and down and his head rolling from side to side. 'Papa! Papa!' he shouted, 'Don't listen to him. Listen to me!'

A few minutes later the boisterous Harry snapped the stem of a beautiful flower. His father rebuked him before gently explaining that Harry had shortened the time of that flower's beauty in the garden. Harry looked down and said, 'Sorry, Papa.' The Prince smiled at his son, who then beamed back.

Children who have cold, distant and unloving fathers don't behave like that with them. Harry's behaviour towards his father, as much as Prince Charles's reaction to it, told any parent that this was a warm and loving relationship. The same could be said of the way he cuddled Prince William as we walked back to the house and he cracked another funereal joke for my benefit. He pointed up to the stone balustrade running along the roof. It was interspersed by urns. He chuckled, 'Those weren't there when I bought the place. I suppose I should have asked your advice before having them erected.'

The Prince asked me if I had any siblings. I replied, 'A brother and a sister, Sir.'

'Are they older or younger?' he asked with genuine curiosity.

'Both younger, my brother by six years, my sister by two.'

'Ah,' he sighed, 'a sister two years younger. I imagine she could be bossy.' And then he laughed. There was no reference to Princess Anne, and I did not presume to mention her name, especially given our little spat concerning cures for the lower spine an hour or so earlier.

Upon our return to the drawing room, via the French windows that lead into the house from the rear hallway, I left my wife chatting about painting in Provence to get something for the Prince from my car. Prince Harry asked if he could come with me. As we entered the car park, he pointed to a gleaming cobalt blue XJS convertible, with its hood down exposing cream leather seats. 'Is that your car?'

'It is,' I nodded.

'Wow! Can I drive it?'

I got in and put the Prince in between my legs and we set off around the car park. He steered while I operated the accelerator and brake.

Then Prince Harry announced, 'We could go out on to the road if you like?'

'Oh, I don't think so.' I replied, and decided that it might be best to terminate the young Prince's driving lesson.

What was worrying, however, was that security was so low-key it seemed to me that if I had been an IRA sympathiser I could have done a runner with the third in line to the throne and have a good chance of getting a couple of miles down the road before anyone noticed. Of course, there may have been MI6 guys up every other tree that I didn't know about, but somehow I doubted it.

Having returned the Prince to the safe care of his father in the pleasant but surprisingly small drawing room, we took our leave of their Royal Highnesses and attended a dinner together with other guests in Tetbury.

My personal relationship with the Prince of Wales wasn't very long, and was certainly of no consequence to him. However, it did enable me to observe that his children adored him and his staff loved and respected him while being quite aware of his frailties. I also found out that some bad as well as a lot of good was done in his name, and that the bad seemed to be without his knowledge.

The Prince, for his part, floated like a butterfly, while occasionally stinging like a bee when disturbed. He seemed to lack focus. He had a hot temper. He did moan on occasion, and his staff told me that he could become both depressed and self-pitying. But he always attempted to hide these insecurities and unwarranted low self-esteem behind an honest self-deprecation.

Moreover, he also displayed both physical and mental courage, and was charming, kind and wanted, above all, not to waste one second in achieving good for the benefit of his fellow countryman. He knew that he was in a position to do so and believed that it was his duty.

Nobody is perfect. We could fill pages with our own faults and those of others, and in the Prince of Wales's case many tabloid journalists do. But to know this man at all is to know that the good far outweighs the bad. I hadn't enjoyed the hours and hours of uninterrupted conversation that Jonathan Dimbleby was to experience a few years later. On the other hand, Prince Charles did not know, when talking to me, that I would one day commit such conversations to paper; therefore I had the benefit of talking to him in a natural and unguarded fashion. And yet I was to draw the same conclusions as Dimbleby: we had both been talking to a very decent human being. And I, for one, have always found it easier to admire the truly honest endeavours of a hard worker who cares for others, than the fake charm of a superstar whose favourite word is 'me'.

The first time I met Princess Diana was in 1991. I was one of several guests of Help the Aged at a large black-tie affair in London because they had endorsed Hodgson Holdings' pre-arranged funeral plan, 'Dignity in Destiny', and as a result received a commission each time we sold a policy. It was a glittering affair and the guest of honour making the big speech was the Princess of Wales.

She clearly had not written the speech herself, and read it without the passion that comes of reading one's own words on a subject about which one is genuinely concerned. Indeed, it was perhaps one of the weakest speeches I have ever had to endure. Nevertheless, it didn't really detract from the occasion because the guests had come to see the beautiful Princess Diana and enjoy being in her presence rather than listen to her speech. Everybody knew that her husband was the committed, brainy one; she was the icon.

John Wheatley of Help the Aged, who was sitting closer to the Princess than myself, leaned round the back of the chair of the lady sitting between us and grabbed my elbow. He mouthed that the Princess would be leaving straight after dinner, but that she would like to meet me. Naturally flattered, I nodded and smiled. A few moments later, the Princess, dressed in a magnificent pink ball gown, was ceremoniously clapped from the banqueting hall and I, along with two or three others, was led by Wheatley to a private room. Apparently this meeting was supposed to have taken place before the dinner, but she had arrived late due to bad traffic. It wasn't mentioned, but I suppose the real reason for the introduction was that myself and the others would be so impressed by it that Help the Aged could count on us for some pretty good corporate or personal donations.

Eventually I was introduced as a 'funeral tycoon' – a description that I was less than pleased with and so was delighted when the Princess laughed that off and commented that I was 'the spit of Robert Redford' (obviously her eyesight was defective!) as she giggled and then flashed her eyes briefly into mine and then down at the ground. For that moment, I thought that I was probably the most important man on the planet. The heady cocktail of her beauty, vulnerability, flirtation and girlish sex appeal made me understand in a flash how men loved her and women admired her.

At the time, I was vaguely aware that the Waleses' marriage wasn't made in heaven. There had been many stories already claiming as much in the national press, saying that she was never at KP when the Prince was, and she certainly wasn't at Highgrove when I went there. But I had no idea of the scale of the problems that she, her husband and their staff were facing as a result of her condition.

The next time I was in the same room as the Princess was some five years later, and by now I had discovered a more accurate picture of her domestic life. The occasion was a large charity dinner in aid of a programme to build a cancer hospital in Pakistan. It had been organised by Imran Khan, the former Pakistani cricket captain who was now pursuing a career in politics, and his beautiful new wife Jemima, daughter of the late Sir James Goldsmith and his former wife Lady Annabel. The guest speaker was to be the Princess of Wales, who was a friend of Jemima's.

Having been most graciously welcomed by Mr and Mrs Khan at the entrance to the banqueting suite, my wife and I proceeded to join the other guests for pre-dinner drinks. There we met my then publishers – Michael Parkinson (and his wife Mary) and Sir Tim Rice, who were on the next table. Tim, Parky and I started talking about a book I was thinking of writing about the relationship between John Lennon and Paul McCartney as both men are Beatle buffs, but we soon drifted on to a topic that fascinates all three of us: cricket.

My wife Christine, who even today is often stopped in a restaurant or even in the street just to be told she looks like Diana, was chatting happily away to the delightful Mary Parkinson. Suddenly they stopped talking and just stood and stared straight through us to a small group of women immediately behind Parky and me. 'Forgive me for interrupting the conversation and just staring at her,' Mary told Christine. 'But I can't help myself!'

'I know,' replied Christine as they both stood transfixed by the sight of the Princess of Wales. Diana was standing with her back to me and our heads were nearly touching. However, such was the heated debate between Parky and me about whether or not Dermot Reeve should be in the England one-day cricket team that we had not only failed to notice that our wives were silently staring at somebody beyond us, the whole room was as well. Before I had woken up to it, the ladies' toilet had been cleared so that the Princess might use it, and then it was time for dinner.

Just before the auction, the Princess made her speech. The difference from four years earlier was most notable – clearly some good had come from the work Peter Settelen, Diana's voice coach, had undertaken with her. She spoke with more authority, diction and conviction, and although the speech was still slightly stilted, it was much better than the one I had heard from her previously.

Christine later explained to Parky that she was glad I hadn't noticed the Princess standing next to me because I had been horrified by the appalling and untrue impression she had given of the Prince and his family and how I was furious with the injustice of it all. Michael, a Yorkshireman who is always looking for his next row, could help himself. 'That wasn't a bad speech,' he called across the table as the Princess left, to much appreciation.

'No, it wasn't,' I admitted, but I couldn't resist adding, 'Not too sure I'd buy a second-hand car off her, though.'

Obviously, my personal encounters with Princess Diana were far fewer and much less detailed than those I had with Prince Charles; I certainly wasn't to have a long and at times personal conversation with her as I did with the Prince. Nor was I to see her in her home or with her children. Nevertheless, such was either her natural charisma or that charisma that famous people acquire as a result of their celebrity that I was completely entranced as she flattered me with her compliment and shy smile. It became easy for me to see how she might, when she had a mind to, persuade people that black was white and white was black. The intoxicating cocktail that was Diana could be a wonderful experience. However, those who stuck around for several drinks seemed to end up with the most dreadful hangover.

It would be completely wrong for me to claim that I knew either the Prince or the Princess well: I knew the Prince well enough for him to know who I was and the Princess only fleetingly. Nevertheless, I did meet the heir to the throne enough times to be able to form an opinion, and in both their cases I saw nothing to dissuade me that the picture I have since built of both of them by talking to people who knew them and were with them throughout the troubled years of their marriage, is right.

Naturally, there are two sides to every story, and certainly the Princess wasn't all bad. Her husband has never claimed that she was. But that's not the point. The point is that she claimed that he was, and lied in order to back up her claim. It is possible for people to have conflicting opinions or even memories, but it is a different matter altogether when stories are invented by one who is then also far from honest about her own behaviour. The only question, the real debate in my mind, remains whether or not these were the actions of a wicked and manipulative woman, or a young lady who was in desperate need of help.

Part Four
Separation, Divorce and Death

Howard Hodgson

Chapter Twelve
The Children (1982–96)

There can be no doubt that these royal parents always loved both of their sons equally and completely. However, this was not always the impression given to the public, especially in the last ten years of the Princess's life and increasingly after their separation was announced in late 1992. This was because the Princess was not above using her sons either as supporting roles in her soap opera, or as a weapon either to hurt their father or even better to discredit him in the public's eyes as a poor parent.

It wasn't until after her death that the public came to see what an exceptionally good father Prince Charles had always been. During her life, the Princess would exploit any opportunity to show herself to be a caring and modern mother who was determined that her boys would be brought up not only with a sense of duty (which was certainly lacking in her), but in touch with modern, everyday Britain (which she certainly wasn't). In addition, she believed every effort should be made to contrast this with the snobby and old-fashioned life of extreme privilege that they received at the hands of their father in remote places like Balmoral. As a result, she would tip off her favourite newspapers when she was going to take the boys to a theme park on a Sunday, so that the Monday press could be full of Wills, Harry and her in jeans getting wet, having a Big Mac and a whale of a time. The press would be encouraged to draw a comparison between these scenes and those of the boys looking serious in ties and suits and going to church with Papa and Granny when it was Charles's turn to have them for the weekend. The general idea was to create the impression that thanks to her the boys were more in touch, and this was in stark contrast to the out-of-date example of boring 1950s discipline that was being dished out by a cold and uncaring father.

The Princess sought to give this impression for three very important reasons. Firstly, she believed that it was essential to get public opinion behind her claim to her sons. She was well aware that the Queen had the constitutional right and authority under common law to take control of both boys' care and education. As such she could become the boys' guardian, or even appoint one: this would probably be their father and that might lead to Diana's exclusion if she finally burned all her bridges with the Royal Family. Of course, the Queen had no such intention, but the Princess, in her disturbed state, believed that Prince Charles and his mother had already hatched such a plot and were only waiting for the right moment to execute it. As the Princess had no legal rights in the matter – the law was last recognised in 1772 and hadn't been changed since – she realised that her best defence against it was a weight of public opinion believing that she was a good mother and that Charles was a bad father. Spin was continually created to further that notion.

Secondly, the Princess wanted to promote the idea that the crown should skip a generation and go straight to Prince William on the Queen's death. By promoting her son as a young man of the people who watched Aston Villa on television while his father stalked deer in the miserable Scottish Highlands, she was giving birth to this idea. Andrew Morton acknowledges that this was her desire, but claims that this was because she believed William was a better man for the job. This is complete rubbish. Diana was well aware that Prince Charles had trained for becoming king of England just about every day since he could first remember. She had resented his dedication to this task and his mother's subjects from the time of their engagement onwards. She was also worried that Prince William might hate the idea of becoming king. Indeed, she is supposed to have confided to Paul Burrell, among others, that William did not want to take on the role. Apparently, Diana believed that Harry was better suited to the job. She told Burrell, 'Harry would see no problem in taking on the job. GKH. That's what we'll call him. GKH, for Good King Harry. I like that.' This story would appear to be true as others were to become aware of the nickname, which wasn't apparently used to Harry's face. It would seem, therefore, that the Princess was attempting to deny the crown to a man who had dedicated his whole life towards that end, in favour of a boy whom she genuinely worried didn't want it. Why? For the good of the people? For the good of William? For the good of the current heir to the throne? No. She wanted to promote her son against his father in order to deliver the heaviest blow she could imagine against her ex-husband. It was bitter spite towards Prince Charles that made her ignore the feelings of Prince William and apparently gave her the right, in her mind, to attempt to alter the accession to the throne.

Her third reason was that anything she could do to promote herself with the children that gave either them or the public the impression that he wasn't a loving father was deeply hurtful to the Prince of Wales.

However, he took comfort from the fact that both boys worshipped him – they were the ones who really mattered, not the tabloids. Moreover, he wasn't prepared to use his sons in public and he wasn't prepared to hurt them by selfish actions in private. The Princess understood this very well and used it to her every possible advantage. She knew he wouldn't fight back in the press, and this gave her a free rein.

A good example of this involves one of her favourite photographs – a shot taken of her aboard the Royal Yacht *Britannia* in Canada in 1991. Her arms are outstretched and her face is a picture of delight as she rushes to greet the children. The photographer also captured Charles, a couple of seconds later, gathering his sons up in his arms and hugging them tightly with his eyes closed in a private moment of bliss. Unsurprisingly the public never got to see this picture. It was Jayne Fincher who took both photographs. That of the Princess became one of the most famous of her that was ever taken. Diana asked Fincher for a copy, which was thereafter displayed in her dressing room at Kensington Palace. However, Fincher was later to admit to Clayton and Craig, 'And then a few seconds behind, Prince Charles did the same thing. He came down; he was hugging and kissing the boys too. But the sad thing was that all the pictures that were used were with her with her arms out, and nobody ever used a picture of him. I think he got a bad press with the children at the time. Everybody kept saying, "Oh this dreadful father" and everything, which wasn't true. He's always been a lovely father. But I think he wasn't seen with the children as she was – and in a lot of high profile places like Thorpe Park. And so people tended to see that and think, Where's he? all the time.'

Another example is how she let it be known that she had stayed at Great Ormond Street Hospital with Prince William after he had been accidentally hit on the head by a friend with a golf club, while the Prince had gone on to host an evening at the opera to hear a performance of *Tosca* at Covent Garden. The result was that the tabloids, now comfortable with their caricatures, ripped into the Prince for being a poor father. The *Sun*, as usual, led the way with the front-page headline, 'WHAT KIND OF A DAD ARE YOU?'

The truth was somewhat different. The Princess had been at lunch in London and the Prince at Highgrove when the news was broken to both of them. William had been taken from school to the Royal Berkshire Hospital. Both parents immediately took off to be with him. The Prince was to comment at the time, 'My policeman said that it was not too serious, but I worried all the way to the hospital until I found him sitting up in bed, chatting away. Then I knew he was going to be alright.' Nevertheless, the Prince had suffered a small indentation at the point of impact and doctors at the hospital decided that he should be transferred to Great Ormond Street to be examined by a group of neurological specialists. After a brief consultation, the surgeons decided to operate. Explaining to both parents that this was a routine and non-dangerous operation, they assured the Prince that there was no need for him to stay as the Princess was doing so anyway. Having been assured that there was negligible risk and that William's mother would be there when he awoke, the Prince of Wales decided that it was safe for him to proceed with his duty and go to the West End where he was host to both the European environment and agricultural commissioners at Covent Garden.

Afterwards, he was told that the operation had been a success; his son was fine and fast asleep. Thus comforted, he boarded the royal train and set off for the Yorkshire Dales to host a visit there by his European guests and their accompanying British officials. The next day he returned to London and immediately went to Great Ormond Street to see his son, who had, by then, made a complete recovery.

The Princess, happy by the tabloids' unfair verdict, wasn't slow to use it to her advantage. A year later, an unnamed friend of the Princess was quoted by Morton as confirming that the Princess believed that the tabloids' view was correct: 'Had this been an isolated incident it would have been unbelievable. She wasn't surprised. It merely confirmed everything she thought about him …'

Diana, who would telephone media friends like Richard Kay most mornings before doing anything else, had used her son's accident brilliantly against his father. 'You're the finest PR operator, man or woman, I have ever met,' a grateful Sir David English of the *Daily Mail* would later tell her. She was indeed.

However, what the public saw in their newspapers and what William and Harry saw in private were two entirely different things. Away from the media, they caught the full effect of her moods, tirades and tantrums just like anyone else. When they were young, these were quite frightening and bewildering to them: they naturally didn't understand what was going on and what they might have done to upset Mummy. The Princess, although she adored her sons, simply did not possess the ability to curb her behaviour in front of them. It was often left to Prince Charles to hand out the hugs and kisses in private as he sought to reassure William and Harry that Mummy would be better tomorrow.

When a friend had suggested that it was not a good idea to rant and scream in front of a young Prince William, Diana had simply replied that the boy was too young to notice and that in any case he would have to come to terms with the truth sooner or later. That remained her attitude throughout the boys' childhood. She was unhappy. It was, in her opinion, her husband's fault and as a result she expected people around her to understand, forgive her and blame Prince Charles.

Trying to keep the lid on such a pressure cooker at home, while still doing his public duty, brought the Prince down to a very low state. As the couple started to live separate lives, he started to recover his confidence and seemed much happier; but then the Princess presented him with a completely new set of problems concerning the children. Not only would she increasingly delight in using them as bit-part players for her own ends in the press, she now also found last-minute excuses to deny Charles access to them, or would make arrangements that conflicted with what had generally been agreed by both of them.

For example, it was only just before St David's Day that Prince Charles's staff discovered that the Princess was planning to take Prince William to Wales for their national day. This went completely against an agreement that they had made concerning the children not having to take on public engagements unless both parents agreed. It was a blatant attempt by the Princess to appear before a large Welsh crowd and present her son to them in the absence of his father. The impression would have been that she cared more about Wales than Prince Charles, and this would have helped her popularity and maybe even the idea that she was a kingmaker and her son should be next in line to the throne. Charles's private secretary only discovered the Princess's plan by chance; luckily he was able to alter the Prince's schedule in order that he might be there with them.

Conversely, on a day when the Prince had been planning to take Harry on board the aircraft carrier HMS *Invincible*, the Princess announced at the last moment that Harry couldn't attend as he had a dental appointment and it would not be convenient to change it. Rather than risk yet another high-profile argument with his wife, Charles did not pursue the matter. Naturally he was disappointed, but the real loser was Prince Harry who was looking forward to watching Harrier jump jets taking off and landing. As time went by, Prince Charles almost came to expect a last-minute phone call announcing some rather lame excuse as to why the children wouldn't be able to do this or that with him.

This is not to say that there weren't many areas of agreement between Charles and Diana about the children – throughout their years together it was perhaps their only real common interest. They were always in total agreement as to how they should be treated and educated. They rarely had a disagreement about them and the Prince did his best to limit their rows in front of them. Both had the interests of their sons at heart. The choice of Ludgrove as a prep school was one they made together, and they were both keen that the boys should attend Eton.

It has been said that the Prince wasn't too keen on Eton and got pushed into it by the Princess. This is not correct. Prince Charles's mentor and drama teacher from Gordonstoun, Dr Eric Anderson, was Eton's headmaster until just before William arrived at the school. In addition the Prince's godson, Tom Parker Bowles, had been happy there, and there were many of the royal couple's friends whose sons were either there or going to be there while the princes would be in attendance.

The Prince and Princess would appear to have made the right decision. Eton played its part in producing two very fine young men, despite the horrors that both had to endure during their time there. Such horrors did not come from within the school as their father's had at Gordonstoun, but from the cards that the outside world was to deal them.

Prince William initially caught the brunt of it. He had become used to his mother phoning him up at prep school and crying hysterically down the phone. At Eton this seemed to get worse as, by this time, his parents had separated and seemed to be waging a war against each other through the press. As he grew older, he became increasingly aware of his mother's problems. It wasn't that he didn't love her – he did, very much – but he wished she could behave differently. He disliked her one-sided and unfair attitude to his father; he hated the press and being put on show by the Princess in theme parks; he didn't want to be some kind of urban kid – he longed to hunt and fish and play polo with his father; and he found his mother's mood swings very unsettling. All in all he found that being with his mother could, at times, be a considerable emotional burden. This is probably one reason why he and Harry took so easily to Tiggy following her appointment to look after them when they were with Prince Charles during the period after their parents' separation.

William confirmed these feelings himself. Prince Charles took the boys on an outing to the Royal Shakespeare Theatre in Stratford-upon-Avon in the mid-1990s with, among others, Bel Mooney and her daughter. The party had a pre-performance supper together, during which the Prince started to chat about his old favourites the Goons. Being of a similar age, Bel Mooney burst into their signature tune, 'The Ying Tong Song'.

'God, aren't parents embarrassing?' said her daughter to Prince William.

'Papa doesn't embarrass me – Mama does,' he replied.

Eton was William's home for nearly nine months of each year during these turbulent times. The school, which totally dominates the pretty town in which it is set, sits on one side of the river Thames, while the other side is dominated by Windsor Castle. Boys all sleep in their own study-bedrooms in one of twenty-five houses with approximately fifty boys in each house. This allowed both princes some privacy. Their housemaster, a historian by the name of Dr Gailey, was a decent man and a source of great comfort to William in particular through the troubled times of his mother's turbulent life and tragic death. The boys were also close to their protection officers, who had been especially chosen with a view to them becoming a cross between an older friend and uncle. But the person they really came to love and were closest to was Tiggy.

After the separation, Prince Charles realised that he would need some practical help with the children when they were staying with him. They were by now too old for a nanny but they still needed looking after and someone who could drive them to the shops or to their friends. He also realised that they would need some form of discipline, and knew how hopeless he was in that department. Hence the appointment of the twenty-eight-year-old daughter of a family friend, 'Tiggy' Legge-Bourke. She was perfect for the job, and the boys took to her immediately. She was a dizzy nursery-school teacher who had a wonderful rapport with all children – indeed, she appeared to be an uncomplicated and overgrown child herself.

William and Harry soon came to treat her like a big sister rather than a nanny or substitute mother: she loved the outdoor life; she loved riding and shooting; she told them jokes, liked their kind of music and watched the same videos as them. Nevertheless, she also managed to keep them in order without ever appearing to be too strict. If she told them to go to bed, they might pull a face at her but they would go. In contrast, if their father told them they would more than likely ignore him or manage to twist him round their little finger and get him to agree that they might stay up for another hour or so.

Diana became extremely jealous of the relationship Tiggy had with her sons: she hated the fact that her boys were having such a good time with another woman. Both William and Harry loved their mother dearly and realised how much she loved them, but Tiggy was like a breath of fresh air by comparison – she was reliable and never irrational or tearful. The Princess became increasingly angry about Tiggy's appointment, and the Prince did not help matters by not being overly sensitive to the situation.

The Prince of Wales had always behaved very correctly concerning Camilla. Unlike Diana's introduction of Hewitt to the boys, Charles had ensured that his children never met his mistress, but he saw no reason why they shouldn't like the woman he had engaged to look after them, and so encouraged the relationship. This infuriated the Princess, and she became even angrier if the newspapers ran stories or pictures of Tiggy fooling around with the boys. It seemed to her that not only was this younger woman attempting to steal the affections of her children, she was doing so in public and thus damaging her image as the world's best mum.

The Princess, herself a serial adulterer, also believed – or at least would have other people believe – that her husband was unfaithful to Camilla. She would write a year before her death that, 'Camilla is nothing but a decoy.' Paul Burrell later claimed that he had been told by Diana that she was convinced, 'Charles had a roving eye and that while Camilla was his principal mistress, she was not the only one. He could not help wandering.' There is no more evidence that this is true than there is that the Prince was planning Diana's death by tampering with the brakes on her car, which the Princess also claimed at that time. She had seen the photographs of Tiggy and Charles kissing on the ski slopes and foolishly, given how she had learned to manipulate the press herself, believed the innuendo that the tabloids were implying. She was mistaken. There was no affair between Tiggy and the Prince of Wales.

Tiggy is a very tactile person who hugs and kisses everyone – including the Prince of Wales, whom she has known since she was a child. In fairness to Diana, there are those who say that Tiggy may have had a huge crush on the heir to the throne, but the very same people will immediately tell you that this was not reciprocated by the Prince, who was at times irritated by the girl and only kept her on because of his sons' great affection for her and the good effect that she had upon them.

Things reached a head at the staff Christmas lunch at the Lanesborough Hotel in Knightsbridge in 1995. The Prince and Princess continued to attend this annual function together, despite the fact that by this time they were divorced. Diana couldn't contain her jealousy any longer. She determined to wreak her revenge on a woman whom she believed had stolen her children and was now having an affair with her estranged husband.

Tiggy had recently been to hospital for a minor operation. At the Christmas lunch, the Princess crept up behind her and whispered, 'So sorry to hear about the baby.' The clear indication was that Tiggy had been in hospital aborting the Prince's child. Tiggy was devastated and was escorted from the room in floods of tears by Michael Fawcett, the Prince's valet at that time. She did not reappear. The Princess stayed and had a good time as the drink flowed freely, and she participated very enthusiastically in the crazy-foam fight as matters degenerated in the way that most office parties do.

However, when Ms Legge-Bourke recovered her composure, her indignation at the way the Princess had treated her was considerable. She instructed libel lawyers and asked them to deny the unfounded allegation and demand an apology. The Prince is said to have been sympathetic to Tiggy's position, but at the same time put polite and gentle pressure on her not to proceed, as he did not wish to see Diana exposed in court in this way. Instead, he promised the matter would be looked into internally. An investigation was launched by Sir Robert Fellowes, by then the Queen's private secretary. It was felt that, as he was Diana's brother-in-law and known to be a just man, the Princess would be forced to accept his findings. In time, Fellowes wrote to the Princess, 'Your allegations concerning Tiggy Legge-Bourke are completely unfounded. Her relationship with the Prince of Wales has never been anything but a professional one. On the date of the supposed abortion, she was at Highgrove with William and Harry. It is in your own best interests that you withdraw these allegations. You have got this whole thing dreadfully wrong.'

Some people report that the Princess was thus forced begrudgingly to withdraw her remark; others claim that she refused and it was left to the Prince of Wales to talk Tiggy out of taking any further action. The latter is probably more likely as it is hard to imagine the Princess apologising, even if a libel action was threatened. She was clever enough to know that the Prince would save her bacon – after all, he always had. She drove him to distraction and at times made him very angry, but somehow he always managed to forgive her, believing that her behaviour was beyond her control. He felt sorry for her even at the worst times, and she knew it.

The Princess's bust-up with Tiggy was not the first she had experienced with a nanny. Barbara Barnes had been the children's first nanny and was also the first of a long list of staff members to be forced out by Diana. Initially she had coped as well as anyone with the Princess's mood swings, but Diana, who was as jealous as she was devoted as a mother, increasingly had 'Baba', as William had come to call her, in her sights. The more the boys loved her, the more Diana rebuked the woman. It came to a head when Barbara took some of her holiday entitlement to attend the birthday bash of her former employer, Lord Glenconner, on the Caribbean island of Mustique. There she was treated as an honoured guest and received almost as much media coverage as other guests such as Princess Margaret, Mick Jagger, Jerry Hall and Rachel Welch.

In Diana's mind, stealing her sons was bad enough, but to steal her newspaper coverage as well was just not acceptable. As she explained to another member of the Kensington Palace staff, 'It's time for her to go. She's forgotten who the star turn is around here.' Barnes, who had not sought the tabloid attention, returned from her holiday tanned and relaxed to find that the Princess had accepted a resignation that she had not tendered.

The very public relationship of Diana with her sons is well recorded and known the world over. Her private relationship was trickier because of her moods, but it was nevertheless loving and there can be no question that both boys adored their mother, even if the sensitive William was at times apprehensive. Less is known about Charles's relationship with his children as he was always less demonstrative in public, has always refused to perform acts of public affection for the media's benefit and hates the idea of using his sons as a way of gaining popular acclaim. Indeed, the more his wife employed this tactic, the more distant he seemed to appear in public. Perhaps it was a subconscious act of disdain for her behaviour.

However, just as the Princess's private persona was completely different to her public one, so it is with Prince Charles. He fools around with the boys and they laugh and joke and kiss and hug a lot more than anyone would imagine from their media image. Examples of their close and tactile relationship are boundless. A typically touching one relates to the last night of their 1997 skiing holiday in Klosters. A twelve-year-old Prince Harry got to his feet and, in front of a table full of people, made a little speech to thank 'Papa' for the wonderful holiday. Then he dashed up to his father and smothered his face in kisses as Prince Charles feigned embarrassment and begged for mercy. When they were small boys they would rush out of Highgrove and into the front field where the helicopter would land as it brought their father home. Sheep graze in that field. Once it was safe for them to do so, they would run across the field and leap into their father's outstretched arms – thus covering his suit in sheep droppings. Suit after suit needed his valet's attention, but that never stopped the procedure being repeated the next day.

It was Charles who personally built them their tree house at Highgrove. They named it Holyroodhouse after the Queen's official residence in Edinburgh. They share his silly sense of humour, as did Diana, and they are both excellent mimics – much better at taking off their father than any of the professionals we see so often on television.

The Prince has aged badly with the strains of recent years, yet despite this and a terrible back, he remains extremely fit. He and his sons have their own polo team, which Prince William insists plays in Aston Villa colours, much to Harry's annoyance as he is an Arsenal fan. They are all accomplished players and play to win. After a match they relax in each other's company over a drink. The mood is nearly always light and both boys, now taller than their father, often indulge in horseplay with him and the Prince can be heard to yell, 'Get off me, you enormous louts.'

At all times, Charles has striven to be a good father, and he has been successful: the living proof is the way his sons have turned out. William has conducted himself with the quiet dignity befitting a future king, having learned as a child from the dangers his mother encountered by flirting with the media and inviting overexposure; and while Harry is more of a Spencer tearaway, he appears to be a normal boy who has not only had to cope with being royal but with his mother's untimely death just as he entered puberty.

However, it would be also quite wrong to leave this subject with the impression that the Princess had only negative effects on her sons' lives; there was another side to Diana the mother, which at times had a very positive effect on them. She was acutely aware that her children had been born into a very privileged environment. She really did see it as her duty to expose them to the rough and tumble of ordinary life where possible. It was Diana who took the lead in this matter, and she was totally supported by Prince Charles who was only too aware that his father's ideas of how a prince should be brought up had caused him much hardship and not done his self-confidence much good. He was determined that this was not going to happen to them, and he never attempted to stop her believing that she, as their mother, had as much right as he did in shaping their future.

Chapter Thirteen
The Greatest Deception (1991–92)

In December 1989, *Vanity Fair* reported on Diana's progress towards sainthood. They were taking their lead from the British press. The *Sun* had been leading the attack on the Prince of Wales, while blowing the fairy dust all over the Princess's image, for several years. Naturally, it was aided by the *Daily Mail*, but the *Sun* was taking things to new levels of absurdity: 'DID CARING PRINCESS DI RAISE YOUR SPIRITS AND HELP YOU AT YOUR TIME OF NEED? Has any royal made your life a little happier when you needed some support and encouragement? If so, share your experience with fellow readers. Write to ANGEL DI, The Sun, London EI 9XP.'

Di's public image had been helped very much by her need to be a celebrity and the tabloids' desire to make her one. She was addicted to this not only as a way of getting at her husband and his family, but as a way of giving love and receiving it without having to endure any of the problems that she associated with a long-term relationship. These were probably natural symptoms of her illness. However, she had also become completely addicted to her own image and, like so many other twentieth-century celebrities thrown suddenly into the limelight, she found it quite impossible to put anything before it. It was her, and she was it.

As a result, her status and the power that she felt came with it started to take over her life. Patrick Jephson has since written that this motivated her every move in public. No smile was too big, no cuddle too tight – as long as it resulted in wonderful coverage in the following day's newspapers. This is not to say that the effect on those receiving the smile or getting the cuddle wasn't wonderful too – it was, and she was brilliant at it – but it became increasingly hard for people like Jephson, who knew what motivated her and how she could behave when the cameras weren't there, to view her behaviour as just saintly goodness.

And this is where it all gets very complicated. There can be no doubt that the Princess used her charity work as a major weapon in her armoury, and increasingly with cynical intent. If you want the world to love you and hate your husband, getting your public image right while harpooning his is important; if you need the world to love you because you will feel terribly empty if you are not a star with the world worshipping at your feet, it becomes essential. Even the simplest soul knows that political manipulation starts and finishes with good deeds, and Diana knew by her late twenties that it was her charity work that would keep her up there as a world icon through her thirties, forties and fifties.

On the other hand there can be no doubt that once she arrived on a visit, whatever the cynical motive for it, the impact on the people she met was superb. Surely there must be an argument that says never mind the motive, just judge the deed and its result. Margaret Jay of Britain's National Aids Trust clearly believes this. She told Clayton and Craig, 'Look, does it really matter to me why she wanted to do this kind of thing? We live in a world in which celebrities have a huge power to help organisations like mine. This one chose to and I'm grateful. End of story. And she didn't have to. Or at least she didn't have to do quite as much and quite as well as she did.'

You can see her point. Dedicated charity people like Margaret Jay are all fighting each other for the public's money. They need celebrity help in order to attract attention. A good day in a clinic with a celebrity results in very positive PR – not just for the celebrity but also for the charity, and that means money, which is the very thing they called upon the celebrity for in the first place. And, in her day, you didn't get a celebrity much bigger than the Princess of Wales. So why on earth should somebody like Margaret Jay worry about Diana's motives?

Were the results of Diana's work good? Unequivocally yes. But that doesn't mean necessarily that the Princess was a good person. To resolve that question it is necessary to look at her motives. To quote journalist and stern Diana critic Christopher Hitchens, 'Where was Madame Ceausescu ever photographed except in an orphanage? Anyone who has the slightest knowledge of the arts of political manipulation knows that's what you do … And it worked on many people who thought, You may say what you like about the Ceausescus, but that Eleanor, she really does her charity work.'

The Princess, while never refusing a distant association with charity work, didn't become enthusiastic about it until she understood the importance of it to her as the vehicle that would enhance her image. Of course, her work had an enormously positive effect on the numerous individuals and organisations that benefited from her patronage. This also explains her mode of operation. As she hadn't been captivated from a young age by the need to do something worthwhile and have her ideas acted upon, like her husband, she wasn't to be found working hard on plans or lobbying politicians as he was. She was all about a quick visit, some great photographs and copy for the press, and off again.

The effect she had was enormous, and very often people thought that they had been visited by a saint. Moreover, sometimes her short visits did more good than Prince Charles's months of hard labour if an idea of his wasn't eventually adopted. But the essential thing to note is this: his motive was to change the life of ordinary people for the better; her motive was to enhance and maintain an iconic existence to which she had become addicted, and then use it to strengthen her position at the expense of her often imagined enemies. Both Charles and Diana did good works, but their motives were driven by very different desires; once the biased reporting has been stripped away and the truth arrived at, it is easy to see whose motive was genuine and who had a hidden agenda.

But that was not how it was reported at the time. After years of sprinkling this fairy dust on the Princess, the tabloids had created an inaccurate picture that a celebrity-mad nation couldn't get enough of. Britain wanted youth, beauty, wealth and celebrity, and the Princess had the lot. Having felt the nice warm feelings created by these pro-Diana stories, and having bought into the idea that she was married to a man who was not only a loony but also a poor father, many wouldn't ever want to hear anything different.

Moreover, the tabloid impression was usually well supported by either grateful recipients of the Princess's immediate affection or grateful charity bosses who didn't mind Diana stealing the limelight as long as the cash rolled in. It's perhaps also important to remember that the real charity workers, like Margaret Jay, saw themselves as the prime architects of their chosen charity's direction. To have a celebrity like the Princess get the publicity that raised the money to pay for this was not only fantastic, but probably preferable than have a man like the Prince come along with his own ideas for a charity's future. Jay probably felt that Diana was helping her obtain her dreams for Britain's National AIDS Trust, whereas Tom Shebbeare always knew that he was helping Prince Charles realise the heir to the throne's own dreams for the Prince's Trust.

However, the Prince, troubled in the mid-1980s by his disastrous marriage at home, his 'loony' image in the press, faltering progress on some of his most treasured projects and poor relations with the prime minister, was, as we have seen, making a comeback by the late 1980s. By then he was living a separate life from the Princess and his domestic day was calmer. Camilla had restored some of his fragile confidence, suddenly his views were in vogue and as a result even Mrs Thatcher was forced to take him seriously. His happiness in these matters only served to destabilise the Princess further, brought her to a new low, fractured the uneasy domestic peace and set her upon a course of action that led to separation and eventually a divorce that she was then to claim she never wanted – just one of numerous contradictions that we come across in the last eight years of her life.

It seems likely that the prospect of Charles finding contentment with Camilla and favour with the people as he struck chords with them on inner-city deprivation, housing, youth education, architecture and the environment, pushed the Princess into an even deeper state of insecurity and neurosis. His apparent resurrection with the British people and thus newfound popularity with their tabloid press as the material 1980s became the caring 1990s seems to have caused her to up the ante and plot her own version of British monarchical history covering the period 1981–91.

By the turn of the decade, the Princess was not only troubled by the fact that her husband appeared less tortured without her and that her tirades at him, when they did meet, seemed to be less effective, she had also been cruelly hit by another emotional problem. While she had been as physically unfaithful to Hewitt as she had been to Charles, he was perhaps the only other man that she had genuine affection for since Mannakee until she became infatuated with Oliver Hoare. Then James Hewitt was posted to Germany and had refused to allow her to intercede on his behalf in order to get the posting cancelled. She was furious with him and believed that he had, just as her parents and husband had before him, let her down. So as the world watched this beautiful icon visiting the sick and the dying, the actual woman was falling closer and closer to her all-time low. She had either alienated or banished those who really knew her and might be able to help her and had replaced them with those who didn't really know her and, in the main, didn't immediately know of her problems. And when they saw them, she was able to lay the blame convincingly at anybody's door but her own.

By now the Princess's life was a series of unconnected and

contradictory styles and actions. At home she loved her sons, but she couldn't control her moods or tantrums whether they were directed at them or otherwise. She could be the most pleasant and kind employer, or so wickedly vicious that if Charles Dickens had written up such a character people would have not accepted it as believable. She could go through lovers with a remarkable sexual appetite, and yet be obsessed by an affair that wasn't rekindled between the Prince of Wales and Mrs Parker Bowles until Diana had committed serial adultery. She could be genuinely consoling to the sick, while cynically cherry-picking the next most media-appealing photo opportunity. She could, as Jephson points out, comfort the dying and their bereaved families brilliantly with genuine compassion one minute, before jumping back into the helicopter with comments like, 'Watch my hat someone. Pass me over the *Mail*, would you. Oooh, hold on to your hats. Wonder what Dempster's written today, something juicy about the Germans I hope. Anyone got any chocolate?'

To be fair to the Princess, no one should have expected her to be totally affected by visiting the dying. She did it often, and funeral directors certainly don't cry every time they conduct a funeral. But that isn't the point. Diana, aided and abetted by the tabloids, wanted the people to believe that she was totally affected in a way that the reserved and cold Windsors weren't. In reality she was just a better actor than any of them. That is not to say that there is anything wrong with that – thousands of people felt a lot better as a result of her visits and millions more as a result of seeing it all in the next day's newspapers. But the truth was that she wasn't as deeply moved as she liked to appear, otherwise the joking conversation that followed once she was out of sight of the cameras couldn't have happened. The problem is the cynical way she sought to use the sick and the dying as weapons against the Queen and Prince Charles. It was the cynical motives behind her actions that were questionable, rather than wonderful things that the mirage she created achieved. She had very questionable ulterior motives, mainly as a result of her illness, that were not held by the other members of the Royal Family who, with the exception of the at times rather silly but less complicated Sarah, Duchess of York, were dedicated to supporting the Queen as head of state. They carried out their duties with this in mind rather than the self-glorification of a self-addicted celebrity who was by now completely self-obsessed and slowly sinking into a state of paranoia caused by an illness that needed serious help.

In February 1992, the Prince and Princess of Wales toured India together but looked increasingly unhappy. While the Prince talked to some industrialists, the Princess went off to visit the Taj Mahal with the press in tow. There she posed alone, sitting sadly in front of the world's most famous monument to love and knowing that the scene was laden with a mischievous potential. The message was not lost on the press, who had known for some time that the marriage was not a happy one and snapped eagerly away. The headlines round the world sang from the same unhappy marriage-hymn sheet that she had wished them to. They knew that this had been the message she had wanted to get across, but they didn't know why. It was only Diana who knew at that time what she had already done, and she knew that all events would have to be carefully managed from now on in order that the press should assist her instead of weakening her position.

Two days later Prince Charles took part in a polo match, and it had been arranged that Diana would hand out the prizes. Charles's team was playing the Indian Cavalry, and the Princess was concerned about what to do if his team won and she had to kiss him in public; with her usual lack of discipline she said so a staff member standing by her on the boundary. She claimed that she hated the dishonesty of it all. In fact, honesty had never been a strong strain in the Princess's character, and by this time she cared little about it. Her real motive was that any kiss with the Prince around Valentine's Day would undo all the good work that she had achieved forty-eight hours earlier.

As she was considering this potential dilemma, the Prince cracked a sixty-yard shot at a wide angle and scored not only a spectacular goal but also one that ensured that his team had won. Even the stoic Prince expected trouble as he walked up to receive the winners' trophy. He had seen that look on her face hundreds of times during the last decade, but he didn't know what she would do or how far she would go. There had been a time when she would reserve her worst behaviour for rows in front of either the children or the staff, but she had become increasingly daring in public as she had refined her PR skills. She presented him with the prize and, as he went to kiss her, she moved her head; he was left missing both her lips and her cheek and rather clumsily kissing her on the neck. The next day was Valentine's Day and this perfect symbol of a lousy marriage was everywhere.

The King and Di

She had cunningly achieved exactly what she had wanted: she had not only reinforced the Taj Mahal story, she had used another photo opportunity to prepare an unsuspecting public for her next move. An exclusive and apparently brilliantly researched book that Andrew Morton was writing and which was due to be published later in the year would be seen to be a true story and not one to be dismissed as pure rubbish. Her silent gestures would lend support to his words when they were published.

On 29 March 1992, Diana's father died. She had recently reversed a decision not to have a skiing holiday with Prince Charles and their sons, and had consequently arrived in Lech, Austria only the day before the awful news broke. Diana adored her father, as he did her. Her sorrow was all consuming, and she broke down. The Prince tried to reach out and help her as he always had and always would to the end of her days. However, she wanted none of it. She didn't wish him to accompany her back to London, and if she had had her way he wouldn't even have attended Earl Spencer's funeral. Nevertheless, he did both – not to annoy her, but because he understood the very bad press he would receive if he did neither. He was right – by making a concession to the Princess and travelling to the funeral service by helicopter while she made her way there by car, he was heavily criticised for failing to do his duty and comfort his grieving wife.

We will never know whether, on learning of her father's death, she felt guilty in the knowledge that she was about to expose him, fairly or otherwise, as a heavy-drinking wife-beater. Thankfully for Johnnie Spencer he died before he had to suffer such indignity. However, the untimely death of Diana's father threw up a real dilemma for the Princess as she realised she had to prevent Prince Charles from appearing to be a dutiful husband during her high-profile bereavement as there was a danger that it might cast doubt on the revelations that she knew were to hit the streets within three months.

Diana had originally selected Andrew Morton, according to him, because she considered him to be a bit of a rebel who would not flinch from firing shots at the Royal Family. In fact, according to one member of her staff, it was because she knew he was flattered by her attention yet clever enough to understand that this was a golden opportunity to get the scoop of the decade. As a result, he would play by her rules of denying that she had anything to do with it while allowing her editorial control. In his mind, such control was a small price to play for the opportunity of making both his name and his fortune. He could be the willing vehicle for her to rewrite a page of British history: she would never have to own up to what she had done, or face the obvious questions about the account's accuracy or her own honesty, and the Windsors would still get the book that they had coming to them.

The Princess had known Morton as one of the journalists who wrote about her and other members of the Royal Family. However, the main reason Diana selected him was because they had a friend in common – an intermediary who allowed her the chance to distance herself from the project and yet exercise perfect control over it. Dr James Colthurst had been introduced to Lady Diana Spencer on her extended skiing holiday in 1979. They became friends and enjoyed the pranks that young, spoiled aristocrats without royal responsibility often get up to. On one occasion they escaped from an après-ski nightclub without paying the bill when he bumped into a pillar on the dance floor and biting into a blood capsule that caused blood to run from his mouth, before being helped out of the club by Diana and another girl.

Colthurst, the son of a baronet whose family have owned Blarney Castle in Ireland for more than a century, came from a similar background to Diana – the aristocracy, a step removed from royalty. Aristocracy has the privilege without the responsibility, but like the outer edges of the Royal Family itself, the effect is often to produce foppish, ineffectual people who are far too fond of themselves and their own pleasures. The problem is naturally caused by human nature and not the characteristics of the individual. Moreover, as familiarity breeds contempt, such people can often be less loyal towards or in awe of the Royal Family than the ordinary man in the street. Many of the aristocracy see the Windsors simply as ordinary people who are perhaps no better than them, and yet they are constantly reminded of their status every time they have to bow or curtsy. Therefore the close proximity of royalty can have a very negative effect, especially if one's values are warped by unearned wealth, privilege, titles and a belief that one's own blood line is just as good if not better than 'the Germans''.

In the late 1980s, Colthurst became the sort of friend Diana could rely on. He was the one she could telephone at any time of the day or night; he was the one who would turn up and then leave when commanded; he was the one who did precisely what he was told and who never questioned her honesty. In other words, he was a devoted Man Friday. Colthurst had little to no personal knowledge of the Royal

Family, so his background and apparent devotion to the Princess led him blindly to believe everything she told him.

In 1986 Colthurst, who was in the process of renewing his platonic friendship with the Princess, found himself relaxing one day in the hospital canteen of St Thomas' in central London where he worked, having just escorted Diana on an official visit to open a new CT scanner in the X-ray department. There he met, by chance, the royal correspondent of the *Daily Mail*, Andrew Morton. Over tea and biscuits, it became clear to Morton that Colthurst was rather more to the Princess than a medic acting as her guide for the day. Morton attempted to befriend the doctor as a possible source of future royal stories. They became friendly and would play squash together on the hospital courts before indulging in large lunches at a nearby Italian restaurant.

In the meantime, Diana and the doctor were renewing their friendship with a succession of cheerful lunches, usually on Fulham Road. Colthurst noticed that the Princess would bolt down her food and then dash to the ladies – a classic feature of the binge–purge symptom that characterises bulimia nervosa. This was confirmed when Carolyn Bartholomew expressed concern to him about Diana's eating habits and they discussed the illness and its dire long-term effects. It was at this point that alarm bells might have been ringing in Colthurst's head. They certainly did in Ms Bartholomew's: it was apparently after this conversation that she decided to make her now famous threat – if Diana did not seek help, she would go to the media and tell them about her bulimia. However, it was an idle threat and I suspect the Princess knew that it was as she took no notice.

Diana's illness psychological, and was much more important to her future health and happiness than pretending that her problems were caused by an unhappy marriage. Many people endure unhappy marriages: they don't all suffer from horrible mood swings, violent rages, persecution complexes and schizophrenia while enjoying multiple affairs before imagining abandonment. It is a great shame that the help the Princess's friends gave was insufficient to deal with her real problems, assisting instead to explain them away or blaming everything on a state of domestic affairs about which they knew little other than what they had been told by a young woman who, by the very nature of her illness, found it hard to discern fact from fiction.

Moreover, and perhaps due to her illness, the Princess seemed to believe, like some extremely spoiled child, that only outrageous behaviour would get her the result she desired – but sometimes she didn't even seem to know herself what that result was. She told Colthurst at the time that she wanted to save her marriage, whereas she told the Archbishop of Canterbury that she didn't; she even told people like Patrick Jephson that she couldn't bear to be in the same room as Prince Charles, while telling Elsa Bowker that really Prince Charles wasn't to blame and that she couldn't help herself when a mood swing occurred.

These are the actions of a young woman in need of urgent help – a help that by now could only be given by friends who really cared about her. They would have probably failed, but at least they should have tried. Moreover, it should have been obvious that the state of the Princess's mind was somewhat disturbed, that her statements might not be one hundred per cent reliable. Colthurst and Morton, apparently did not see it that way.

In his 2004 book *Diana: In Pursuit of Love*, Morton, while admitting that the Princess had been less than honest with him, still clings to the original concept of why his 1992 book was written. He explains, 'By degrees Colthurst began to catch glimpses into the true nature of the life that Diana was trying to come to terms with. Her marriage had failed, and her husband was having an affair with Camilla Parker Bowles, the wife of his army-officer friend Andrew, but she was expected to keep up appearances, required by the Royal Family, and live a life of pretence.' Her living at Kensington Palace meant she was surrounded by courtiers who she felt preferred her to be seen – looking quintessentially attractive – and not heard. Her sense of claustrophobia was made worse by the fact that everyone from the Queen downwards, was somehow colluding in the duplicity. For Diana, conspiracies were not theories but her reality.

This statement is rendered of little value as much by what it fails to say as by the pathetic attempt to hold on to a view that was constructed by someone clearly suffering from paranoia. Indeed, Morton goes on to admit that at no point during the writing of *Diana: Her True Story* did the Princess admit to having any affairs – she even insisted that Hewitt was only a friend. Amazingly Colthurst and Morton appeared to give her the benefit of any doubt despite all the available evidence to the contrary, and took her word for it. Actually, as she was always going to have editorial control, they could hardly have done anything else. Morton recalls that despite her dependence on Colthurst, she did not tell him everything. 'While she was raging against her husband's infidelity she was hiding the fact that she had enjoyed a long if sporadic love affair with Captain James Hewitt from 1986 to 1990; and a dalliance with James Gilbey, who was later to be exposed as the male voice on the notorious "Squidgygate" tapes, a telephone conversation illicitly recorded over New Year 1989–1990.' In conversation with Colthurst, she would dismiss Hewitt merely as a friend, always speaking of him in less than flattering tones, until, that is, she needed Colthurst's help.

'The first indications of her relationship with James Hewitt, which was alluded to in a Sunday newspaper in 1991, came during the Gulf War when the dashing but indiscreet tank commander borrowed a news reporter's satellite phone in the Gulf to call the Princess at Kensington Palace. Diana was so alarmed by the prospect of Hewitt being confronted on his return from the war by newsmen who would link her romantically with him she asked Colthurst to draft a statement for Hewitt to read out to the media. "She was worried because she couldn't trust him to open his mouth and come out with joined-up sentences," Colthurst said. "Understandably, she was never explicit about the true nature of her relationship with him."

'Hewitt flatly turned down our request for the book and with Diana passing the relationship off as a friendship there was nowhere else to go with the story. We did not have the faintest inkling either about her infatuation with the art dealer Oliver Hoare who was the object of her love and devotion by early 1992.' For the Princess was never one to disclose absolutely everything, no matter how close individuals thought they were to her.

Notwithstanding that, twelve years later Mr Morton apparently still knows nothing of the Princess's relationships with Barry Mannakee or Philip Dunne, to name but two. Not only is Morton excusing himself for being so easily legged over, he makes a virtue out of the Princess's deviousness in the process. I can hardly image him being as kind to either the Queen or the Prince of Wales as he has been to the Princess and himself.

However, either unable to see this, or hoping that we wouldn't, Morton continues to explain how the book came into being: 'Dr Colthurst reminisced, "It was obvious that it was an issue that she had discussed with others and that it preyed constantly on her mind. The first and simplest solution was for Diana to confront her husband. But she had tried that ... she had seen the Queen who sympathised, had seen what was going on but had nothing to offer ... the second scenario was to continue her silence and seek psychiatric help. She had already tried that. The problem was that she knew that she wasn't ill ... no amount of psychiatric counselling would change the circle of deceit ... the third scenario was to go public and to reveal to the world what her life was truly like. But how could she smuggle her story out?"'

The thinking behind the three scenarios was of course essentially flawed. The first scenario was never going to work as the Princess knew perfectly well, even if Morton and Colthurst didn't, that the Prince was well aware that she had been a serial adulterer before he had been reunited with Mrs Parker Bowles. The Queen had refused to intervene because she now knew that both Charles and Diana were having affairs, as the Duke of Edinburgh's correspondence with the Princess proves. Therefore, as long as both remained private matters, she didn't intend to interfere or side with either. However, her daughter-in-law, with a typical lack of justice or realism, wanted the Queen to prevent her son from seeing his mistress while leaving her alone to enjoy her various affairs in private.

The second scenario is laughable, and the lamest of excuses is given for the third scenario being the only option. Colthurst claims that the Princess knew that she wasn't ill. In the history of mental illness surprisingly few people suffering from any form of it believe that they are actually mentally ill. Usually they – just like the Princess of Wales – believe themselves to be right and sane and the rest of the world wrong or insane.

So in the absence of wise counsel from Dr Colthurst, and in the face of the ambition of a man who wanted to reveal himself as a great investigative journalist, the plans were laid by the Princess to use these two men to deceive both the British people and the rest of the world. Eventually she and Colthurst came to the conclusion that she would have to choose between a series of newspaper articles, a radio or television interview or collaboration with someone on a biography. The articles were rejected on the grounds that while their contents would be sensational, their longevity would be limited, whereas the interview was rejected, as Diana believed that there was an incestuous relationship between Buckingham Palace and the BBC. This gave rise to fears of censorship or worse exposure. Therefore, the collaboration with a biographer was the chosen route.

The King and Di

To start with, Diana decided to initiate one or two sneaky leaks of confidential information from the Prince of Wales's office. She gave the information to James Colthurst and ordered him to pass it on to Andrew Morton. Morton used them effectively and the Princess was pleased. As a result, Morton was finally selected as the unofficial biographer of what was in fact to be her autobiography. However, before making the final approach to him, Colthurst asked the Princess if she really wanted to try again with Prince Charles. Later Colthurst was to recall, 'She was very clear and said, "Yes." That response conditioned my approach to the book.' Morton interpreted this to mean that Colthurst would always put Diana's well-being before any consideration concerning the book.

Did Colthurst and Morton really believe that the contents of the book they were going to publish were designed to help the Princess repair her marriage? And did not such a statement completely conflict with her other statements about wishing to escape with her sons from a dead marriage, or her constant refrain of 'I've had enough, I've really had enough.' And couldn't Colthurst see that such contradictions made by a woman whom he knew was suffering from bulimia should be questioned for the Princess's own sake, especially as he suspected that she wasn't always totally frank with him? Apparently not.

Morton continued that, 'In keeping with the undercover nature of the whole operation James and I met to discuss her thoughts in the incongruous surroundings of a working men's café in Ruislip, North West London, close to the place where he was, at the time, attending a course. What I heard changed my life for ever.' Colthurst tripped out some of the apparently alarming facts that made up the Princess's life. Morton, despite having worked closely with the Royal Family day after day for the last ten years, was amazed and somewhat bewildered that he had followed the royal couple around the world and had never once sniffed this story, which was apparently taking place under his very nose. Nevertheless, he was keen not to pass up on this incredible scoop.

However, Morton's American-born publisher Michael O'Mara was deeply sceptical when Morton reported these discussions to him. He demanded to meet Colthurst and, not unsurprisingly, asked him why the Princess, if she had been so very unhappy, always looked so radiantly happy in the thousands of photographs that had been taken of her in public. But in the end, O'Mara concluded that as Colthurst hadn't asked for any money (even though he was eventually to receive a small fortune for his part in the deception) he wasn't a con man and therefore there might just be some truth in his story. Consequently he insisted on a test: a tape recording of Diana's 'memoirs' would be made before the three of them met again.

So far Morton's publisher had come up with just two possibilities: either the Princess had said these things, or she hadn't. This was to be a recurring theme throughout the following scandal, encouraged by the Princess's insistence that she hadn't collaborated with Morton, but confused by her refusal to refute the contents of his book.

However, there was an obvious third possibility: that she held these views and had said these things, but that she was not being truthful. Given the unstable nature of her personality, the fact that Colthurst suspected she was being less than honest with him on certain issues and the fact that neither Morton nor the rest of the press had suspected any of this despite their constant attention, might not a real investigative journalist have smelled a rat? Morton didn't. So, armed with an old tape recorder and a list of questions prepared by Morton, Colthurst arrived at Kensington Palace in May 1991 for the first in a series of interviews that would continue through the summer and the following autumn. The great deception was underway.

Colthurst was immediately surprised by how 'well practised' the Princess's answers were, but nevertheless he was concerned for her, feeling that she needed to be protected most of all from herself, 'So in the early months there were several issues, such as suicide attempts, which I rather soft-pedalled on … her potential for taking her own life was always there.'

Here Colthurst finally damns himself in his own words: he knows the Princess has bulimia, he suspects she is not always honest, apparently she wants to save her marriage but he also believes she could be suicidal – and yet he continues to aid and abet her in a course of action that would eventually expose her to many people as a manipulative fraud, or a madwoman, or both. In addition her actions, which he apparently did nothing to arrest, would lead to a separation that she later claimed she did not want, a divorce that made her life even more miserable, and eventually a car ride that killed her. Of course neither Colthurst nor Morton could have predicted any of these events. With a friend like Colthurst and a conspirator like Morton, the Princess didn't need enemies, imagined or otherwise.

The King and Di

As 1991 progressed, the Princess got her secret scheme off the ground. The tape method that had been demanded by O'Mara as a test was used as the permanent method of creating the book. For obvious reasons Morton – a well-known royal hack – could not keep turning up at Kensington Palace, so it was decided to continue with Colthurst who, as a friend of Diana's, could. From Diana's point of view this tightened her creative control without having to meet with Morton directly, and yet she was, understandably, nervous of having Colthurst riding around London on his bike with these explosive tapes in his pocket. One day he was knocked off his cycle and came very close to spilling the beans.

In many ways, Colthurst was just the fall guy. He put Diana first before either his career or his personal life, and was permanently at her beck and call. His devotion to her, for whatever reason, was complete, and while he advised her very badly, he was, in his defence, no match for the wilful and manipulating Princess and does not seem to have initially sought any financial reward for his part in the deception. The question of Morton's role is not so clear. Was he a hack whose career was going nowhere and who just got lucky by having written about Diana and then getting to know Colthurst? Was he a man who was sensationally outwitted and manipulated by a dishonest princess? Or was he a man who went along with Princess Diana's story, suspecting that large parts of it were very unreliable but leaving that to her conscience? Either way, and especially since her death, he has been quite prepared to use her name in a strange cocktail of attempting to justify the account while at times pretending that there was no distortion of events at all, despite the evidence to the contrary.

As the Princess and her fellow conspirators were inventing their own Gunpowder Plot and were enjoying the intrigue as if they were acting out a James Bond story, the rest of the unsuspecting world went about its business. John Major, who had been prime minister for a little over a year, called an election for early April 1992. His Conservative government had come within three months of running a full five years in an attempt to regain popular support and win a fourth consecutive term in power. However, the Labour Party, with Neil Kinnock as its leader, was hot favourite as the campaign got underway. Indeed, they were so confident of victory that they kicked off with a victory-style rally in Sheffield several weeks before polling day. A reserved British electorate wasn't impressed.

'Honest John', as he was affectionately known by some of his party – a kind of backhanded compliment to a grey man who perhaps had more integrity and compassion than ability – rejected such an American presidential style. His approach was to concentrate on taking his soapbox into the towns and cities, getting on it and talking to the people. He was the sort of politician who was vastly more impressive in the flesh than he was on the television. He seemed taller and better looking, and more importantly his genuine interest in people shone through. A senior PR agent employed by the Tories at the time declared that if he could get John Major into every front room for just ten minutes, the prime minister would probably die in office. On the occasions that I met him, it occurred to me that this was a more sensible statement than it first sounded. Moreover, Major himself obviously took this advice seriously and decided to conduct an old-fashioned meet-the-people campaign as a result.

The Tories started to recover ground in the opinion polls, but still the pollsters gave them little chance as they believed the gap was too wide to narrow in a mere three weeks. However, little by little the gap was closed. On the eve of the election, Mr Murdoch, who would in later years be persuaded to support New Labour by Mr Blair in a media carve-up deal, must have smiled as his *Sun* newspaper featured Mr Kinnock's head as a light bulb accompanied by the headline 'IF KINNOCK WINS TODAY, WILL THE LAST PERSON TO LEAVE BRITAIN PLEASE TURN OUT THE LIGHTS'.

As the results started to come in, it became clear that Major would win with a reduced, but nevertheless clear, working majority. Honest John had pulled off a miracle and I suspect that his close friend the Prince of Wales was probably secretly pleased for him – even if he was far too professional to let it show.

The next morning the stock market shot up by over 200 points as the city demonstrated with glee its relief. Kinnock, having now lost two elections, resigned, and the Labour Party chose John Smith to lead them. Smith was a grey, decent man attempting to lead his party to an electable position further to the right, while Major was attempting to pull his party further left from the far right of Thatcherism. As a result, both wanted to sit in the middle ground of politics, and in reality their policies seemed to get closer and closer as the opposition started to jettison socialism because it was being told by bright young men like Tony Blair that the only way to get elected was to steal the Tory clothes. The Tories and the Labour Party started to sound like each other.

Thus the country, reassured that the election result must be OK if even the opposition was saying the same kind of things, went back to sleep, and a very quiet media period followed – so quiet that my own marriage breakdown hit the headlines with the *Daily Mail* and the *Sun* siding with my wife, while the ill-fated *Today* supported the young career woman with whom I was associated. A rather nasty game of domestic football was played – I seem to remember with my head being used as the ball – for a couple of weeks before Diana came to the rescue. The post-election peace was to be shattered by news that the Royal Family itself was collapsing...

During 1991 and the early part of 1992, *Diana: Her True Story* took shape. The modus operandi remained the same. Morton would try and focus the direction with questions and Diana would record her life on tape under such guidance: her life as she saw it was captured and then smartened up by her ghostwriter.

The Princess wanted the world to know that her childhood had been deeply traumatised by her parents' violent rows before Mummy 'legged it' and abandoned her. As a result she became an elective mute for a period and totally failed at school. She had always been attracted to Prince Charles, but he had married her purely for the purpose of providing a son and heir. He had never loved her and had continued his affair with Camilla Parker Bowles throughout their courtship, engagement and marriage. She had been forced to bring up her two sons single-handed as her husband was a cold, distant father who preferred polo and the company of his mistress to her and their children. He was a stiff, old-fashioned man who was obsessed by duty and was out of touch with modern British life, a man who had expressed bitter disappointment at the birth of their second son as he wanted a girl and, worse, the boy she produced had red hair. All of this was made even more intolerable by everyone from the Queen downwards taking Prince Charles's side, not appreciating her contribution to the royal image and conspiring behind her back to protect Camilla Parker Bowles and her relationship with the Princess's husband.

We now know that this strange cocktail of fact, partial fact, exaggerated fact, twisted fact and plain fiction does not stand up to any form of scrutiny. So how did Mr Morton, a brilliant investigative journalist according to his publisher, get it so wrong? Firstly, he did not research the book sufficiently; it was dictated by the Princess. Secondly, upon its completion, each chapter was delivered to her for scrutiny. Thirdly, as the spirit of the book was extremely underhand and Diana's involvement top secret, Morton had no way of verifying what Diana said other than reading any evidence she provided or talking to people she said he could talk to. She showed him some post-1986 letters from Camilla to Charles, which she had stolen from her husband's briefcase, and directed him towards people that she had primed. And in order to dispel the Hewitt question, she told Morton that he could approach him but then absolutely forbade Hewitt to tell her fellow conspirator anything. This was Diana at her animal-cunning best and Morton, whether he knew it or not, was being duped.

So Morton saw some recent love letters from Camilla and talked to some of the Princess's friends, who told him that Diana had also told them the same stories. Amazingly, he took this to confirm their validity. It apparently did not occur to him that none of her friends could verify any of it in their own right as they had not been there, nor that Prince Charles might have gone back to Camilla as a result of his wife's own infidelities and vile behaviour. All the evidence was there.

Morton could have properly verified everything. Indeed, it would have made the whole scam seem more realistic and the Princess's actual involvement less likely. However, Diana would never have allowed this as it would have thrown up many more awkward questions than provided pleasant confirmations, and the real truth would almost certainly have raised its ugly head. Morton therefore had no choice but to accept that he was a sort of ghostwriter. The Princess dictated what went into the book and edited out anything that she didn't like. Given Diana's state of mind, this meant that the work roamed into areas of spite and fantasy.

As time moved on, the Princess became increasingly edgy. She was desperate to get her version of her life on to the streets, but equally she was petrified that her involvement might be found out. She wanted her version of her life to be believed, but hadn't the courage to put her name to it, not least because she was well aware that large parts of it were simply untrue: if someone popped up to confront anyone, they would have to confront Morton and not her. This put her fellow conspirators out on a limb and made life difficult for them at times. For example, when Colthurst, Morton and O'Mara took Camilla's letters to a leading libel lawyer, they were duly treated with some distaste and told that they were insufficient evidence to prove that the Prince and Camilla were actually lovers. The Princess flew into a furious rage when she learned this: her daring act of theft had been in vain. Nevertheless, the lawyers said that if Morton described the relationship of Prince Charles and Mrs Parker Bowles as a 'close friendship' often enough, readers would assume that they were lovers.

Just before Christmas 1991, Morton claims that Patrick Jephson added to all the pressure by telling Diana that the 'men in the grey suits' knew about the book and her involvement in it. This is unlikely, as not only did the book take both the Prince's staff, Buckingham Palace and the government completely by surprise when it was eventually published, it also caught Jephson off guard – otherwise why was he, as we shall later see, surprised when she refused to sign a joint statement with the Prince refuting the book's content. And the fact that Colthurst, Morton, O'Mara and the Princess – hardly the KGB – could write this book by dictating it at Kensington Palace and discussing it on their mobiles and landlines and remain completely undetected goes along way to dispelling all the ridiculous and paranoid conspiracy theories with which Diana loved to fill her head and which have grown to idiotic proportions since her death. By this time the Princess of Wales believed that everyone's mind worked just like hers; she thought up new conspiracy theories daily – it would have been absurdly amusing if it hadn't been so sad.

The book gradually became a race against time for a number of reasons. Sarah Ferguson was secretly seeing her American lover, Steve Wyatt, in Texas. She wanted out of her marriage and thought it might be a good idea for Diana to jump ship with her – but if she didn't, would Diana look after the Princesses Eugenie and Beatrice for her? Diana's fellow conspirators could see that either way, the Duchess of York's influence could have a bad effect on the Princess, and thus damage the smooth passage of the book in some way.

Moreover, Diana was becoming increasingly worried that she was losing ground in a largely imagined PR war with her husband's camp and the Palace. The feeling was made a lot worse when in February 1992 Lady Colin Campbell published a book called *Diana in Private: The Princess Nobody Knows*. Neither Prince Charles nor the Palace had assisted the author in any way, but the book had been apparently well researched by a woman who had access to many at court. She took the view that any problem with the Waleses' marriage should be laid at Diana's door; much worse, she strongly hinted that the Princess had romantic interests with other men. This was what Diana had always feared – the real story getting out before her propaganda did. She was both furious and extremely concerned. Ironically, Lady Colin Campbell, while only touching the tip of the iceberg, was at least investigating the right iceberg, whereas Morton, wittingly or otherwise, was at the wrong pole. What the brilliant investigative journalist also didn't know was that a great amount of Lady Colin's information had come from Diana herself. The Princess neglected to tell anyone that she had gone to Lady Colin first with the idea of her 'true story'.

Originally, Lady Colin Campbell had approached the Princess in order to write a book about Diana's charity work. The Princess seemed to like the idea. But by August 1990 she had changed her mind and wanted Lady Colin to write a different story. 'Had Diana told me that she wanted me to produce a panegyric, I would have turned her down cold. However, she did not. She led me to believe she wanted me to "write the truth of my life," to quote her. "The fairytale is killing me," she said, "If I don't escape from it, I'll die." I agreed to write what became *Diana in Private* on those conditions, thinking that I would have the liberty of producing a balanced account of her life. Only later, after contracts were signed, did I appreciate that we had misunderstood one another's positions. She did not want a truthful account of her life, but a heavily slanted version with which she could gain a separation from Prince Charles, whereas I told her, "I'm not about to trash your husband when he doesn't deserve it."'

Unsurprisingly this caused the Princess to fly into a rage: she and Lady Colin parted company and didn't speak again for three years, by which time Morton had become 'a creep' in the Princess's mind – someone to be blamed for a book that she no longer liked.

Not long after learning about the impending publication of Lady Colin's book, Diana also became aware that it was to be serialised in the *Sun*. This could not only seriously damage her reputation; it could also render her largely imagined version of events useless. Urgent action was called for. Morton recalls, 'The Princess immediately passed on her fury to James Colthurst, who phoned me on the "scrambler". I too was deeply concerned but, as I told James, there was little I could do – the only thing that could remove Lady Colin's version of events from the front pages would be an even bigger royal story and there were none available (that is, not until my book arrived in June). Colthurst relayed the information to Diana, who to my astonishment instantly provided the blockbuster story we required. She had recently learned that Fergie had visited the Queen to talk about a separation from Prince Andrew; after much discussion the Queen had agreed that a separation was the best option in the circumstances.

'When Colthurst passed the story on to me I was dumbfounded. I had not dreamed for a minute that a royal scoop to blow away Lady Colin's account could materialise – but here it was in spades. I duly wrote the front-page story for the *Daily Mail*, which the Queen's press secretary, Charles Anson, later described as "inch perfect". As we had nail-bitingly hoped, Lady Colin Campbell's Diana stories were submerged by the new feeding frenzy in the tabloids.'

Sarah Ferguson thought the Palace had leaked her unhappy news. 'They needed to send a warning to Diana, to keep her in the fold and shore up the monarchy. My public vivisection would be a pointed reminder: "This is what happens if you cross us." (They did indeed scare the daylights out of my sister-in-law, who was now afraid to be seen with me, and I could not blame her.)' Poor Sarah, she had no idea that here was another Palace conspiracy dreamed up by Diana: it was she who had shopped Fergie and that was why the Princess suddenly didn't want to see her sister-in-law out of pure guilt. Eventually, Sarah worked it all out. She later commented, 'I had no idea that she was using me.' But she was rightly very angry when she did, and stopped speaking to her sister-in-law.

It is most interesting that Morton sees himself as Diana's spin-doctor rather than an investigative journalist. Laughably he adds, 'Our main objective, however, was to ensure that the book measured up to Anson's assessment of the article – that it reflected Diana's life, both in words and in pictures, as accurately as possible.' We now know that not only did Mr Morton's book bear very little resemblance to Diana's life, but also even now he has failed to correct his errors in the face of the facts and simply ignores elements of her life. He remains a spin-doctor, a mere tool in the Princess's great deception. Perhaps as a result of the enormous boost to both his professional status and financial security, he has sought to hide behind the mirage and preserve as much of her deception as possible.

His book *Diana: Her True Story – In Her Own Words* not only confirms her deception but also the fact that the Princess was devious, dishonest and mentally unstable. It did perhaps more harm to her reputation by allowing the world to see through the mirage to the real Diana than any fair-minded book that sought to correct the inaccuracies of his original work. By using her own words it confirmed her as a liar. Morton has done more to expose the Princess's fallibilities since her death by allowing the world to read the transcripts of the original tapes.

As the manuscript was finalised, Diana and her fellow conspirators, having survived thus far undetected, now had to ensure that the book was serialised, or it would just disappear. The conspirators knew that with Diana refusing to put her name to the book it would be dismissed as pure tabloid rubbish unless a serious newspaper could be persuaded to put their name to it. However, neither the *Daily Mail* nor the *Sunday Times*, the two best vehicles, were interested. Andrew Neil, editor of the *Sunday Times*, was particularly opposed to the idea, having been previously criticised by both readers and executives for serialising an earlier royal effort of Morton's that was considered to be lightweight.

They decided to ask Diana's friend Angela Serota to speak to her friend and Neil's boss, Andrew Knight, the CEO of News International, and assure him that the book was authentic and met with Diana's approval. This did the trick and the *Sunday Times* changed its mind.

Just before the serialisation started in June, Murdoch rang Neil from New York to warn him of the forthcoming onslaught from the Establishment. 'Be careful: they are not nice people and you are about to become their number-one enemy.' He was right about the number-one enemy bit. When the first instalment appeared, the Archbishop of Canterbury warned about the damage to the boys, something their mother had failed to consider in her self-obsession; the Labour politician Peter Mandelson complained that the book was 'scurrilous' and that there were 'no longer any boundaries between fact and fiction'. These were but two of the typical comments as the great and the good lined up to heap criticism on the book. Max Hastings tore Andrew Neil limb from limb on Radio 4's *Today* programme, adding that the story was 'a deluge of rubbish and a farrago of invention' that lacked a 'single reliable fact'.

Following Neil's mauling, he started to wobble and phoned Morton for help. He had to take on Lord St John of Fawsley on the ITV lunchtime news and wanted to avoid being humiliated again. He told Morton that he needed more ammunition to back up his paper's position. It was decided that James Gilbey, whom – unknown to Morton – the Princess had added to her list of lovers, should be asked to issue a supporting statement. Happily for the conspirators he agreed. Morton cobbled together something to the effect that the Princess had often told Gilbey about her suicide attempts, and that he had seen fit to tell Morton this in an interview that he had given freely and for which he had not received any payment.

Neil wasn't the only one wobbling like a jelly in a high wind. Diana, whose devious little plan had now escalated into a national scandal, had experienced a bad weekend. Prince Charles had received a faxed copy of the article on Sunday morning at Highgrove. Although he had known about the forthcoming serialisation, the contents of episode one were far worse than he could ever have imagined. He was understandably horrified and immediately went back upstairs to confront his wife. She denied any involvement and, feigning extreme offence at the accusation, burst into tears, dressed and left for London. The Prince was confused. He wanted to believe the Princess in her adamant denial, but on the other hand Morton had been so true to Diana's tapes that he couldn't help but notice that some of the expressions used were typical of her and perhaps only her. He was later to tell a friend, 'She says that it has absolutely nothing to do with her. I want to believe her, but when I read the article I can hear her voice.'

Murdoch, with typical cynicism, having allowed the *Sunday Times* to run the serialisation, now decided to back both horses. *The Times* was amazingly unconvinced about the veracity of the book, and ran the headline: 'ROYAL BOOK SERIAL PROVOKES DISTASTE'. Harrods, major bookshops such as Hatchards in London and James Thin in Edinburgh, as well as supermarkets such as Tesco and scores of independents throughout the land, refused to stock the book.

In the run up to the serialisation, the chairman of the Press Complaints Commission, Lord McGregor, had come under intense pressure from politicians and members of the public alike urging him to condemn mounting press speculation about the state of the Waleses' marriage as rival publications desperately tried to spoil the *Sunday Times*' big scoop prior to the publication of episode one. On Monday, 8 June, the PCC responded by preparing a press statement denouncing this 'odious exhibition of journalists dabbling their fingers in the stuff of other people's souls in a manner which adds nothing to legitimate public interest in the situation of the heir to the throne'. McGregor rang

Sir Robert Fellowes and read him the statement before adding that he had heard rumours that the Princess had either directly or indirectly collaborated with Morton. Fellowes, having read the article the previous day, had already confronted his sister-in-law. She had vehemently denied any involvement, just as she had to her husband. Accordingly Sir Robert gave, in good faith, his assurance that she hadn't been involved, and so the PCC's statement was issued.

Now some of Diana's friends were panicking. It was all very well for the Princess: she was tucked up behind large palace gates while the wrath of the media and an infuriated public bore down on their private homes. Many now feared that she was having second thoughts and would sit back and just leave them exposed to the media's mercy. Following many tearful telephone calls, when not all were convinced by Diana's rather glib assurances that the pressure would ease once Morton was out promoting the book, it was decided that something would have to be done. She suddenly realised that if just one cracked under the pressure and gave the game away, she was done for.

So the Princess had to find a way of giving the public a sign that she stood by what her friends had apparently told Morton, without giving the impression that she had encouraged Morton, let alone collaborated with him. It was OK if the nation thought that here was a brave little trouper who had suffered in silence and whose close friends couldn't bear to see her pain any longer without speaking out; it was not OK if they believed that the Princess had not only been involved but had actually masterminded the whole project.

Princess Diana knew that that would be a disaster for her image, as she would be seen as having behaved in a devious and dishonest fashion – which of course she had. Worse, as a result there would be serious questions asked about the accuracy of the book, and the long-term damage to the Princess would be enormous. This is what worried her – not the trouble she would get into with the Establishment, as was so often promoted by writers like Morton. Just like many people suffering from her condition, she was frightened of being found out, as she would then be forced by others to confront her dishonesty – something she had never forced herself to do.

The conspirators decided that, although it was not without some risk, the Princess would have to be seen publicly with one of her friends who had cooperated with Morton. It was decided that the obvious choice was Carolyn Bartholomew, as Diana was due to visit her and her husband William at their Fulham home anyway. Diana lost her nerve and wanted to pull out, but Carolyn, backed by Colthurst, managed to convince her that it was absolutely imperative she pulled herself together and kept the appointment. The Princess, like her mother, was fond of portraying herself as a strong and brave woman. However, in both their cases the reality was somewhat different: both women were more likely to run away rather than face the music in a crisis.

Morton and Colthurst had quite rightly realised that a photograph of Diana embracing Carolyn said vastly more about the authenticity of the book than anything Andrew Neil or Morton himself could ever say. Reluctantly, and apparently having forgotten how much her friends had risked on her behalf, the Princess agreed to take the chance. On Wednesday, 10 June, Morton called Stuart Higgins, the deputy editor of the *Sun*, which was due, as another Murdoch newspaper, to serialise the book after the *Sunday Times*. He told him to send a couple of discreet photographers to Carolyn's home where they would be able to get some very interesting shots. Throughout the day, the Princess remained very fearful of going, and it wasn't until seven in the evening that she left to make the journey. At that time, Morton got a frantic phone call from William Bartholomew to say that he had walked up and down his road a couple of times and was sure that there were no photographers around. Morton couldn't get hold of Higgins, but desperate measures were called for. He picked up the phone again and this time called his old colleague from his days at the *Daily Star*, Ken Lennox, who was by now at the *Sun*'s rival, the *Daily Mirror*. This was a very risky thing to do, not because Lennox couldn't be trusted, but because it wouldn't take a bright journalist too long to put two and two together and come up with the fact that as this was a surreptitious photo opportunity, Diana, famous for tipping off the press, was behind it, its message, and also the book. Morton had not consulted the Princess, who would more than likely have turned the car round and gone home.

Lennox only lived in nearby Chelsea and was there in good time to photograph the Princess as she embraced both Carolyn and William before leaving. The photographs bear all the signs of being staged-managed. In one, William is looking pointedly into the camera instead of at Diana as the Princess kisses his cheek; in another, the couple's son, dressed in his pyjamas, points at the cameraman as Diana starts to walk away. It is amazing that no bright journalist realised that the

Princess had tipped the press off herself. However, they didn't, and another mini crisis had been averted.

That night Lennox resisted the *Mirror* editor's pressure, as he demanded to know who had tipped him off. Lennox refused to tell Richard Stott, who the next day called in their own royal correspondent, James Whitaker. Stott was more than a little keen to find out what was really going on, as he had relied on the Princess's comment to photographer Kent Gavin that she had 'absolutely not' cooperated with Morton, and had run a headline to say as much. Now he felt exposed. Later he was to say that, in hindsight, as Diana had said she wasn't, he should have known that she was.

For his part, Lennox would never tell anyone who tipped him off, and many writers went on to make numerous claims that it was a woman with a smart voice, perhaps even Diana herself. All Lennox would tell people was, 'Well, only I know who phoned me – and I'm not telling you!'

Whitaker, who had been taken to task for missing out on the scoop of identifying Diana as Charles's latest girl all those years ago, was once again on the back foot. Stott again demanded to know where Lennox's tip-off came from. 'He hasn't got any royal contacts,' protested the portly correspondent.

'Well, he seems to have one more than you,' replied Stott tartly. Even this sarcastic comment didn't jolt the veteran reporter into any action, and the true nature of what had happened remained secret. In fairness to Whitaker, none of his colleagues did any better. One can't help but think that if they had all spent years trying to investigate and write true stories as opposed relying on tip-offs from people like the Princess, their ability wouldn't have been found to be so wanting at this moment. Without the conspiracy being exposed, the photograph of the Princess with Carolyn did the trick and the flow of unrestrained criticism was slowed.

Diana might have got away with it with the public, but she was summoned nevertheless to see her brother-in-law Sir Robert Fellowes, who was starting to understand what was going on. He seriously admonished her for the visit to the Bartholomews' home. Then she left for a visit to Liverpool where a woman in the crowd stroked her cheek and the Princess started to cry. Morton years later dismissed what turned out to be just another devious act as merely being clever: 'As ever, Diana had been much cleverer than anyone truly suspected, her tears to some extent premeditated. While she had given her friends support, through her show of tears in Liverpool she had also distanced herself from the book while winning over public sympathy.' Of course he was right: this was typical Diana.

However, all of the Princess's theatrics would have counted for nothing if Michael O'Mara hadn't bought off another of her friends who seemed intent upon something close to blackmail. O'Mara received a call from a man acting for photographer Terence Donovan, who was a friend of the Princess. The man explained that a picture of Diana used by the *Sunday Times* and attributed to Patrick Demarchelier had in fact been taken by Donovan, who had not given his permission for its inclusion. He now wanted £70,000. O'Mara explained that it had been an innocent error, but this was immediately rejected. It was pointed out to O'Mara that Donovan had given the picture personally to Diana and that unless his very high price was met – the normal cost of using a photograph for a book then was a mere £500 – legal action would follow before a revelation to the world's press of who had supplied the picture to the publishers.

One silly error by the normally impeccably dishonest Princess was about to prove her complicity. Once again Diana had lain down with dogs and was about to get fleas.

It was a worrying time for O'Mara. On the one hand he wanted his author to be seen as having pulled off a masterly piece of journalism and be vindicated so that the book would sell and sell. He also didn't want his publishing house associated with the dishonesty of a deliberate conspiracy. On the other hand, £70,000 was a large sum to find, and if serialisation was not forthcoming and the book flopped, it might not be earned back. There was a standoff, during which O'Mara even contemplated getting staff to remove the wretched photograph from the printed copies of the book by the use of razor blades. In the end, he yielded to Donovan and paid him a five-figure sum that granted permission for the photograph's use.

As letters of support started to flow in from a deceived public, and the Eating Disorders Association reported that there had been an increase in people contacting them for help, the conspirators congratulated each other that this was due to the fact that the Princess had been courageous enough to make public her private difficulties. But of course she hadn't. She was still sticking to the story that she had nothing to do with the book. If the Princess had written an accurate account of her life, explained about her eating disorder and had been brave enough to put her name to it, this would have been very courageous indeed. But she hadn't done that: instead she had written a largely fictitious account of her life, had not been brave enough to put her name to it, and blamed everybody from her parents onward for her own failings.

The success of the Carolyn Bartholomew photograph did more than just silence the attacks on Diana's friends; it also helped the *Sunday Times* and silenced the PCC. On the same Monday that Max Hastings had savaged a troubled Andrew Neil, whose defence was to invite Hastings to deny the strength of his sources, Morton had been obliged to appear on the ITN and keep his promise to the Princess of Wales to lie about her involvement. He told millions that the Princess hadn't helped him in any way. As a result, the Palace and the PCC seemed vindicated, and that had only caused the *Sunday Times* to be exposed to even more vilification as their decision to run the serialisation was completely ridiculed.

The following day, Andrew Knight, knowing that he had to pull a rabbit out of the hat and having already played his part in the Diana and Carolyn photo plot through his connection with Andrew Neil, duly contacted Lord McGregor. He later recalled that, 'I did write probably a rather pompous letter to him saying, "Look, we know that this book is true and moreover we know that it does have the willing sanction of the Princess of Wales." And he rang me and we had a conversation about it, which he was surprised by. "Well," Lord McGregor said, "I don't believe you, Mr Knight." So I said to him, "Well, look, Lord McGregor, if you don't believe me, just look at tomorrow's newspapers, because in tomorrow's newspapers will be reported an event which has not yet happened. Later today the Princess of Wales is going to visit Carolyn Bartholomew, who's one of the sources for the book, and that story will be reported with photographs in tomorrow's tabloid newspapers." And he said, "How extraordinary. I'm amazed."'

When all of this came true on the following day, McGregor understandably felt very let down. He could hardly hide his anger because he knew those around Diana had wilfully misled him, and the fact that it seemed the Palace press office had also misled the media only made matters worse. But his greatest anger was reserved for Sir Robert Fellowes, who had given him personal assurances that his sister-in-law had nothing to do with the book.

This now appeared to be a dreadful deception that had made the PCC look ridiculous. Lord McGregor rang Lord Wakeham, the leader of the House of Lords, and Lord Mackay, the Lord Chancellor, and asked them to ensure that the government intervened to stop this awful downward spiral of relations with the media. By this time, Diana's desire to have a domestic dig at her husband and his family was becoming something of a constitutional crisis. As a result, Wakeham phoned Sir Robert who was with the Queen on an official visit to Paris. By now Sir Robert had realised that his sister-in-law had lied to him. Her word was worthless, and he was truly embarrassed. Being a man of great integrity, he rang Lord McGregor immediately, offered his profuse apologies and promised that he had given his word in good faith. Lord McGregor accepted this apology, believing now that Sir Robert was just another of Diana's victims.

Fellowes was so mortified by what had happened that, as further evidence surfaced about the Princess's involvement with the book, he offered his resignation to the Queen. However, Her Majesty quite rightly believed that Sir Robert had only acted in good faith and refused to accept it. Later in 1993, he also offered his apologies to the Prince of Wales, who with characteristic good grace, especially as he and Fellowes had not always seen eye to eye, accepted. Lord McGregor might have genuinely forgiven Fellowes, but the whole episode had deeply upset him. One of his colleagues at the PCC, David Chipp, commented that he didn't think he was ever quite the same again.

Andrew Knight now looks back on that time with mixed feelings: 'I had second thoughts when my mother cried when we ran this book, and I realised that we'd hurt her and millions like her. And yet I knew it was true. And for that reason I also felt hurt that good people – because I think the Prince of Wales and the Princess of Wales are good people – I felt hurt that they were hurt.' The likeable Mr Knight gets close to admitting that he might have made a mistake – something very rare in the newspaper world. Nevertheless, and I can only assume in all innocence, he was still confusing authenticity with truth. He should have said that he knew that the book was authentic, because he certainly didn't know that it was true.

Lord McGregor was also to reflect later that, 'I felt as I have always felt, that the protection of the privacy of public persons turns in part on their prudence, and the observance of proper standards of behaviour and partly on their truthfulness. And I felt that in this particular instance, on all those counts, there had been a serious failure.' These are strong words of criticism; some have said they are unnecessarily harsh and only so because his Lordship was so bitter. I do not agree. The Princess had actively sought the help of a journalist in order to deceive the world by writing a fictitious account of her life and had then attempted to cover up her involvement. She had done so in order to serve serious and unwarranted character assassinations on many people, including the heir to the British throne. With typical hypocrisy, she expected the PCC to protect her from articles that she saw as invasions of her privacy – ones that she hadn't had a hand in manipulating – while she expected to get away with this sort of shabby and underhand behaviour herself.

Not long after the serialisation, a PCC report into the affair was leaked. It quite rightly concluded that Diana had been guilty of invading her own privacy. From now on she could expect very little sympathy and not too much protection from a PCC that was thereafter sceptical of any complaints she made as it had serious doubts about her ability to tell the truth.

On 5 July, Diana's masseur Stephen Twigg got in on the act telling the *Sunday Express*, 'The situation has to end ... otherwise there will be a tragedy.' The Prince read the article over breakfast, before asking Diana if she actually knew anyone who wasn't talking to the press on a daily basis. His feelings of betrayal must have been immense. It was not just the one-sided bias, the exaggerations or even the out and out lies, but the lengths that the Princess had gone to in order to distort the truth.

By now, the Prince must have understood the extent of his wife's treachery, and it must have been very difficult for him to confront the fact that he was married to a woman who seemed hell-bent on destroying him and the monarchy by employing any dishonest tactic at her means, and without the slightest regard for their children in the process. At the same time, even some of Diana's circle of conspirators was starting to have second thoughts, realising that this was a scandal they wished they hadn't got involved in. Before the final decision had been taken to go ahead with the Morton book, Diana was starting to have doubts herself. Colthurst, who at this point seemed determined to push her into it for reasons best known to him, came up with yet another piece of strange advice.

He suggested that perhaps the Princess should consult an astrologer to see what sort of reaction the public and the Royal Family would have to the book. Diana had for many years been an avid reader of star-sign predictions at the back of the magazines. She took to the idea immediately, but realised that she could hardly visit one of her regulars as they might blow the whistle on her. Luckily, Colthurst just happened to have a friend who was an astrologer. His name was Felix Lyle. Diana consulted him and on the back of that consultation the decision to proceed was finally taken. Lyle was to continue to be in the inner circle throughout the planning and writing of the book. But after he saw what had happened, he had some regrets: 'I think that it satisfied her need for revenge; it undoubtedly showed the Royal Family in a very unfavourable light and to a lot of people this was long overdue. I just felt it didn't get to the heart of it. I felt it had too much of an axe to grind, to be honest, and part of me felt a bit ashamed of that actually, and I just felt that maybe I should have rethought my strategy originally.'

Morton and O'Mara's initial reaction to the Princess's tale had been sceptical. Morton, as a royal correspondent of ten years' standing, had wondered if there wasn't something slightly Walter Mitty about the story that Colthurst had told him. O'Mara had insisted that the Princess commit some of it to tape before he proceeded. When the book was published, and especially before they knew of her involvement, this was also the general reaction of Diana's more sensible friends who hadn't been part of the deception. The vast majority of these people, who had known her as a child, teenager and even as a young married woman, didn't recognise her as this doomed, deeply unhappy, downtrodden person. Her close friend Janet Filderman spoke for them when she insisted, 'I know from Diana herself that she wasn't as unhappy as the book purported her to be. It made it seem as though she was in misery all those years, and it wasn't true, because I knew her in those years, very closely and very well. It's exactly what would happen in any marriage if you take the wife's and the husband's side totally separately. You will go one way or t'other, and I think that is what it was all about.'

Unfortunately, the Princess hadn't sought the advice of Filderman or her loyal society friends. Lord Palumbo confirms that those known to him would have decidedly advised her against doing such a book if she had ever asked them: 'If she'd come to somebody like me or others and said, "Do you think we should do this, do you think this book is a good idea?" we would've all said, "No" – or I would've anyway – and that was not what she wanted to hear. So she went ahead anyway because she was an instinctive creature.'

Even Diana herself had eventually had second thoughts, and she was continually to tell people over the last years of her life that Morton had damaged her relationship with many people, the most important of whom was her eldest son who quite rightly had been horrified by the whole affair. This seems to me to be a very harsh judgement on a man who merely wrote what he was told to. Unashamedly, she was proclaiming that he had got it all wrong just before her death, when she also claimed that she had known that the Prince of Wales had loved her when he married her and that it was ridiculous to suggest otherwise.

However, not all of her more intelligent friends saw it quite that way. David Puttnam defies Diana's statements to others when he claims that she never regretted her involvement in the book. He was to tell Morton, 'She owned what she had done. She knew what she was doing and took a calculated risk even though she was scared shitless. But I never heard one word of regret, I promise you. With all her faults she was a good woman.'

After a jittery start, *Her True Story* became the second best-selling British book of the 1990s. *In Her Own Words* was the best-selling book of 1997 as Morton and his publishers couldn't resist cashing in on her death. Millions of copies of both versions and his sequel *Diana: Her New Life* have been sold worldwide, and *Her True Story* has been translated into more than thirty-five languages. As a result of this stunning publishing success, Andrew Morton received numerous awards, among them Author of the Year, Investigative Journalist of the Year and Scoop of the Year, as well as a special award for services to journalism.

However the Princess came to view the book, the damage it did to the Prince's reputation could scarcely have been greater. It was made worse by reports that friends of the Prince had been emulating friends of the Princess by briefing the press against her. There is very little evidence to support these claims, and it seems likely that it was just part of the spin being put about by Diana and her supporters to excuse their continuing devious behaviour. In some cases this would appear to have worked, as many biographers, including the open-minded Clayton and Craig, seem to have accepted her camp's explanation of this. But the actual evidence suggests that such claims were a myth, an effective tactic created by the Princess that would help excuse her if she was found out as she could then claim that she was only fighting fire with fire.

All the Prince's friends, however, knew that it was a fundamental rule of their relationship with the Prince that nobody was ever to talk to the press without his consent, which was not usually given – and certainly not during these troubled times. One or two may have broken this rule, but I have found no evidence to this effect and I have discovered a lot to the contrary.

There was supposed to have been a widely reported conversation between Lord Rothermere, the owner of Associated Newspapers, and Lord McGregor, during which Rothermere was supposed to have claimed that both the Prince and the Princess had sought to use national newspapers to get across their side of the marital nightmare. How this came to be reported is not clear to me, but later Lord Rothermere was to repudiate it anyway. And other than this, the PCC has never been offered any information to suggest that either the Prince or any of his friends sought to use the media against the Princess.

However, none of this was that clear at the time and the rumours appeared to be correct when an article appeared in the *Sunday Times* after Morton's serialisation had concluded. It was entitled 'THE CASE FOR CHARLES' and claimed to contain input from many of his close confidants such as Patricia Brabourne, King Constantine of Greece and the Diana-disliking Romseys. The article claimed that it had sought these people's help to present the 'other side' of the Waleses' marriage. The claim was completely misleading, which was eventually admitted by senior Murdoch executives.

What had actually happened was that Andrew Knight had met Charles's cousin Norton Romsey during a test match against Pakistan at Lord's cricket ground. They had a private conversation, during which Norton Romsey expressed his dismay at how shabbily the *Sunday Times* had treated the heir to the throne. He told Knight that the Morton book was biased, in many cases inaccurate and gave a very unfair impression of Prince Charles. Knight, perhaps because he was still aware of how upset his mother had been by Morton and impressed by the genuine anger displayed by Romsey, returned to his office and repeated the gist of the conversation. However, he insisted that if a reporting team was assigned to the story, it could only proceed if, and only if, Romsey and other close friends of the Prince agreed to talk to them. By this time several of the Prince's friends had already contacted Aylard and asked for permission to speak out against the lies in the Morton book and put the record straight. Aylard, on behalf of the Prince, made it perfectly clear that if they wanted to help Prince Charles they must remain silent and not say anything about the marriage or the Princess. The Prince believed that to do so would only make a terrible situation worse. It was bad enough that the Princess was employing such unreasonable gutter tactics; for him to be seen joining her would not help the position.

Richard Aylard had become a late convert himself to his master's opinion. On the eve of the serialisation of the Morton book, Buckingham Palace had an inkling, not least from the heavy advertising campaign being run by the *Sunday Times*, that this book was not going to be fair to the Prince of Wales. Aylard consulted the Queen's assistant private secretary, Robin Janvrin, and came to the conclusion that the Prince could no longer stay silent as the media unfairly tore his reputation to pieces. Charles was initially unsure that this was a very good idea, but was eventually persuaded by Aylard that he had no alternative, so Aylard drafted a statement that the book was in many ways inaccurate and distorted to the point of fabrication. It stated that the Prince and Princess both regretted its publication, which could damage their family life and make the carrying out of joint official duties all the more difficult. However, when Jephson and Philip Mackie read the statement to the Princess, she stated that the book wasn't inaccurate and refused to put her signature to anything that said it was. As a result the statement wasn't released.

This was an amazing slip by the Princess: she wasn't supposed to know what was or wasn't in the book as it was not yet available in the shops, and as only the first part had been serialised, she could not have known that the whole book was accurate. Some at Buckingham Palace took this to be pretty conclusive evidence that she had, directly or indirectly, collaborated with Morton on the book. Unfortunately for him, this did not at that time include Sir Robert Fellowes.

Now the Prince's original opinion was reinforced. Everyone should say nothing – as one of his closest friends was to note at the time, 'He wants all of us to say NOTHING and nothing is what we will say.'

Thus, when a reporter from the *Sunday Times* telephoned all of the Prince's friends, they all refused to comment. A senior executive at the paper was later to admit that the reporter couldn't get a single quote. He went on to say that, 'My impression was that they were all under instructions not to talk.' Andrew Neil, not exactly known to be a friend of the monarchy, nevertheless confirmed this saying, 'We did have terrible problems because we were led to believe that Charles had put the word out that he did not want his friends to reply because it would be seen as retaliation.'

However, despite this wall of silence, and against the instructions of Andrew Knight, the article went ahead based simply on his exchange of confidences with Romsey at a cricket match. Now Knight realised what it was like to be a victim of the inventive Murdoch press himself, and he was deeply embarrassed. More seriously, and quite understandably, the article gave exactly the impression that the Prince had wished to avoid – namely that he was involved with the Princess in a mud-slinging competition backed up by their respective private armies of friends.

This was made worse by Penny Junor, a balanced writer who saw the injustice of Charles's position. Her 1991 book *Charles and Diana: Portrait of a Marriage* concluded that the marriage, as a working partnership, was a healthy one. On 6 July 1992, the *Today* newspaper published a four-page article by her under the headline 'CHARLES: HIS TRUE STORY'. The paper claimed that Junor had been contacted by a circle of his friends determined to put the record straight. No doubt they would have loved to line up to do exactly that, but the Prince had forbidden them to do so. Although the article was entirely sympathetic to the Prince and a lot more truthful than Morton's book, he was nevertheless furious when he read it, especially with Romsey whom he now suspected – this article having followed the one in the *Sunday Times* – of being the prime suspect. The Prince once more instructed Aylard to ask his friends to keep silent and remember the effect this would all be having on his sons.

Until the publication of the Morton book, the Prince had taken the view that his marriage, although not a loving one, would survive. It certainly was not what he had expected when he had asked the bouncy, friendly girl who apparently loved anything he liked and seemed devoted to him to accept his hand; but they did have two wonderful children, and they owed it to them and to the nation to keep the marriage going. Moreover, although they hadn't been domestically very close for some years, they had still managed to do a good job together on foreign tours. He hoped that they would be able to rekindle a good friendship. Even after the serialisation of the book in the *Sunday Times*, he rather foolishly clung to the idea that she was innocent of any collaboration in such malice. He was hoping that such vile rubbish had been uttered by her silly 'Sloane' friends. It was only when Sir Robert Fellowes apologised for misleading the PCC and offered his resignation to the Queen that Charles was finally forced to face the grim reality of what his wife had done, and whom she had become.

Some historians have considered that it is curious that the Prince never replied to the accusations made against him in the Morton book, and didn't even take the cowardly way of letting others do it for him as his wife had done. His reasons were virtuous and sensible: he did not believe that two wrongs made a right, did not wish to prolong his children's torment and still genuinely did not want to do anything that would hurt Diana. Also, and most sensibly, he knew the best way to stop this terrible spiral was not to give the Princess a further excuse to do more damage. However, in the absence of any spirited defence of his own position, the ordinary man and woman were left with little alternative but to suppose that the Princess's account of his callous behaviour was correct. Moreover, he knew that the press were always going to give her the benefit of the doubt and that he wouldn't even get a fair hearing. This added to the above reasons and his virtuous – if somewhat naïve – view that in the end actions speak louder than words led him to keep his counsel, while he struggled to understand why his wife had embarked on such a destructive and devious course of action.

For Diana's part, her venture into this fabrication of her life perhaps owed as much to the need for a pre-emptive strike as it did to the desire to lash out in revenge against people whom her condition ensured she now saw as enemies. There had been a rumour floating around Fleet Street that she had been taped having a late-night conversation of an indiscreet nature with a man who was not her husband. She had apparently been made aware of this by one of her journalist friends, who knew nothing more than that. Naturally she had denied that it was possible, but the prospect of such a tape being published must have filled her with fear because she knew it was true. She had already been alerted by James Gilbey, who had been confronted by *Sun* journalists outside his home in Lennox Gardens, west London, and told as much. Eventually her worst fears were realised when the National Enquirer in America mentioned the tape and excerpts were published. By then she knew that exposure in Britain was just a matter of time: the race was on.

Diana had lived a charmed life as far as the tabloids were concerned. Given the number of men who came and went by day and night to Kensington Palace, the number of letters she had written to both Hewitt and Waterhouse while they served out in the Gulf during the first Gulf War (she wrote over 100 love letters to Hewitt alone), the number of men she openly had dinner with in London restaurants and the number that she chatted to endlessly on the telephone, she was courting disaster. She knew the *Daily Mail* would continue to turn a blind eye to the less flattering side of her personal life, but what about all the other tabloids? Although she had embarked on a major charm offensive with other editors and key correspondents by inviting them to lunch, flirting with them and giving them the odd exclusive, she knew that this would not save her if a really big story about the true nature of her devious and promiscuous life broke in just one tabloid paper – the others were bound to follow and the damage to her image would be huge. She believed that the net was finally closing in on her, and this was the final motivation for her to release her version of her life – a fantasy version with its sensational contents of bulimia, attempted suicide and Cinderella-type treatment at the hands of the cold and wicked Windsors. A version that would paint such a vivid picture of unkind oppression that anything else would be lost.

She may have failed every exam she had ever taken, but this was Machiavellian brilliance at its best – or worst.

Chapter Fourteen
The Separation (1992)

Over the years, the Prince's unsuccessful marriage had not been a matter for his family's discussion, but they were of course aware that all was not well: they had witnessed the Princess's tirades, tantrums and at least one feigned suicide attempt. Her undisciplined behaviour was obviously a cause for concern, but as she was by no means like this all the time, and given their reserved nature, they took to averting their gaze and saying nothing in the hope that this was just a phase she was going through. Charles had never enjoyed a close enough relationship with either of his parents to feel able to confide in them, and so had suffered in silence. All three of them put the nation first, and their overriding concern was that the show must go on.

The Morton book changed all of this. After the first instalment in the *Sunday Times*, a number of the Prince's closest friends who, having been denied access to the press by Prince Charles, now felt so strongly about the injustice of what had happened and how unfairly it was being reported that they took it upon themselves to write to the Queen and point out how stoical her son had been throughout the long roller-coaster ride of his marriage. This intervention, and the shocking and hysterical way that the media were now reporting the book and its main characters, spurred the Queen and Prince Philip into action for the first time.

Now this all changed, and for the first time they rallied to the Prince's side. The Duke, who had never been that supportive of his eldest son, not only entered what he saw as a useful correspondence with the Princess, he also wrote the Prince a long and sympathetic letter in which he praised him for possessing saint-like fortitude. Naturally, this letter remained private, whereas Paul Burrell made ones to the Princess public. It is in this context that one might assume that the Duke's comment to the Princess that no one in his or her right mind would leave Diana for Camilla should be taken. It is probable that, in his attempt to pour oil on very troubled waters, the Duke was humouring a young woman whom he now understood was running dangerously out of control and was capable of doing great damage.

It was in this atmosphere that the Queen and the Prince of Wales sat down together and discussed for the first time whether it might be better for all concerned if he sought a separation from the Princess.

John Major wanted to be made aware of the latest developments. Consequently he was fully briefed as, having been so dismayed by press speculation that he felt it could lead to him having to address the House of Commons, he wanted to ensure that the country wasn't heading towards a constitutional crisis because of an imminent break-up of the Waleses' marriage. In more than one meeting with those closely involved, he became fully acquainted with the scale of the problem. Among others called upon for assistance was the Archbishop of Canterbury. He concluded that the Prince was more genuine than the Princess in wanting to save their marriage and, as a result of Diana's manipulation of the press, that he was much more sinned against than sinning.

Soon afterwards, the Prince authorised an approach to be made to Lord Goodman, a senior British lawyer, to see what his legal position was. He was still not totally convinced that his marriage could not be salvaged at some level, but with the Princess talking openly about a separation, he was advised that this would be the prudent course of action. Little did he realise that the next bombshell to explode on the front steps of Buckingham Palace would make any idea of saving the marriage seem impossible.

The busy lifestyles of the Prince and Princess of Wales demanded that they were always equipped with the latest mobile phones. The Princess, who had become increasingly convinced that her landlines at Kensington Palace were being tapped, chose to use her mobile phone when making personal or sensitive calls. Despite assurances by a senior member of the Queen's household staff that the Buckingham Palace switchboard wasn't eavesdropping on her, Diana continued to imagine that people were talking about her behind her back and listening in on her telephone calls. In 1989, mobile technology was still new and had one very serious drawback: it was possible, for the investment of a few hundred pounds, to acquire a portable scanner. Amateur radio enthusiasts had used these machines for years to eavesdrop on the police, air traffic control and the ambulance service; they could be retuned to pick up nearby mobile-phone signals. People began to listen in to other people's private conversations in order to hear something that might titillate them – a good measure of what it takes to amuse certain elements of the British population. At the end of 1989, two men recorded royal conversations that were more than just titillating: they were illicit, salacious and in places just very silly. Naturally they smelled money.

As a result, in January 1990 one of the men, a radio ham named Cyril Reenan, approached the *Sun* with a tape of a private conversation between the Princess of Wales and another man who clearly wasn't her husband. The recordings had been made on the previous New Year's Eve. The *Sun* sent Stuart Higgins to Oxfordshire to meet Reenan. Higgins was later to recall that, 'We went to Didcot railway station and he came and sat in our car. We put the cassette in and listened to it almost mesmerised for twenty minutes. My gut instinct was that it was absolutely her. The content was explosive and we knew we had a major, major story.'

Quite so. However, this was an illegal tape of a personal conversation and one that was mainly talking about private lives. Therefore, shouldn't the tape be handed back as it wasn't fair on the Princess to expose her in this way? And was such a scoop really in the national interest? Naturally the editorial staff and royal correspondents at the *Sun* wanted to run with the story; but Andrew Knight didn't and according to him he was, surprisingly, backed by Rupert Murdoch. Knight claims that he and Murdoch took the responsible view that these stories were too explosive to print: 'The irony is that by the time these events started coming out, Mr Murdoch had come to the belief that the Royal Family, although it was the pinnacle of a system of snobbery that he didn't relish, nevertheless on balance was a good thing, and he was reluctant to see it undermined. I don't think that's ever been believed … but it's true.' Murdoch was only too aware that Middle Britain, the sort of stalwart core of Britain who buy so many of his papers, is pro-royalist and he reluctant to undermine it.

Andrew Knight has always claimed to be a true royalist himself; so now, with Mr Murdoch on his side, what did he do next? Did he discreetly return the tape to the Princess with a little note warning her not to be so frank on her mobile in future? Did he destroy the tape and pretend that it never existed? Or did he keep the tape in a safe place so that the story might be run when the time was right? I'm sure no one needs me to confirm which option Murdoch and Knight chose. Once it was sure that it had the genuine article, the *Sun* paid its source and hid the tape in a safe place.

Personally, it has always been my belief that News International, perhaps on lawyers' advice, didn't run the story initially in case it was a stitch-up. If the *Sun* had got this story wrong, it would have faced public anger, ridicule, PCC censure and perhaps a huge legal bill. Then, when the Morton book came out, it all fell into place and so the story was run in the confidence that it was indeed Diana. And by that time they had known for two years the identification of the man.

The tape that had mesmerised Higgins but Murdoch had put on hold, certain that he would find a better moment for its use, would have been a fairly normal one between lovers if one of the parties hadn't been married to the future king of England. The man was James Gilbey, the apparently purely platonic friend who had managed to fly to the Princess's rescue over the authenticity of the Morton book. He called Diana 'darling' fifty-three times, and 'squidgy' or 'squidge' fourteen times, and so the tape became known as 'Squidgygate'.

The Princess exchanging terms of endearment with a lover, bad as that might appear for a woman who had portrayed herself as an excellent mother and a good wife to a cold husband who took his sexual pleasure elsewhere, was bad enough, but it didn't end there. She also talked about how her husband made her life a real torture, and described a lunch at which the Queen Mother had given her a strange look. 'It's not hatred, it's a sort of interest and pity ... I was very bad at lunch and nearly started blubbing. I just felt really sad and empty and thought, Bloody hell, after all that I have done for this fucking family ... It is just so desperate. Always being innuendo, the fact that I'm going to do something dramatic because I can't stand the confines of this marriage.' A top London doctor, who attended the Princess of Wales at this time and who cannot be named for obvious reasons, says that there is compelling evidence of BPD in just those few sentences. The belief that others thought she was mad, the anger at imagined ingratitude, the persecution complex, the feelings of emptiness and yet the slight admission that she was 'very bad at lunch' are, according to him, clear indications of her illness.

When the illegal recording had been made, the Princess had been at Sandringham with her husband and children; the lover had been in a parked car in Oxfordshire. Higgins and Co knew, or at least felt sure, that it was the Princess of Wales, but they weren't certain who the man was. They would need to bottom that out if the tape had any chance of becoming a major scoop. So they set about finding out who he was as the debate raged as to whether the story should run.

On the tape, Higgins and Co could hear that the Princess had been speaking to a man called James. Apparently he was looking forward to wrapping her in his protective arms in a couple of days' time, while Diana responded to say that she was not keen to get pregnant. Higgins and his team had heard the rumours about the Princess's affair with James Hewitt, but knew that he couldn't be the man on the tape, as Diana had complained to this James that she had dressed Hewitt from head to foot. The man then declared that he had been obsessed with the Princess for three months. Higgins, with a lot more investigative skill than that shown by Morton, decided that this was the line to follow – find the right James and he would get to know if the tape was genuine.

He later recalled, 'Eventually we managed to pin down the man who called the Princess "Squidgy". It was James Gilbey. He lived in Lennox Gardens and we went to his house early one morning and confronted him when he was just about to go to work. We told him face to face, fairly aggressively, because we wanted to be provocative, "We have got a tape which we believe contains a private conversation between you and the Princess of Wales in which you repeatedly call her 'squidgy' and it is a fairly intimate conversation." At which point he went completely white, got in his car and drove off. That doesn't amount to him signing a piece of paper saying, "Yes, it is my voice on the tape," but clearly we had the right man.'

Gilbey hadn't kept in touch with Diana after she had ruined his car's paintwork all those years ago. In those days, when she was a slightly chubby cleaner and he was a man with a nice car, she had fancied him more than he had her. Now she was the most successful media star in the world. In this second affair, he was besotted by her but she blew hot and cold as she enjoyed taking her revenge on him. She confessed to a friend that she often led him on to the point of penetration before refusing to have sex with him. The more she did, the more he was like putty in her hands.

Naturally, the first thing that Gilbey did was to warn Diana about the apparent mess they had got themselves into. The news must have terrified the Princess, as this kind of revelation, especially if taken in isolation, would surely damage her image. Worse, the Princess didn't know what to expect. Which conversation had been recorded, and what had she said about whom? Had she sworn, or said something pornographic or very rude about the Queen? The Princess wasn't to know that Andrew Knight had decided not to run the story for the time being, and so her first reaction was to ensure that if she was going down, her husband was going with her. Immediately following the

The King and Di

Princess learning of what had happened from Gilbey, the *Sun*'s sister newspaper the *News of the World* started to receive blackmail-style cut-and-paste notes alleging an affair between Prince Charles and Camilla Parker Bowles. I have not been able to find anyone who helped the Princess do this, but as she had the strongest motivation and the timing is just too close to be brushed off as merely coincidence, there must be a very good chance that these notes were cut and pasted by the Princess on her own. This secret was just too dark to share with anyone as they were bound to question her sanity as a result, and that remained her greatest fear.

By this time the Princess of Wales was consulting some unorthodox practitioners of alternative medicines. Despite this, or some might say because of it, she didn't feel any better, and this had the effect of making her manically search all the harder. She saw every kind of therapist: she had aromatherapy, reflexology, colonic irrigation, acupuncture, massage, chiropractic treatment; she consulted astrologers, mediums and even a doctor who ran magnetic pulses through her body. None of it seemed to do her any good, but it cost a fortune. When added to her other passions of clothes, holidays and working out at the expensive Harbour Club in Chelsea, her bills were topping £3,000 a week – a fortune in 1992. And yet none of it helped dispel her feelings of emptiness.

The Queen, having considered the advice of the archbishop and the prime minister, decided that the couple should give their marriage one last try and ordered them to take a holiday together. Diana agreed to go, but looked as miserable as possible when the press were about and this completely undermined Charles's attempt to present their vacation on Greek billionaire John Latsis's yacht as a second honeymoon. She could hardly do otherwise, as to do so would have completely wrecked the image that she had so painstakingly put together as a defence against the eventual publication of the Squidgygate tapes.

As usual, the entire Royal Family was at Balmoral for their summer holiday in August. Neither Diana nor Sarah Ferguson were by now very popular with the others: not only were the rest of the family shocked by the public disgrace and humiliation that they had both heaped on them, they were also pretty fed up with their rude and juvenile behaviour. The previous summer they had managed to annoy family, guests and staff alike by their antics. They had made loud and destructive motorbike rides across a nearby golf course. They had made handbrake turns in the Queen Mother's Daimler which had gravel flying everywhere. They could be heard to be referring to other family members as 'the Germans', Prince Philip as 'Stavros' and Prince Charles as 'Boy Wonder'. The Princess had been politely rebuked for being bad-tempered and rude to the staff, and the Duke of Edinburgh had even felt it necessary to ask Sarah not to flirt with them. But all of this paled into insignificance when compared to the summer of 1992, as huge scandals hit both of these undisciplined and spoiled young women.

Fergie, whose marriage to Prince Andrew had continued to go from bad to worse, brought the name of the House of Windsor into serious disrepute when, on 15 January 1992, the *Daily Mail* published photographs of her with Steve Wyatt. Apparently the photographs had been discovered in Wyatt's London flat. It was clear that this was not a platonic relationship, and the resulting media frenzy became intense. After six days the pressure really got to her, and she suggested to her husband that perhaps a separation would be the best thing. The next day the couple went to see the Queen who, alarmed by the way her daughter-in-law's affair was being treated by the press and having witnessed the deterioration in the marriage herself, didn't need too much persuasion to give her permission. It had been agreed that the news would be withheld until after the April general election.

However, as we have already seen, in order to blow the Lady Colin Campbell book off the front pages, Diana had betrayed her friend and confidante by giving Andrew Morton the story and so, in February 1992, he had written the front-page story for the *Daily Mail* and made poor relations between Fergie and her in-laws all the worse, as each thought that the other had leaked the revelation to the press.

So Fergie was still smarting from what she mistakenly thought had been a royal leak about her proposed separation, while the Queen thought that Sarah had broken her word to keep quiet, when they both arrived at Balmoral for the summer vacation. Naturally, things had been made even tenser by the Morton book's revelations about the Princess, and her apparent endorsement of them. The atmosphere was already hardly conducive to a happy family holiday, but then Sarah managed to shake Balmoral to its very foundations. She hit the headlines for all the wrong reasons again, this time in a graphic way that left no doubt about her infidelity and her unsuitability to be a member of the Royal Family. The *Mirror* had managed to get its hands on several photographs of a bare-breasted Duchess of York having her toes sucked by her financial adviser, a friend of Wyatt's who was also American, bald and called John Bryan. The whole of the media went into overdrive, and the Queen must have wondered what on earth was going to happen next. Princess Anne's marriage hadn't been successful, but at least her husband Captain Mark Phillips had left the household with good grace, just as Princess Margaret's husband, Lord Snowdon, had. This couldn't be said of these two Sloane Rangers, who seemed determined to bring the Royal Family down.

Unsurprisingly, the silly and now thoroughly humiliated Sarah fled Scotland. But the Queen and her family didn't have to wait too long for the next awful revelation to buffet the Windsor reputation. They must have felt that things couldn't get much worse. They were wrong.

Patrick Jephson was on holiday with his family in Devon at this time. He was Diana's private secretary and in many ways not blameless for the sad outcome of the Princess' story. Naturally, Jephson was only an employee, and the Princess was a very wilful woman when the mood took her. However, Jephson was well aware of the her failings as well as her strengths, and knew only too well that her accusations of cruelty and coldness against the Windsors were more about her attempts to cover up her own shortcomings than anything else. He knew that the Princess was quite prepared to use her 'work' as a weapon, would never put the people or anyone else before herself and that she knew perfectly well, especially in calmer moments, that the Prince didn't have a cruel bone in his body. He was well aware that the Princess, for reasons of ill health or otherwise, unfairly sought to tarnish the Royal Family's reputation as a way of excusing her own inability to do the job. He was clever enough to see all of this and yet, as a servant to the nation's Royal Family, he failed to attempt to guide the Princess down a sensible and reasonable road. Instead he appears to have aided her and abetted her in some of her schemes in a perverse way – as some sort of immature competition with his erstwhile friend, Richard Aylard, who was his opposite number in the Prince of Wales's office. However, perhaps Jephson didn't sufficiently take in to account that Aylard wasn't intending to destroy the Princess; in fact his orders from the Prince were quite to the contrary.

As a result of his attitude, he played a full part in the growing animosity between the now separated offices of the Prince and the Princess of Wales. He saw that there was some sort of competition afoot and that it was his job to recast the Princess as a royal celebrity – a kind of modern performer who made the Prince look old-fashioned; if he could wrong-foot his old chum Aylard in the process, so much the better. In effect he was playing power politics and without sufficient focus on the actual institution of monarchy and what was needed to help it through such a difficult period.

In August 1992, with Sarah, Duchess of York banished from the castle for appearing in the newspapers like no other princess had before or happily has since, Mr Jephson was standing, by the royal command of the Princess, at dawn in a Devon telephone box, reading out the morning headlines to his boss so that she might decide whether she could dare go downstairs to face breakfast with other members of the family.

By now Fleet Street was sure that the Princess had in some way assisted Morton with his book. They now regarded her as fair game. The *Sun* had been sitting on the Squidgy tape for two and a half years. Now, faced with the *Mirror*'s sensational shots of Fergie's breasts, Murdoch had second thoughts, just as anyone who really knew him always believed he would. On 25 August 1992, the *Sun* printed the whole story under the huge headline 'MY LIFE IS TORTURE'. Stuart Higgins was acting editor on the day: 'Apart from some of the material at the beginning of the tape, which we thought was rather tasteless and offensive, we published every word of the tape and we put it on an 0898 number for people to listen to as well ... She had had her say if you like, and clearly part of her aim in writing this book [Morton's] was to dilute or stop Squidgygate ever appearing if she could.'

To a large degree her plan was successful: it now seemed to many people that the Princess might be forgiven anything if her life was as bad as the Morton book had said it was, and in a way some of her comments on the tape supported the picture that the book had painted. Her position was perhaps further helped by the fact that Princess Anne and Prince Andrew's marriage breakdowns appeared to confirm Morton's assertions about the Royal Family; and at least this daughter-in-law wasn't baring her breasts in public – even if her language left a lot to be desired. So to a certain extent, even Fergie's blunder also helped deflect attention from the outrageous nature of Diana's comments and the fact that she was having an affair.

Squidgygate would clearly have been viewed in a different light, one that was a lot more critical of Diana, if it had appeared a year earlier. Thanks to the order in which these events where presented to the public, and by promoting a mainly fabricated version of her own life, the Princess had managed to portray herself as a victim, whereas Fergie had become a trollop. How ironic that in fact Sarah was miles behind Diana in the infidelity stakes.

Somehow Diana didn't see the Squidgygate tape as her fault or something that she should feel sorry for. In fact, she took out the excruciating distress that she felt on the Royal Family instead, and announced that she would not be accompanying the Prince of Wales on an official trip to Korea. Initially the Prince, displaying the patience of a saint, gently tried to persuade her, but she would have none of it. Then the Queen intervened and advised her daughter-in-law that it was her duty not to let the nation down – a discussion that was billed as a 'showdown' by the press once Diana had leaked the story to them. But the Princess did not yield even to Her Majesty. In the end, and with his patience finally exhausted, the Prince bluntly told his wife that she would have to come up with her own explanation to the nation as to why she was staying behind. At this point the Princess finally relented and meekly explained that as the Queen had asked her to go, she would accompany him after all.

The trip was, from a PR perspective with the people back home, a disaster. The only thing the press were interested in was the royal couple's marriage, and for the first time Diana made no attempt to disguise her feelings. The normally brilliant performer now acted out a very different part. She went out of her way to look extremely miserable, and frequently appeared to be on the edge of tears. She was genuinely depressed, but now seemed determined to flag that fact up rather than put on a wonderful performance as she had so often done in the past. Despite this the trip, as all trips undertaken by these seasoned ambassadors of Great Britain, was a great success in terms of trade deals and government ties. As usual the man in the street, or at least some of them, would come to benefit from the economic advantages derived from this goodwill mission.

But all of this was just lost under the coverage that clearly spelled out that the couple could no longer bear to be in each other's company. The fact that both the Prince and the Princess were aware that this was the only story being told back home only served to make matters worse. The trip was a dreadful experience for both of them. The Princess seemed close to a nervous breakdown, while the Prince frequently looked shattered by his brave attempts to paper over the cracks and save the nation's pride. When they stood side by side in a moment of solemn silence at a military war memorial in the national cemetery, the tabloids seized on the image as proof that here were two people who had come to loathe one another's presence.

Peter Westmacott, the deputy private secretary who was accompanying the Prince and Princess on the trip, was upset that none of the good news regarding trade deals was being reported and decided to take James Whitaker, the portly royal correspondent of the *Daily Mirror*, to one side and complain about the nature of the coverage. He apparently sympathised, before adding that it was obvious that the marriage wasn't exactly made in heaven. 'I'm not saying it is,' replied Westmacott. 'What I am saying is that you guys are getting it so grossly wrong, you're misreporting what's going on and ignoring the substance of the visit.'

Whitaker, so often the bridesmaid and never the bride when it comes to royal scoops, now decided to produce one of his own. But somehow he didn't succeed as it was his rivals at Sky News, part of News International, which was interrupting broadcasts within two hours to say that 'Palace official confirms that marriage is on the rocks.' Whitaker defended himself to his own editor for the lost scoop by saying that he thought it was his duty to share what he had been told with the other journalists on the trip. Westmacott was seriously unamused by the fact that he had been misquoted, while Whitaker's employers were furious that his inability to keep his mouth shut had shared the story with the competition. By the next day all the tabloids were running the piece.

This followed days of speculation about deteriorating relations between the Princess and her parents-in-law. There had been reports back in the UK that the Duke of Edinburgh had been writing to the Princess to admonish her for her selfish behaviour. Before she died the Princess indicated that the Duke had intended his letters to be a constructive help and as we can now read them courtesy of Paul Burrell, we can see that this was the case. However, that doesn't explain how the press got to hear about such private correspondence in the first place and why they should choose to interpret them in such a way. The obvious answer, given that the letters were confidential, was that either the Duke or the Princess leaked them. Only one of these people had a history of secret press briefings, and only one at that moment would have wanted the press to put that connotation on the story. Therefore it doesn't take a great deal of intelligence to realise how they came to be in the newspapers.

At the end of the tour there was the usual prize giving from the Prince and Princess to their aides, when tradition has it that the royal couple should hand out small gifts to each member of the team. By now the Princess appeared to be in an even more severe state. She was unable to speak and didn't seem able to stop herself from appearing tearful. According to one of their staff who was very fond of both of them, the Prince 'was marvellous. He did all the talking, all the smiling, covered up for her. He was very protective, very professional.' Nevertheless, it was still obvious to everyone there that this would be the very last time they would do a tour together as husband and wife.

From Korea the couple flew to Hong Kong. On the flight Westmacott did his best to talk the Princess out of her planned separation. She had always liked him and had flirted with him to such an extent when he first arrived that it was rumoured in the corridors of the Palace that they were having an affair. They weren't, but the unhealthy amount of attention that Diana paid Westmacott perhaps cost him the top job of replacing Sir Christopher Airy, which went to Richard Aylard instead. Westmacott pointed out that the boys needed to have two parents, she was good at her job and she could always have her own friends and her own private life if she wished. He implored her to try and find a modus vivendi that could work for her. But she was adamant that she wanted a separation, and so he knew, as he and the Prince disembarked for a three-day visit to the colony while the Princess stayed on board in order to return to London, that this was finally the end of the line.

By the time the aircraft arrived in Hong Kong, the storm in London concerning 'PALACE OFFICIAL IN GAFFE' and 'PALACE OFFICIAL CONFIRMS MARRIAGE OVER' had broken. It was Westmacott's unenviable task to go and wake the Prince with faxed copies of the British press and explain to him how this latest media feeding frenzy had started. The Prince listened to Westmacott's tale and his profuse apology with a tired smile. He accepted the apology and was understanding, telling Westmacott that in his opinion it was a waste of time trying to talk sense to people like Whitaker. The Prince has always been gracious to those who took their problems to him rather than letting him hear about them from others, and this case was no exception, despite the fact that he was by now thoroughly worn down by it all and seemed emotionally exhausted.

When he eventually returned home, the Prince's mood collapsed into one of total gloom. He had finally come to realise that his marriage could not be salvaged in any form. He wrote to one of his closest friends describing his despair now that he understood that even friendship with Diana was out of the question. He admitted that he had to fight against a serious temptation to cancel his public engagements. 'The strain is immense and yet I want to do my duty in the way I've been trained ... I feel so unsuited to the ghastly business of human intrigue and general nastiness ... I don't know what will happen from NOW on but I DREAD it.'

He made arrangements for one of his annual weekend parties at Sandringham. It had become the custom for the Prince and the Princess to invite eight or so couples each year at around this time for three days of shooting, walking and long and usually amusing dinner parties. The weekend had been timed in order that William and Harry could come home from school and join their parents. Diana had always made an effort on such occasions to adhere to her husband's wishes that the children should be spared as much of the trauma surrounding the crisis in their marriage as possible. However, the Princess often undid much of this by then telephoning William up at school to complain about his father – a trait that she had taken from her mother. Unaware of that, the Prince believed the Princess would put the children first on this occasion as she had in the past, and so was looking forward to having his sons home and saw the weekend as a possible oasis in a period of his life that by now looked to him to be unimaginably bleak.

Therefore, it was to his astonishment that less than a week beforehand, he discovered that his wife had decided to stay away from Sandringham and take their children to stay with the Queen at Windsor Castle instead. Totally dismayed by this fresh piece of miserable news, the Prince complained to the Queen who tried hard to dissuade Diana but nevertheless felt unable to deny her as this might only make matters worse.

In the meantime, the Princess had made a remarkable recovery from her tearful state in Korea and had made a very successful solo trip to Paris where she had been accorded a forty-minute meeting with the French president, François Mitterrand – an honour never extended previously to a lone Princess of Wales. In France she had delighted in seeing the French magazine *Paris Match*'s cover with a photograph of her by Patrick Demarchelier (genuinely so, on this occasion) and the accompanying headline that simply read 'COURAGE PRINCESSE!' Now her pantomime turned in the other direction and she performed with flawless composure, only days after appearing to be a nervous wreck, and she revelled in all the rapturous attention that the French heaped upon her.

Unperturbed by the effect that she might have on the children, the Princess ignored all pressure brought to bear upon her and stated that if she wasn't welcome at Windsor then she would take the children to Highgrove for the weekend. She even joked to Patrick Jephson that Nicholas Soames could eat all the food bought for her. Soames, by this time a member of John Major's government, was and still is an extremely large gentleman.

The Prince pointed out that he couldn't cancel their guests at such short notice. Not only would it be extremely rude, but also the newspapers were bound to get hold of the story and their treatment of it would only fuel more speculation about their marriage. He both wrote and spoke to the Princess on the phone in a final attempt to persuade her to attend. In the end he argued that while he couldn't force her to be there, he wanted his sons to be with him and therefore they should still come to Sandringham even if she wouldn't attend. Again she refused to listen, and took the children to Windsor.

As it happened, the castle was an unfortunate destination. On Friday, 20 November, a terrible fire swept through a part of it. It had started in the private chapel and spread quickly, causing anything up to £40 million of damage. On the advice of Michael Peat, then the Queen's accountant, the castle had not been insured. This is usual practice with very large buildings of this nature as the annual premiums and excess payments are so high that it is considered to be uneconomic. Indeed, many insurance companies don't insure their own buildings as a result. However, the public was unaware of this, and when the heritage secretary Peter Brooke offered to pay the bill from the public purse, there was a general outcry. For the last two years there had been a deep economic recession, and the public were hardly in the mood to bail out a family who apparently didn't even bother to insure their homes safe in the knowledge that the taxpayer would pick up the bill. This seemed all the more unsatisfactory as the royals didn't even pay tax themselves either. Naturally, no tabloid pointed out that they didn't pay tax as result of a perfectly legitimate arrangement arrived at in the past. Dissatisfaction with the monarchy was now reaching a height not seen in the United Kingdom for over a century.

A few days following the fire, and with Windsor Castle still a smouldering ruin in places, the Queen made an anniversary speech at the Guildhall in London. Unusually she didn't deliver a typically impersonal speech of national aspiration, but instead launched into a talk about her own recent experiences. Her tone was also more emotional than usual, and this was heightened by a voice made husky from the combination of a cold and the amount of time she had spent walking among the smoking ruins with her eldest son, who had raced to Windsor in order to comfort his mother before returning to Sandringham in the early hours of Saturday morning. '1992 is not a year on which I will look back with undiluted pleasure … In the words of one of my more sympathetic correspondents, it has turned out to be an annus horribilis … No institution – City, Monarchy, whatever – should expect to be free from the scrutiny of those who give it their loyalty and support, not to mention those that don't.' Two days later, on 26 November, it was announced that the Queen and the Prince of Wales would pay tax on their private incomes from 1993, and that five members of the 'outer' Royal Family would be excluded from the Civil List. 'THE QUEEN PAYS TAX AND IT'S VICTORY FOR PEOPLE POWER', blared *The Sun*'s headline as Murdoch sensed a twentieth-century British version of the French Revolution might be underway. Motivated by his antipathy to the British Crown, he seemed to be getting his way. He had used the Duchess of York's stupidity and the Princess of Wales's devious dishonesty to attack a monarchy struggling to cope with the impossible life it had created for itself in the royal goldfish bowl, a life made all the worse by two untrained and extremely selfish women who in one year seemed to have managed to rupture a deep relationship between the Royal Family and the nation.

The fact that so many people didn't seem to notice that it was neither the fault of the Queen or Prince Charles says a great deal about a British public who had apparently shed most of its national qualities of respect, decency and Christian kindness in favour of a lawless march towards atheism, materialism, a compensation culture and the vulgar hero worship of shallow celebrity. The Queen and most other members of her family had, after all, only been attempting to do their duty as normal, and so they had every reason to feel more than a little hurt by public reaction and somewhat resentful of the damage done by these two women, which seemed to have destroyed years of dedicated service.

The Princess, who had been telling her friends for years that she wanted to break free, even now couldn't make up her mind what she wanted to do and her behaviour remained as erratic as ever. But suddenly the decision was made for her. The Prince, furious at his wife's attempts to deprive him of his children, horrified by her lies and deceptions, tired of her tirades and tantrums, sickened by her continued use of the press in an attempt to destroy an institution that he had been brought up to serve, now snapped. On 25 November he demanded a separation. He had given up friends to try and please her, he had given up his dog because she hated animals and was jealous of it and he had let perfectly reasonable members of staff go because she had taken against them. In return he had received no love or companionship, his children had been traumatised by her behaviour, he had been embarrassed and even humiliated by the completely biased and often untrue Morton book and she had almost caused huge humiliation of the British nation by her singularly selfish behaviour in Korea – a behaviour that she had all too easily managed to correct the following week in Paris.

The fiasco over the weekend incident with his sons and the complete sense of loss he felt over the damage at Windsor had focused his mind. He had at last come to the conclusion that she could perhaps do more damage if the sham went on, and as he was by now thoroughly fed up with her scandals in the press and her private blackmail regarding his children, he decided that it was best for all concerned to give her what she had said on occasion she wanted but had never had the courage to claim.

He removed his effects from Kensington Palace as she did from Highgrove. She later told her financial advisor Joseph Sanders that, before she left the marital home for good, she chucked some of her husband's favourite clothes on a garden fire. She was fond of destroying or abusing other people's personal belongings – after all, it had only been twenty months since she had packed her stepmother's clothes into bin bags and thrown them about before kicking them out of the back door of Althorp.

On 9 December 1992, John Major rose to address a packed but silent House of Commons. He read out the following statement: 'It is announced from Buckingham Palace that, with regret, the Prince and Princess of Wales have decided to separate. Their Royal Highnesses have no plans to divorce and their constitutional positions are unaffected. This decision has been reached amicably and they will both continue to participate fully in the upbringing of their children. Their Royal Highnesses will continue to carry out full and separate programmes of public engagements and will, from time to time, attend family occasions together.'

A person close to both of them who was aware of the negotiating that was necessary in order to agree such a statement told me that what had surprised him at the time was the importance that the Prince placed on the upbringing of the children, while the Princess wanted it emphasised that her constitutional role would not be affected and that she would be able to carry out her own public engagements. Upon reflection, I tend to disagree – it was quite natural that the Prince, as a father, especially as he had been unfairly painted as a poor one by his wife, should want a statement that confirmed access to his children, while it was also understandable that the Princess wanted to know that she was going to keep her status and modus operandi, as without them her celebrity status might fade. Nevertheless, within a year, a princess who had fought so hard to obtain the right to have a separate programme of public engagements was to change her mind and retire from public life.

The Prince was on a Business in the Community visit to Holyhead on the day that the separation was announced. Later he was to attend a Prince's Trust board meeting. The news had started to leak, and there were lots of jostling reporters and photographers waiting for him as he arrived at the airport to return to London with the Business in the Community CEO Julia Cleverdon, who was amused to be described as 'an unknown woman in green'. On the plane back to London, the Prince told Julia about the separation announcement that was being made by Mr Major, and she later recalled that this was the most deeply miserable that she had ever seen him or was ever to see him until the Princess's death occurred, which seemed to throw an even deeper shadow across his life.

After the announcement, the Prince's senior staff quickly divided the household in two. The staff were asked if they had any preference; eighty-five per cent said they would prefer to remain with Charles. The Prince wanted to have a small staff that he felt could be trusted in order to minimise the chance of further embarrassing revelations being dished out to the press. He decided to keep number-three butler, Bernie Flannery, to himself, and he let the two senior butlers, Harold Brown and Paul Burrell, join the Princess. The former was already at Kensington Palace; the latter was at Highgrove and apparently very reluctant, according to his wife, to be sent to London to join the Princess as he saw it as a serious demotion.

And so, to all intents and purposes, ended a marriage that had captured the imagination of a nation when it had begun some eleven years earlier. No one thought it would reach this state, but then no one understood for a minute who Diana really was or what she had done.

Chapter Fifteen
The Divorce (1993–96)

In February 1993, Anthony Holden, who had originally been a supporter of the Prince and had complained that the tabloids' obsession with the Princess and her obsession with both them and herself were deflecting from Charles's good work, had changed his tune. Having fallen out with the Prince – why or how Charles has to this day been unable to fathom – the journalist had written extensively against the Prince. He penned a cover story for the American publication *Vanity Fair* entitled 'DI'S PALACE COUP' It read, 'There is a new bounce in her step, a cheekier smile on her face, a new gleam in those flirtatious blue eyes ... at long last the sham is over.'

As we now can judge by watching the Settelen tapes, this was not the case; the Princess was actually lapsing into a serious neurotic condition. Indeed as American readers feasted on this dreamed-up picture of Princess Diana by a man who was totally unaware of her real predicament, the Princess was in fact going through the very worst months of her life. Nevertheless, in her battle to protect her image while doing as much damage as possible to that of the Royal Family, Diana was grateful for his words, as he would soon discover. 'I got a phone call from a friend saying, "Be at San Lorenzo at 12.40 p.m. next Wednesday." I met him and we noticed that the table next to us was the only one with flowers on it. At one o'clock in she came with the boys and a nanny and she saw us and said, "Oh, what are you two doing here, why don't you join us?" And this was the beginning of a process that recurred quite a lot over the rest of her life. And the gist of it was that she was saying thank you to me for being supportive in what I'd written in *Vanity Fair*. And I have to say I thought, "Well, this is some measure of the difference between them as human beings." Because for at least ten years I thought I was a better PR man for Prince Charles than the ones he actually paid – for most of the eighties in fact – and there wasn't the slightest note of thanks from him.

'She was very funny, very smart, very good company. OK, she wasn't going to win the Nobel Prize, she was not an intellectual, but she was very savvy about people, which I liked. Very candid, surprisingly candid – particularly about other members of the Royal Family to somebody that might quote this stuff in books or journalism. And there was this unspoken thing – she never said once, "For God's sake don't print that!" She called Buckingham Palace the "leper colony", and if you want to know what she thought about the Queen Mother, she called her the "chief leper".

'If I was being manipulated, well it was a very nice way to be manipulated, and as long as I was aware of it, I didn't see the harm.'

However, Holden was right about one thing: this did tell us reams about the individual personalities of the Prince and Princess of Wales – but not in a way that had even occurred to him.

Nor does Mr Holden seem to have realised that it might not be in the best interests of the young princes to hear their mother describe their grandmother's home as a 'leper colony' or their great-grandmother as the 'chief leper' to a journalist, in front of them and their nanny, and in the middle of a public dining room.

Nevertheless it also should be added in fairness to Holden that Diana knew who he was and would always act accordingly. Whatever her mood, however great her desire to throw a tantrum or fall out with him, she never would: he was a journalist, so she needed him. Therefore he must never be allowed close enough to her to get a glimpse of the flawed personality that she really was. On the other hand, Vivienne Parry was a very close friend and assistant for twelve years. She was genuinely fond of and loyal to the Princess, and remained so despite her understanding of who the Princess really was and how certain aspects of her behaviour did not improve in the slightest after the separation had taken place: 'There wasn't one friend that she hadn't fallen out with at one time or another and I think part of it was that she felt difficult in the company of people who were very close to her, particularly if they started to criticise. And what she didn't understand was that sometimes people criticise you because they love you, not because they don't.'

I am told that this is a classic symptom of Borderline Personality Disorder and is why so many sufferers end up hating their family, their friends and even their psychiatrists, all of whom are only trying to help them.

Parry continued, 'For a time there would be a friend that was there all the time that she would ring at all hours of the day and night, and then suddenly that person would be dropped. And it would usually be because they had been truthful, or because Diana had tested their loyalty in some way and she felt that they had not lived up to her test. I don't know why she felt the need to do that, but she did do it and it harmed her. I saw her doing it and it broke my heart. There were countless people I knew who were friends of both Diana and myself, who would come weeping to me because Diana had dumped them.'

But this sort of self-obsession and self-indulgence is another common feature of BPD. A sufferer will want to spend an almost claustrophobic amount of time with a new friend, do anything for them and expect a 'drop everything and come to me' loyalty in return. If that friend or lover can't keep up with such an obsessive relationship, for whatever reason, they are rejected for not loving the sufferer. As the Princess's greatest love was her husband, it was only natural as a result that he would also become her greatest hate for this very reason.

The more astute of Diana's busier friends, like financial advisor Joseph Sanders, became quite cautious about getting too close to her: they had no desire to end up on the phone to her continuously before eventually being rejected. He recalls, 'She thought I was looking after her, making her money, and she respected my opinions. So from time to time she asked me about things that were troubling her. But I didn't take it upon myself to ask her if there was anything troubling her, she would've been on the phone twenty-four hours a day. And she did have a lot of other people that she asked about things.'

Wise words that James Colthurst, the Princess's faithful friend throughout the great Morton saga, would have done well to heed. As time had gone on, the Princess had become more and more demanding. His wife had become increasingly distressed by the nightly disturbance of extremely late and long phone calls from the Princess, while he had become increasingly frustrated by Diana's angry reactions to what he saw as constructive criticism. From her point of view, he was dead once she found out that he stood to gain maybe as much as £500,000 from the publication of the Morton book. Joseph Sanders points out that, 'She felt that he should've run her errands for nothing. She couldn't forgive him for doing her a favour and profiting at the same time. Even though he needed the money and she knew it. She was very protective of herself like that.'

Colhurst's friend Felix Lyle recalls, 'It became too much for him.' Their inevitable parting was a painful one. 'She turned on him. She had a little bit of a problem with loyalty… and he became a sort of pariah. He said that she used to refer to him as "that shit", which I think was a great shame and the end to rather a sad story.'

Another casualty was Carolyn Bartholomew, her friend since

childhood who had done so much to help Diana publish her version of her life, a woman who had helped paint Prince Charles as a faithless husband. She was relegated to a mere acquaintance once the book was out. Her husband, William, remains extremely angry about the way the Princess treated his wife. He believes that the Princess just couldn't see enough of Carolyn while Morton was preparing his book for publication; she hardly ever saw her again thereafter. However, that was later put down, by Diana herself, to the fact that when asked by the press, Carolyn had denied that Diana had actually tried to commit suicide. She had only sought to protect the Princess's reputation, but from Diana's point of view it was the wrong answer and so her friend must be punished.

James Gilbey, another conspirator, was also edged out forever once the Squidgygate tapes hit the press. He had tried very hard to gain favour by faithfully forgetting that he had been a lover of the Princess when delivering her messages to the press as his opinions and perceptions, but it wasn't to save him.

So, as usual in such matters, they didn't live happily ever after. By this time Diana was also referring to Morton in less than flattering terms as she came to blame him for her predicament, and she was to fall out seriously with another Morton 'source' – her brother Charles, who wrote in a letter to her that he hoped that she would seek help for her mental condition as a result.

Colthurst is perhaps the only one who still counts himself today among one of Diana's strongest admirers, is proud of his role in her life and remains a critic of the way he still believes that the Royal Family treated her. The Morton book also caused Diana to fall out with her middle sister Jane. She had been torn between standing up for the husband she admired and loved and a sister who had nearly lost him his job by lying to him, but whom she also loved. She chose her husband, and a vindictive Diana would never quite forgive her for it. Another family member who refused to stomach the Princess's behaviour was Lady Fermoy. The old lady, who had worked so hard to help Diana get offered the chance to marry Prince Charles was appalled by her granddaughter, denounced her and refused to receive her until just before she died.

Diana also fell out with Rosa Monckton at this time as her friend had the courage to tell her that she must stop being pathetic, pull herself together and remember that she was representing Great Britain while on that tour of Korea in October 1992. Diana blanked her out for a year as a result, before phoning her up as though nothing had happened.

But the Princess reserved her cruellest and most selfish behaviour, if one excludes what she had done to Prince Charles, and therefore by implication their children, for James Hewitt. She asked him to give an interview to the *Daily Express* denying the assertion by Lady Colin Campbell that they had been having an affair. Although Hewitt had hardly any contact with the Princess since his return from the Gulf, he rather foolishly agreed to her request and lied to the paper in an article written by Anna Pasternak. The other tabloids, furious that they hadn't got this exclusive, turned on Hewitt and accused him of making money at the Princess's expense. They labelled him a cad. This was quite unfair, as Hewitt hadn't earned a penny, at this stage, out of any newspaper story. Now Hewitt realised that he was being engulfed in a tidal wave of media criticism that could end his army career and make getting an alternative job difficult. He turned to Diana and asked her to issue a short supporting statement that he had only talked to the press to protect her. She refused and never spoke to him again. His career was over and his reputation ruined. He went on to make some foolish mistakes in his own right, but it should not be forgotten that Diana placed him in that position in the first place and then refused to lift a finger to help him. Effectively, the episode ruined his life.

Having laid the blame for Hewitt's 1992 predicament as an ex-army officer with a reputation as a cad at Diana's door, one cannot but help comment that from the time of his cooperation with Anna Pasternak on *Princess in Love*, Hewitt spent a not inconsiderable amount of time living off his affair with the Princess, to his eternal discredit. And despite having amassed a fortune for this, he seemed unable to hold on to either his poorly gotten gain or any semblance of dignity befitting an army officer mentioned in dispatches.

When his apparent 'celebrity' status finally began to wear thin, and his creditors – not least the Inland Revenue – began to close in on him in 2005, Hewitt, by now a badly ageing forty-seven-year-old with a self-confessed drink problem and a drug-related arrest, finally decided to let the world know that he was every bit as much the knave as he had ever been the fool. Now he dramatically changed the story that he had been living off for the last decade to one that might rekindle interest in his part in this royal fantasy.

In September 2005 the well-known publicist Max Clifford released an autobiography. In it he claimed that Hewitt confessed to a new version of his affair with Princess Diana that was completely at odds with what he had previously sold as 'true revelations'. Now his affair with the Princess started in 1982, within a year of her marriage to Prince Charles, and not in 1986 as he had previously claimed. He even agreed to go on television and be hypnotised in order to regress to his 'Diana days'. Under hypnosis he claimed that he had met Diana in 1981 and had began an affair with her, at her behest, in 1982.

The book's publication coincided with Prince Harry's twenty-first birthday. It naturally brought up the question of who Harry's actual father might be all over again. Previously Hewitt had always claimed that he couldn't have been Harry's father, as he hadn't even made Diana's acquaintance until Harry was a toddler. Now he was supplying Clifford's publishers with photographs of him as a child that might be compared to ones of Harry at a similar age.

A desperate act – but perhaps desperate measures were called for as the foolish playboy apparently had neglected to direct any of his wealth towards HM Revenue and Customs, who took him to court in October 2005 claiming that he owed them £2.7 million.

It would appear that only Mr Hewitt, Mr Clifford (who claims that he knew about the affair as early as 1984) and the late Princess really know the truth. As hard as I have tried, I cannot find anyone to verify it. In any event I believe that, despite the confessions being repeated under hypnosis, the Princess should, in the absence of any corroborating evidence, be given the benefit of any doubt. Moreover, whatever Max Clifford would like the world to believe, the overwhelming evidence is that the close bond between Prince Charles and Prince Harry is not solely built on the affection of a doting father and an admiring son, but a relationship that has never been scarred by doubt.

Nevertheless, the Princess's claim – that she had truly loved Hewitt as the man who had consoled her as she had been forced to come to terms with Charles's unfaithful affair with Camilla Parker Bowles – lies in complete tatters.

As the Princess's mental state drifted dangerously close to a serious case of paranoia, and her friends increasingly banished as a result, so she replaced them with a growing army of alternative counsellors. These people, happy with what association with the beautiful Princess would bring, were naturally less inclined to be critical of her. There was psychic Rita Rogers, therapist Susie Orbach, colonic irrigator Chryssie Fitzgerald, acupuncturists Oonagh Toffolo and Lily Hua Yu, energy healer Simone Simmons and fitness trainers Carolan Brown and Jenny Rivett. Then, on Brown's advice, she also engaged actor Peter Settelen as her voice and speech coach – a move that we now know was not only to benefit him greatly financially when he sold his videos of her to NBC in America, but which was also to betray her by showing America a side of her that had always been explained away previously as just the exaggerated and biased opinions of the Prince's supporters.

Now largely surrounded by therapists and healers who did their best to please her, the Princess still remained restless and sought the advice of new ones continually. She would present herself as a damaged and unhappy woman, harmed by a traumatic childhood and the behaviour of vile in-laws and heartbroken by a failed marriage. There would then follow an intense period during which she was highly dependent upon her new counsellors before she would say she was making good progress only to drop them and move on and repeat the whole process again with someone else. In other words, Diana was repeating with her medical advisors the same behavioural pattern that she did with her lovers and friends.

As a result, there are several people who claim that they cured the Princess's bulimia; in their mind they are right because Diana had told them that she was now cured and didn't need them any more. In reality she was merely dumping them in order to repeat her tale of misery to the next therapist. It seems that it was the need to tell this story that drove her, and not a desire to find a cure for an illness that was but a symptom of a much more serious mental disorder. Her beautician, Janet Filderman, knew that the Princess made herself sick occasionally when depression had driven her into a comfort-eating binge, but adds, 'I don't think she had bulimia as I know it. I have two or three clients who really have been like that, and believe me there is no comparison because Diana had a super figure, wonderful teeth, good-quality hair, skin was good, eyes were bright. I don't think you can have those signs if you have bulimia badly.' It would appear that either for reasons of attracting attention, or to point the finger of blame at her parents, her husband and his family, or even because to a degree she somehow found it romantic, Diana's bulimia, which she would freely admit to anyone who would listen, was nothing like as serious as she liked to make out.

It certainly did nothing to inhibit her public performances, which were triumphant in 1993 and gave no clue to the fact that her private existence was becoming more stressful rather than less following her separation from the Prince of Wales. Patrick Jephson was proud of her performances in public where, in the Princess's contradictory life, she seemed always to be able to put matters behind her and shine. He was nevertheless alarmed at her private life as he saw increasing numbers of quacks introduce her to a bizarre variety of physical and emotional stimuli. In addition, he worried about the contents of her medicine cabinet, which was on hand to supplement her alternative cures with Prozac and sleeping pills. The Prozac only seemed to deepen her depression, and sleeping pills around one so disturbed can be an obvious danger. Diana, however, did not attempt to take her life. Her previous bids during her marriage had all been feigned, and one concerning pills had involved emptying a bottle of them down her throat before reporting the fact to Prince Charles. As he had just taken two aspirin and had left only two in the bottle, he was not inclined to treat her attempt as anything but a cry for attention. And as there was no longer anyone close at hand whom she wished to impress with such pleas, she seems to have lost interest in suicide attempts. However, Jephson could not be certain of this, and therefore his concern was well placed.

The public engagements of the Princess were carried out with great professionalism. She knew how important they were to her worldwide army of admirers, and she knew how important they were to her. She realised only too well that if she failed she would play right into her detractors' hands; if she succeeded it was a magnificent platform to keep alive the deception that had been sent across the world with the success of Morton's book. Her game plan was to use her celebrity status as much as possible in her continuing war against the House of Windsor, and happily the beneficiaries were the people she visited and the millions of lives she brightened up as a result of the ensuing media coverage.

It seemed to be a life that she could cope with. Moreover, if used positively, it was something the British government felt it could harness for the national good. In March 1993, Diana accompanied the minister for overseas development, Lynda Chalker, to Nepal. The trip was a great success. Jephson saw this as an opportunity and recommended an increased involvement with the International Red Cross, while Chalker reported to John Major that the Princess still had a role to play on behalf of Britain.

Jephson has since claimed that Major agreed despite representations from the Palace that as 'a demonised inadequate' she should not play any such role. This is completely wrong. John Major and the Prince of Wales enjoyed a close relationship, and when asked, the Prince encouraged the prime minister to engage her – a fact supported by the fact that the Prince became furious with his estranged wife when she decided to give up public life at the end of that year despite her successes. Nevertheless, although her husband gave internal encouragement, it appeared that the royal establishment was being externally petty, driven on by protocol and precedent. There were reasons for this, but as they were neither explained to nor understood by the public, it was understandably felt that Buckingham Palace was merely attempting to demean an innocent young woman and punish her for being more popular than any other member of the Royal Family. As a result, actions like taking her out of the Court Circular and not playing the national anthem to greet her were despised by the people and a serious PR mistake by the Palace, which played into the Princess's hands while inviting her to up the ante in her war with them.

Diana was travelling light: she only had herself to worry about, whereas Buckingham Palace had to worry about the constitution, precedent and the monarchy's responsibilities to uphold the status quo without regard to the personal needs of any one member. This made it hard for them to manoeuvre and often made it seem as if they were attempting to isolate her and even remove her from public life.

Naturally, Diana exploited this for all it was worth. When she learned that Prince Charles planned to visit the peacekeeping troops in Bosnia, she decided that she wanted to make a separate trip there, confident that the soldiers would give her a warmer welcome. Buckingham Palace, seeing the ridiculous and damaging nature of such an infantile competition, refused to allow her to go. They also blocked her from visiting Northern Ireland for security reasons. And when the Queen chose the Prince of Wales to represent her at the funeral of the two children killed by the IRA's bomb attack in Warrington, something the Prince wanted to do as a mark of solidarity against an enemy who had murdered his great-uncle, Diana was furious. She was livid that such a high-profile funeral would be seen the world over with her not being there. She responded by calling the grieving parents and then visiting them at their homes – after ensuring that the press had been tipped off.

When the Queen didn't invite her to Royal Ascot, in the way that most mother-in-laws don't invite estranged daughter-in-laws to family gatherings, Diana took her revenge by using her trump card – the princes. She arranged to take them to Planet Hollywood on that day, having tipped off the press; she captured all the tabloid front pages in the process, and rejoiced at the prospect of how angry that would make the Queen. In fact it didn't, as the Queen, unlike the Princess, didn't have the neurotic desire to be on the front pages every day. However, it did yet again further the idea that the Princess was one of the people – she was in jeans at the glitzy, fashionable burger bar, while her enemies were dressed up like nineteenth-century toffs. The Princess never missed an opportunity to present herself as a thoroughly modern mum, who was also a wonderful humanitarian and beautiful with it, but nevertheless a woman saddened by the harsh treatment dealt to her by the uncaring Windsors.

All of this served to create the impression that there was a terrible war being waged between the Waleses. This was partially true. There was a war being waged by Diana, and given some of the actions of Buckingham Palace it appeared at the time that they were fighting back, whereas they were actually spending most of their time trying to work out how to respond to her latest exploits. In reality, however, there was no campaign afoot to discredit the Princess. In fact, in August 1993, when the Prince declared independence of Buckingham Palace and set up his own press office at St James's Palace, he gave very clear instructions to his staff that they shouldn't say or do anything that might reflect badly upon the Princess. He knew that she was continually briefing journalists against his family in the manner that Anthony Holden alluded to; but he also knew that the monarchy could only lose from such public squabbles, and that such press coverage was hateful for his sons, who were at boarding school. He remembered only too well just what a cruel environment such places could be, and how his sons might be taunted over embarrassing press coverage. He felt that if he didn't respond, things would blow over, so he left no one in his office in any doubt that no matter what she did or said, they must always remember that the Princess was the mother of his children and anything that would hurt her would also hurt them.

If 1992 had been an 'annus horribilis' for the Royal Family, 1993 didn't start off much better. This time it was the Prince of Wales who was causing the scandal, and apparently doing so without any assistance from the Princess.

For a man who protects his privacy and that of his children obsessively, the Prince must have suffered the ultimate humiliation when, in January 1993, an intimate late-night conversation between himself and Camilla Parker Bowles was published by the *Daily Mirror*. Back in the autumn of 1989, another radio ham had managed to eavesdrop on a second private royal conversation. He had also taped it. Having read the Squidgygate story in the *Sun*, he decided to take his tape to the Manchester offices of the *Daily Mirror*. It quickly found its way on to editor Richard Stott's desk in London. He had to balance up in his mind what to do.

On one hand the tape would cause the heir to the throne terrific embarrassment at a time when the monarchy was already struggling following the topless photographs of Fergie, the Morton book and the Squidgygate tapes. Worse, this was something that he had brought upon himself and which didn't involve either of the two silly girls who had done so much damage in the previous year. Moreover, as this was a private conversation that had been illegally recorded, what would happen when the Press Complaints Commission came down on the newspaper? On the other hand, what a scoop this would be over the *Sun*.

By the following January, having checked out by various methods that the tape was genuine, the *Mirror* felt ready to let its readers know what the Prince of Wales and his mistress talked about on the phone late at night. It was a private conversation, just as Diana's had been, and naturally neither should have been published. From that point of view, there is no difference between them. However, the contents are very different. Whereas Diana was dominating her conversation with James Gilbey by spitting out venom and bad language against her in-laws, Charles and Camilla are having the sort of silly conversation that two slightly drunk lovers might have in private while they are in bed, alone, relaxed and behaving like two silly teenagers.

CHARLES: ... He thought he might have gone a bit far.
CAMILLA: Ah, well.
CHARLES: Anyway, you know, that's the sort of thing one has to beware of. And sort of feel one's way along with, if you know what I mean.
CAMILLA: Mmmmmm. You're awfully good at feeling your way along.
CHARLES: Oh stop! I want to feel my way along you, all over you and up and down you and in and out.
CAMILLA: Oh!
CHARLES: ... Particularly in and out.
CAMILLA: Oh, that's just what I need at the moment.
CHARLES: Is it?
CAMILLA: I know it would revive me. I can't bear a Sunday night without you.
CHARLES: Oh, God.
CAMILLA: It's like that programme *Start the Week*. I can't start the week without you.
CHARLES: I fill up your tank!
CAMILLA: Yes, you do!
CHARLES: Then you can cope.
CAMILLA: Then I'm all right.
CHARLES: What about me? The trouble is I need you several times a week.
CAMILLA: Mmmmmm. So do I. I need you all the week all the time.
CHARLES: Oh, God, I'll just live inside your trousers or something. It would be much easier!
CAMILLA: [laughs] What are you going to turn into? A pair of knickers? [both laugh] Oh, you're going to come back as a pair of knickers.
CHARLES: Or, God forbid, a Tampax, just my luck! [laughs]
CAMILLA: You're a complete idiot! [laughs] Oh, what a wonderful idea!
CHARLES: My luck to be chucked down the lavatory and go on and on forever swirling round on the top and never going down!
CAMILLA: [laughing] Oh, darling!
[end display text]

This must have been toe-curlingly embarrassing for both the Prince and Mrs Parker Bowles. However, the puritanical outburst that followed was both hysterical, hypocritical and out of all proportion. A nation who most likely had similar private conversations with their own lovers was horrified, and instead of Charles being a hero as he would no doubt have been in France, he was vilified from every direction. There were lurid headlines and cartoons, widespread condemnation from republicans, questions about the Prince's fitness to become the next king of England and, amid the mounting fever pitch, even demands from various Conservative cabinet ministers that the Prince must give up Mrs Parker Bowles – ironic considering what we now know about their own sex lives.

But why was the nation being so tough on the heir to the throne? Hadn't the tabloids been painting him as stuffy and out of touch with his people and yet, horror of horrors, here he is behaving just like any of them might and probably most do when in private. In 1993, when none of Diana's domestic behaviour was really known and her affairs certainly were not in the public domain, this tape seemed to confirm what she had been telling the world through Morton – that her husband had never given up his mistress and had ruined her marriage to him by continually refusing to do so. The deceit and deception of Diana's largely imagined autobiography was yet again raising its head.

Even the *Mirror* tried to justify its publication of the tape on the basis that it had caught the Prince out lying and that Diana had been right all along. This statement is rubbish on two counts. Firstly, the Princess had not been right all along but had deceived the lot of us, and secondly the Prince had never lied as he had neither confirmed nor denied an affair with Mrs Parker Bowles as no member of the press had ever dared pose such a question to him.

The episode became known as Camillagate. Amid all the fury and outrage, the heir to the throne was often portrayed as a rather crude adulterer not fit one day to take his place at the head of the Church of England. What people failed to detect was that the Prince had found in Camilla what he had expected to find in Diana when he asked her to marry him. It was clearly a loving relationship – easy, friendly, close and free from the suspicion, tension and jealousy that marred not only Diana's relationship with Charles but also those with all her other lovers as well. The Prince and Camilla clearly took pleasure in just being able to speak to each other and, most importantly, they made each other laugh. It is now a well-known fact within his household that however miserable the at times self-pitying Prince becomes during the day, a call to Camilla at night, from wherever he may be in the world, always has the effect of cheering him up. It doesn't spur him on to greater efforts – his drive and determination are constant – but it does lighten his mood, and for this his staff members are grateful to her.

Charles has always had a ridiculous sense of humour and likes to be around people who are fun to be with. But there was more to his relationship with Camilla than just laughter: she was interested in him, she gave his ego a much-needed boost, she liked listening to his proposed speeches, she believed in his work, she genuinely shared his enthusiasms, she made no demands of him and she understood who he was and why he must put the country first. She was also interested in him sexually, and out of that close relationship came a giggly banter that allowed her to tease him when he was being pompous or angry, but only in a way that never bashed his fragile self-confidence by putting him down.

She had by now become not just a lover and friend, but had filled Mountbatten's shoes and was both the mother and partner he had never known. He had at last found the relationship that he needed to sustain the strange cocktail of traits his personality had become as a result of his background. The warm glow of love mixed with genuine affection and maternal protection must have seemed very attractive to one whose life we have followed through much loneliness.

The Prince had tried harder than the vast majority of men might be expected to in order to make his marriage work. If the Diana that turned up initially, determined to get the job of being the future princess of Wales, had remained the cheerful, fun-loving young woman who apparently loved Balmoral and horse riding, then most people that I have spoken to who knew them have no doubt that the marriage would have worked and endured the test of time. As we now know, she didn't, and following five mainly unhappy years of tantrums, black moods and feigned suicide attempts, and having discovered her affairs with other men, the Prince retreated to the security of an older and more stable woman. He might have chosen another, but luckily for him he didn't. To be fair to Princess Diana, once the Prince had returned to Camilla, their very compatibility was bound to mean that she would never be able to win him back again. This must have been very sad for her, as by her own actions she had lost the one man she had convinced herself was the only one she ever really wanted.

There remains even now some controversy as to how the Camillagate tape came to be recorded in the first place. The *Daily Mirror* still sticks to the original version and claims that the radio ham from Cheshire didn't come forward earlier as he was terrified of being 'thrown in the Tower' for making the recording. However, the government felt that one radio ham recording one member of the Royal Family was one thing, but two different ones recording separate members of the family – especially as it involved the two who were going through the most serious matrimonial problems – was just too much of a coincidence. They ordered an investigation at MI5 and other intelligence agencies, but nothing was found.

Penny Junor in her book *Charles: Victim or Villain?* hints that Diana herself might have been behind the recording. She concludes, 'The Princess was one of the very few people who knew the Prince's mobile telephone number, and it was known that she had been worried about bugging on her own account and had installed some sophisticated equipment at Kensington Palace.' Lady Colin Campbell supports this theory, and goes further by suggesting that in 1989 the Princess appealed to a man in the protection services to 'help me win my husband back'. Faced with a most appealing Princess, the man agreed, without realising that her real agenda was to blackmail her husband with the tape she asked him to make by bugging Prince Charles's mobile phone.

Lady Colin asserts that the power she would possess if she could get her hands on such a tape was not lost on the Princess. The Prince would have either to give up Camilla completely and return to her domination, or face the consequences. The tape was duly recorded on 17 December 1989. Now Diana had what she wanted, but would have a problem explaining how she came by it. That meant that it had to be broadcast in order for a scanner to pick it up, and this was done on 18 December. This is supported by the fact that during the conversation, Camilla refers to her son's birthday as tomorrow, when actually the tape was broadcast on his birthday. According to Lady Colin's unnamed source at court, this gaffe gives the game away and would come back to haunt Diana.

Eventually Diana waved a copy of the tape in the Prince's face and told him either to abandon Camilla, or give her a separation. Apparently, he replied by telling her not to be so ridiculous. Soon afterwards, the secret services laid a trap for her and were rewarded with the Squidgygate tape. They then broadcast this three times in a two-week period, confident that it would be picked up by a ham somewhere, and it was.

The truth is still shrouded in mystery. However, as everybody, including Prince Charles and Mrs Parker Bowles, agrees that the tape was recorded in late 1989, I believe that it has to be unlikely that the Princess had any involvement in its making. I don't doubt for a minute that she would have jumped at the opportunity – that would have been quite in keeping with her personality – but holding on to it for over two years as she plotted the Morton book while being fearful of being exposed by Squidgygate would have been quite out of character. Moreover, when Andrew Morton said only a major royal scandal would blow Lady Colin Campbell's book away in the spring of 1992, Diana responded by sacrificing Fergie. Why would she have bothered if she had this gem in her safe?

In addition, it would be completely out of character for the Prince of Wales to encourage the secret services to organise a revenge recording, and he has no power to order them to do so anyway. He has not only always protected the Princess's reputation, but by causing her that embarrassment he would surely also have guaranteed that she would use her tape of him and Camilla, which is the last thing he would have wanted.

Indeed, when the whole business came out, it had proved to be a terrible agony for the Prince. He felt that he had let down so many people. His parents, his children, the rest of his family, those in the nation who loved and wanted to look up to the monarchy, Camilla, her children and her elderly parents, all of whom would all now be the butt of dirty jokes. He even felt that he had let down Andrew Parker Bowles, who was a friend of his and Camilla's despite their separate lives. Andrew would happily remain friends with both of them, despite the fact that the tape's publicity made his position as her husband untenable and so forced the couple to divorce.

Even today the episode troubles the Prince. He knows that people not sympathetic to him or the monarchy will recall it at the time of his coronation and at all other meaningful moments in his life. He remains deeply ashamed of the embarrassment that he caused his mother, deeply sorry for the pain it caused both his and Camilla's children and deeply angry with the press for printing a private conversation that meant nothing to anyone other than the two people who were enjoying a light moment together.

Squidgygate and Camillagate show our society up in two different lights. The cruel and totally unwarranted exposure of private conversations between both the Prince and Princess of Wales and their respective lovers, with all the misery that this brought to everyone concerned, was only undertaken by Britain's gutter press because it knew such stories would find a huge and ravenous appetite among its readers. On the other hand both, Charles and Diana were treated very kindly while going about their public duties by the large crowds that greeted them immediately following the publication of both tapes. On the morning of the Camillagate publication, the Prince was due in Liverpool. He had to summon up all his courage to get out of the car and face a crowd of people, not at all sure what sort of reception he would receive. He acted as normal, and so did they. There were no placards, sniggers, clever one-liners from some unseen cheeky Scouser at the back; best of all, there was no absence of people. Indeed, throughout this troubled time, the people who ventured on to the streets to see the Prince showed him nothing but love and enthusiasm. None of his staff can even recall even the faintest of jeers.

Nevertheless, despite his brave exterior, the day had been one of his worst to date. As he returned south, he wondered when and if things might ever return to normal for the monarchy, him and his children. In particular he remained concerned how they would be treated at school because of the press coverage, and he was only too aware that it was their father and not their mother who had on this occasion been responsible for their misery. It had been a ghastly twelve months. He prayed that things would now get better.

The damage done by Camillagate would have been serious in its own right. However, following on from what now seemed to be the correct revelations in the Morton book and the Squidgygate tape, the damage to the Prince was enormous. The high standing that he had built by the end of the 1980s by his genuine good works had been virtually destroyed. It seemed so very unfair.

What could be done? The Prince could put his head down and withdraw from public life and just wait to become king. But would he agree to such a thing given his passionate beliefs and sense of duty? Nobody who had spent any time with Prince Charles believed for a moment that he would. Moreover, would it not be a crime to interrupt or even truncate the genuine difference that he had made over the last twenty years to the less well-off youth who had been largely neglected by their parents and the state alike? The Prince's Trust could continue without him, but it would desperately miss his enthusiasm, leadership and magnetic pulling power. And wouldn't those opposed to the monarchy only complain that the Prince of Wales was failing to fulfil his duties to the nation in favour of leading a life of laziness, painting and polo.

Those around the Prince, mainly led by his fiercely loyal private secretary Richard Aylard, decided that the 'seeing is believing' concept so often used by the Prince in order to sell the need to support the good works of either the Prince's Trust or BITC was what was now called for. Consequently, they wanted him to agree to make a long and in-depth television programme about his work and what it was like to be the Prince of Wales. They believed that if the nation could see the Prince at work and at play, they would see the man they all loved and respected. They would witness his compassion, dedication and kindness at work, and they would see what a decent dad he was at home and how his kids really loved him. They approached the Prince, who initially wasn't at all sure – he was by now extremely cautious about having anything to do with the media. He worried that the programme would only be seen as a rejoinder to the Morton book and might even invite another vile broadside of lies and innuendos from the Princess. There was support for his thinking. Max Hastings came to hear that such a programme was under consideration and strongly advised against it. He later recalled, 'And I remember one of the Prince of Wales's closest aides saying, "But we've got to do something." And I said, "But this is a fundamental huge mistake at the heart of your thinking – that this is a sort of public war which can be waged by public relations means."'

Sir Max had a point, but Aylard and Co ignored his advice: they didn't wish to wage a war against the Princess, they were only seeking to show the nation what the Prince of Wales was really like. Furthermore, they knew that they would never be allowed by the Prince to attack the Princess, although it has to be said that by now some of them held her in low regard. Perhaps naively, they didn't appreciate that the mischievous tabloid press would not allow them to achieve this aim. Max Hastings did, and warned them that the only thing that the nation would want to focus on was the marriage of the royal couple.

Aylard finally persuaded the Prince to take part in a professionally made documentary that concentrated wholly on his life, without any criticism of the Princess stated or even implied. He was therefore able to offer Jonathan Dimbleby eighteen months of unprecedented access to the royal household, to the royal archives and to Charles, his advisors and friends. It was to be a serious and respectable programme to celebrate the twenty-fifth anniversary of Prince Charles becoming the Prince of Wales. It would have no ulterior motive and would attempt nothing more than to show what Charles did and why he did it.

Nevertheless Diana, who had rewritten history with great cunning and to date had got away with it, was loath to see this programme made. Not only did she not believe the assurances that nothing would be said against her, even if that was the case, the programme was bound to show the Prince in a good light and this would contradict her version of their life together. It might even bring into question some of the doubts that she had so cleverly placed in the public conscience. She immediately started briefing journalists against the programme, claiming that it was yet another attack on her in the ongoing war of the Waleses. As she was by now seeing conspiracies everywhere, this wasn't altogether surprising. One only has to see the Settelen videos to know that the making of the Dimbleby programme was bound to run a serious risk of annoying the Princess whatever it said or filmed. Therefore there would always be a chance that the good it achieved might be outstripped by the harm a beautiful and popular princess with a tormented mind and little discipline might inflict by way of an uninvited reply.

Arthur Edwards, the *Sun* photographer and journalist whose working life had been to follow the Prince round for years, wrote in November 2004, 'For many years Charles has been a figure of fun, taking all the criticism in his stride … If you think of all of the negative things said about Charles over the years – from the marriage crisis years with Princess Diana to his love for Camilla Parker Bowles – he has never once hit back. He kept his dignity and forbade his oldest friends from speaking out on his behalf. Even when his views on organic farming, architecture and health were ridiculed Charles kept his silence – and has been proved to be right. You cannot move in supermarkets for organic produce, the ugly buildings around St Paul's are being torn down and more people than ever are turning to alternative medicines. You could call him a visionary …'

These words, written over a decade after the Dimbleby programme was being researched, are a true testament to the Prince's attitude then and are totally supported by those who worked with him on the project at that time. The Prince believed that it was his role to speak up for the people and give voice to his passionately held views. However, he also realised that if he wanted the monarchy to remain above the destructive madness of British politics, he must not take public debate involving things in which he believed down to a level of trading insults in the way politicians and newspaper editors do daily. Therefore, having made his views clear, there would be no response to the insults that might fly his way. Sensibly he had understood that if 'tit for tat' was inappropriate for his dealings with government ministers, they were even more so with members of one's own family, and naturally that included his wife.

Dimbleby himself reports that, 'The one thing that the Prince implored me to do, the only thing, was that I should do nothing to hurt the Princess, whatever I might hear from those of his friends who might be indiscreet enough, despite his injunctions to them that they would cease to be his friends if they spoke poorly of the Princess.' Editors, journalists, authors and even the fairly balanced Clayton and Craig have either ridiculed this statement as a lie or at least said that it should be taken with a pinch of scepticism. They wished to believe Diana's assertion that this was a counter-attack against her. As a result they drew the incorrect conclusion that Dimbleby was playing the role of Morton – in other words, Charles's words would be coming through Dimbleby's mouth just as hers had come through Morton's pen, and he would be in a position to deny them should he so choose.

This thinking is totally flawed. Firstly, the programme contained no attack on the Princess whatsoever. Secondly, the subject of the programme, the Prince, is on camera virtually throughout and could hardly deny his involvement in the making of the programme in the way that the Princess did with the Morton book. Thirdly, independent individuals working on the making of the programme all confirm that this was also Dimbleby's comment to them at the time. Fourthly, as a result, the programme is simply an honest and genuine celebration of the Prince's work and in no way can it be vaguely regarded as a propaganda film against his wife.

So why did these scribes seem so keen to tar the Prince with the same brush as Diana? Why did they wish to insult an international journalist of high acclaim and hitherto unquestionable integrity by doubting his word? The answer comes in three parts. If the Prince was only telling the world who he was and what he did, this made the Princess's past behaviour seem unacceptable and paranoid and took away her excuse for future behaviour along the same lines. By showing the world who he really was and what he did the Prince would receive public acclaim (which he did) and this might prove the Prince's detractors in the press wrong, or at least bring into question the Princess's picture of her husband that she and Morton had painted. And lastly, in Diana's mind, and it has to be said in the minds of many of those journalists whom she had sought to enrol on her side, good publicity for the Prince was a victory for him and therefore, by implication, a defeat for the Princess, and so had to be attacked. Charles's mind worked totally differently. Of course he had been annoyed throughout his marriage that his wife lunching at a Knightsbridge restaurant might get more publicity than a speech that he was making on the same day, but he never considered media coverage to be a competition and certainly not a weapon to be used against Diana.

Dimbleby also wrote a biography of Prince Charles. Many detractors of this relationship between the Prince and the veteran broadcaster seize on this fact as further proof of a surreptitious attack on the Princess by claiming it was all part of a master plan – a two-pronged attack. Again this is nonsense. The book was not part of the original package as many previous writers have claimed, and only came to be discussed as enthusiasm for the project grew and the Prince came to trust and like Dimbleby. Eventually Dimbleby was to express his frustration with and dislike of the way the tabloid press had treated his work when he wrote in 1998, 'The first edition of *The Prince of Wales* was published in October 1994. At the time, eminent critics hailed it as a unique and important work of biography and history. However, in the foetid atmosphere created by the tabloid media, a significant number of commentators preferred to draw attention exclusively to that small proportion of the text in which I explored, somewhat gingerly, the collapse of the royal marriage.

'In the resulting furore, even fair-minded observers found it difficult to disentangle my account of the role, the life and the character of the heir to the throne from the travesty offered to the public by the majority of newspaper editors who chose to view him through the cruel prism of their own cheap but circulation boosting prejudices. In the process, truth (let alone respect, understanding or compassion) almost invariably yielded to the contrived banalities of a soap opera in which the scapegoat – to the evident indifference of his persecutors – happened to be a real person with real feelings. If he responded with reciprocal disdain, it was hardly surprising.'

Not only is the Dimbleby book a fine work of history that is now happily in the public domain forever, but also his impression of tabloid editors is more than justified. However, any fair-minded person concerned with the nation's direction still has to worry whether his work will not be lost under the tons of complete nonsense that the tabloids produce and which no longer becomes tomorrow's chip papers but are stored on computers for posterity.

The Morton and Dimbleby books are not comparable. One is a lengthy, detailed, well-documented and accurate account of our future king's life, written perhaps affectionately but nevertheless honestly. Moreover, it had no intention of recording history but was obsessed with rewriting a small but exceedingly vain part of it. As a result, Dimbleby has every right to feel that such comparison is insulting both to the Prince of Wales and himself: 'My book and my film contain not a single word of criticism by the Prince of the Princess. No single word of criticism from any of the friends. Everything about the Princess that I have published was recorded – as we now know – with her approval, by others, beforehand.' Indeed Dimbleby, at the request of Prince Charles, cut out a lot of very damaging material that had come to his attention while the book was being researched, and he dropped altogether a chapter dedicated to the Princess's Borderline Personality Disorder.

Nevertheless, Sir Max Hastings claims that his virtuous attitude towards the boycotting of royal marriage books softened when he heard that Dimbley's book was also being offered to the *Sunday Times* for serialisation just as Morton's had before: 'When one found that both the Prince and Princess of Wales were willing to flog enormously valuable commercial properties to the Murdoch press then you feel "What's the point?" ...' If Hastings had read the Dimbleby book he would have soon realised that it was a true biography of a future king that gave an accurate account of the man and balanced his strengths against his weaknesses. The book is a worthwhile publication by an intelligent journalist and worthy of serialising in any quality newspaper.

On 29 June 1994, fourteen million British television viewers tuned in to watch Jonathan Dimbleby's documentary about Prince Charles. The programme, like the book, concentrated on the life, views and personality of the Prince. Like the book it made little reference to the Princess. However, most unwisely, the journalist in Dimbleby couldn't resist asking the Prince about his private life, perhaps because not to do so after the Camillagate tape had been published the previous year would have seemed to be a cop-out. The Prince told the truth – in light of Camillagate he could hardly have done anything else – when he explained that he had committed adultery once he had been certain that his marriage had 'irretrievably broken down'.

The immediate tabloid reaction was as predictable as it was hostile. 'NOT FIT TO REIGN' was the *Mirror*'s headline, and the newspaper claimed that that was the verdict of its readers in a poll taken immediately after the programme finished. The *Mirror*'s interpretation of its own poll is somewhat misleading. In fact a modest thirty-two per cent had said that; forty-six per cent had said that the Princess should divorce him; fifty-five per cent said that his confession had made no difference to the monarchy; fifty-four per cent had said that he was right to make the confession and sixty-one per cent said that he was indeed fit to be king – almost double the amount that had said he wasn't. But unbelievably, whatever the public really thought seemed to be almost immaterial as the tabloid editors fell over themselves in the rush to defend the Princess.

The true picture that Aylard had wanted to portray of his master had been somewhat soiled by a question that had only occupied moments of an otherwise highly successful production. That moment was seized on by the tabloid editors who, even though by now some realised that Morton's book may be flawed, still believed that it was the public's wish that they stand by the Princess. The poll in question makes that quite doubtful, but they had been doing it for years anyway and Diana's wooing of the media hadn't yet begun to wane and was thus, at this point, still paying dividends.

If there was a failing in Aylard's thinking, it was that he had believed that by showing the Prince of Wales as he really was he might dispel the false impression given by the Morton book and the field day Andrew Neil and other editors had had in promoting it. However, the combination of Camillagate and Squidgygate in the wake of the Morton book, and Dimbleby's question in the programme about the Prince's private life, gave the impression that at least that bit of the Morton book was right and therefore the rest might be also. The Prince's refusal to fight back after *Diana: Her True Story* had been serialised in the *Sunday Times* had condemned him in some people's minds as guilty; their suspicions were further confirmed when he admitted in front of 14 million people that he had committed adultery.

The programme and book were, in their own right, a good idea and were certainly in the public interest. Both were objective and truthful and were being made by a respected journalist who kept his own professional integrity. But the mistake lay in attempting to shed some light on the Prince's domestic situation. To do that justice one would need a dedicated book or TV programme that portrayed the Princess as she really was. As the Prince was never, quite rightly, going to cooperate with such a programme or book, it would have been much better to remain silent on the subject. By bringing up Charles's adultery, Dimbleby turned his programme down to the Princess's level and played right into her hands. No doubt Dimbleby would answer that charge by pointing out that he had the journalistic right to ask whatever he wanted to, which is true. After all, the deal that he had struck with Aylard had given him 'sole discretion' regarding the contents, and he wasn't going to damage his reputation with his peers by failing to ask that very important question. So some of the blame for this slip-up must be laid at the Prince's door: he should have refused to discuss his private life on public television. He had never talked about his domestic arrangements before; a throwaway answer about it on national television was clearly not a good place to start. His honest candour and naivety had, not for the first time, played right into the hands of his enemies.

But if the book is an important contribution to modern monarchical history, and the television programme was only soiled by a moment of madness, the real problems were created by the serialisation in the *Sunday Times*. Aylard had negotiated with Dimbleby and had received no firm assurances that the journalist would surrender any rights of editorship. Worse, Dimbleby's publishers didn't restrict the rights of the *Sunday Times* in what proportion the book should be serialised or the impression given by the serialisation as a result – why should they? They naturally wanted to allow editor Andrew Neil to maximise circulation of the paper and therefore get them maximum exposure for their product.

But Andrew Neil, who has always been anti-establishment and a republican, saw another great opportunity to twist the knife into the Royal Family and therefore not only sought to sensationalise the serialisation, but to do so at the expense of Prince Charles. The lasting impression of the pieces in the *Sunday Times*, once the headline writers had finished, was of a whinging Prince whose parents had missed most of his childhood, who had loved Camilla most of his adult life, who had never loved his wife and who had been forced into marrying her by a bullying father. The tabloids picked out the bits that suited their cause and the Prince's enemies at the *Daily Mail*, the *Sun* and the *Mirror* had another field day as their columnists gave him yet another beating.

If one sits down and reads the 700-page labour of a meticulous journalist, which remains the handbook of royal fact concerning the Prince's life, one gets a very different impression of Charles as a boy, a man and a prince. Moreover, Dimbleby was horrified by how the *Sunday Times* and consequently the tabloids had trivialised and distorted his book in order to attempt to make it follow a Morton pattern. As a result of the *Sunday Times*'s treatment of the serialisation, it is easy to see how people might have got the wrong impression and believed that the Prince was now giving his version of events. Unfortunately, this was exactly what he had thought might happen when he had said that such a programme and book would be seen as a rejoinder to the Morton book. He had now been proved right and was somewhat furious with Aylard. A book and a programme that were originally seen as vehicles that would produce definitive, comprehensive and authoritative work from an independent and well-respected journalist, in order to correct the false and unfair positions of the Morton book and the tabloid press, had gone sadly wrong. They had ended up being more damaging than anything else, much to the horror of friends and family who had contributed eagerly in order that the tabloid impression of the Prince of Wales might be dispelled once and for all.

Was Aylard solely to blame? It had been his project and he had kept all of the negotiations very close to his chest. This meant that when disaster struck he didn't have too many friends around to support him. However, as the final decision to go ahead had been taken by Charles himself, the Prince must accept the responsibility for the outcome. Also, Dimbleby, who had every right to write what he wanted, as long as it was factually accurate, should have paid more attention to the serialisation issue if he wanted the *Sunday Times* to reflect what he had written. He knew only too well how distasteful and devious the Murdoch press could be.

While Dimbleby had been busy making his programme, the Princess had been busy stealing the headlines. In July 1993 she visited Zimbabwe and behaved extremely professionally. She managed to charm the inhumane president Robert Mugabe, and she was photographed with children dying from AIDS. She also attended other projects run by Help the Aged and the Leprosy Mission.

By now Max Hastings' traditionally royalist *Daily Telegraph* was covering the trip favourably as a result of an apparent change in attitude towards Diana. Hastings himself years later explained this was as a direct result of the Dimbleby book being serialised by his rival Andrew Neil at the *Sunday Times*. This is a strange comment as the serialisation was over a year away at that time. I am troubled that Sir Max has seemed less than open on this point, but haven't been able to discover what or who really changed his mind about the royal marriage. This is all the more intriguing when one considers that he must have known by this time of Diana's involvement with the Morton book and therefore her deceit must have been clear to him. Nevertheless, support from a serious newspaper was welcome and no doubt encouraged other diplomatic and establishment circles to take the Princess more seriously. As a result she made many worthwhile appearances during the autumn of 1993.

Things seemed to be going well for her. However, this was Diana the mirage and, as we now know, matters were very different in private. Once away from the cameras, she remained very depressed and paranoid. In November of that year this was well emphasised when she appeared to be disturbed by a nasty privacy scandal. The *Daily Mirror* published unauthorised and fairly candid photographs of her in a leotard. She was still using Carolan Brown as her fitness instructor and the two of them had taken to working out together at the LA Fitness Centre in Isleworth, where Ms Brown worked. The gym owner, one Bryce Taylor, planted a camera in the ceiling and sold photos taken from it of the Princess to the *Daily Mirror* for £100,000. The paper published them with the pathetic excuse that they wished to expose a serious flaw in royal security. Diana's long-serving, loyal and effective detective, Ken Wharfe, who perhaps became a little too close to the Princess for her good as he was later also to make a fortune cashing in on his experiences with her, had by now left her service. No one detected the camera, which had been planted after the initial security sweep had been done.

Every other tabloid, which no doubt would have done exactly the same thing if it had bought the photographs, poured scorn on the *Mirror* in an act of communal hypocrisy, but the Press Complaints Commission, despite its mistrust of the Princess herself, was genuine in its condemnation of the rag. Diana, who told Carolan Brown that she felt as if she had been raped by the owner through the lens of his camera, appeared to be extremely traumatised by the affair and announced that she intended to sue the *Mirror*. Most people in the country sympathised with her.

But the gym owner Bryce Taylor stood his ground and insisted that Diana had colluded with him in the taking of the photographs, pointing out that she wasn't sweating and was wearing full make-up in them. Diana was furious and responded by launching into a lawsuit against Taylor claiming breach of trust. These proposed lawsuits sent a wave of panic through her friends and supporters, and this was heightened when they learned that the *Mirror* had selected Geoffrey Robertson QC, one of the most aggressive courtroom barristers in town. His team was now doing its research and was rumoured to have dug up many recent occasions when supposedly private events had been photographed with the Princess's help. Worse, they were thought to have also uncovered a number of relationships between Diana and men that she had met at the same gym.

Initially, the Princess refused to back down, but following the revelations of her affair with Oliver Hoare and her nuisance calls to his wife, she started to listen to advisors like Joseph Sanders who pointed out that she certainly could not afford to run the risk of being humiliated further by more sexual revelations being exploited by Robertson's team. Eventually, Diana agreed that Sanders should approach the chief executive of the *Mirror* and arrange a meeting. In the end Taylor being paid off with a six-figure sum by an unknown admirer or admirers of the Princess, 'to spare her the indignity of entering the witness box', settled the matter in February 1995. But surely if someone launches a lawsuit with herself as the star witness, might she not consider that a court appearance is on the cards?

Absolutely – but the truth was that the Princess in the end simply could not afford to run the risk of further scandal. She had been exposed as both a marriage-breaker and a stalker in the period between announcing her intention to sue and the eventual-out-of-court settlement.

The Palace officially and openly supported the Princess in this scandal, but there were several courtiers, well aware of her previous deceitful behaviour, who were inclined to believe that Taylor was actually telling the truth. They were only too aware of how vain she was and to what ends she would apparently go in order to manipulate the public's perception of her. Their opinion was further supported when Taylor was eventually paid off. Perhaps the truth will never be known. However, Patrick Jephson has since said that behind the scenes the Princess behaved very differently to her public protestation. The episode allowed her once more to play the victim, and it also provided her with the excuse that she had been looking for in order to retire from public life. Moreover, he has claimed that far from being horrified by the photographs, she was actually quite proud of them as they showed her body to be fit and sexy.

Jephson was aware that she had been wishing to stop the duties that he had been arranging for her for some time and understandably, having gathered allies around him to help her cause, he had been struggling to keep this wish suppressed. But the *Mirror* photographs gave her the excuse she needed and she grasped it with both hands. Yet again the Princess had failed to complete something that she had started. This pattern, which had always dogged her life and would do so until her death, is but another symptom of a mental illness that was the root of her erratic behaviour. Now an embarrassed Jephson had to make apologies on her behalf. He felt she had wasted the opportunity he had provided, could lose the allies he had created and had left him with egg on his face in his competition with Richard Aylard.

But Lady Colin Campbell disputes Jephson's analysis, and claims that Diana retired because she believed her engagements were drying up as the Establishment was shunning her for fear of embarrassing the Prince of Wales. Lady Colin credits Diana with understanding that she was bound to be edged out in favour of a 'born royal'. She was jumping before being pushed, and the Princess did give the *Daily Mail* a story to that effect when she retired. Nevertheless, while it is true that 'born royal' is where the power really lies, I have found nothing to suggest that charities were backing off her, and in any case Diana sincerely believed, however stupidly, that it was Charles who should step aside in favour of her and their eldest son William – a belief that she would rather unrealistically harbour until just before her death.

Either way, many of Diana's new admirers were shocked and even angry when Jephson told them that the Princess now needed a break. They had booked her and now literature would have to be binned and a replacement found. But at least they had been forewarned. The vast majority of Diana's less important charities had no idea of her intentions until they read about them in the press.

The Princess decided to make her announcement on 3 December 1993 during a speech that she was to give to a conference for Headway, the National Head Injuries Association. Jephson became extremely nervous as the day loomed and still Diana refused to let him see the text. In the end she showed it to him with only a few days to go. Jephson knew his boss well and therefore realised that as she hadn't stuck at her job, she was equally unlikely to stick at her retirement – especially as she would soon miss all the adulation that went with it. He realised that this was yet another act of histrionic behaviour that she would soon regret, and he secretly advised an increasingly frustrated Buckingham Palace and 10 Downing Street of his considered opinion.

As soon as he could, he showed the Queen's office the text. They were rightly alarmed that they would be blamed again. At the last minute, Jephson and the Queen's deputy press secretary, Geoffrey Crawford, persuaded Diana to alter the text in order that it should sound less theatrical. Nevertheless, all concerned feared even then that this undisciplined and dangerous woman was just about to cause another major row.

The day arrived and the Princess of Wales bade her adoring public a sad farewell: 'I hope you can find it in your hearts to understand and to give me the time and space that has been lacking in recent years … When I started my public life twelve years ago I understood that the media might be interested in what I did. I realised then that their attention would inevitably focus on … our private lives … But I was not aware of how overwhelming that attention would become, nor the extent to which it would affect both my public duties and my personal life in a manner that's been hard to bear.'

It was definitely the most emotional personal statement by any member of the Royal Family since the abdication of Edward VIII over fifty years previously, and quite naturally it was major news. Her charities were shocked, and many were furious that their patron would just withdraw without any notice, which was bound to cost them revenue. Some privately exploded in serious anger at her selfish behaviour, while others expressed sincere sadness in public realising how much she would be missed. Some of the tabloids blamed the *Mirror*'s gym photographs, but most took their lead from the *Daily Mail* and blamed the Prince of Wales. The *Mail*'s headline declared 'CHARLES DROVE HER TO IT'. How did they come by this information? Diana had taken the trouble on this difficult day personally to brief the newspaper on her 'real' reason. So on the same day as she was making a tearful speech about how the tabloids had caused her retirement, she was nevertheless still secretly briefing them about a private life they were supposed to have intruded upon. No wonder Sir David English thought that the Princess was the best person alive when it came to personal PR.

The greatest irony was that the person who was most angered by this retirement was her husband. He knew the value of her work; he also knew how it kept her going; and he thought it was an absolute dereliction of duty to stop.

The Princess had negotiated her separation agreement with great tenacity and more than a little skill. She had been determined not to be 'buggered about' like Fergie had been, according to her. She had known that, thanks to Morton, Squidgygate and Camillagate, public opinion had swung against the Royal Family, and she knew that they were not keen not to have to endure any more public rows or scandals. The Prince in particular was keen to avoid pouring more fuel on the fire, for the sake of his sons and the monarchy.

Public washing of dirty laundry had always been the Princess's speciality. She had no shame, and this gave her a distinct advantage. Add to this her animal cunning and secret media deals, and it is clear that Charles knew he was batting on a very sticky wicket. Diana made it quite plain to him that if he didn't agree to her demands, she would cause a new scandal that would make those of 1992 pale into insignificance. As a result she got most of what she asked for, including his promise that he would not seek a divorce and that she would indeed be crowned queen upon his accession.

Most of what she wanted had been referred to in the prime minister's statement to Parliament, including her demand that she would be crowned queen when Charles became king. She believed that this would make it harder for the Queen to wriggle out of any of it, and that the matter was cut and dried. It was not. She had failed to take Parliament's reaction into account, which was adverse in the extreme. Major had hardly finished making the announcement when it was evident that Parliament on all sides was rumbling with both disbelief and disapproval. This was a matter of considerable constitutional importance, and Parliament made it clear that it would not be trifled with. By the next day, there was general agreement that Diana had no right to be queen if she did not wish to remain a fully participating wife of the Prince of Wales. Her position brought into serious question the sanctity of marriage and the example set by the Royal Family. As far as they were concerned, the Princess couldn't have her cake and eat it.

The Princess was shocked and completely distressed by this reaction. Her financial advisor Joseph Sanders later said, 'She cried and cried and cried and cried. You'd have thought that one of her boys had died. She really felt the loss acutely.' Realising now that she would never be queen, and spitting bile with the uncontrollable anger that she now felt by being unusually denied her own way by MPs at whom she knew she could not hit back, her vengeful side went into overdrive. She would explain to friends, 'We'd have been a good team as monarch and consort, but if I can't be queen, why should he be king? ... I don't see why my husband doesn't step aside and let me and the boys carry on the Wales name.' She made it plain that in her opinion Charles should give up his position as Prince of Wales and with it his right to be the next king of England.

She seemed to have forgotten that the throne was his by birthright, while she had only married into the Royal Family. She seemed to have forgotten that he had dedicated his life to upholding this birthright and honouring it. She seemed to have forgotten that her eldest son had told her that he hoped it would be a 'long long time before I take over from Papa'. She seemed to have forgotten that she had always found it difficult to stick at anything for long. She seemed to have forgotten that the Queen would never have agreed to this and nor would the Prince of Wales, who would have put up with a miserable existence as a child and a forced change of character for nothing. And most importantly, she seemed to have forgotten that the monarchists from the government to the man in the street knew that the succession should never be tampered without having the most serious of reasons to do so – and her reason wasn't about anything except her unreasonable envy and a resulting desire to bring Charles down.

'She was suffering from an acute case of what psychologists call envy. It's not creditable, but there's nothing abnormal about it. All sorts of normal people suffer from envy,' was how Dr Basil Panzer described it to Lady Colin Campbell.

Nevertheless, it was not until shortly before her death that Diana finally gave up her campaign to make William the heir to the throne. Camillagate, the Dimbleby programme and best of all the mischievous *Sunday Times* serialisation of his book had helped encourage her, while the *Times*, demanding to know whether 'she jumped or was she pushed' when she retired from public life, just added further weight to her belief that she might achieve this vindictive dream. As a result she relentlessly attempted to manipulate public opinion by briefing her stooges at her favourite papers, and when that didn't work she went on television to explain her opinion to the world in her *Panorama* interview.

As Jephson and Prince Charles had rightly predicted, retirement didn't suit the Princess. She had time on her hands and seemed to withdraw further into herself as she came to trust fewer and fewer people. She still had four protection officers available to her, but in the main she declined to use them and even had her chauffeur wash her cars rather than drive them. She would spend hours either sitting in her sitting room window with her mobile glued to her ear, as she called her flavours of the month incessantly, or just wandering around Knightsbridge on her own, where she made an easy target for the paparazzi. They would lie in wait for her on her way back from the gym or when she was out shopping, and pounce. Some days Diana could cope, enjoying all the attention and proof that she was still a beautiful star, and she would pose for them; on others, when she was really feeling down and tearful, didn't feel that she looked great or was just having a bad day, she would understandably refuse to cooperate. But now there were no protective policemen to ward these animals off, they would easily corner her, and if they weren't going to get a photograph of her smiling, one of her crying would do just as well. Given her mental state and the level of their taunts and insults, this was easily achieved. Jayne Fincher, who had been photographing the Princess for over a decade, was horrified by this behaviour: 'They would be right up close in front, so that she couldn't walk one step, so she's got to keep dodging. It's physically oppressive. It would be like being hunted by a pack. And they would be verbally aggressive to her, they would say, "Take your clothes off because we need to earn some money." They'd use foul language at her and be completely abusive and horrible.'

One could argue that the Princess had brought a lot of this upon her own head by refusing to use the security services that she clearly needed, and by her own desire to be on the front pages of the tabloids daily for many years, as well as her attempted manipulation of the press. However, this in no way excuses the behaviour, and only goes to prove that our society is so concerned with celebrity and money while being totally unconcerned with right or wrong. She may have been a princess, but on such days she was just a girl in deep distress and they couldn't have cared less – and nor did the editors who were so keen to buy the photographs.

For the first time in many years, Diana's old magic with the press seemed to be wearing thin. Articles started to appear that questioned her motives for doing certain things. People started to question her outings with the boys to theme parks, and asked whether her real motive was just to use the boys as a way of manipulating the press and scoring points over her husband. Diana immediately thought that the Palace was briefing against her in the way that she had spun against Prince Charles. It is true that people like Sir Robert Fellowes no longer moved quickly to support her, nor were they inclined to show any trust in her. Some courtiers even made it plain that she was going through a difficult period of her life and needed space; others expressed regret at her lack of emotional stability. However, their comments were extremely minor by comparison to the rumours and lies that she herself had spread about the Royal Family, and they were certainly not the reason for the Princess's new and less attractive media image. Nevertheless, Diana confronted her brother-in-law and complained bitterly that she was being used by the Palace in the newspapers. This led Lord Charteris to comment, 'It was ironic. She who had taken her dirty linen to the public for a good airing, complaining that they had no right to say she must be treated with love and understanding. Of course it was patronising, but it was a damned sight nicer and fairer than any of the accusations she'd made against the Prince of Wales and the rest of the Royal Family.'

The real point was that the press needed a new angle on her; without the cuddly photos of a fairy-tale princess, they needed something else. She had given it to them by having been found out by many of the editors to be deceitful, and then by appearing to be a neurotic woman thanks to certain vile elements of Britain's paparazzi.

But this was just part of the most complex area of Diana's life – her relationship with the press. No one becomes as famous as she did without a permanent campaign being waged on his or her behalf in order to attract the coverage that she achieved. The Princess didn't have a team, but she worked on her own campaign both relentlessly and with a brilliance bordering on genius. Sir David English, editor-in-chief of Associated Newspapers, the owners of the *Daily Mail* and employer of Richard Kay, was aware of the mutually beneficial relationship between his papers and the princess and thought he understood the position perfectly. He concluded, 'Diana liked the tabloids. She had no quarrel with any of their staff photographers, most of whom she knew by their first names. She regularly met with tabloid editors. Indeed, she had ongoing contact with all editors. She was – perhaps by necessity – a media groupie.'

English, who knew the Princess very well, was a great fan of her media skills. He once told her, 'If you were not the Princess of Wales, you'd be running your own commercial public relations company. And it would be the best in the world.' He also knew that Diana was capable of 'scheming, of obsessive manipulation, that whole frightening and distressing picture of a beautiful and terrified creature at bay.'

This opinion – that she was a brilliant media operator who was totally in control of image creation unless she was unfairly attacked in the streets by rude and threatening paparazzi – is not strictly correct. Firstly, the Princess could only have ever been brilliant at creating an image for herself. She was, to herself, the all-important obsession. It have would have been most unlikely that she would have ever shown the same animal cunning or interest in creating commercial PR for anyone else. Secondly, this obsession with herself led her at times to make serious errors of judgement when dealing with the tabloids, and when things went wrong, she would be furious and blame the newspapers for this rather than herself. She would be very rude behind their backs, but never to their faces, as she never forgot that she would need them again in the future. If they wrote things that she didn't like, she wouldn't forgive them, but neither would she alienate them. Instead she would even increase the charm offensive in the hope of getting a better result next time. Thirdly, her relationship with the paparazzi hadn't been that very different from the one she had enjoyed with other areas of the press for many years. She had become quite brilliant at engineering photo opportunities, and had used them endlessly to further her image. Things only really started to change with the paparazzi in 1993 when she made the mistake of thinking that she could manage without protection officers, while some parts of the media were tiring of her image to a certain extent, and her behaviour was becoming extremely unpredictable. This tilted the balance of the less favourable paparazzi and journalists against her, and gave those whom she didn't court and flirt with a new angle to her story.

And as no one can give exclusives to everyone all of the time, it was to a certain extent inevitable that sooner or later those who felt short-changed by her would turn on her as a way of writing something new and original. Moreover, they would care no more about the truth of any of it than anyone had done when writing what she wanted written.

This all meant that a Diana denuded of police support, paranoid of the way her image was presented and in a state of severe depression, was still able to get by in her convoluted relationships with the journalists who supported her and whom she felt she needed to cultivate in order to manipulate her coverage. But there were now days when she could no longer control the position on the street, her mask slipped and the paparazzi and journalists smelled blood. And it wasn't just them who squared up for the fight – the Princess could behave every bit as badly and as dangerously to them as they did to her. It became almost as common for the Princess to scream, 'Fuck off!' or 'Get lost, bastards!' as it was for her to smile and joke with the paparazzi. The pattern seemed to be that if she had tipped them off, she obviously wanted them there and she would be charming; but if she hadn't requested their attendance, she believed that they had no right to invade her privacy. She simply refused to accept that press relations don't work that way and that the more abusive she became, the more the paparazzi lost respect for her, and so the war hotted up.

The result of this breakdown of diplomatic relations between the Princess and the paparazzi became more than exchanged insults: it became a dangerous game of race and chase that could have cost lives. Mark Saunders and Glenn Harvey were part of the paparazzi pack that used to follow her around at that time. One day they were trailing her up the M4 motorway. Diana was driving in the fast lane, with their car not far behind. Suddenly the Princess pulled over and let the two photographers pass. This done, she then pulled back into the fast lane and speeded up behind their vehicle. Now both cars were travelling at around ninety miles an hour, and the Princess started to ram the car in front of her. Saunders accelerated while Harvey gestured to the Princess to back off. Diana was by now driving with one hand on the wheel, while gesturing back wildly with the other. There were just millimetres between the cars before Saunders managed to shake her off at 120 miles per hour. Then he slipped into the middle lane, and Diana sped past without a glance in their direction.

There are countless other tales of chases through the residential areas of London at ninety miles an hour, jumping red lights, driving at high speed through narrow streets at night with lights off, and even deliberately swerving into paparazzi vehicles. Perhaps this area of her life became a tragic habit, a dangerous game of cat and mouse that would end so horribly in a Paris tunnel. Either way, this was a war that Diana could not win and her behaviour over this period did nothing to promote her own image, while it only continued to damage the Royal Family's reputation.

There is no doubt that the Murdoch press had an anti-royal agenda, and over this period the undisciplined behaviour of the Princess of Wales and the Duchess of York played right into their hands. Having both women left free to their own devices was clearly a major problem to the monarchy, but a gift from heaven to the tabloid editors. Neither woman realised that, as powerful as they saw themselves, they were never going to be a match for the media; attempting to manipulate it was a very dangerous game to be playing.

However, while the Princess seemed unable to sort out the turmoil created by her courting the paparazzi one minute and then literally wanting to drive them off the road the next, she remained very careful to court most tabloid editors and their journalists; no matter what they wrote, she became ever more keen to make friends with them. She continued to believe that if she could charm them, they would write exactly what she wanted. She had varying degrees of success, dependent upon her target's intelligence and professional integrity. The most notable scalp was Richard Kay, whom she met when she went to Nepal in 1993. Kay was a public-school boy, so the extremely class-aware Princess saw him as a gentleman and 'one of us'.

The Princess had known Andrew Morton before the book, but she never befriended him; she even ridiculed him to anyone who would listen during the last years of her life. Morton had done his job and could be dispensed with. Moreover, any ongoing stories leaked to him would only draw attention to their collusion. And there was another drawback: he came from working-class origins, which meant that in Diana's mind he was not worthy. With Richard Kay things were different, and as she gained confidence in him, so she began leaking private information, often invented or exaggerated, to him. As a result, exclusive stories about the Prince and Princess of Wales began to appear in either the *Daily Mail* or the *Mail on Sunday*. Such stories read so much like propaganda for Diana that it became well known in media circles that Kay was the Princess's messenger. When Kay wrote 'friends of Diana', Fleet Street suspected that he really meant Diana herself; following her death, Kay confirmed that this was indeed the case.

Either blinded by her charm or not aware that he was being manipulated, Richard Kay picked up the baton where the Princess had ordered Morton to lay it down. His association with Diana did not have the range or depth of Morton's; but swiftly he became her new media vehicle. Her almost daily exclusives leaked to Kay, which was done with David English's knowledge and approval, enhanced his position at the *Daily Mail* and created a pro-Diana and anti-Charles feeling among the paper's readership. However, it also served to lose the Princess any remaining sympathisers that she might have had in Palace circles. It was assumed at the time that the Princess was doing this in order to strengthen her position in what she saw as an ongoing war with the House of Windsor. However, following her death, Kay let it be known that not only had Diana spoken to him on a daily basis, she had also confided in him – for publication – the most private aspects of her life with Dodi Fayed, even though there was no need to do so. What compelled her to do this?

The psychiatrist Dr Michael Davies provides the answer to that question. He not only knew the Princess, he was well aware of her medical history. He concluded that the Princess of Wales was a true narcissist. 'People think a narcissist is someone who is in love with her own image, but that is not so. In lay language, a narcissist is someone whose sense of self is so shaky that she exists only when others are reflecting their impression of her back to her. That is why the Princess of Wales was so sensitive to criticism and so dependent on the good opinion of others.' That is the reason she needed the constant attention of the media, and why she so often complained of emptiness. 'It's a frightening condition to have,' continued Davies, 'because sufferers have such voids within their personalities. I am convinced that was her true problem, and that everything else that followed as a consequence – the weak sense of self, the feelings of emptiness, of alienation, the maladjustment, the eating disorder, the depression, the fear. As she matured and developed a sense of her own existence, the corollary was a firmer sense of self. That's when her problems started lessening, when Diana the individual started to blossom.'

Dr Davies's opinion, which is built on his knowledge of the Princess's symptoms and which mirror those of any BPD sufferer, is that as a true narcissist Diana was addicted to the acclaim of others as her only way of feeling any self-worth. This would explain why her media image was at times more important than her children, why she was so delighted when the coverage was good and furious when it wasn't, and why above all else she felt that she had to have total control over it. Moreover, he would appear to be correct when he states that her problems lessened when she matured, but this can only really mean during the last two years of her life when she seemed to find a calm from some of the good works that she had undertaken and as a result attempted to develop a better relationship with her ex-husband and his family.

Nevertheless, she hadn't been totally cured – if she had she wouldn't have been telephoning Richard Kay with inside information about her affair with Dodi Fayed on the very night that she was killed. Neither would she have tipped off the paparazzi that she was going to be in Paris unexpectedly that evening. And as a result of that tip-off, it was her media-junkie habit that set off a chain reaction that killed her in the end.

In the midst of all of this turmoil and twilight gloom came a ray of pleasure and hope: Diana had a new man in her life. His name was Oliver Hoare. Hoare, although Eton-educated, came from a fairly modest Norfolk family and certainly wasn't assured of his seat at the table of high society. He had had to make his way up there by his considerable charm and good looks. A *Daily Mail* article of the time even rumoured him to have slept with either sex in his desire for self-advancement before eventually allowing the immensely rich Iranian heiress Hamoush Bowler to take him under her wing and call him 'my protégé'. Hoare was in his twenties while Bowler was twice his age. She encouraged his interest in Islamic art and even took him to Tehran.

Once back in London, Hoare established himself as an Islamic antiquities dealer. In 1976 he married Diane Waldner. She was French, extremely rich – an heiress to a great French oil fortune – and the daughter of Baroness Louise de Waldner, who counted the Queen Mother among her friends. Hoare had arrived. They set up home in the most expensive part of west London, and through Diane's connections moved in the highest social circles. As a result they eventually became friendly with the Waleses, and it was Diane's mother's home in Provence that Prince Charles visited for a period of recuperation when he broke his arm playing polo in 1990.

Most men would have been extremely grateful for their good fortune in marrying one so good-looking, rich and well connected, but apparently not Hoare. The same *Daily Mail* article accused him of conducting numerous affairs, including a four-year fling with Ayesha Nadir, the twice-divorced wife of the fugitive Polly Peck tycoon Asil Nadir. It would not be long, however, until he turned his wandering eye towards the Princess of Wales.

The effect that Hoare was to have on the Princess was extraordinary. This was not only because he was the older man that always seemed to attract her, but because she found it hard to possess him – a problem that she had also encountered with the Prince of Wales. For Hoare, this relationship probably meant little more than a deliciously exciting and dangerous fling. He certainly gave that impression. But Diana was so consumed with passion that she not only took to smuggling Hoare into Kensington Palace in the boot of her car, something that she had often done with other men over the years, but even once went round to his house, when she knew that his wife was away, dressed in only a fur coat, diamond earrings and high-heeled shoes, which she described to journalist Ross Benson as 'my tart's trotters'. Burrell relays this story, but believed that his mistress was on her way to see another lover – heart surgeon Hasnat Khan. In fact the Princess didn't even meet Khan until September 1995. It was Hoare that she hoped to surprise, but when she got there he was out and so, with her ardour dampened, she was forced to return home feeling rather silly.

The King and Di

Hoare became worried that Diana's passion and constant need for attention was getting out of hand, and he became most concerned that news of the affair would get back to his wife. This led him to agree with the Princess's wish to get rid of her protection officers in an attempt to keep matters secret. This became all the more urgent to him once he had been discovered by them half-naked, smoking a cigar behind a potted bay tree in a corridor at Kensington palace. Ken Wharfe recalls, 'Hoare did not like having us around. He told the Princess to get rid of us. He was more concerned that his wife might find out than he was about the Princess's safety.' Of course, Hoare got his way and there was to be a much more serious consequence than just Diana being jostled by the paparazzi in the street as a result. Wharfe has always believed that this dismissal of her officers led indirectly to the Princess's death. He claims, 'If I or one of my colleagues had been on duty, she would never have got into that car.'

However, in the small circle that makes up royal society, Hoare was never going to keep the affair secret. The Prince became aware of it very quickly, but provided that it caused no public scandal or embarrassment to the Royal Family, he seemed quite content to ignore the affair, and has even remained friendly with Oliver Hoare since. Not surprisingly, Diane Hoare did not treat the matter so lightly. Harsh words were exchanged and serious threats of divorce made. He immediately promised to end the affair if she would give him one last chance.

But getting rid of Diana was easier said than done. Lady Colin Campbell writes that the Princess was suddenly hit by two awful pieces of news: Hoare wanted to end their affair, and she was pregnant. The combination finally sent her over the edge.

Diana knew she would have to have an abortion. She wanted to keep the baby, and drove herself crazy imagining that it might be the little girl that she had always wanted. But how could she avoid an abortion? She wasn't divorced, and an illegitimate child would ruin a public reputation for which she had sacrificed everything. When Hoare finished their affair, he was most likely unaware that she was pregnant, but there was no certainty that the child was his as the Princess was seeing other men at the same time. The combination finally drove Diana to a state where she could no longer control her actions.

Lady Colin Campbell writes that just before the abortion, and immediately after, Diana was unhinged with grief and misery. It was reported she reverted to her nuisance phone call habit. She might make over fifty silent calls a day. Diane Hoare called in the police, who traced all the calls back to Diana's private line, her mobile, call boxes near Kensington Palace and her sister Sarah's telephone. Oliver Hoare asked the police not to proceed with the case and so it was closed. However, the news was bound to leak out, and when it did a furious Princess accused her husband's staff of tipping off the press. In fact the leak had actually come from a boy who was at school with one of the Hoare children; it became more graphic when Hoare's chauffeur Barry Hodge sold his story about his boss's relationship with the Princess to the *News of the World*. The mortified and totally humiliated Diana was forced to admit that she had made some of the calls once a story that she tried to float through some of her media friends that she was actually shielding a member of her staff was met with incredulity by the nation. However, she continued to deny that she had made all the calls, and still claimed that there was a conspiracy against her. But for once nobody believed her. She, who had shown no mercy to others when vindictively ruining their reputations, was now receiving some of her own medicine and would receive the same lack of sympathy that she had shown to her victims. Ironically, she would have received a lot of sympathy from some of the public if they had known what had finally pushed her over the edge – but news of her aborting an illegitimate child would have damaged her prized reputation even further and so remained a closely guarded secret.

Following her exposure as a stalker, the burden of mass humiliation only added to the weight of her other problems. She became obsessed with the idea that the police would prosecute her for making the nuisance calls, despite the fact that they had agreed to drop the case and the fact that advisors like Joseph Sanders assured her – as Lady Colin Campbell recounted in *The Real Diana* – that princesses of Wales didn't get prosecuted for such minor offences. Initially she refused to believe him, and confided that she had made over 400 calls to the Hoares' home, but insisted that she did speak if Oliver answered the phone. It took months before she finally accepted that she had got away with it and would not be brought before a court.

What finally helped Princess Diana come to terms with the abortion, Oliver Hoare and the possibility of a police prosecution was the arrival of yet another man in her life. Unfortunately, this man was also spoken for. Will Carling was the strong, masculine and highly regarded captain of the England rugby team. He was engaged to, and living with, a very attractive PR girl, who became a television presenter, named Julia Smith. Both Carling and the Princess were members of the exclusive Chelsea Harbour Club. The Princess had taken to working out there with her fitness trainer Carolan Brown. 'I bet I could get Will Carling to ask me out,' Diana told her trainer, before adding, 'I might be able to stop that marriage happening.' Carling was due to marry Julia Smith in a couple of months' time. Carolan Brown, in her ignorance of the realities of the Princess's sex life, put this apparently cruel and selfish comment down to Diana's youth and lack of sexual experience, and didn't really take it seriously.

But Diana had other ideas. She started a relentless flirtation, and soon Carling was bowled over by the Princess of Wales's interest in him. He just couldn't believe his luck, and was completely flattered by her attention. Diana, as she did with all her men, immersed herself in whatever interested them. However, on this occasion, and quite unlike the pursuits of Prince Charles, which she had no genuine interest in, the Princess was actually keen on Carling's interest in physical fitness. It helped her maintain an attractive body, which she rightly saw as an important part of both her image and her ability to attract the men whom she wished to seduce. Carling was dedicated to his weight-training and exercise regimes, and soon Diana upped her own programme to impress him. He was what she needed at the time – a flirtation and a conquest that made her feel better about herself. She never fell in love with him, but was delighted to encourage him to become besotted with her without regard for the effect that this might have on the lives of Carling or his fiancée.

Meanwhile, the pin-up boy of English rugby married his pretty bride, who knew absolutely nothing of her husband's relationship with the Princess, even though Carling was talking about it to many of his friends, and such stories started to become well known in rugby circles. The new Mrs Carling believed that her relationship with her husband was strong and passionate and that her marriage was working well. In reality, Will Carling was seeing the Princess several times a week, usually at either Kensington Palace or at the Chelsea Harbour Club, where he now acted as her exercise advisor.

After more than a year of this amazingly going on without either the tabloids or Julia Carling suspecting anything, exposure came from another woman whom Carling had allowed to know too much. This was his personal assistant, and when she and Carling parted company amid much vitriol, she alerted the press to her boss's affair. Julia was surprised to learn that her husband and the Princess were even friends, never mind lovers. She confronted him with the newspaper reports; he denied them and claimed that he barely knew the Princess and that she only knew him as a result of princes William and Harry admiring him as captain of the successful England rugby team. Julia Carling was duly convinced that her husband was telling the truth and issued her now famous public warning to Diana that she had 'picked on the wrong married couple to try and break up this time'.

However, within days poor Julia was humiliatingly forced to eat her words: Carling was spotted by a now alerted press entering and leaving Kensington Palace. He claimed that he had only popped in to drop off some presents for the two young princes. An angry Julia issued him with an ultimatum – never see Diana again, or risk the break-up of their marriage. When the newlywed Mrs Carling opened her newspaper a few days later, she saw a very guilt-ridden Carling and Diana stealthily leaving the Harbour Club following an early-morning meeting.

The Carling marriage was over. Now the Princess was faced with a new anxiety: would she be named as co-respondent? Not only would this continue the embarrassment of her exposure, but also the resulting court hearing would put her down in history as a marriage-breaker. For a while Mrs Carling, who by now realised that this possibility allowed her the pleasure of wreaking a little vengeance, said nothing, which led the tabloids to speculate that she might. The Princess was once again on the receiving end of a public humiliation that would damage her reputation. Left to her own devices and without an heir to the throne either to blame or hide behind, she seemed to be increasingly exposed as the deeply troubled and flawed personality that she really was. In an act of amazing self-denial, she refused to accept any of the responsibility for her latest misfortune, choosing instead to blame the press and Julia Carling. 'Why can't they leave me alone?' she moaned to her friends. 'It's hardly my fault if that bitch can't keep her man.' This might be considered to be a fairly one-eyed view from a woman who had made a career out of playing the victim to Camilla's vamp. By comparison, Julia Carling appeared generous, commenting, 'It would be easy to say she ruined my marriage, but it takes two to tango and I blame Will for getting involved in the first place.'

For the Princess of Wales, it was a sad fact of life that people who constantly court the press by holding secret daily briefings can never hope to control a media image that such celebrity interest and exposure creates. She had been playing with fire for years, and now her fingers were well and truly being burned.

A few months after her retirement from public life, Jephson managed to persuade Diana to go back to work on a part-time basis. With the help of Mike Whitlam, she was induced to become a British board member of the advisory committee of the Red Cross. She managed to attend some meetings in Geneva in the summer of 1994, but as the serious nature of these became plain to her, Jephson 'watched my boss's eyes glaze over' and she duly quit in September.

In the 1980s she had convinced herself that her problems stemmed from her marriage and the confines of royal life as dictated by the Palace. She dreamed of being free and having her old life back again. But freedom hadn't bought her happiness. She felt unable to work. She had seriously damaged her reputation, which would have by now been in complete tatters had it not been for the lasting impression that the Morton book had made in the public consciousness that her problems were somehow Prince Charles's fault. She was more fragile mentally than ever before, and more likely to be on the phone in the middle of the night to someone whom she might drop next week in a sudden distress about an imagined slight.

But in Dianaland, none of this was her fault. Just as her problems during her marriage had been the fault of either Prince Charles, his family or his staff, now all her problems were down to the press, Diane Hoare, Julia Carling, Tiggy Legge-Bourke, Andrew Morton, other Morton conspirators, Sarah Ferguson, Elton John, her brother Charles, her sister Jane, her brother-in-law Robert, Buckingham Palace, St James's Palace or anyone else that she happened to fall out with – a list far too big to record here. The Princess had cut herself off from those who wanted to help her, and surrounded herself with people who only told her what she wanted to hear; when they didn't, they were discarded.

There could be no doubting that 1993, 1994 and 1995, her years of freedom, had been awful years. The Princess felt that she had been given a terrible battering by the media in general and by the tabloids in particular. The exception was the *Daily Mail*, who had remained as loyal as possible, balancing any criticism with an equally sympathetic article in the same edition, in exchange for their continuing hotline from the Princess to Richard Kay. But however important the *Daily Mail* was to Middle England, it was not enough to counter the bad press that she had been getting from the other tabloids. Diana understood this, and knew that she must mend fences with the other press barons. Top of her list was Rupert Murdoch. Luckily an opportunity soon presented itself. Murdoch was on the board of the United Cerebral Palsy Fund. They were looking for a celebrity to honour at their New York annual dinner. Murdoch rightly guessed that the Princess needed some good press to counter all the stories his papers had been running about her sex life, nuisance phone calls and marriage-breaking antics. He wrote to her, 'I would be personally appreciative if you would consider this. Love, Rupert.' Murdoch knew his American friends would be impressed if he could land a huge celebrity like the Princess of Wales. Year after year they had struggled to get someone with half the profile. He also knew that she was smart enough not to turn him down and that she would revel in all the 'Saint Di' photo opportunities that would obviously present themselves as a result of her acceptance. And of course he was right.

But despite this, these first three years of freedom had taken their toll. Not only had her mental state deteriorated further as she bounced from one PR disaster to another, but it was probably made worse by her lack of any consistent goals. On the one hand she wanted to remain the Princess of Wales, enjoy the privileges and even talked on occasion of getting back with Prince Charles both as a royal partner and as a wife; on the other hand, she had days when she expressed a desire to meet a man she could marry and have more children with – especially a daughter. Joseph Sanders told Lady Colin Campbell, 'She was definitely on the lookout for men. She wanted love and she wanted to find someone to share her life with, even to marry.' The Harbour Club was somewhere to meet attractive men, and Diana was reportedly not backward in introducing herself, which would explain her penchant for exercising in full makeup. Sanders told Lady Colin Campbell of her most enduring relationship from the Harbour Club was with Christopher Walley, an imposing property developer she saw until shortly before she died.

Sanders' comments raise two most interesting points. Firstly, and he is well supported by others who were close to the Princess, he asserts that we will never know just how many men Diana had sexual relations with. If he is correct, some have said that it might be considered to be surprising that so many have been 'gentlemen' and remained silent despite the lure of the tabloid shilling. On the other hand, I remember as a founder member of the Harbour Club, prior to the Princess joining, the credentials needed for membership. A man selling his story about Diana to the press might expect to lose such membership and become a social leper in Kensington and Chelsea, as well as receive the same life-wrecking treatment from the other tabloids as the unfortunate Hewitt did; moreover, anybody who could afford the club's debenture and fees didn't need the tabloids' cash anyway, and as most would more than likely be married anyway, they had their own personal and highly financial reasons for staying silent. To get a £100,000 from a tabloid in order to gain notoriety while losing more than a million and custody of the children is not a sensible thing to be doing.

The second point concerns Christopher Walley. If Sanders is correct, which he might well be as again there are many people who support him in this assertion, it serves to confirm that Diana didn't consider sexual fidelity to be an important part of her behaviour towards men she claimed to love. Sanders states that she continued to see Whalley until just before she died. This means that she was seeing him while carrying on a love affair with the man she told many was the only person she had ever wanted to marry since her break-up with the Prince of Wales, Hasnat Khan. This is not only a further example of her voracious sexual appetite and infidelity, but also of her double standards when it came to the rules she applied to others, in particular Prince Charles.

Fitness trainer Carolan Brown explained that, 'She was the sort of person who didn't like being out of a relationship. She didn't like being on her own because she needed constant reassurance that she was loved. That was her ultimate dream – to find a perfect husband, have more children and settle down. She was looking for the right man.' She might well have been, and was apparently trying out half of Kensington and Chelsea in the process – whether available or otherwise. Moreover, the perfect husband seemed to be, in Diana's mind, one who didn't mind sharing his wife with several other lovers and a media habit. This was always Diana's ultimate problem with relationships – her simple inability to consider the other party or put their needs on a par with hers. It was a symptom of her illness that while she could have feelings for others in all extremes, she could never understand their feelings, and from such a lack of comprehension came a lack of consideration.

The Princess met Dr Hasnat Khan by accident in September 1995. He was one of a team of specialists who performed a triple heart bypass operation on Joseph Toffolo, the husband of Diana's acupuncturist Oonagh, in London's Royal Brompton Hospital. The Princess met Khan while visiting Joseph, and soon started to visit her friend's husband and other patients daily in order to meet up with the doctor. Naturally, a lot of convalescing heart patients couldn't quite understand what on earth they had done to deserve all of this wonderful attention from the Princess. Nevertheless, they weren't complaining and must have been extremely cheered by her. Then, one night in December, Diana was discovered leaving the hospital by a *News of the World* photographer. Instead of running away, she stayed and posed for photographs, and then phoned the newspaper's royal correspondent to announce that she regularly visited the hospital at midnight on a mercy mission in order to dispense comfort to the sick and the dying.

Some believe that the Princess made the best of being caught leaving the hospital by a hostile tabloid; others think that this is too much of a coincidence given her normal reaction during this period to an unwarranted intrusion by the press and the fact that following the Carling fiasco Diana knew she had to pull off a coup with that particular newspaper in order to redeem her tarnished image with its readers. On balance, the second line of thought seems the most likely. Either way, she was indicating an intention to put her media image ahead of her personal happiness or any consideration for her new lover. Initially she was more than pleased when her scheming worked and the *News of the World* readers swallowed her propaganda and so forgot about the complaints of Diane Hoare and Julia Carling.

Hasnat Khan was a thirty-seven-year-old heart surgeon from Lahore in Pakistan. He was a member of the world-famous Professor Sir Magdi Yacoub's cardiac team. The Princess confessed to her hairdressers Nathalie Symonds and Tessa Rock as well as the long-suffering Joseph Sanders that it was love at first sight and that she found Hasnat irresistible. He was indeed an attractive man, if somewhat tubbier than her usual preference at the Harbour Club and a lot less lean than Prince Charles's physique that she had originally so admired some fifteen years earlier. The Princess explained to Sanders that she intended to get her man. 'She set out to get him. She told me so herself. She said had a thing about doctors. The fact that he helped sick people fascinated her. She really admired him. All the hours he worked, and the sacrifices he made for his profession.' This might have been the case at the outset, but it wasn't too long before she came to resent his devotion to his calling as she had with Prince Charles before him. In both cases she quickly lost admiration for both men's sense of duty when she realised that it prevented them from giving her their undivided attention. Again I am assured that this was a natural symptom of the insecurity her illness created within her.

However, initially she set out to win Khan, just as she had the Prince of Wales, not only by expressing her admiration for his devotion, but by showing immense interest in all the things that interested him. Moreover, as an older and cannier woman, she didn't just fake it as she had when she was young, but she read up on heart surgery and the Muslim religion in order to appear genuinely at one with him – she even asked if she might attend operations that he and Sir Magdi performed. Natty, as the Princess had nicknamed her surgeon, got his boss's consent and so Diana started to watch them at work in the operating theatre. She confessed to friends that this made her feel quite sick but believed that it was worth it as her presence impressed Hasnat.

Diana then made another serious media blunder that did her reputation further damage. A television news crew were filming a piece on Sir Magdi and his team: Diana wore make-up, gold hoop earrings and had her fringe attractively shooting out from underneath her surgical cap. In a sterile operating theatre, all of this is forbidden. When the item was shown, the result was a media outcry that even the faithful *Daily Mail* joined in. She was accused of self-promotion and of ghoulishly invading a patient's privacy in order to be seen at a gory operation looking beautiful while appearing saintly. Given her publicity over Hoare and Carling, some people actually started seriously to question Diana's mental state openly for the first time. The resulting publicity showed the midnight mercy visits to the hospital in a new and less flattering light, and thus undid all the positive PR she had sought to affect with that story.

Joseph Sanders later claimed, 'Diana was upset. She hadn't intended to get publicity. She was looking at her man at work.' What did the Princess expect? Here was a film crew doing a piece on a heart operation and looking on, not only in the theatre but right up by the table, was one of the most famous and beautiful women in the world. Was she so naive that she really believed they would ignore her presence? Or was it that, despite her lover's concern for no publicity regarding their relationship, she simply could not resist her insatiable craving for it – but had this time got it horribly wrong?

Hasnat Khan, while finding Diana very attractive and being flattered by her attention, was already starting to feel the pressure of her demanding nature and the unwelcome proximity of a media that she bemoaned but seemed unable to discourage. It is doubtful whether he knew at this stage that she was actually secretly encouraging the press and initiating coverage that was eventually bound to blow his cover and throw him under the spotlight. Diana, either unaware or unconcerned by Khan's worries, pushed ahead with the relationship. She got closer to Jemima Khan, wife of Imran but no relation of Hasnet, believing that she could help her win and then keep an eastern man. Now starting to dream of a new start as she had occasionally with James Hewitt, the Princess threw herself east with energy. She started to burn joss sticks at Kensington Palace. She ordered an array of Pakistani traditional clothes and made quite a fashion statement by wearing them. She visited Pakistan twice, secretly visiting Hasnat's family on the second occasion when she tried to lobby them for their support of her. They were kind to her, but certainly had no wish for Hasnat to tie his future to a non-Muslim, non-Asian princess who didn't really share their values however much she protested that she did. She found them to be a much tougher nut to crack than she had the Windsors. Nevertheless, the Princess convinced herself that they would come around to her way of thinking eventually, and told friends on her return in May 1997 that, 'They love me and I love them.'

However, the affair with Hasnat had already become strained. Khan had been enraged on 3 November 1996 when the *Sunday Mirror* published a detailed account of his affair with Diana. He was convinced that she had leaked the story to the paper as he was not only well aware by now of her habit of doing such things, she believed that some of the detail could only have come from the Princess. They had been arguing increasingly about his refusal to make the sort of commitment to her that she was demanding, and Khan believed that Diana had leaked the story in order to force his hand. He was probably right: the whole incident seems not too dissimilar to the 'mystery blond on the royal train' story that had finally pushed Prince Charles into proposing to her sixteen years earlier.

Diana, panic-stricken that she might lose the surgeon, enrolled Joseph Sanders to help convince him that she had had absolutely nothing to do with the article. She also got valuable assistance from her old friend Richard Kay at the *Daily Mail*. His Monday article described the *Sunday Mirror*'s piece as 'bullshit'. Once again the *Daily Mail* had taken the Princess's word; once again it turned out to be a lie. In the end Khan was persuaded, but things were never quite so idyllic again and by the time the Princess had returned from visiting the Khan family in the spring of 1997, she realised that she was now facing the same problem that she had encountered with Prince Charles: duty. She admitted to friends that while she admired the work that Khan did, it got in the way. 'But he has so little time for me. It's become a problem. We're always arguing over it. He puts his work before me. If he really loved me, he'd put me first.' Nothing in Dianaland had changed.

As the rows with Hasnat escalated, the Princess felt increasingly rejected. Characteristically, she responded by becoming even more obsessed and argumentative, which only served to drive Khan away from her. Diana then decided to change tack and attempted to make her lover jealous. She had been secretly seeing other men throughout her relationship with the surgeon, but now she decided to see some of them publicly. Suddenly it was all right for Christopher Whalley to take her to lunch, and she was also seen dancing seductively with Gulu Lalvani, the electronics tycoon, at Annabel's in Berkley Square. Initially the plan worked, and Khan was made to feel very jealous. However, in the end, such feelings ebbed away as he came to understand that her manipulative personality and media obsession would have inevitable effects upon both his career and his relationship with his family. Diana was important to him, but not important enough for him to damage either.

By the time the Princess set off on her first holiday with the Fayed family in July 1997, her relationship with Khan was strained to breaking point. On that holiday she met Dodi Fayed, and almost immediately started an affair. Some have claimed that she only did so in order to make Khan jealous, others that when she met Dodi she immediately realised that he would put her first and foremost in his life in a way that neither Prince Charles nor Hasnat Khan would ever have done. No one can be sure. However, a very upset Hasnat Khan hid his obvious grief behind dark glasses at her funeral. He might not have wanted to marry her, and he might have come to see how flawed she was, but he clearly still had very strong feelings for her.

Despite all these other distractions, the War of the Waleses had remained a major issue in the Princess's mind. She had realised that, while a constant trickle of sympathetic information in her loyal newspapers was more than useful in sustaining a media position, it was not big enough or strong enough to alter public perception on its own. She worried that the media impression created by the adverse Hoare, Carling and Brompton Hospital publicity had created a picture that cute little stories from Richard Kay, however frequent, could not correct. It was only a matter of time before she would want to relieve all of her pent-up emotion and reach the masses with her version of all these recent events in order to attempt to restore her long-term reputation. If possible – and given a big enough stage – she would be able to deal a blow to her husband and appeal to the public directly that the accession was best left to her son (with her as the power behind the throne).

Intoxicated by such a heady cocktail of insecurity, ambition and media addiction, the Princess started to hint that it might be possible to make either a television programme or perhaps even a series of programmes about her and her work. The major US stations were quick to take the bait and, given her love of America and her realisation that American news was world news, she was tempted to go with them. She even had lunch with both the queens of American chat shows – Barbara Walters and Oprah Winfrey – and both were prepared to give her whatever she wanted in order to obtain the interview of the decade. But however impressed Diana was with either of them – and she was most impressed with both – she realised that it was realistically only going to be a British programme that would hold sway with the British public. If she really wanted to reach out to them, it must be through a British television company.

This in itself presented major problems. Firstly, the major British channel, and certainly the one with the highest global respect, was the BBC. However, the Princess did not trust the corporation, and regarded it as the media arm of Buckingham Palace. Her opinion was further enhanced by the fact that the chairman of the board of governors, Marmaduke Hussey, was married to the Queen's lady-in-waiting, Lady Susan Hussey – the woman who had tried so hard to help Diana during her engagement and early married life. Lady Susan had genuinely liked the Princess, but had been forced to witness more than just the occasional Diana tantrum and so was suspected of being part of an imagined Palace plot against her.

On the other hand, the Princess found the prospect of either ITV or Channel 4 less daunting. Moreover, she was friendly with both Sir David Frost and Clive Allen, and was prepared to consider either of them as suitable to interview her if their existing contracts permitted them to work with either of those independent channels. However, she remained quite rightly concerned that both would value their journalistic and broadcasting reputations enough not to give her the poetic licence that she needed in order to make a Morton style info-mercial. The Princess was PR-savvy enough not to want to be caught out, and understood only too well that no programme at all would be better than one that might lead her into the difficult ground of her sex life and mental health problems.

It was a hard decision full of danger, and one that Diana realised she would have to get right. As she considered her position carefully, a little known and even less-acclaimed broadcaster by the name of Martin Bashir came to her attention. Bashir, a son of Pakistani parents who had emigrated to Britain, was born in 1963. As a boy he showed a strong determination to succeed, as first-generation immigrants often do, and this was perhaps helped by a troubled family background – his father suffered from psychiatric problems and his brother died of muscular dystrophy. Bashir graduated from Southampton University with a top degree in English and History. He became a sports reporter and then a political journalist with a reputation for being left wing and chasing stories that rarely turned into anything concrete. After nine rather unexceptional years at the BBC, he eventually graduated to the prestige *Panorama* programme as a reporter.

However, en route he had perfected an ability to become a smooth and clever operator and as a result enlisted some fairly impressive support. On joining *Panorama*, he approached Tom Mangold, at the time the top investigative journalist that the BBC had to offer, and asked if he might be permitted to shake the great man's hand, explaining that the last wish of his dying brother was that he should emulate his style. Mangold was impressed, and determined to put in a good word for an Asian immigrant in the white man's, middle-class world that the BBC had become. He was somewhat less impressed when he learned that Bashir had told the same story to John Humphrys, the much-feared grand inquisitor of BBC's Radio Four, as well as the equally famous war correspondent Michael Nicholls.

In 1993 and 1994, Bashir had vaguely come to public recognition by making two controversial documentaries about the financial dealings of the former England football manager Terry Venables. As a result he also gathered a libel writ from Venables, who complained that some of the documents used in the programmes had been fabricated. Apparently, Bashir had employed the skills of a graphic designer to recreate material that he believed had originally existed but had been unable to lay his hands on. However, he presented them as genuine in the programme and so soiled the BBC's reputation, according to the Venables legal team, by having commissioned forgeries and then passed them off as genuine. This was something that a tabloid newspaper might get up to – but had Bashir brought the BBC this low? When Bashir confirmed his conduct on *TV-am*, there was naturally more than a little sympathy for this opinion in many quarters. Venables himself remains angry about the whole affair over a decade later because of the inaccuracy of both programmes and the fact that there was a second programme despite his complaints that the first was a tissue of lies. Moreover, he was only asked to comment on them, without having any knowledge of what would be said in them, the day before transmission. He sees that as making media sensationalism rather than fair reporting and most people would agree with him.

Therefore, we can safely assume that by the time the ambitious Bashir had come round to the idea of doing a Diana interview, he was more than capable of bending the truth and flattering to the greatest degree in order to get what he wanted. By the summer of 1995, when the BBC had been forced to worry about the fallout from the Venables programmes, Bashir had already moved on. He had heard that the Princess of Wales was looking to do a programme or even a series in which she might be persuaded to reveal the 'dirty tricks' campaign that she claimed was being waged against her by certain elements of the media and even from within Buckingham Palace itself. He realised that he was at the back of a high-calibre media queue, but nevertheless he remained undaunted. He went to work. Bashir is known to be both charmingly persuasive and cunning, as his programme on Michael Jackson has since proved him to be. But it should be noted that he got to meet the Princess only because she wanted him to. The fact that she was in her 'Pakistani period' thanks to her affair with Hasnat Khan was probably helpful, but perhaps not as helpful as the fact that he represented the prestigious *Panorama* programme and Diana rightly believed, despite her mistrust of the BBC, that if *Panorama* said something to the nation, it was accepted as gospel.

Bashir, thinking that he was the only one playing mind games and that he would have to persuade a reluctant princess to talk, got his graphic designer friend Wiessler to forge documents that he persuaded Charles Spencer were authentic and which proved that the Princess was being stalked and constantly watched by MI5. As a result Morton now claims that Diana, convinced by her brother of the validity of these documents and in fear of her life, was reluctantly persuaded by Bashir to speak out following many theatrical and frankly comical clandestine meetings – including one in an underground car park that imitated a scene from a Hollywood movie. It was complete theatre and utter nonsense: Bashir's 'forgeries' hadn't persuaded Diana to speak out – she did so because she had always planned to, and when she did her motive wasn't self-protection, it was self-justification and revenge. These were the subjects that the Princess theatrically addressed through her sorrowful eyes and dark makeup while sitting in the young princes' sitting room in KP and being interviewed by Bashir. And the main reason that Bashir was selected was that he agreed to terms that she had always doubted other presenters would find acceptable. Bashir was not only prepared to offer Diana total secrecy, but he also agreed to allow her control over what was filmed and what would and wouldn't be included in the final cut. Jackson might have been tricked by Bashir, but the Princess of Wales certainly wasn't. As usual when it came to the media, the Princess wished to be the puppet master and in Bashir's case, just as in Morton's before him, she had succeeded.

Max Hastings, who had somehow by this time become beguiled by the Princess, was asked for his advice and responded by counselling her not give such an interview. He was joined by Lord Palumbo, Lord Puttnam and many others. Vivienne Parry recalls, 'Of the people that she did talk to, those with media experience said very firmly, "Don't do it." But she ignored them.'

She went further than that and actually lied to most of them by telling them that she had no intention of doing the interview anyway. As part of her demand for total secrecy, she had made Bashir promise that the contents of the programme would not be shown to top BBC executives or the board of governors. Bashir agreed. How he hoped to keep such a promise if the top brass got wind of what was in the programme is a matter for some speculation. On the evening of 5 November, the Princess, who had unexpectedly given her staff, including the 'rock' Burrell, the evening off, ushered Bashir and his crew through a rear entrance to KP. She was about to give an Oscar-worthy performance.

On 20 November, the programme was broadcast to 23 million viewers in Britain alone. Looking mournful, dressed for bereavement and with saucer eyes that attempted to yell sincerity through layers of exaggerated black make-up, this was pure theatre. She talked through her eating disorders, her attempts to harm herself and her miserable marriage. She turned on Camilla and claimed that her marriage had always been a crowded place with three people in it. Next it was James Hewitt's turn for a bashing. Apparently she had loved and adored him, but he had let her down. Then came the most spiteful cut of them all – she suggested that Prince Charles might not really want to be king and might not be up to the job anyway; this implied her son Prince William might be a more suitable heir. As for her, she was happy just to be 'queen of people's hearts'. Then she finished this off with a chilling message for the Royal Family: she would not 'go quietly; I will fight to the end.'

With Diana acting as director, take after take was shot of certain questions until she was completely happy with the contents. She intended to portray herself as a trapped soul who had been damaged by a cruel and brutal Palace that had brought about all her problems and then taunted her with accusations of madness. The impression cleverly created was that the Palace might have tried to destroy her by driving her mad, but she was not, and was strong enough to survive. She believed that by addressing her mental problems in this way, she could dispel the claim that she was mad by openly referring to it and then explaining it was all part of a miserable plan of persecution that she had had to endure at the hands of the Windsors since she fell into their clutches in 1981. Naturally, this had all been made much worse by a hideous media that made her life a living hell.

To the less well informed, it appeared to be a frank and open account of her life. Of course it was not. There was no mention of her scores of lovers, many of whom came before Camilla returned to the scene; no mention of her cruel treatment of staff; no admission that she really knew that her husband had given up the greater part of his life to be the next king, was well prepared and keen to play his role; no admission that she knew Prince William wasn't even too keen to be king after his father, let alone instead of him; no explanation of why she made nuisance calls to Diane Hoare; no explanation of why she had accused Tiggy Legge-Bourke of having an abortion; no explanation as to why she had broken up Will and Julia Carling's marriage; no explanation as to why she was ghoulishly peering into a man's innards while being dressed inappropriately in an operating theatre; and quite naturally she neglected to say that she briefed the press most days, and even tipped off the hated paparazzi when it suited her.

The Princess certainly did not want to address these issues, so she quite rightly ignored them. This way, she could excuse her attempts to harm herself and have eating disorders by laying the blame at the door of her husband while still appearing to be frank. Her thinking was that if her *Panorama* interview kicked up as much of a storm as her Morton book, the other stories, which were of course much harder to explain away and certainly couldn't be blamed on Prince Charles or the Queen, would get forgotten just as Lady Colin Campbell's book had in 1992. And for the most part she was right.

She astutely admitted to the affair with Hewitt because she knew he held hundreds of letters from her and pictures of them making love in the garden of his mother's home in Devon – she knew a denial might be dangerous given the way she had treated him. But, in the end, it was when her unpleasant envy got the better of her and she attempted to deprive the Prince of Wales of his birthright to what she described as the 'top job' that she made a tremendous mistake. This was the final straw for the Queen, and resulted in a divorce that was to have very serious repercussions on the rest of her life.

On the night the interview was shown, a group of courtiers gathered in the Buckingham Palace press office to watch it together. Among them were Charles Anson and Philip Mackie from the Queen's press office, Richard Aylard, Allan Percival and Sandy Henney from the Prince's press office, and Geoff Crawford, who was Diana's press officer and just as much in the dark as everybody else. He was to resign as a direct result once he had understood the nature of the interview and the fact that it had been conducted without his knowledge. Understandably, he considered his position untenable. Philip Mackie, a likeable Scot who loved to assert that he had the inside track on every royal story, told the others before the programme began that he already knew what was in it and that there was nothing to worry about. He bet the others a bottle of champagne that he was right. After some fifteen minutes of transmission, Richard Aylard informed him that he owed the rest of them a whole case already.

Patrick Jephson arranged to watch the broadcast with Anne Beckwith-Smith. Diana had only told him about the interview after it had been recorded and less than a week before transmission. Fearful of what she might have said, he tried to smooth things out in advance with Buckingham Palace – it was after all, according to him, only the 'inner child' stamping her feet as usual and demanding attention. Not in his worst nightmares could he have believed how far she would go. After watching the programme, he also concluded that his position was untenable and was to resign soon after.

Interestingly, the Princess, who had used the programme as a brilliant propaganda effort to settle old scores and perhaps even seize the crown for her reluctant son, never made an issue about her safety. Why? It would have been the easiest thing to do – a few well-chosen lines about 'dark, secretive forces' would have alerted the public, and the Princess was a polished enough media performer to know how to get that across most effectively.

Newsnight, the BBC's late-night news magazine famous for its tough questioning and rather smug pseudo-intellectual status, had hurriedly put together a discussion group. Anthony Holden and Nicholas Soames had agreed to appear. By the time *Newsnight* went on air, Soames was shaking with rage. He could no longer disguise his disgust at the unfairness and injustice of it all. He had witnessed years of what had really happened. He could no longer help himself and, despite the fact that he was a government minister and therefore not supposed to criticise a member of the Royal Family, and had been ordered by the Prince to hold his tongue, he tore into the Princess and accused her of being 'in the advanced stages of paranoia'.

Lord Palumbo watched Soames's outburst with some sadness as he realised that Diana had finally burned all her boats: 'I'm sure that those people who were advising the Prince of Wales said, "I told you so, that's what she's all about." It gave ammunition to those people who opposed her, unnecessarily. It had a pretty devastating effect. It made the situation irretrievable …'

Naturally, some people saw through the act and believed they had seen a theatrical appearance from a vindictive woman hell-bent on revenge; but it has to be said that they were in the minority. The majority of the public believed that they had been appealed to by a defiant victim. The *Panorama* programme cemented what the Morton book had written in the public's mind. Myth had finally become fact, history was rewritten and from that moment on Diana had an army of devotees who found it quite impossible to believe the facts as and when they were to emerge in the future. The BBC had inadvertently provided the Princess of Wales with the best possible platform with which to preach a sermon against her husband. She had gleefully accepted it, without regard for either the truth or the feelings of her children. In her vindictive determination to repay her husband for refusing to concentrate wholly on her at the expense of his duties, she had not only hurt her children, she had damaged the monarchy, which included her sons, especially Prince William as a future king. It also unfairly hurt the vast majority of the British public who wanted to love and believe in the Royal Family as a focal point of British patriotism.

Now the Queen realised that she had reached the end of the road with her daughter-in-law. Her tolerance and kindness had been treated as a weakness that made the Princess believe she was now unstoppable. Finally, Her Majesty had had enough. She was concerned about William and Harry, and was no longer prepared to put up with Diana washing her dirty linen in public. It was not only undignified, it was increasingly damaging to the institution of monarchy. The time had come, in her opinion, to bring this marriage, which had started with so much hope and produced two fine sons, but latterly had only produced grief and heartache, to an end. After consulting the prime minister and the Archbishop of Canterbury, she wrote officially to her son and daughter-in-law and asked them to divorce immediately.

Diana was in New York fulfilling her promise to Rupert Murdoch. There, in the Hilton grand ballroom, guests paid $1,500 a plate to see Henry Kissinger present her with the United Cerebral Palsy Humanitarian of the Year Award. A press baron had called in a favour, a princess needed the good PR, and there was good old Henry to oblige. The evening had been a great success for all concerned. However, the Princess's upbeat mood was soon brought down on her return when she received the Queen's letter. A tearful Diana phoned Patrick Jephson and complained bitterly that this was the last thing that she wanted to happen. A grave Jephson just shook his head at the other end of the line. The Princess had, by her own actions, made it inevitable.

However, it didn't take the Princess too long to dry her tears and steel herself for the battle ahead. She certainly had mettle and didn't appear phased by the Queen's request once she had got over the initial shock. She didn't even acknowledge Her Majesty's letter and took over a month to reply to it. People simply didn't treat the Queen this way but Diana, who was nevertheless most concerned that she was accorded her dues as the Princess of Wales, made a point of doing so.

Eventually negotiations commenced and, at the request of the Princess, a confidential meeting took place between her and Prince Charles at St James's Palace where only preliminary details were discussed. It was therefore to everyone's complete surprise when they discovered Diana had breached her own request for secrecy and put out a press statement entitled 'THE SADDEST DAY OF MY LIFE': 'The Princess of Wales has agreed to Prince Charles' request to a divorce. The Princess will continue to be involved in all decisions relating to the children and will remain at Kensington Palace with offices in St James's Palace. The Princess of Wales will retain the title and will be known as Diana, Princess of Wales.'

The Queen had never encountered such impertinence during her forty-year reign and, quite uncharacteristically, issued an immediate response: 'The Queen was most interested to hear that the Princess of Wales had agreed to the divorce. We can confirm that the Prince and Princess of Wales had a private meeting at St James's Palace. At this meeting details of the divorce settlement and the Princess' future role were not discussed. All the details on this matter, including titles, remain to be discussed and settled. This will take time. What the Princess has mentioned are requests rather than decisions at this stage.'

Now it was Diana's turn to be livid. She had become unaccustomed to being thwarted in her desires, and to be so in such a public manner made it all the more humiliating. The Princess determined that if the Queen wanted to play it this way then that would be all right by her. She knew that she was able to be more economical with the truth and fight a dirtier game than ever the Palace would descend to. She just needed one chink in the Windsor armour. She didn't have long to wait.

George Smith was a veteran of the first Gulf War; it was perhaps as a result of this that, when he came to be a member of the Prince of

Wales's staff, he had come to suffer from both alcoholic and mental problems. Prince Charles, characteristically, had been sympathetic to his problems and had given him every opportunity to continue in his job; but it became clear that Mr Smith was unable to carry out his duties and would have to receive a period of hospitalised treatment for his mental disorder. However, as he left, the corridors of St James's Palace were echoing to a claim of his that he had been raped by Prince Charles's valet.

Upon hearing this, the Princess of Wales, armed with a tape recorder, went to visit Smith in hospital. There she lavished both praise and sympathy upon him and soon had the rape allegation on tape. Having turned the tape recorder off she then skilfully suggested to Smith that the man who raped him could also have been the same man that Smith might have discovered in bed with the Prince of Wales when he had served Prince Charles his breakfast one morning. Smith readily concurred, either through illness or a willingness to please Her Royal Highness, and so repeated this story back to her, which she duly also captured on tape.

In the following years Smith was to repeat what Princess Diana had done to many people; he even offered to give a full account to a Sunday newspaper provided that he received a large five-figure sum. Somewhat surprisingly, the publication and Mr Smith couldn't agree terms and so the nation was spared yet another sordid tale from one trying to make money from a royal association.

Diana, like anyone else with even the basic knowledge of how the Palace works, knew that this story could not be true, for the very simple reason that George Smith was not in a position within the royal household, nor had he ever been, to be allowed to serve the royal breakfast. He simply could not have caught Charles in a compromising position with his valet. However, this salient point did not deter Diana from utilising her recording as a tool in her attempt to get exactly what she wanted as her divorce settlement.

Anyone who knows the Prince of Wales realises that the idea of him being gay is completely laughable. So why didn't the House of Windsor simply laugh this accusation off? The answer to this question lies with the mischievous attitude of the British tabloid press. The Queen and the Prince of Wales believed that they could not afford such a scandal, however untrue, to be aired and see it go down the same 'there's no smoke without fire' route that Diana's other inventions had.

Indeed, when this story eventually surfaced in 2003, it was whipped up into a media frenzy that forced Sir Michael Peat, on behalf of Prince Charles, to seek restraining orders on the press.

Diana continued at very low ebb as she strove to come to terms with a divorce that she had caused to happen but now claimed she had never wanted. She complained to the departing Jephson that someone had taken a shot at her in the park and that the brake wires had been cut on her car. Jephson had both claims investigated but failed to come up with anything that might support her claims. Nevertheless, the Princess continued to see conspiracies everywhere, and so started a new phase of leaving rude, accusing and highly disturbing messages on her staff's answering machines. Jephson himself was pleased to leave the Princess's employment by late January 1996.

Richard Aylard handled the divorce for the Prince, whose busy schedule didn't allow him to sit locked in rooms with lawyers for days on end. Thus Aylard, who already had to follow a hectic schedule of his own, was additionally closeted away with lawyers for several hours a day, almost every day for months. For the dedicated Aylard, this had a very bad effect on his own marriage, which started to fall apart as a result of his continuing determination to put Charles first at all times. Aylard didn't mention this domestic problem, and it didn't occur to the self-absorbed Charles. His marriage eventually failed.

The Princess had engaged the high-profile Anthony Julius of Mishcon de Reya, while the Prince was represented by Fiona Shackleton from the royal solicitors of Farrer & Co. Negotiations were both difficult and acrimonious. The Princess started out demanding some £35 million and gave Julius the instruction to go for her husband's jugular. The air was thick with innuendo and surreptitious references to the George Smith tape. Prince Charles had finally learned that it simply wasn't possible to trust his wife, and therefore any deal would have to include a confidentiality clause that prevented her from ever again talking about their marriage or anything else that might be damaging to the monarchy. This became an inflexible condition that initially the Princess, seeing how it might restrict her future axis of power, resisted. But Charles was adamant. He now knew that the only way to protect himself and the institution that he had been raised to inherit was by silencing her, and the most effective muzzle would be the law by way of a binding agreement that would impose severe financial penalties if she broke it.

The King and Di

Julius behaved as instructed; the Princess wriggled and her legal team often appeared to the other side to move the goalposts and were occasionally accused of 'unagreeing' previously accepted points. However, by the end of July they had agreed a settlement, which was widely perceived as generous to the Princess. This had always been the Prince's financial intention from the outset provided that she agreed to be prevented from inventing further fabrications against the Royal Family. It was thought to be worth more than £17 million although, as both parties had signed the confidentiality agreement that the Prince had insisted upon, the actual details were never published. (The publication of her will following her death indicates that the figure would appear to be correct.) They retained equal access to their sons and continued to enjoy equal responsibilities in the children's upbringing. The Princess was still to be regarded by both the Queen and the Prince of Wales as a member of the Royal Family, and as such would continue to be invited to most state and national occasions. She would be allowed to continue to live in Kensington Palace and, at her request, her office would also move there. She was forced to agree not to work for financial gain as the Royal Family were not pleased with Sarah York's commercial activities, rather unfairly forgetting that they were entirely due to the poor settlement forced upon her. Indeed, the rather shabby way the Royal Family had dealt with the Duchess of York had only emphasised to Diana how she must stand up to the Queen and the Palace. Nevertheless, she felt no apparent sympathy for her one-time friend and sister-in-law. 'That cow! Thanks to her, I'm having to give up the right to make money,' said Diana rather hypocritically – unlike Sarah, she had never shown any inclination to stick at a job at any time during her life.

Despite this and her enforced silence on royal matters, by and large the Princess got almost everything in the end that she had prematurely announced and had been rebuked by the Queen for doing so. However, there was one detail that she hadn't counted on, and that was that she was to be stripped of the title Her Royal Highness. This was not the Prince of Wales's decision, but had been insisted upon by the Queen. It has since been said that the Princess also wanted this. Given that it is known that Diana stopped talking to her own mother for the last year of her life as a result of Mrs Shand Kydd telling *Hello!* Magazine that she thought that her daughter was better off without the title, this seems very unlikely. Either way, in PR terms it turned out to be a serious blunder by the Queen.

Originally Diana had suspected that the Queen would offer her a new title of HRH Princess Diana; she determined to hold out for the title Princess of Wales. She believed that after Queen of England, the title Princess of Wales was the best in the world and she intended to keep it. The Queen took her at her word and agreed. Diana never thought for a moment that that would involve losing her HRH. 'I didn't think they'd do it. Who ever heard of a princess of Wales who wasn't a Royal Highness,' she later complained. Reeling from the shock, while trying to save face by claiming that Prince William had talked her into accepting the position, she actually knew that she had no choice in the matter, and now no ability to counter-attack sneakily through the press. She concluded that a queen who was determined to teach her a lesson had personally motivated her diminution in rank.

It is true that her relations with the rest of the Royal Family were hardly cordial. Princess Margaret of Hesse and the Rhine told Lady Colin Campbell, 'The Queen had lost all patience with her. So had Prince Philip and the Queen Mother, who viewed Diana as the greatest danger to the monarchy – Wallis Simpson included.' Nevertheless, the Queen and Prince Philip were mindful to keep open the lines of communication open and remain civil and understanding.

However, Charlotte Pike, the former editor of *Almanach de Gotha*, did not believe that it was quite as straightforward as Diana believed. 'Royal life is governed by precedence. If you're the Princess of Wales you rank before the Duchess of York and after the Queen. There's a sense to it, an inevitability. So basically once you're out your status is demeaned.' This public aspect might seem like humiliation to the person being divested of their status, and not being in the Court Circular or invited to things that you would have been before would seem to somebody like Diana as a personal attack.

Although Ms Pike undoubtedly has a point, it should not be forgotten that by now the Queen and her advisors, Prince Charles more than any other, knew what a completely unstable and vindictive woman they were dealing with; they should have realised that the stripping away of such a title was bound to be like a red rag to a bull. It was a poorly thought-out decision in light of the fact that they now craved a period of calm more than anything else. 'They punished me for not settling for HRH Princess Diana,' she complained time and again to friends, refusing to accept that she had in fact been granted the title she had originally asked for. That said, the acceptance of the title HRH Princess Diana would have guaranteed her the same status as if she had been born a royal princess, and she would have been free to marry whomever she wished in the future and still retain her royal rank; this was not the case with the title that she had chosen.

As the dust settled, there was one very positive result that was gained from the settlement. Now forbidden by a binding contract to involve herself in any further fabrication and distortion about her marriage and her relationship with the Prince of Wales and his family, the Princess was forced to abandon such intrigue. As a result she turned her guns on to unfortunate women like Victoria Mendham, Tiggy Legge-Bourke and Jane Atkinson, and made their lives pretty miserable. However, accepting that Charles was now out of bounds, she made a genuine effort to improve relations with a man who had shown her much kindness and a lot more love than she had ever admitted to publicly. As a result, she enjoyed the best relations with him that she had had for many years during the last year of her life. This was a godsend for their children, and something that all three princes were able to cling on to as a great comfort following her death.

Chapter Sixteen
The Dynasty and the Destiny (1996–97)

While the Princess's domestic life had been spilling on to the pages of the tabloid press in the early to mid-1990s, the Prince had been keeping himself busy by his continued running battles with the Establishment on questions of architecture, education and the loss of traditional values in British society. Often the press ignored his pronouncements, but when they did pay attention to him it was generally from a negative perspective, although there were notable exceptions when he appeared to have caught the mood of the people and thus forced the tabloids' approval. As usual their attitude, either way, did nothing to influence his beliefs, which he increasingly saw as his calling to publicise. This made him much admired in some quarters and frowned upon in others where it was believed that he was abusing his constitutional position.

He had controversially, if to some wholly properly, continued to criticise a state of British architecture where he believed the modernists and post-modernists had ignored the wishes of the people and had only sought to impress each other with their designs. The architectural establishment responded with a clear resentment for the temerity of the Prince to challenge their certainties with his own. His old friend Lord Palumbo, the land developer who had proposed the Mansion House skyscraper that Charles had condemned as a 'glass stump', had been forced to comment, 'God bless the Prince of Wales, and God save us from his architectural judgement.' Richard Rogers, whose design for Paternoster Square had been described by the Prince as having failed to 'rise to the challenge' was more direct: 'Time and again the Prince has singled out individual architects for criticism; in so doing he is violating the principles of a constitutional monarchy.' And it has to be said that many British architects had some sympathy with such a statement. Peter Ahrends, the architect whose work the Prince once famously described as a 'carbuncle', perhaps understandably felt the need to retaliate and went even further: 'He has done nothing to further the debate on modern architecture ... [the Prince's views] are out of step with the country as a whole.' This last statement proved not to be the case.

As usual, a profession under attack from the Prince had questioned his constitutional right to speak out against them, but also they had made the mistake of claiming to speak for the people; it soon became clear that it was the Prince who was speaking for a people who could not be heard by a profession that had been deafened by its own arrogance. Public opinion sided time and again with the Prince and so, slowly but surely, the new buildings that were erected in the 1990s and came to dominate the centre of British cities had a more traditional feel and were generally accepted as being better for it. However, this failed to silence a hard core at the very centre of avant-garde British architecture, and from them there were constant mutterings that if the Prince was so bright, why didn't he use his influence, land and wealth to build something that practised what he preached? Why hadn't he put his money where his mouth was?

Richard Rogers was particularly scathing: 'Sadly, in recent years our Royal Family has had a poor record as patrons of the arts and sciences. As yet there is little to suggest that the Prince is an exception in this respect. As a man with strong views about architecture, a high public profile and enormous wealth, he has an extraordinary opportunity to commission buildings for his large estates. But he has yet to produce a noteworthy construction ...'

Rogers' words clearly show the dislike he had built up for the Prince as a result of Charles's criticism of his work. Unfortunately for the architect, the Prince was about to do what Rogers had implied was beyond him. The Duchy of Cornwall was preparing a development plan for a site on the outskirts of the town of Dorchester where it had owned land for over 600 years. A plan was presented to the Prince for this development, but he rejected it as he clearly felt that it didn't meet his requirements for urban development in a rural surrounding. Instead, he grabbed the opportunity to put his ideas into practice while delivering a huge broadside to Rogers and Co.

It was here that Poundbury was born. Its passage through the planners was slow, and the obstacles created by warring factions within the duchy and the classical designer Leon Krier made for difficult times. Moreover, the Prince insisted that the local community should be involved, so it was decided that a weekend of consultation would take place. The thinking was that it was important for the Prince to bring two strands of the his vision together: the idea of classical ideals as contained in Krier's master plan, and the wishes of the people who would come to live in Poundbury. Naturally, there were those who were employed by the duchy who were not sold on the Krier concept as being practical to start with, and believed that if the project proceeded it could even bankrupt the duchy. The idea of then asking the public to get involved had them worrying that this would cause costs to lurch even further out of control.

But the Prince held his nerve and rode a middle course through years of discord before the project was eventually built after it had been scaled down and modified by consultant Sarah Oborn, who had been brought in by the duchy and had convinced a most disillusioned Krier to accept most of her reforms. It had been worth all the aggravation and, upon completion of phase one, it received wide acclaim from many architects around the world. The people who lived there appeared to be extremely happy, and the thousands of visitors who continue to come and see the small town every year leave with a very favourable impression. As a result, scores of new urban developments built on the edge of rural England have come to resemble Poundbury far more than the awful 1960s developments that a lot of the Prince's detractors had designed. It had been a difficult road, and the Prince had been demanding while not always being terribly practical, but by sticking to his guns and insisting most of his concerns were addressed, he had struck a blow for the people and ensured they were more likely to be housed on estates that had some individual rural village character rather than the faceless Luna boxes that either met the economic criteria or pandered to the whim of an architect who would never be required to live on his design.

On 16 February 2005, just days after the announcement of his engagement to Camilla Parker Bowles, the Prince proudly showed the chancellor of the exchequer, Gordon Brown, round phase two of the development. By then his ideal of an urban extension with the integration of affordable, social and privately owned housing built around the concept of the diversity of a rural village was accepted as wisdom, and the ideas of the architectural avant-garde of some twenty years earlier had long since been discarded as a result of their tendency to cause social problems rather than assist social cohesion.

However, back then, whatever bad feelings the Prince had generated among the nation's leading architects paled into insignificance when compared to the outrage that was to be felt by the Conservative government when he turned his eye from architecture and on to the educational establishment. At the end of 1989, he had delivered a speech as patron of the Thomas Cranmer Schools Prize. 'The fear of being considered old-fashioned seems to me to be so all-powerful that the more eternal values and principles which run like a thread through the whole tapestry of human existence are abandoned under the false assumption that they restrict progress.' Then to make his point he added in a touch of ridicule. 'Looking at the way English is used in our popular papers, our radio and television programmes, or even in our schools and our theatres … [I and others] wonder what it is about our country and our society that our language has become so impoverished, so sloppy and so limited that we have arrived at a wasteland of banality, cliché and casual obscenity. It leads me to wonder, for instance, how Hamlet would deliver his great "To be or not to be" soliloquy in the language of today … What about this: "Well, frankly, the problem as I see it at this moment in time is whether I should lie down under all this hassle, or whether I should just say OK, I get the message, and do myself in. I mean, I'm in a no-win situation, and quite honestly I'm so stuffed up to here with the whole stupid mess that I can tell you I've just got a good mind to take the quick way out. That's the bottom line …"

His audience roared with laughter, and his widely reported speech was largely applauded by a public that once again seemed to agree with him. However, the modernists in the broadsheets were much less impressed. He was rebuked by the editorial in the *Independent* for sounding like 'a rather reactionary club bore', and the literary editor of *The Times*, Philip Howard, attacked him for talking 'unhistorical and reactionary rubbish'. This speech might not have caused quite such a stir if it had not just come on the back of some off-the-cuff remarks that had somehow found their way into the newspapers, which the Prince had made to a private gathering of businessmen. He had complained that none of his own staff could either speak or write English properly, and that this was because English was no longer taught properly in school. Hardly surprisingly, both teachers and the education secretary were affronted. However, a survey conducted by the *Sunday Times* and a readership poll conducted by the *Sunday Mirror* suggested that the Prince's sentiments enjoyed great support among the people.

The general response to his Thomas Cranmer speech overwhelmingly confirmed this impression. The *Daily Telegraph* reflected upon this when it editorialised, 'On architecture there may sometimes be room to differ from the Prince. On the decline of the English language there is none … When we realise that what the Prince of Wales is attacking has persisted through ten years of Conservative government we get some idea of just how far the road back will be.' The *Telegraph* had flagged up that the government was, at the very least, partially to blame. As a result, Charles found himself being once more dragged dangerously close to the edge of a political arena where he was not supposed to set foot.

Sixteen months later he delivered the Shakespeare Birthday Speech at the Swan Theatre in Stratford-upon-Avon. Now the Prince took off the gloves. He bemoaned that several GCSE courses in literature had no Shakespeare at all. There was at least one A-level English literature syllabus where Shakespeare was not compulsory. Thousands of children were leaving school having been denied the right of seeing a single Shakespeare play on film or the stage. He wondered why this was. Perhaps it was a symptom of the nation's great flight from our great literary heritage. 'Are we so frightened and cowed by the shadowy "experts" that we can no longer screw our courage to the sticking place and defiantly insist that they are talking unmitigated nonsense? You forget – I have been through all this before with the architects! I've heard it all over and over again, and it is high time that the bluff of the so-called "experts" was called …'

He then acknowledged the difficulties faced by hard-pressed teachers in the classroom before returning to his onslaught on the 'experts' whom he held accountable for the worsening standards of education in Great Britain. They were purely following fashionable trends towards the exclusively contemporary, the immediately palatable and the apparently relevant – to such an extent that we were now in danger of ending up with future generations being culturally disinherited. He then sympathised with what he suspected were thousands upon thousands of parents who felt utterly powerless in the face of yet another profession – the educationalists – who thought that they knew best and were no longer willing to listen.

Now the Prince had most definitely crossed the constitutional line. Already he had gone further than even the Queen would have deemed wise, and even his outspoken father, the Duke of Edinburgh, would perhaps have stopped here. But the Prince merely paused to draw breath before broadening his attack to extend it beyond the educational establishment that he obviously had so little time for and directing his fire on government policy as well.

'Here in Britain, we seem to get it wrong almost before we have begun. In France, Italy and Belgium, every child under five receives nursery education from the state. Here, less than half our children have the right ... It is almost incredible that in Shakespeare's land one child in seven leaves primary school functionally illiterate ... In most schools, children are deemed incapable of learning foreign languages before the age of eleven – yet by the age of fourteen half of them have given it up. As if that wasn't enough, present indications are that after the age of fourteen children will not be required by the National Curriculum to study any aesthetic subject ... Perhaps most alarming of all, only one third of our sixteen- to eighteen-year-olds are still in full-time education. In France, the figure is sixty-six per cent, Japan seventy-seven per cent, the Netherlands seventy-seven per cent. Forty per cent of our children leave full-time schooling with no significant educational qualifications at all.'

But he did concede that the government's concept of a national curriculum did seem to enjoy cross-party support, and therefore he hoped that all sides would join together to ensure that matters improved, before finishing by insisting that the nation should vigorously resist the temptation to ignore cultural heritage due to expediency, a desire for a utilitarian approach or a mistaken sense of political correctness. 'After all, there is little point in becoming technically competent if at the same time we become culturally inept. In pleading for a restoration of sanity, I have to admit to a feeling of profound sadness that a great deal of damage has already been done ...'

The speech was as unpopular with the Establishment as it was popular with the public. A furious National Association of Teachers immediately denounced it as 'nonsense', and the secretary of state for education, Kenneth Clarke, was privately seething with rage. However, the headline writers in both the broadsheets and the tabloids sensed that the Prince had yet again struck a chord with a people who shared his sense of outrage, and so supported his stand.

As a result, Kenneth Clarke was rounded on by journalists from all sides and asked to comment on the royal rebuke of his department. He cleverly reminded the press of the issues where Prince Charles was clearly in favour of government policy, and generally diffused the situation rather well. However, in private he allowed his feelings be known in the bluntest of language, even asserting that the Prince had offended against constitutional propriety and that the matter had been made all the worse by the Prince's office having failed to send over a copy of the speech until the morning of its delivery, which had prevented him from reading it until after it had been made and the news hounds were closing in. The Prince's office strenuously denied this charge, claiming that he did not finish the speech until the early hours of the morning that it was delivered, and that they had rushed a copy round to the Department of Education as soon as it had been typed. However, privately they were to admit that that had resulted in an inadequate amount of time being allowed for Clarke's people to study the contents, and some secretly believed that Prince Charles had finished the speech late on purpose so that no one could complain officially to him prior to it being made – it would have caused a far bigger constitutional row if he had then refused to be guided by the secretary of state for education.

Things were eventually smoothed over a month later. On Prince Charles's return from visits to Brazil and Czechoslovakia, where he had made powerful speeches in support of the environment and against communism, he wrote personally to Ken Clarke to apologise – a letter that he almost ruined by reiterating that he was totally unrepentant about the contents of the speech in any event: 'The speech was very much a personal statement about Shakespeare and the deeper values that underlie a study of our great literary heritage. I tried my best to minimise anything that could be construed as "party political" and I consulted very widely indeed. The positive letters I have received from all sides – Labour and Conservative, teachers and university lecturers, pundits and "experts", academics and members of the public, have certainly encouraged me. The last thing I wanted to do was to make your life any more difficult than it already is, but at the same time I believe there are profound values at stake which I feel it is my duty to emphasise.'

There can be no doubt that the Prince saw this as his role just as sincerely as he held such views on education in the first place. However, this does not make the opposing view – that as a constitutional monarch-in-waiting he should keep such political views to himself – any less valid. The fact that the Prince has been able to get away with such interference in political matters is largely because he has always been lucky enough or shrewd enough only to speak out on matters when it quickly becomes clear that the silent majority are with him, and thus his detractors are forced to back off. This occasion had been no exception, and the speech was been endorsed from all quarters just as he had reported. Indeed, St James's Palace was awash with letters of congratulations. Characteristically, the Prince did not let matters rest there: over the coming years, many initiatives and schemes were launched as a result of the speech, but by far the most important point was that the national curriculum, which was eventually inherited from Ken Clarke by John Patten, who openly supported the Prince's views, was directly influenced by the Stratford-upon-Avon speech. The Prince had won a greater victory than he could ever have imagined. Shakespeare was, after all, to be taught in all schools to all children. If, as Clarke had supposed with some justification, the Prince had indeed trespassed across a constitutional dividing line, then he had done so to great effect.

As the 1990s progressed, the Prince continued to show keen interest in his chosen themes of freedom, education, protection of the environment, improving the lot of inner-city children and giving the disadvantaged a better start in life. In addition, his pet projects of Poundbury and the Mary Rose Trust took up a lot of his time when he was not carrying out state duties. Unfortunately, the Mary Rose was affected by wrangles, arguments and bitter disputes between the architect – the American Professor Christopher Alexander – the Trust's officials, planning officers at Portsmouth and the Prince's office.

The Mary Rose was Henry VIII's flagship. It had sunk in 1545 about a mile and a half outside Portsmouth Harbour. Mountbatten had first explained to Charles when the ship had been discovered in 1973 that there was a plan to raise her. Immediately the Prince became passionate about the national-heritage value of such a project. By 1982 the ship had been raised, and from then on the Prince of Wales got caught up in dispute after dispute concerning the ship's restoration and the plans for a museum in which the wreck might be housed. Many of the ensuing arguments were leaked to the press, much to the Prince's embarrassment and annoyance.

By late 1992 the Prince was becoming concerned that the rifts with Krier and Alexander over the Poundbury and Mary Rose projects respectively might threaten a much bolder project that he hoped to launch in order to silence his critics and which would also realise his architectural vision of the future. He wanted to establish a national institute of Architecture in his own name. Prince Charles had already run a summer school at the Villa Lante, a palazzo owned by the Italian government just outside Viterbo, in both 1991 and 1992. Both had been great successes and so he decided to press ahead with the establishment of a permanent institute and took on a lease from the Crown Estates at 14 and 15 Gloucester Gate in Regent's Park. He established an academic board and designed a foundation course. With finance provided by the Prince's own charitable trust and some support from a few individual benefactors, the Prince of Wales's Institute of Architecture was launched. It was received with the expected scepticism from the architectural establishment, but got an unusually fair hearing from the media.

In May 1992, the Prince replied to a letter from his 'secretary in architecture', Brian Hanson, saying, 'I hope you can keep in mind the overriding need for the Institute to act as a catalyst to bring together the profession associated with the built environment so that we can emphasise the need to rediscover a kinder, more appropriate approach … I want the Institute to teach its students reverence – reverence for the landscape and the soil; for the human spirit which is a reflection in some small measure of the divine; and for the 'grammar' of architecture which, as a language, enables an infinite variety of forms to be expressed within the context of harmonised sentences …' Somehow, and probably without meaning to, Prince Charles had woven together in these few words the themes that had been with him and had been welling up inside him since puberty. Man's identity within the natural world; the relationship of that natural world with the idea of God; the expression of God within the human spirit; and the potential of design and building to express and rejoice in such a holy alliance of God with mankind upon the planet. In a more virtuous and reverend period of our history, more people might have understood what he was about. It is to his sadness and our loss that this was not the case. Nevertheless, he was proud and happy when the first full-time students enrolled for the foundation course in the autumn of that year. It was but a moment of fleeting happiness as his irritation with so much fabrication, exaggeration and downright lies gave way to a humiliation of almost unendurable proportions as *Diana: Her True Story* was serialised by the *Sunday Times*.

Throughout the 1990s the Prince never lost his enthusiasm for the Prince's Trust, BITC, education, the environment, architecture, national heritage, the armed forces or the thousand other things that he saw as his duty to protect or nurture on behalf of the nation. However, a lot of his energy and hard work has gone unrecorded as the press preferred to follow Diana's lead and majored on issues of family gossip, intrigue and scandal instead. As a result, there can be no doubt that the image of this caring and mostly virtuous man was lost under the fabrications of Morton, the humiliation of Camillagate, the scandal of Squidgygate, the indignity of the *Panorama* interview and the heap of idiotic stories of brake cables, homosexual rape and death conspiracies.

Following her divorce, Diana blamed the loss of her title on her immediate decision to drop her involvement with a hundred charities, including some previous favourites of hers like the Red Cross and Help the Aged. Her PR assistant Jane Atkinson warned her against the idea, explaining to the Princess that it would be judged as being petulant and sulky. Diana refused to listen, and instead believed that the people would sympathise with her and blame the Queen for having removed her HRH status in the first place.

The Princess explained that she was having a clear out of her 'old' life and wanted to lighten a workload that few on her staff thought was exhausting as it stood. Nevertheless, she was determined to go ahead despite much advice from friends to think again. The six charities that were retained were the National AIDS Trust, Centrepoint, the Royal Marsden NHS Foundation Trust, the Great Ormond Street Hospital for Children, The Leprosy Mission and the English National Ballet. A former assistant of that time was to comment, 'She kept the first five because they provided her with the best propaganda and photo opportunities, and the last one because she genuinely loved it.'

Jane Atkinson just waited for the bad press to hit her desk, and the Princess to hit the roof: 'I don't think that I ever thought there was a good time to do it. We always knew that it was going to be a negative media story. She tried to do it as a story, which gave her some sympathy for losing the HRH title, and it backfired! We all knew it wouldn't work. It seemed a like a cold-hearted thing to do …'

Centrepoint was particularly grateful for Diana retaining an interest in them, as they were heavily reliant on the publicity she afforded them and believed that if she had walked away, it might have sunk them. Mike Adler's National Aids Trust had also survived, despite the fact that he had recently accused the Princess of attempting to hijack his charity and use the publicity for her own ends. It was felt by some at the trust that Diana had made such a point about being the only royal to identify with AIDS and be seen (as were many Hollywood celebrities) as caring about AIDS victims that she couldn't withdraw without a serious loss of face. At the time, governments seemed somewhat coy to highlight a sexually transmitted disease that many people mistakenly believed was spread solely by homosexuals, whereas the celebrities who supported AIDS charities were seen by the young as politically correct and caring, and the ever-astute Diana realised this.

Those who believed that the Princess had only retained this charity for PR reasons may have a point as, although the National Aids Trust was kept on, Mike Adler recalls that it was at this time that the Princess seemed to lose interest and disengaged from the association: 'To be quite honest, by the end of her life we hardly asked her to do anything. It was better to plan to do things knowing that she wouldn't be there. We began to operate as a charity with a patron but without her.'

Despite a successful trip to Chicago with Jane Atkinson that summer, where the Princess had a great success raising money for the treatment of breast cancer – she had behaved impeccably and the Americans had totally fallen in love with her – Atkinson's day were numbered. One or two articles had appeared about Jane and other members of the Princess's staff. Diana hadn't liked them and believed that Atkinson had engineered herself into a starring role, so she became mistrustful of her. Then Diana started to withdraw the help that she had freely given to her PR advisor when she had first taken up her position: 'She'd always helped me considerably with background things that had happened before. And then just suddenly I would ring her and say, "Can you explain about this?" and she would just be unhelpful and say, "Well, tch, you should know that!"

'When she resigned the charities, she had already written the press release and discussed how it should be handled. Then later in the day she rang me and was very angry because of the way that the media had treated the story. She felt it had been very negative to her. I explained that I'd only answered the questions in the way that we'd agreed, but she accused me of not doing so. And then one of her friends was on the ten o'clock news saying almost exactly the same things that I'd said. And when I rang the Princess and asked if she knew that her friend was on the news she said no, she didn't know. I think her words were, "You can't always stop your friends talking."

'It was impossible for me to do my job in an environment like that. I thought, well that's it. I can't continue to function properly as a media adviser, so I ought to resign.'

And so yet another of the Princess's staff bit the dust: she was the second PR advisor to go within a year. Thereafter, Diana came to rely on the PR advice of her friends, which meant in reality that she advised herself. However, she still had one last amazing PR triumph to come – one that would shape the way that she would be remembered and help give her a saintly and caring image that shines from beyond the grave.

Despite lightening her workload, the Princess was still a very high-profile character on the British and world stage, mainly thanks to the six charities that she had retained, but now she had a lot more time to devote to herself. She would rise at seven and, following breakfast, make her way over to the Harbour Club for her daily workout. Then she would return to Kensington Palace and chat to friends on her mobile while her hairdresser did her hair as she planned her day. There would almost certainly be the obligatory phone call of intrigue to Richard Kay at the *Daily Mail*, but these were slightly more guarded and considered now that she was bound by a legal document that would hit her very hard financially if she blundered. Then around would come her army of therapists, whose skills she believed would help her recover her mental well-being and overcome other illnesses – one of which was a constant feeling of tiredness that was continually aggravated by insomnia, which Diana had suffered from since childhood and had battled for years by taking large quantities of sleeping pills.

    Slowly, as the novelty of having this extra time to herself wore off, the Princess became bored and so once more wanted her life to lurch back in the direction of commitment, just as she had so many times before. She had long wanted to be given a role as a roving ambassador, and blamed the Queen for blocking this. In reality, it is most unlikely that anyone at Buckingham Palace would have ever been consulted as it is extremely doubtful that anyone in the Major government would have treated her aspiration in this regard very seriously. To send this beautiful and popular princess on selected goodwill missions as a royal ambassador with a government minister in tow was one thing; to let her represent the country on complex political and diplomatic issues was quite another. As one former minister put it, 'The Princess lacked the training, the consistency, the discipline and I'm bound to say the intelligence to be trusted with such tasks and as such was never considered for such a post. Moreover, as far as I am aware, she never formally requested us to consider her for a position in the first place.'

As 1996 progressed and the Princess became more resentful that government opinion seemed to think of her as insufficiently well informed, astute and disciplined for a serious role like roaming the world as an ambassador at large, her friend Lord Palumbo told her to make the best of the time on her hands by targeting certain specific issues that interested her. For once, the Princess listened to the sensible advice of a true friend. The veteran politician and journalist Bill Deedes had been involved in the anti-landmine campaign since 1991.

Deedes, whose excellent charity pedigree includes work for UNICEF, had quickly appreciated the problem of landmines. Promoted by the arms industry as a cheap and effective form of defence, millions had been laid wherever there had been armed disputes since the Second World War. When these finished and the soldiers went, often with the only maps of where their mines had been laid, the mines remained as dangerous bombs that maimed and killed innocent civilians, many of who were children. In addition, and as a result, the concerned land could not be farmed, which only served to cause further poverty and misery.

Now a major effort was underway to clear existing minefields and prevent new ones from being laid. It was a difficult issue to tackle because powerful corporations, and even some governments, were opposed to any form of a ban on their use. Deedes realised that Diana would bring about huge publicity to his cause and at the same time prove to herself and any doubters how she might negotiate the difficult political situations that would almost certainly arise as a result of dealing with this urgent and extremely tricky issue.

However, there was a problem: the Red Cross was the charity that had focused on this issue. It was also one of the charities that the Princess had recently dropped. Despite this, Deedes managed to fire her imagination and made her see how important a job she could do. Nevertheless, when she called up Mike Whitlam and said that she wanted to talk to him about landmines again, he must have been surprised and slightly sceptical; but still, if she really meant it this time, he was delighted. He decided to put her to the test and told her that she would have to go and see the effects of landmines for herself, and therefore suggested that she should go and visit a country that was clearing up after a recent war.

Understandably, Whitlam was concerned that if the Princess flirted with the issue and then dropped it, as she had with other Red Cross issues before, this would do more damage than good. However, Diana assured him that she was most concerned to help and he knew as well as the next charity boss the brilliant effect that she might have on media attention if she really got involved. With any luck, this might generate some progress on a planned global landmine treaty that was bogged down in supposed bureaucracy with several nations who rather hypocritically said that they supported it. This wasn't just a collection of the predictable Third World dictatorships: their number included Britain, Canada and the United States of America.

At first Whitlam decided to take the Princess to Cambodia, but this was considered by the Foreign Office to be too dangerous, as was Bosnia. In the end, Angola was settled on. There were thought to be 15 million landmines scattered among a population of only 12 million people. A documentary team from the BBC, allegedly encouraged by Diana herself, asked if they could come along and make a film. The Princess was delighted when Whitlam informed her, and so he agreed. There were two benefits to be gained from having the BBC present: a magnificent promotional documentary, made by the internationally respected broadcaster, would be shown throughout the world, and their presence as a fly-on-the-wall unit would ensure that the Princess's behaviour would be impeccable.

However, Whitlam still had to convince the top brass in Geneva that this wasn't going to be an expedition that was simply too dangerous for the Princess. In the end he was forced to fly to Geneva and attend meeting after meeting to reassure them that he would be able to get round some of the obvious difficulties of taking a princess to such a place without the protection of the British Government on hand.

Diana also saw that this adventure was more like a trip her hated sister-in-law Princess Anne might make for Save the Children than the usually glitzy sorties she herself made. Her fashion wardrobe wouldn't be appropriate. She even asked Whitlam for advice on what clothes to take – Chino trousers and open-necked shirts were his rather sensible if somewhat predictable recommendations. But the fact that the Princess had asked in the first place not only indicates how keen she was to please him and how grateful she was for the opportunity he had given her, it also shows how dedicated she was to setting the stage absolutely right for a great documentary performance. She had learned from the mistake of dressing incorrectly in the operating theatre and was not going to be caught out like that again. If she were going to be taken seriously, she would have to dress more like Anne and less like a fashion icon on this trip. Her natural touch in this matter has to be admired – especially as her commitment to getting it right had such a positive effect and did so much good.

The trip was set for January 1997. There was complete chaos at Heathrow as Diana, Whitlam and his assistants tried to check in alongside an army of journalists who were going to join scores of others already out in Angola to cover the trip. Eventually, the Princess was given some VIP treatment by airline staff, but once on the plane she was again surrounded by journalists, as she was when they changed planes in Brussels. But Diana didn't mind one little bit: she was on stage, tapes were recording, cameras were flashing and film running. She was focused, fired up and ready. She chatted easily, seriously, charmingly and, when appropriate, slightly flirtatiously.

However, as the plane landed at Luanda Airport, Diana looked out of the window and could see a massive reception party. There were thousands of journalists and soldiers all milling around, and at the front were dozens of local dignitaries lined up ready to be presented to the Princess. Understandably she panicked, and thought that Whitlam had got it all wrong and that she would have to change into something more formal. But Whitlam held his nerve and reminded her that this was a Red Cross affair and not a royal visit. It was up to them to set the tone and call the shots. Diana immediately calmed down and said, 'OK, you're in charge.'

The airport was a complete wreck. The terminal was barely a shell of a building, the runway was short and bumpy, it was extremely hot, dusty and there were a lot of flies. The journalists there were surrounded by soldiers either to protect or intimidate them, or perhaps both, as this area was still a war zone. Mainly these professional writers fell into two camps: tough war correspondents and those who had the rather softer job of following the Royal Family around and making up snubs and slights between them if no real ones could be found. The first lot took such conditions in their stride; the second thought that they had woken up in hell.

The next day, the 100-strong party of officials, charity workers, die-hard journalists and whingeing royal correspondents left the centre of Luanda and made their way through shanty town after shanty town in order to reach one of the Red Cross health centres. It was very hot, very dusty and flies, which were everywhere, collected around the children's eyes, perhaps giving rise to an infection that can cause blindness. They ran after the convoy, with their hands stretched out for money, as it trundled slowly over the appalling roads. This was the sort of poverty that is common as you travel further south into Africa, and it was not particularly unusual to the people from the Red Cross or the war correspondents; but the number of amputees struggling on homemade crutches did shock them. There are apparently more amputees per head in Angola than any other country in the world.

The convoy eventually found its way to the health centre. Sewage was running down the centre of the street. The royal correspondents weren't impressed, but the Princess thanked Whitlam for forcing her to see it as it really was. She said that it made her feel like a real helper. Moreover, Diana had come prepared: she had done her homework. At one point Whitlam explained that the British had left 10 million mines in the North African desert following their famous victory over the Germans during the Second World War. The Princess corrected him and told him that if he cared to look into the matter he would find out that it was actually 23 million. He did and she was right.

Diana wanted to visit Cuito, reputed to be completely ringed by minefields and almost in ruins. This town was still virtually cut off and judged to be extremely dangerous. They had planned to visit it as part of a trip to nearby Huambo, but the government said that such a visit was too dangerous and refused them permission to enter the town. The Princess refused to accept the decision. She pestered officials, and when that didn't work she brought the matter up with the president's wife. She even sent one of her staff to check the place out. He reported back that it was possible – a little dangerous perhaps, but possible. It was eventually decided to take a reduced party there in a small plane.

While the problems associated with this were being worked out – including locating a plane – a row erupted in London when a group of Conservative MPs criticised the Princess's visit, saying that she was on a collision course with government policy. Whitlam put in calls to ministers and eventually, in the early hours of the morning, after Whitlam had actually read excerpts out from the government's own paper on their policy on landmines over the phone, he eventually convinced them to put out a joint statement from the foreign secretary and the Ministry of Defence saying that there was no conflict between the aims of the Red Cross visit and government policy.

The trip to Cuito went ahead. They had hired two small planes instead of one; once in the air, everyone was told that the plane with the Princess on board was going to Cuito while the other one would fly straight to Huambo as planned. Some journalists on the plane not going to Cuito felt cheated, but as it was agreed that those that did go would share their material with those that didn't, it was smoothed over without so much trouble in the end. The Princess had pressed to get her way, and for once it had been for a very useful effect: it is generally recognised that the visit was one of the highlights of the trip, and it only took place as a result of her determination.

Then Jennie Bond, who had been lucky enough to be travelling with the Princess to Cuito, suddenly demanded to know what was the Princess's reaction to the story coming out of London. Diana fended her off easily enough, but appeared to be angry in the Land Cruiser afterwards when she exploded at Whitlam. 'Why is this being said? Why do people want to do this? What do I have to do?' The BBC crew filmed it and of course they were pleased, thinking that in her anger she had forgotten about them, as so many people do when they have a film crew with them every minute of the day. They were wrong. It was precisely *because* they were there that she had said what she did. Nor was she angry with Whitlam, She knew that she wasn't going to get a right of reply against those MPs, so she used this opportunity of having the BBC film a private conversation to portray herself as a victim once more and make her point. In PR terms, it was quite brilliant.

Ironically, in the end Huambo was perhaps the more dangerous of the two visits. It was still in a disputed area and therefore very much still part of the war zone. From the airport the group had to walk in a single file into town behind an anti-mine engineer, such was the danger from landmines. The town itself was like a ghost town as they made their way through it to the little hospital, which had no equipment and hardly any drugs. The staff had obviously done their very best to present it as best they could to their very important visitor, but they couldn't disguise how very basic it really was. There weren't even enough beds, so many people had to make do with lying on the floor.

As the Princess toured the wards, the patients had no idea who she was. This war-ravaged country had no newspapers or television, and only a radio station that told them what Luanda wanted them to think and believe. They had never heard of the Prince or Princess of Wales, and some probably hadn't even heard of the Queen. But it didn't matter. As the Princess travelled through the hospital, she did so with great majesty.

Christina Lamb, an accomplished war reporter for the *Sunday Times* who had come on the trip as a 'Diana cynic' but who was now impressed by a side of Diana that she hadn't expected to see, movingly recalled years later to Clayton and Craig, 'And there was this little girl who was clearly in a terrible condition. She'd gone to fetch water and had stepped on a mine and basically had her insides blown out. It was horrific. And the hospital said that she wouldn't survive – they were just making her as comfortable as possible. You could see that she probably wouldn't last, maybe even the day.

'As Diana moved on, I stayed and just asked the girl a few questions, because I thought I would write about her. And she said to me, "Who was that?" And it was quite hard trying to explain Princess Diana to somebody who didn't know. And I said, "She's a princess from England, from far away." And she said to me, "Is she an angel?" And I found that really moving. This little girl probably died a few hours after that – I know she died – and it somehow seemed nice that that was the last thing she saw, this beautiful lady that she thought was an angel.'

Following the visit to the hospital, the Princess was scheduled to walk through a half-cleared minefield. The Halo Trust, the organisation that actually cleared the mines, wanted to show her an array of cleared mines and just how important and dangerous their work really was. Here they could show Diana some exposed or half-extracted mines, and how they went about dealing with them. In Cuito she had been told how a group of children had been playing on a football field that was supposed to be cleared. Unfortunately, one mine had been missed and as a result seven of them had been killed and others badly injured when one child trod on it. So she knew what to expect, and that even cleared areas weren't always entirely safe. The Halo Trust workers walked her through a cleared area until they came to the 'coal face', and she listened with great interest as they showed her a recently de-fused mine and explained how this was actually done. Next she walked back from where she had come on her own for the benefit of the photographers and film crew. It was actually perfectly safe, but in her body armour and visor walking alone through a minefield she made a powerful image – one of immense strength that could benefit both the Red Cross and the Princess personally the world over. When some photographers complained that they hadn't got a good shot of her, she smiled and did the walk again. It was a breathtaking shot, and not only helped bring the Red Cross crusade to the world's attention but won the Princess a lot of new friends also.

The Princess had very much wanted to win her spurs back with the British public, and had grabbed this opportunity with both hands; but there can be no doubting that whatever else Diana had got up to in her life, however else she had behaved in irrational, unfair, cruel and dishonest ways, this was her at her best and her very finest hour. Whether she had really turned a corner and would have gone on to champion this cause by adding staying power to her obvious ability to show unknown people great compassion while bringing their plight to the attention of the world's press, we will never know.

And yet, on this triumphant trip that would do more than anything to convert a princess into a saint following her death, Diana was using her time in between visits and photograph opportunities cruelly to bully a member of her staff, Victoria Mendham, and insist that she paid back the cost of accompanying her to the Caribbean. It was yet another defining paradox in a life full of them.

So how is this possible? How could this princess be so completely schizophrenic as to appear to a little girl as an angel one minute, while a moment later appearing to a devoted staff member as a devil? There can be no doubting the sincerity of Christina Lamb's observations: the Princess did appear like an angel, and while her time in Angola had only been short, and she hadn't dedicated years of her life to this kind of work as hundreds of unsung heroes and heroines had, she had made a difference by bringing the matter to the world's attention. Surely this was valuable use of her position, time, beauty and celebrity status. Sometimes over the last fifteen years she had used these talents very well in highlighting the plight of the poor, the sick and the dying.

So who was the real Diana? Which person should we believe in, the angel or the devil? The answer is both, because both existed. And here lies the real problem. Those who love Diana can only see the angel and refuse to accept that the other Diana really existed in any form but in the imagination of her detractors' minds. Equally, the Princess's detractors, horrified by her dishonest behaviour that brought such heartache, pain and damage to the Royal Family, can't see beyond this and therefore judge any good that she might have achieved as just being an act of one who is only attention seeking and wanting to manipulate the media. There is a lot of evidence that her detractors have the stronger case, but does that really matter when it comes to the effect that her intervention was to have in cases like the Red Cross campaign against landmines? In just eight days she had caused a media sensation. Just by her very presence, she had ensured that her trip was covered by virtually every news bulletin in most countries of the world. She had used her media position to good effect, and as a result a lot of good had been done – and that is a fact, whatever her real motives might have been and however long she might have stuck at it had she lived.

Of course anti-monarchists like Christopher Hitchens have a point when they claim that the real heroes are the people who dedicate their lives to these campaigns, and that Diana's most celebrated good works resulted from her jumping on an already rolling bandwagon (and off again when it suited her) and just posing for some rather well-rehearsed photographs. A work of no real substance, just the glitzy froth and not the real drink of dedicated goodness. It is certainly true that without the efforts of these unsung heroes, the Princess wouldn't have had a cause to turn up for and glamorise. She certainly never showed the dedication to initiate a good cause and stand by it through thick and thin at home or on the public stage in the way her husband has all his life. But should this be allowed to detract from the good that she did do? The effect was enormous, even if her work and genuine dedication were not. It was all a mirage really, but to those people, just like that little girl in the hospital in Huambo, it was a vision of goodness and that is what really matters.

So in the end, the good happened for whatever reason, and it was genuinely good. The bad also happened, and sometimes it cruelly affected people's lives. Either way, the Princess had even less control over any of it than anyone. Her illness saw to that. Nevertheless, the Angola trip helped confirm the mirage that became Diana's legacy.

In May 1997, the Tories were thrown out of office after eighteen years in power. A lot had been achieved during that time, and Britain's standing had risen dramatically as Margaret Thatcher had become something of an icon for tough economic reality and equally tough foreign policy. But, after eleven years, she had fallen victim to her proposed and much hated poll tax bill, and John Major had become her initially very popular successor. However, a downturn in both the British and the world economies, party in fighting over the EU and a series of Tory sleaze scandals had seriously weakened his position both within his party and with the electorate.

To make matters worse for the Conservatives, the old Labour Party had been taken over by men determined to modernise and reform it so that it wasn't really a traditional socialist party any more. It is perhaps the greatest achievement of Mrs Thatcher that she forced the old Labour Party to recognise that if they ever wanted to take office in the foreseeable future, they would have to move massively to the right. New Labour had started under the leadership of Neil Kinnock and progressed under the likeable John Smith before really taking shape under the young leadership of the totally ruthless Tony Blair. He understood, perhaps more than anyone, what was needed. He was intelligent, well educated and above all hadn't had working-class socialism driven into him. As a result, he had no love affair with nationalisation, trade unions or class warfare.

When Thatcher was prime minister, Blair had seen the writing on the wall. People whom she had made homeowners and shareholders by allowing them to buy their council houses cheaply and shares in the de-nationalised industries at knock-down prices weren't going to return a party to power that sounded more like the now deeply unpopular communist parties of Eastern Europe than a modern democratic British party. He and a number of his allies, some of whom had started on the left of the Labour Party, knew that the only way back to 10 Downing Street was to steal the Tory clothes.

This is precisely what they did. New Labour was, economically at least, a lot more Conservative than Edward Heath's Conservative government had been in the early 1970s. But it also promised to be more modern and presentable, and claimed that it had an almost presidential, youthful leader who was in touch with the nation's young families. The public were tired with the Tories after their eighteen years in power, and all the recent sleaze scandals and in-fighting, but not tired enough to elect an old socialist-style government. Now they didn't have to, because there was New Labour.

Originally, the Princess had been a staunch Conservative. She had admired Mrs Thatcher, although she thought that she wasn't right wing enough, especially when it came to crime. However, she had become less enamoured with the Tories during Mr Major's reign. She found it harder to charm him than she had expected, and had suspected that this might have something to do with his friendship with the Prince of

Wales. As a result, she had also suspected that the prime minister had vetoed many of her PR sorties immediately after her marriage break-up. She made a point of getting to know the Blairs, perhaps in the belief that they would be the new inhabitants of 10 Downing Street anyway, and thought that Tony might be more susceptible to her charm. She apparently liked them, and was keen to jump on their bandwagon of Cool Britannia. She often boasted that Cherie Blair asked for her advice on matters of fashion; indeed, the *Daily Mail* has more than once printed photographs of Mrs Blair evidently copying a Diana outfit.

Moreover, Diana was now moving in a social set where many had changed their political allegiance. One was her close friend Gulu Lalvani, who had been a Tory Party donor but was now backing New Labour. He had invited her to join him at Labour's late-night victory party at the Royal Festival Hall but, although tempted to go, she knew that, as a royal, she should remain impartial in public. More importantly, she knew that any open support for New Labour would seriously annoy many of her friends in the press – especially her long-term allies at the *Daily Mail*. So instead she remained at home but stayed up late, cheering Blair and Co on as she watched the results come in on her television set. And the Princess did have a genuine reason to be pleased as Robin Cook, the new foreign secretary, announced a ban on landmine sales within a month of taking up his post.

The new prime minister also invited Diana to Chequers and told her that he was considering giving her the ambassadorial role she had told him she wanted; he had apparently already spoken to Bill Clinton about it. But, as with so many of Blair's easily given promises, nothing ever happened. The Princess had told him that she could see herself playing a peacemaker's role, and was confident that she could achieve success by mediating in Northern Ireland. Tony Blair is not stupid: her pronouncement must have scared the living daylights out of him, and made him think again.

Piers Morgan records in his memoirs *The Insider* that on Monday 28 July 1997 Blair had explained to him during an interview that Diana needed to keep going at her landmine work, saying, 'She earns a lot of respect around the world for her work on landmines and I want that to continue.' So he seemed to have made up his mind about her request for another job, but just hadn't quite got round to telling the Princess that she was stuck where she was. And by Wednesday, 30 July, Diana's fate was certainly decided when Blair, in an act of amazing indiscretion, told Morgan that the Queen had given him 'a bit of a kicking' at their weekly meeting following Morgan's headline 'BLAIR BACKS DIANA'.

Since her divorce and forced silence on matters concerning the Royal Family, relations with Prince Charles had steadily improved. He took to dropping into Kensington Palace for tea from time to time, usually when he used the nearby helipad. On one such occasion, he reminded her what great legs she had, and this pleased her so much that she was still telling friends about it days later. They looked very relaxed together at Prince William's confirmation and Prince Harry's school sports day. Charles even invited the Princess and Prince William to accompany him to Hong Kong, where he was due to hand over the colony to the Chinese. She was very tempted as she liked Hong Kong and they had a mutual friend out there, David Tang. She said she would think about it.

Following on from her triumph in Angola, the Princess appeared more relaxed in public. In March, *Vanity Fair* commissioned the celebrated New York photographer Mario Testino to shoot a number of portraits of her for their July cover. The results were excellent – among some of the best pictures ever taken of this strikingly beautiful woman. Under the headline 'DIANA REBORN', she looked serene, confident, lovely and relaxed. The public might have been forgiven for believing that Diana had at long last put all her troubles behind her and had now found peace of mind. Unfortunately this was not the case.

Behind the scenes her personal relations remained as stormy as ever. Both her acupuncturist Oonagh Toffolo and her energy healer Simone Simmons had made the mistake of filling emotional gaps left by the banished and had become Diana's friends. Initially they had both been a source of comfort to her as her roller-coaster relationship with Hasnat Khan lurched along; but inevitably she quarrelled with both of them and so they were also discarded.

In June 2005, Simone Simmons published a new account of her private conversations with the Princess. The book, entitled *The Last Word*, caused a major stir among the tabloids: it was serialised in the *Sun* and was therefore rubbished in all the other tabloids. Simmons made many extraordinary claims: Diana had had a one night stand with JFK Junior; she had taken cocaine; she thought she was going to die and that this convinced her to go on her drug crusade; she had seriously tired of Paul Burrell and was going to sack him. The *Sun*'s opponents dismissed these and other stories as rubbish. The *Sun* responded by putting some of Diana's messages to her former friend on a premium-rate number. However, the three recorded messages said nothing whatsoever to support Ms Simmons' claims.

So did Diana sleep with JFK Junior? My research indicates it to be unlikely. It would certainly have been quite out of character for Diana to tell Ms Simmons about it in such language and detail and, as it was supposed to have happened at about the time she was being banished by the Princess anyway, it does seem hard to believe. In addition, her statement that Diana was very circumspect in her other courtships, given the Princess's actual behaviour with scores of other lovers, indicates that she really hadn't understood or got that close to the Princess anyway. On the other hand, Ms Simmons wouldn't have been the first person to whom Diana told something very private – or even lied – and then regretted her actions, subsequently dropping the individual stone dead.

Either way, the idiotic tabloid frenzy that greeted these rather weak, in some cases rehashed and in other cases fanciful revelations some eight years after the Princess's death was a fine testament to the shallow standing of British tabloid journalism. The *Sun* wasted its lead editorial two days running and even defended its decision to run with this nonsense on the laughable grounds that it was nice for the young princes to realise that their devoted mother had found great happiness in a one night stand.

The Princess also pursued her ongoing vendetta against Tiggy Legge-Bourke, who by now had surpassed Camilla Parker Bowles as public enemy number one in Diana's mind. Convinced that this younger woman was determined to replace her in her sons' affection and marry their father, she continued to plot against the children's nanny despite serious advice from her true friends to drop the matter. Her office issued a hostile statement about the nanny after she was photographed pouring champagne at an Eton School picnic that Prince William had wanted his mother to stay away from in case she arrived – as she usually did – with the tabloid press in tow. To Diana's horror, the press sided with Ms Legge-Bourke and criticised the Princess. Unable as usual to accept responsibility for her actions, Diana immediately deflected the blame on to her new secretary Michael Gibbons, and then attacked the editor of the *Sun* Stuart Higgins, who later told Clayton and Craig, 'We ran the story about what the Princess had said about Tiggy Legge-Bourke, which came from the Princess's office ... [Later] her aides ring up and say, "How could you do that? It's totally untrue." They had clearly been told by the Princess, "Get on the phone and give that Higgins bloke a bollocking, now!" And I said, "But you know it's true. You told me!"'

Of course, this might be a case of who do you believe – a princess who has a serious problem telling the truth or a tabloid editor whose newspaper is hardly famous for caring about the truth? Interestingly, Stuart Higgins's big rival at the *Daily Mirror*, Piers Morgan, unwittingly becomes the man to clear his name and damn the Princess. Some three weeks earlier, a patient from the famous Priory Clinic had phoned the *Mirror* and told them that the Princess had made a secret visit there and told a group of thirty or so patients about her own eating disorder. Morgan could see that this might be a good scoop. He immediately faxed Kensington Palace the story for the Princess to verify. Diana phoned him back and went through the story line by line. Morgan, flattered that he had now opened up a relationship with this beautiful and powerful woman, faithfully took all her alterations down. Diana was keen for everyone to know that she was now completely recovered but that home life was usually the cause of such an illness – this was about as close as she could get to blaming Prince Charles without risking breaking the confidentiality agreement. Morgan told the Princess that he would personally see that her wishes were carried out before faxing the revised version. She thanked him before adding, 'Please remember we have a chance to help other people.' Within the hour, every alteration had been attended to and her office had phoned back to say that she was both happy and grateful. Headlines were even agreed before Morgan headed off to celebrate a great scoop.

The next day, Morgan awoke to his story making the news and was pleased that he had done so with the Princess's help and agreement. Perhaps now the *Mirror* might be able to break up that cosy little arrangement that Diana and the *Daily Mail* had enjoyed for the last few years. It was therefore to both his horror and amazement that he learned that the Princess had issued a statement ferociously attacking the story as a shameful invasion of privacy. Diana went on to declare her deep disappointment that such a story had been leaked to the press. Whether the Princess had just changed her mind or had worried about the confidentiality agreement with Prince Charles is not clear.

Nevertheless, Morgan was flabbergasted and must have felt a little silly in front of his staff, as they all knew what had gone on. His thoughts swung between rage and revenge. He very nearly put a tape of their conversation on an 0898 number under the banner 'DIANA – WE NAME THE SOURCE'; but in the end he didn't, realising that she would reward him by freezing him out if he did and that would only play right into the hands of the *Sun* and the *Daily Mail*. He recalled in his memoirs, 'I will have to play by her rules. And if I don't, it's permanent Siberia for me, like so many of her friends and media contacts before.'

Nevertheless, he couldn't help but call her office and speak to Michael Gibbons about how this had happened. Gibbons explained that the Princess had thought about it and changed her mind overnight as she didn't want the article to be seen as a signal for a free-for-all on any future visits that she may wish to make to clinics. Morgan was furious: 'I replied, "Michael, I don't understand, no, it's a bloody joke. She went through every word with me, laughing and joking throughout. What will she do when I put the tape in the paper?"

'"Oh, the Princess doesn't think that you'll do that now that you are getting on so well."

'I'm trapped on Planet Diana, a crazy place where she still calls all the shots and is famous enough and important enough to newspapers to get away with it. You have to hand it to the little minx. Even by her standards, this is breathtaking behaviour.' Not to mention devious and dishonest – but perhaps that wouldn't occur to a tabloid editor. But it would before too long, as Morgan's memoirs recall on Wednesday 8 May when he noted the Eton Tiggy story in all the newspapers and then got a call from Gibbons to tell him that the Princess would like him to be aware of her views on the matter: 'I could actually hear her dictating them in the background. "Erm, the Princess feels very deeply hurt and angry that Ms Tiggy Legge-Bourke would behave in this idiotic way. Clearly she is a bad influence on the boys, as the Princess has been fearing for some time."

'I make the story the splash in tomorrow's paper. The *Mail* and the *Sun* have it, too – with the *Sun* taking an even harder line than we have. Diana had clearly got herself nicely worked up by the time Michael Gibbons called their editor.'

Two days later he records, 'Diana's lost it. Her views on Tiggy dominated the news but she was getting a lot of flak for being too nasty. So she issued a statement denying saying anything unpleasant about Tiggy, insisting that she was "delighted" she went to Eton in her place, and blaming an "employee in her office" for speaking without her consent. For God's sake, I'd heard her in the background giving Gibbons specific adjectives to describe Ms Legge-Bourke. Now she was dumping on him in the most disgusting manner. I rang him outraged, but was told he will no longer be taking calls from the press. Unbelievable – she's not only dropped him right in it, she's banned him from defending himself. Michael's far too loyal and decent to return the favour, but he must be bitterly hurt. I finally got to speak to him on his mobile and he sounded petrified of saying anything. I told him: "Don't let her get away with this." But he replied sadly: "Piers, you know what the Princess can be like, you remember that stuff with the clinic. It will blow over, it always does." Nobody should treat a good guy like this. It's cowardly and horrible. I splashed on "Queen of fibs", I know she'll freeze me out for a bit now, but I don't care. Diana's got to learn that you can't behave like this.'

Despite her appalling behaviour, the Princess remained unrepentant. She raised further eyebrows when she let it slip to *Le Monde*, the serious French daily, in answer to a question about Tony Blair's attitude to landmines, 'Yes, it's terrific. It's what he promised and he's doing a terrific job. The last government was hopeless.' This was an uncharacteristic gaffe on Diana's behalf, but luckily for her the Conservative Party was still distracted by its own in-fighting and failure to launch a serious complaint, and in any case the comment was largely lost under the praise that the interviewer Annick Cojean heaped upon the Princess for her dedication to good causes. The journalist's admiration knew no bounds as the Princess explained, 'Wherever it is in the world that someone calls me in distress, I will run to them.' Diana's fans sighed in admiration.

On 16 June 1997, the Princess was off to the US with Mike to launch the American Red Cross anti-landmine campaign. She arrived in time to attend Katherine Graham's eightieth birthday party. The publisher of the *Washington Post* had become a friend of Diana's, and not a bad friend to have as the proprietor of one of the world's leading newspapers – a fact not lost on the media-conscious Princess. The next day Diana gave a press conference with Elizabeth Dole, the president of the American Red Cross. That night she also attended a dinner for 500 at the Museum for Women in the Arts, and her presence ensured the evening was a total sell-out and raised an impressive $650,000.

The King and Di

While in the US, the Princess wanted an audience with President Clinton. It was her intention to bring up her future with him. Wisely Clinton palmed her off with a breakfast meeting with his wife Hilary instead. Then she jetted off to New York to meet Mother Teresa in the Bronx. This was brilliant PR, and Diana expertly used the opportunity to ring a kind of Mother Teresa endorsement of her out of the occasion. She returned to Washington still hoping to meet Clinton and carry out the rest of her Red Cross commitments before returning to New York once more on 24 June for the preview party of a charity sale of some of her dresses. This had been a rather clever fundraising idea thought up by Prince William. The 800 guests all parted with £100 for the privilege of attending, while the actual sale itself raised an amazing $3.26 million. The proceeds were split between several charities, with the lion's share going to the Aids Crisis Trust.

Following a quick trip home and a couple of rows with the troubled Hasnat Khan, it was back to New York again to lunch with two of the city's most important and influential women – Tina Brown, editor of the *New Yorker*, and Anna Wintour, editor of *Vogue*. They met at the highly fashionable Four Seasons restaurant. There, Diana told her luncheon companions that Tony Blair was about to send her on 'missions' so that she would be 'sorting people's heads out' and spreading love and peace in the process. Her two guests were incredulous and sneaked a glance at each other that said, 'Did I just hear what I think I heard?' as the Princess's conversation flashed from Angola to secret visits to hospices in the middle of the night and back to Tony Blair again. Using a discretion that would have been completely lost on a British tabloid editor, the two wise women of New York chose not to exploit the situation and share all of this private conversation with their readers.

While the Princess of Wales's life had been a roller-coaster affair through the 1990s, her former husband's had been more mundane. He had neither received the accolades nor the criticism that Diana had. Instead, and with the steady support of Camilla Parker Bowles, he had gone about his business. His confidence and self-esteem remained fragile, and he had not lost his capacity for self-pity. However, neither had he lost any of his dedication to make a difference by his hard work and selfless commitment to just causes.

The Prince's Trust had continued to grow. By the mid-1990s it was reaching more than 12,000 individuals each year, with a programme of grants and training delivered by over 1,400 volunteers. Turnover had grown to a very substantial £10 million per annum. Moreover, the Prince's Trust Volunteers Programme was giving more than 5,000 youngsters every year the chance of attending an intensive six-day course to discover the value of team building by working together on various community projects. After much cajoling from the Prince, the secretary of state for employment established an inter-departmental group involving twelve government departments to find ways in which government might assist in the expanding of the programme. In opposition, the Labour party had borrowed great swathes of Charles's ideas for their own thinking on the young – something Mr Blair would appear to have forgotten a decade later. In fact key aspects of the Volunteers Scheme were adopted by Labour for the party's Commission on Social Justice. As a result, the Prince of Wales could justly claim that his ideas and initiatives had seeped into the social thinking of both major political parties.

Indeed, it would not be unreasonable to claim that Prince Charles's work for the young and disadvantaged throughout the last thirty years has exceeded, in both imagination and execution, anything attempted or achieved by Margaret Thatcher, John Major, Neil Kinnock, Michael Foot, Gordon Brown, Tony Blair, Michael Howard or any other British politician. For this he should be very proud, and the nation grateful.

By the mid-1990s the Prince's Youth Business Trust had become a model that was copied in the US, Canada and India among other places. As a direct result of the Prince's personal interventions in 1993, the employment secretary dramatically increased the government's commitment to the PYBT by announcing that he would give £10 million in matching grants to that raised in the private sector, which ensured that a three-year expansion programme got off the ground. In Scotland the Prince's Scottish Youth Business Trust was launched in 1989. By 1995, and despite operating in some of the most challenging areas of the United Kingdom, it had invested more than £8 million in 3,000 young people; more than seventy per cent of these were surviving in business after three years.

In Wales, the Prince of Wales Committee, which had been chaired by the Prince personally since the 1970s, was also prospering. By the mid-1990s it was funding some 350 projects each year on a budget of nearly £1.25 million and with 15 project officers. Under the Prince's direction the Committee had successfully got the Welsh Joint Education Committee to agree to include Environmental Studies in their syllabuses. In 1994 its School Landscape project attracted over 600 children to work on 15 sites across Wales.

Business in the Community, the first organisation set up in the UK to develop partnerships between business, government and the community, had expanded to boast a membership of over 450 companies, and this included 80 of the country's 100 largest businesses. By now it had a staff of nearly 150, and about a third of these were on secondment from member companies. It had a turnover of more than £5 million per annum, 8 regional offices and 5 campaign teams. In addition, Business in the Environment had been launched by Charles in 1989 and, 7 years later, was linked to some 2,900 companies and 50 environmental networks promoting good practice through environmental management publications for small- and medium-sized companies.

In Scotland, by 1993 the Scottish Business in the Community was responsible for 44 Enterprise Trusts, which had helped to establish over 16,000 new businesses and created almost 29,000 new jobs in the process. In that year, these Trusts raised around £14 million.

Prince Charles had launched the Business Leaders Forum in 1990. By 1994 it had held 17 International Forum meetings that had involved more than 4,000 business leaders from just about every corner of the globe. In Poland, the Czech Republic and Slovakia, the BLF had by this time established networks of nearly 100 business leaders to help regeneration programmes through education, training and environmental projects. Also in 1994, as president of the Business Leaders Forum, he launched a project called Inner-City Action, which linked community leaders in the US and the rest of the western world with community leaders in the developing world in order to tackle jointly the problems of youth unemployment, shortages of housing, lack of skills, ethnic minority conflicts and environmental pollution.

By the summer of 1994, the Prince of Wales's Institute of Architecture had seen some 150 students pass through its doors. By now the institute had the necessary validations and accreditations to offer professional qualifications and postgraduate degrees. However, it would never raise the £40 million needed to secure a long-term future. Nevertheless, in 1993, six years after the Prince's now famous 'Luftwaffe' speech at the Mansion House, he was informed that the secretary of state for the Environment had approved a planning application for Paternoster Square that included the designs by John Simpson for which the Prince had argued so tenaciously. Consequently Charles wrote to the developers, 'It is a great relief that after all these years of effort and planning there is a chance that this scheme may come to fruition. You can rest assured that I will continue to take a very close interest in the whole project and will no doubt drive you all mad in the process.'

Building at Poundbury also finally got underway in 1993, and by the mid-1990s the first section was completed and occupied by Guinness Housing Trust tenants and private buyers in equal measure. Meanwhile, the Prince started another battle to save Britain's architectural heritage. Disconcerted by the heritage secretary David Mellor's decision to veto a scheme devised by the English Heritage and the National Heritage Memorial Fund to buy the Elizabethan mansion Pitchford Manor for the nation, the Prince summoned the most powerful conservationists in Britain. This led to a private presentation being made to John Major on behalf of the newly formed Pitchford Group by Simon Jenkins, the former editor of *The Times*. John Major was impressed, and this forced a change in government policy. In addition, and led personally by the Prince, the Pitchford Group lobbied successfully to increase the level of support that they might expect from the National Lottery.

While the national tabloids had been blowing hot over some of Diana's charity work but holding up their hands in cold disapproval of her little scandals, the Prince had taken an ever-increasing interest in the Duchy of Cornwall. He had by now completely woken up to the fact that he had land where he could prove that being kind to the environment did not necessarily mean that one had to make a financial loss. His managers' somewhat understandable scepticism about the virtues of organic agriculture had been destroyed by the fact that the Prince had converted the 1,000-acre Highgrove Estate to organic farming. Not only was it profitable, it had become one of the largest organic farms in Britain, and certainly the most admired. Also around this time, the Prince, aware that not many farmers enjoyed his wealth, had helped lobby the Ministry of Agriculture successfully for a five-year incentive scheme to help farmers meet the costs associated with conversion to an organic regime. Once more, with the sympathetic John Major at the helm, government was being more helpful and green than the Prince had ever dare hope under the early years of Thatcher.

In 1992 Prince Charles formed a charitable company for Duchy Originals, organic biscuits made from oats bought mainly from the organic produce of Highgrove. Charles took a keen interest in their packaging and labelling, sometimes to the consternation of his marketing people. He had become convinced that the duchy and its tenant farmers could dramatically increase profits by cutting out the middlemen and marketing their own products including biscuits, cheeses and ice creams. He was convinced that such products would do very well in the US and, following the 1992 introduction of the single market in Europe, there also. By the mid-1990s Duchy Originals were available at more than 1,000 independent outlets in the UK and were also becoming strong performers in the multiple grocer sector. Exports were also being shipped to France, Germany, the USA, Ireland, Canada and Japan, with sales increasing month on month.

Some products added later, such as soups and soft drinks, could not be produced organically because the necessary ingredients could not be bought in bulk. This was a serious disappointment to Prince Charles, but they were added nevertheless to the profits of the charitable company. From time to time Labour MPs complain of the extent of the duchy's profits. They tend to forget that, as a result of the duchy's success, the government does not pay the Prince of Wales anything for his work or his upkeep, that the Inland Revenue receives millions in taxes from the duchy and, thanks to his belief in the organic ideal, his hard work and enterprise, and the charitable status he gave Duchy Originals, millions have also been raised to support those in Great Britain who need a hand-up and haven't been getting it from those very same MPs.

Also in the early 1990s, the Prince had responded personally to a plea from the Czech president and established the Prague Heritage Fund. The fund was set up to finance three projects in Prague and was promised that if it raised £700,000, the Czech government would match the amount. £1.4 million could pay for quite a lot in the Czech Republic in the 1990s. It was decided that the principal revenue would come from a concert held within the grounds of Prague Castle. The Prince took out his fountain pen and wrote personally to artists like Murray Perahia and Dame Kiri Te Kanawa and asked them to perform. He then wrote to the crowned heads of Europe as well as heads of state and governments in order to secure patronage. In 1994 the concert took place, was televised by the BBC and was eventually shown in more than 30 countries. As a result, the £700,000 target was exceeded by £100,000 and the restoration work commenced.

Despite all of this, which was all accomplished alongside his presiding over state occasions and official trips to represent Her Majesty abroad, the Prince still found time to support complementary medicine and chair the Royal Collection Trust on behalf of the Queen. In an average year the Prince attends about twenty state functions; he attends more than fifty events on behalf of his charities; he makes well over fifty major speeches in support of his causes; he attends around twenty Duchy meetings and literally hundreds of other meetings with government ministers and his own courtiers in order to lobby for and support his charities, causes and intercede on behalf of his people. In addition, he visits around ten cities or towns on his 'away days', and usually makes around six international state visits. Thereafter he can be found very often working late into the night writing letters by hand to the great and the good, or simply to one of his mother's subjects. It is a travesty that as a result of a continued determination by the majority of the tabloid press to give a false account of what he does or who he really is, there are far too many of his future subjects who have absolutely no idea about any of it.

Despite somewhat chaotically working his way through this hectic programme in the 1990s, he was still finding time to harass government ministers. The environment secretary, the agriculture minister, the employment secretary and the trade minister were his usual targets as he pressed his causes regarding the environment, organic farming, the long-term unemployed and the need for greater collaboration between all government departments so that more advantage could be taken from royal visits overseas. He was especially mindful of the Middle East where he was becoming increasingly concerned to improve relations between Islam and the Christian West.

Unlike many politicians, the Prince had taken the trouble to learn about Islam and had attempted to understand the religion and therefore see its good as well as how it might be hijacked by extremists for the purpose of recruiting young men to join a 'holy war'. In 1993, before his departure to visit the Gulf, he made a speech to academics in Oxford. It had been written on the basis of much expert advice, and had been passed by the Foreign Secretary despite its controversial contents. In it, the Prince launched an attack that went further than any international politician had in expressing his 'despair and outrage at the unmentionable horrors being perpetrated in southern Iraq [by] Saddam Hussein and his terrifying regime.' Referring to Hussein's claim that the destruction of the March Arabs' habitat was solely for agricultural purposes, he continued, 'How many more obscene lies do we have to be told before action is taken? Even at the eleventh hour, it is still not too late to prevent a total cataclysm. I pray that this might at least be a cause in which Islam and the West could join forces for our common humanity.'

Inevitably, this impassioned outburst had the headline writers in the West reaching for their pens. But in the Arab world it was the remarks that the Prince went on to make about the suffering of the Bosnian Muslims that had the greater impact, as did his pleas to the West to overcome their prejudices about Islam. He distinguished between revivalist Muslims and extremists. He pointed out that extremism was not the sole preserve of Islam and that other religions, including Christianity, had extremists as well. He recalled the important part that Islam had played 'in our past and our present, in all fields of human endeavour. It has helped to create modern Europe. It is part of our inheritance, not a thing apart. More than this, Islam can teach us today a way of understanding and living in the world which Christianity itself is poorer for having lost. At the heart of Islam is its preservation of an integral view of the universe. Islam – like Buddhism and Hinduism – refuses to separate man and nature, religion and science, mind and matter, and has preserved a metaphysical and unified view of ourselves and the world around us ...'

The response to the speech in the Islamic world was united in its ecstasy. Newspapers across the Middle East reprinted the speech in full, and their editorials marvelled at the Prince's wisdom while radio and television commentators looked into its meaning with great enthusiasm. The leaders of the four Gulf States he visited offered him both their praise and gratitude. The king of Saudi Arabia paid the Prince the very unusual and even unprecedented compliment of visiting him in the house that had been provided for him, rather than summoning Charles to attend his own palace. This was seen as an act of great political homage.

Reports were sent back to the Foreign Office from wherever he travelled in the Gulf of his success and how his speech and subsequent goodwill visit had driven Britain's standing to the highest level – a matter of no little importance in either political or economic terms. Indeed, the regard that Prince Charles is held in the Gulf today, well over ten years later, has in no way diminished, and he is generally thought of very favourably for both his intelligence and fair-minded nature.

Given the unstable political nature of the region and the wealth of the oil-rich Arab nations, one would have expected the newspapers to have been reporting such a success on page one, just as they would a few years later with Diana's Angola trip. In fact, only the *Financial Times* bothered to send a correspondent on the tour, and as a result the rest of the British press gave scant coverage to this considerable achievement. The simple truth was that trips like this were now considered to be just too insignificant, too repetitive and too banal to warrant the sort of extended coverage that Robbie Williams, the Spice Girls or Princess Diana might expect for their new hairdo. As one tabloid columnist of the time put it, 'Give them chips every day if that is what they want. Fruit might be better for them, but that's not our job. Our job is to give them what they want and if they demand chips so be it.'

This is the real nature of the problem for the heir to the throne. He is dedicated, works hard, shows compassion and wants to do the best for his future subjects in particular, and mankind in general. He sees it as his duty – even his calling – to have the right to be consulted, the right to encourage and the right to warn. But in a tabloid world that is only interested in new wealth, new celebrity, new fashion and new gossip, none of this cuts any ice, and his efforts are either cynically made fun of or even ignored altogether. It is not surprising that the Prince is only really known to many people in Britain and most in America as the man who preferred the horsy Camilla to the beautiful Diana. This is hardly a fair reflection of any of their lives; in particular it is grossly unfair on the Prince. But where can he go and what can he do to get a fair hearing? It would appear that in the shallow country that was once an admired nation, there is nowhere.

Therefore it is hardly surprising that he believes that Islam can teach people a code of decent human understanding and principle that Christianity knows about but no longer has the power in this heathen and selfish land to administer. Britain has become a place where many say they want to see the return of 'family values' – provided that such values are not applied to their family. They want to see less crime as long as it is not their child who is arrested. They want to see more hospitals as long as they don't have to pay for them. They want to see less drunken violence on the streets as long as they can have as much to drink when and where they want. Given this state of affairs, only a fool would fail to realise that in such a place a competing tabloid press is bound to promote a flawed celebrity like Diana in place of a man who seems to come from another planet like Charles.

If we have turned our back on this man's values, it is hardly surprising that we do not wish him to remind us of virtues that we don't appear any longer to have the self-discipline to obtain. Therefore his virtue must be ridiculed in the name of modern reform, political correctness and republicanism. The fusion of sixties selfishness and arrogance and the greed of the eighties have produced a cancer that Prince Charles does not have the chemotherapy for, and I seriously doubt if anyone else does either. Perhaps we really are on the road to destruction.

Chapter Seventeen
The Last Summer (1997)

Some commentators have taken the view that by the last summer of Diana's life, her success with landmines, her improved relationship with Prince Charles and her celebrity status across the world had somehow combined together and miraculously cured her of the illness that had so affected her personality for the last sixteen years. They point to her selfless behaviour in Angola, the positive and complimentary comments that she began to make about her ex-husband and how she seemed so at ease as she jetted around the world for either work or pleasure.

Their view is supported by the Prince himself. He had always believed that if he refused to retaliate against her fabrications and lies, eventually she would return to being the fun-loving and kind girl he had been so impressed with when he first met her. His relief when relations improved was also shared by Buckingham Palace, and that is why Diana was rewarded by being given permission to go to Angola with the Red Cross. However, all the medical opinion I have consulted appears united that it is extremely unlikely that the Princess was by then on the road to recovery, and the facts tend to support their view, not that of Prince Charles.

Angola was a triumph, and it did show that the Princess had a big heart and some profound humanitarian instincts. But she also knew that she needed something to blot out the scandalous revelations of nuisance calls and ghoulish photographs. Moreover, she knew that she had to be much nicer to Prince Charles and the Royal Family and stop leaking untruths about them to the press if she wanted to hold on to her financial settlement. In addition, she had come to realise that her deceit in the Morton book and the *Panorama* interview had resulted in the last Conservative government viewing her as a self-publicist and loose cannon. If she wanted to enlist the support of the new Labour government and secure its agreement for the ambassador status she so desired, she would have to avoid making the same mistake with Tony Blair, especially as the Prince counted Peter Mandelson as a close friend and advisor and Diana knew Blair rarely did anything without consulting him. Therefore she knew very well that she would have to build bridges with her in-laws.

So, as the Princess jetted around the world associating herself with

Mother Teresa and other good causes, one might have been forgiven for thinking that at last her health had taken a turn for the better. The reality was, as we now know, somewhat different. Shocking treatment of many people including Jane Atkinson, Victoria Mendham, Tiggy Legge-Bourke, Oonagh Toffolo, Simone Simmons and Michael Gibbons all occurred in the last six months of Diana's life. Circumstances had changed, and therefore so had the targets. The Royal Family might have breathed a great sigh of relief as the Princess suddenly turned from a vindictive and scheming nightmare into a charming family member who had turned up just before Christmas 1996 at Eton for Prince William's carol service and kissed Prince Charles, much to his surprise, in front of the world, but the truth is that while her ambitions dictated kinder behaviour towards the Windsors and a less scandalous public image, her behind-the-scenes behaviour to people who were mere friends or employees and with whom she had no need to curry favour hadn't improved at all, as many independently verified accounts confirm.

    The cessation of the Princess's dirty-tricks campaign against the Royal Family should have made life easier for all concerned, but ironically it was to involve the Princess herself in a mini-storm as a direct result of her changed attitude. Elton John had organised for Diana to write the foreword for a coffee-table book *Rock and Royalty* by his friend Gianni Versace. John had also obtained the Princess's agreement that she would attend the book's launch at a fundraising dinner for his Elton John AIDS Foundation on 18 February 1997. By 10 February, more than $400,000 worth of tickets had been sold when Diana eventually got to see an advance copy of the book. Given the title of the book, and the author's reputation, she was perhaps a little foolish to have left it until so late in the day – but when she had agreed to write the foreword and attend the launch she couldn't have cared less about how the Royal Family might have regarded such a publication. But now this had all changed, and when she finally got to see a copy she was horrified. Photographs of nude males were juxtaposed with those of certain royals, including the Queen. The book was not pornographic by modern standards, and would in many quarters just be viewed as artistic expression, but she knew that it would not appeal to the more old-fashioned sensibilities of Prince Charles or his mother. So the Princess, by now aware that ongoing hostilities with the Royal Family no longer suited her purpose and keen to build bridges with them, panicked that her association with such a book could damage her cause. She realised that, while it couldn't be construed as having broken her confidentiality agreement, it might be seen as endorsing people poking fun at the monarchy, and that was hardly a way of furthering her new ambition by persuading either the Royal Family or both political parties that she was now a reformed character.

Consequently, she promptly disassociated herself from both the book and its launch, and in typical Diana style went public about her decision to do so – although having a quite word with the now sympathetic Prince of Wales to explain her concerns and quietly withdrawing from the gala dinner might have been a fairer way of dealing with Elton John and Gianni Versace. But the media junkie in the Princess saw this as an opportunity to turn disaster into triumph and actually ingratiate herself with both the Prince and his mother. 'I am extremely concerned that the book may cause offence to members of the Royal Family,' she told her public. 'For this reason I have asked for my foreword to be withdrawn from the book, and I will not attend the dinner on February 18th, which is intended to mark the book's launch.'

Naturally, her actions brought about an unmitigated disaster for Elton John and Gianni Versace, as they would any other charity fundraiser faced with the same fait accompli. Diana knew this only too well as someone who had been around charities for a decade and a half, but she gave it no consideration. A charity bash for AIDS victims was not going to stand in the way of what she wanted, so John and Versace had to be dumped. Once she had done this, the gala dinner was doomed and they had to cancel it or face the humiliation of a public rout as other guests followed the Princess's lead. Versace had the good grace to reimburse the lost revenue to the AIDS Foundation, but understandably he was very angry with the Princess and a highly embarrassed Elton John stopped speaking to her. Ironically, this feud would only end when the Princess made a very public move to comfort a distraught John during Versace's funeral service. The outside world marvelled at her compassion without knowing what had preceded her public act of sympathy.

However, in February that year this act of loyalty towards the crown was seen as another step in the right direction, and the Princess had clearly accomplished her goal. Increasingly, the Prince and Buckingham Palace saw Diana as being now both cooperative and at last behaving as a princess should. This was crucial to her plan to develop on the international stage. She not only realised that neither Major nor Blair or even Clinton would give her anything to do without royal affirmation, she had also not forgotten that the terms of her divorce settlement restricted her freedom to leave the country. As she intended to grow old gracefully as a beautiful international humanitarian star, she could see the dangers ahead if the Queen refused to give her consent for the Princess to travel. Sacrifices had to be made, and that just happened to be Elton John and Gianni Versace's bad luck – as well, of course, as all those dying people they were attempting to help.

Mohamed Al Fayed is a tough businessman and is used to getting his own way. In 1987 the Co-operative Wholesale Society and my business, Hodgson Holdings plc, paid Mr Fayed £31 million for the House of Fraser Funeral Division and so I got to see how he operated. I can say that it would be hard to find a man further removed from the character of Prince Charles or one with a greater desire to climb to the pinnacle of global society. Underneath his brash manners and glittery lifestyle is a man with burning ambition. Like the Princess of Wales, he does not believe that truth should come between him and his ambition.

He had seen for some years the cultivation of royalty as an important part of both his social ambition and his desire to be granted British citizenship. Harrods, which was originally part of the House of Fraser and which he retained when he sold the rest of it, prominently displayed its many 'By Royal Appointment' crests, and he also sponsored the annual Windsor Horse Show. Somewhat disappointed that the Windsors in Buckingham Palace, Clarence House and St James's Palace seemed happy to accept his money for their charities but paled at the very idea of mixing with him socially, Al Fayed turned his attention towards Princess Diana and her sons.

Like Murdoch and others before him, Al Fayed viewed Diana as the chink in the royal armour. Her late father had been a friend of his and he had known Diana for many years. The Princess used his store frequently and increasingly he made it his business to support generously her favourite charities. Moreover, he had made Raine Spencer, Diana's once despised stepmother but by now apparently a close confidante of hers, a non-executive director of Harrods. It was through Raine that Al Fayed discovered that the Princess had made no firm arrangement for her summer holiday with her sons. He was seated next to the Princess at a dinner at the Churchill Hotel when he took the opportunity to invite her and her sons to join his family holiday in St Tropez. He assured her that no expense would be spared concerning her privacy, security and enjoyment.

This was not the first occasion that he had asked the Princess to join his family on holiday. On previous occasions Diana had politely declined having taken the advice that to do so could harm her image. But now she was tempted. She was frightened that William and Harry would have a better time during the summer holidays with their father than her. After all, he still had access to many fine yachts around the world and could take them horse riding, fishing and hunting on the massive Balmoral Estate. She realised that they had inherited their father's love of country life, and as they grew older it had become increasingly difficult to keep them from becoming closer to him. The Princess was not good at sharing anything with anyone, and least of all her sons with their father. She might have appeared more reasonable in order to gain her in-laws' support, but in reality nothing had really changed, and the existence of Tiggy Legge-Bourke only made matters worse. Her presence as the children's nanny made Diana sincerely believe, however wrongly, that a perfect family was developing around her boys' father, with Ms Legge-Bourke playing the role of mother better than she ever had. She felt excluded – even though she had wanted the separation – and extremely vulnerable. In a perfect world she would have had custody of the children, but she knew neither Prince Charles nor his mother would have ever agreed to this, and nor would she have got her extremely large financial settlement if she hadn't agreed to be much more reasonable about the Prince of Wales having proper access to his sons.

In the Princess's mind, the summer holidays had become something of a competition for the hearts and minds of William and Harry, and she worried that the Prince of Wales, aided and abetted by Tiggy, was going to romp away with it. So it was natural that a holiday at Al Fayed's luxury villa in the magnificent Gulf of St Tropez was tempting, and she also felt sure that having his four youngest children there would make it even better for the boys. Then Al Fayed announced that he was about to add the new £20 million luxury motor yacht *Jonikal* to his small armada of boats that would be moored in the gulf within easy distance of the villa. It seems that this news made the Princess's mind up and, against the advice of many of her closest friends, she decided to accept Al Fayed's invitation.

One person who was not offering negative advice about going on holiday with Mohamed Al Fayed was his grand employee Raine Spencer, and her views were by now well respected by her stepdaughter. Diana had not only fallen out with most of her friends during her separation and divorce from the Prince of Wales, she had also become alienated from most of her family. Relations with her sister Jane had never recovered, and she had had angry exchanges with her brother Charles due to his withdrawal of an offer for her to have a house on the family estate. Matters were only made worse when he then questioned her mental state and expressed hope that she would seek medical help. In addition, she was not speaking to her mother as a result of the latter telling *Hello!* magazine that her daughter was better off without her HRH. Having cut all communications with her mother, Diana turned to her stepmother and waved an olive branch in her direction. Amazingly, Raine put Diana's insults, rudeness and fabrications behind her. She even apparently forgave the way Diana and her brother had trashed her belongings after their father's death.

'She was closer to Raine at the end than she was her mother,' was Joseph Sanders' assessment. Two decades of cruel and atrocious behaviour were simply wiped away by a forgiving Raine, who had much to be forgiving about: in addition to verbal insults, the Princess had even on one occasion launched a physical attack and pushed her hated stepmother down a flight of stairs at Althorp just before Raine's sixtieth birthday celebration. When she was told that she could have killed her stepmother, she simply replied, 'Who's going to charge the Princess of Wales with murder?'

But now they were friendly, even close, and the Princess had come to respect the wisdom of the older woman and began to admire how Raine got results. Raine told her to go on holiday with Al Fayed, and have a great time. Not for a moment did she have any idea what the consequences would be.

On 11 July 1997, the Princess of Wales and the young princes were collected from Kensington Palace by a Harrods helicopter and taken for lunch to the Al Fayed Elizabethan mansion, Barrow Green Court, at Oxted in Surrey, before flying on to Stansted Airport. From there they took a private jet to Nice. At Nice a private limousine ferried them to the small harbour of St-Laurent-du-Var where they boarded *Jonikal*.

The luxury yacht then cruised sedately west for two hours along the French Riviera and into the setting sun. Eventually they arrived to stay with the Al Fayed family at their eight-acre property, which looks across the Gulf of St Tropez towards St Maxime. Mohamed, his wife Heini and their children were staying in the main villa, while Diana and her sons enjoyed the privacy of a small separate guest villa. It had been an exciting start to the holiday for the boys, and Diana was pleased that she had accepted Al Fayed's invitation.

As they travelled, the Princess must have mulled over her career options in her mind. Things were starting to look up. Her improved attitude towards the Prince of Wales was paying dividends and a grateful Royal Family seemed keen to reward her. Her trip to Angola, her association with Mother Teresa and her immense popularity in the USA had improved her standing with the British public and gone some way to erasing the embarrassing memories of the Hoare, Carling and Tiggy Legge-Bourke fiascos. She was hopeful that Tony Blair would find an ambassadorial role for her that would surely keep her face on the front pages for years to come. And if he didn't, she had other ideas of self-publicity that could act as plan B. These included an autobiography for publishers Random House about her charity work. Contracts had been drawn up but remained unsigned while the Princess considered the offer of an alleged $500,000 advance. She was also considering whether or not to join Ivana Trump's former husband Riccardo Mazzucchelli in a venture that would sell clothes and jewellery on shopping channels under the name 'House of Diana'. And she had also been in negotiation for nearly a year with American screen actor Kevin Costner who wanted her to play herself in a sequel to *The Bodyguard*. She had accepted thirty pages of script written especially for her, and had even dined with the studio bosses at Warner Brothers. After her death many claimed that Costner exaggerated the story in order to bolster his career with some much-needed publicity. However, both David Tang, a friend of mine and a good friend to both the Princess and Costner, and the Duchess of York have since confirmed that Costner was telling the truth.

In all three cases the Princess would have to have given her share of the proceeds to charity as her divorce settlement precluded her from earning money for her own personal gain. But she was well aware of that and saw all three possibilities as potential opportunities to keep her publicity machine rolling along. So why didn't she finalise any of these deals? The reason is simple: none were part of plan A, and signing up to any could ruin her chance of becoming an ambassador. As a result, she vacillated and signed up to nothing, extremely conscious that she mustn't upset the Royal Family even though, given her addiction to celebrity, she must have been seriously tempted to take the film role.

Once there, the boys might have been expected to love spending their days either swimming off *Jonikal* in the clear, warm Mediterranean, lounging by the villa's pool, jet skiing, sailing or scuba diving. It was all perfect save for one thing – the press and paparazzi had arrived en masse only a few hours behind them. It appeared that their privacy might become seriously impeded once they ventured from the security of either the villa or *Jonikal*. It is most unlikely that anyone on either Al Fayed's staff or the Princess's would have tipped the press off. Al Fayed's staff had been made well aware of how important it was for the holiday to be private, and they did not dare disobey their employer. Moreover, the only person who dared leak things out of Kensington Palace was the Princess herself. We will never know but, given that the Princess was still tipping off the press and the paparazzi almost daily about where she was going and what she was doing until the night she died, there must be a very good chance that she was the one who actually spilled the beans to them on this occasion as well.

But if it was her, why did she appear to be displeased with their arrival? The probable explanation is that given Prince William's loathing of media attention and the trouble Al Fayed had gone to in order to protect her sons' privacy, she could hardly do anything else. Moreover, it was common for Diana to tip off the press and then appear angry at their presence. It was part of her planned image – a beautiful woman being so famous and irresistible to the world that the press would simply follow her anywhere and everywhere just to catch the briefest of shots. The press chasing a reluctant Princess was, in Diana's mind, an appealing impression, whereas a princess chasing the media was not.

Three days after her arrival, and for reasons best known to the Princess, she decided to take matters into her own hands and approach the press. She jumped into a small motorboat and made for the media boats stationed some way away. On the way she provided some graceful and elegant pictures as she sailed through the air, her arms spread-eagled dramatically. Then she gave an impromptu press conference at sea to the British contingent in which she said, 'My sons are always urging me to live abroad and be less in the public eye. Maybe that is what I should do, given the fact that you won't leave me alone. I understand I have a role to play, but I have to be protective of my boys. William gets very distressed, and he can get freaked out with all the attention. But you are going to get a big surprise with the next thing I do.'

What did she mean? We will never know. Nevertheless, it was a great pity that she had never previously paid attention to William's distress – which was real enough. The truth is that the Princess had had a series of rows with her sons over the last few days. The importance of such disputes should not be underestimated. As a result, Diana felt the need to shift the blame for this media intrusion from herself to the media in a vain effort to make peace with them. From the boys' point of view the holiday had become everything that they didn't want. The Princess had genuinely wished to make it a memorable time for them before losing them to their father for six weeks. However, her idea of a good time surrounded by the Al Fayed family and a media circus was not theirs, and they couldn't wait to get away to the peace and calm of their father and Balmoral.

They weren't enjoying their holiday with Diana one bit. They hadn't taken to Al Fayed, and they simply hated all the publicity. The Princess had been telling the truth when she had said that her children had told her to live abroad. What she hadn't articulated was that it had been said in anger and that they had added that they wouldn't be joining her. In fact there had been one massive row between Prince William and his mother, when harsh words were sadly exchanged – a terrible tragedy given that she was never to see her sons again once the holiday was over. For the young princes, the whole week had been an extremely uncomfortable time in spite of the beautiful weather, the warm sea and the wonderful Al Fayed toys. Without the press presence, the Princess might have won them over, but she had been unable to put them before her addiction. Her obvious guilt and attempt to shift the blame on to the media is perfectly reflected in her tirade at them. But even this wasn't the whole story: the Princess also had an ulterior motive for the impromptu press conference.

Naturally enough, the exquisite photographs and clever outburst guaranteed her all the press coverage she craved, especially as by now she had one eye on the fact that Prince Charles was going to throw a birthday party at Highgrove for Camilla on the eighteenth and the

The King and Di

Princess, in her time-honoured fashion, intended to grab and keep the headlines for the next few days. According to Diana's friend, the astrologer Debbie Frank who assisted Kate Snell in her book *Diana: Her Last Love*, 'Dodi was someone who came into Diana's life in that July when she really needed an out. She needed to get away from her feelings of despair that were coming back about Camilla and the possibility that Camilla and Charles would end up together.' This opinion is poorly formed. Firstly, Diana had understood only too well for a long time that Charles and Camilla were bound to be a publicity item. Secondly, as a result she was offended by the attention they might attract and her competitive nature resented being unable to control that. Thirdly, she was currently far more concerned emotionally about the threat of Tiggy Legge-Bourke than Camilla.

Nevertheless, the press were confounded by her unexpected outburst. Many had suspected that it was the Princess who had tipped off the media about the holiday, and this view seemed to be have been confirmed by her initial attitude to their presence. For the previous two days both the Princess and Mohamed Al Fayed had seemed very relaxed and had been giving the impression that they were enjoying all the attention. They were obviously posing for photo opportunities from a distance and providing them when none were requested. Moreover, if she had really wanted privacy, it was but one burst of *Jonikal*'s powerful engines away. The older heads among the press corps suspected this was nothing more than a plan to outshine Camilla, and they reported as much.

On the morning of 18 July, the British tabloids were overloaded with Diana's holiday snaps just as she had intended. But the words that accompanied them weren't those that she had intended. The photographs were fine, but the press hadn't taken kindly to her tirade, and the tone of the articles suggested that she had set the whole thing up to deflect from Camilla's big birthday milestone. Diana, as sensitive to criticism as ever, had a statement issued from her Kensington Palace office denying that she had made any such comments to the media. This, and her similar denial of comments she had made to the French publication *Le Monde* but now regretted as she realised that ambassadors weren't so indiscreet, did her reputation with the media no good whatsoever, and reopened the wound that had been festering before the Angola visit.

This press criticism also made her fear that she might have

overstepped the mark with Prince Charles, which might undo all the good work she had undertaken in order to obtain her ambassadorship. She didn't want this, and nor did she want to ruin her recently improved standing with the media – although how she thought that calling them all a bunch of liars was helpful is unclear. Nevertheless, she wisely withdrew from public view, something that she could have done from the beginning of the holiday if she had wished to, and let Camilla have her birthday party on the centre stage.

In France, 14 July is Bastille Day, when the French celebrate revolution, genocide and regicide. Dinner was taken on *Jonikal*. The yacht had been strategically moored so that the aft dining deck could get a good view of the firework displays from Port Grimaud, St Maxime and St Tropez. As Al Fayed had promised, no expense was spared as hideous amounts of food were placed before the guests on silver plates, and then whisked away with the majority untouched. Apparently, this very much impressed Prince William, who was used to royal thriftiness where food is never wasted – he had never seen such luxury before. He was in particular taken aback when a whole fish was removed to the galley untouched.

At this dinner, the party was joined by Al Fayed's eldest son Dodi. He had been ordered there by his father, who apparently felt that the Princess would benefit from the company of someone nearer her own age. Born Emad Fayed, Dodi was forty-two years old. He was known to the wider world as a film producer, and had invested money in a number of films, including the Oscar-winning *Chariots of Fire*, while still in his twenties. However, a *Vanity Fair* article reported that since then he had developed a nasty cocaine habit and this tended to limit his ability to settle his bills. Sadly, such were his insecurities that he believed he needed to do this in order to retain their friendship. Most people who knew him would agree that he was a pleasant man who was lazy, woefully insecure and terrified of his father – a complicated cocktail of kindness, gentleness and generosity to people whom he wanted to please and a wicked cad to people to whom he owed money or just didn't need any more. Discarded women came into the latter category.

Diana knew she was on to a certainty with Dodi. They had first met in 1986 at a polo match, then again briefly in 1992 at the London film premiere of *Hook*. In the spring of 1997 they had attended the same dinner party, and as long ago as the beginning of the year she had told friends that Mohamed Al Fayed had told her that she and Dodi were made for each other, and how Dodi admired her. It was inevitable that Al Fayed, with his own plans firmly settled in his mind, would invite his son to arrive unexpectedly and meet the woman who held the keys to everything he wanted. He knew he could rely on Dodi – his son's gentleness and willingness to please made women overlook his puppy fat and find him attractive, and of course he was always keen to follow his father's wishes.

However, Al Fayed, like so many before him, had underestimated the complex character of Diana. As usual she had her own agenda. She needed to rekindle her romance with Hasnat Khan; she would need to recapture the front pages following Camilla's fiftieth birthday bash; and she was in need of male attention, flirtation and probably sex. And here was Dodi – the perfect answer. A public romance would make Hasnat jealous, grab the headlines from Camilla and make her feel alive. It was Diana rather than Dodi who took the lead in the seduction.

As the dinner concluded and the fireworks were launched and exploded into the balmy night sky, Dodi picked up fruit to eat and dropped some. Diana picked it up and threw it at him. He recognised the sign and the look in her eyes. He threw the fruit back at her. Diana then let Dodi have a mango in the face and another on the back. An enormous fruit fight ensued, with both of them chasing around the deck after each other like children. A crewmember was later to comment, 'They were chasing each other and laughing and giggling like a couple of kids. Then they wrestled a bit and stopped – just staring at each other.' As that contact was made and those looks exchanged, it mattered not what was going through the mind of Dodi or, for that matter, his father: the Princess had made up her mind.

The following day, Diana learned of Versace's murder. Proving that she could reduce the media access to nil if she really wanted to, she kept out of view, made arrangements to attend the designer's funeral and pursued her new love target. However, once Camilla's party was out of the way, the media junkie in Diana re-emerged and was quickly back on deck, in full view of the telescopic lenses and keen to get her fix. She created interesting poses that she knew the paparazzi couldn't resist. She got a child to hose her down, and then swung on a rope from one of the ship's davits in full view of the press launches before plunging into the sea. Next she was off on a jet ski with Prince Harry, before introducing Dodi by being photographed swimming with him.

Naturally, all of these photographs were published around the world.

Dodi spent the days and evenings with his family, Diana and the princes either on board *Jonikal* or at the villa. But at night he retired to sleep aboard another of his father's ships – the schooner *Sakara*. There was a reason for this: Dodi was not alone. Not only was he not alone, in three weeks' time he was due to marry the girl who was accompanying him – the former *Vogue* model Kelly Fisher who had been going out with Dodi for a little over a year. Ms Fisher had arrived on 16 July, and remained on board the *Sakara* while her fiancé made his excuses by saying that he had to attend to business with his father. If a passion ignited between Dodi and Diana, Kelly could be dispensed with; if not, Dodi could go ahead with the marriage. Just as Prince Charles had been the ultimate spouse for the young Lady Diana, so the Princess of Wales was the greatest catch possible for Dodi and, of course, his father. The scheming Fayed hadn't got where he was by passing up such opportunities.

During the five days spent on board *Jonikal*, Diana used the same seduction tactics that she had used on Prince Charles all those years ago and scores of men since. There were the long intimate conversations about lonely childhoods and the need to be loved. Dodi was receptive. He was gentle, loving and wanted to be liked. And to be fair, his childhood and Diana's had a marked number of similarities: they were both from broken homes, each had been separated at an early age from their mothers and, perhaps as a result, both suffered from deep insecurities.

On 20 July, Diana and the princes flew back to London on the Harrods jet. That evening an excited William and Harry were on their way to their beloved Balmoral. It might not have been Diana's idea of heaven, but the boys had their father's blood running through their veins and, for William in particular, the idea of having a proper holiday rather than performing in a media circus was particularly appealing. Diana was quite understandably sad to see them go – a feeling made much worse not just by the fact that it would be six weeks before she saw them again, but also by the insecurity that their happy departure brought about.

The next day, Dodi sent his new princess a huge bouquet of pink roses and a solid gold Panther watch worth £7,000. Diana was not necessarily impressed: she craved adoration and attention much more than gifts that she was quite capable of either buying herself or being given every time she made a foreign visit. In addition, such a gift, while it might sweep most girls off their feet, which is clearly what Dodi and his father wanted, was not in the same league as the $200,000 watch King Juan Carlos of Spain had bought her from the upmarket jeweller Bijan over a decade earlier.

On 22 July, Diana jetted off to Milan, this time in Elton John's private jet, to attend Versace's funeral. The bitterness that had erupted between them as a result of the *Rock and Royalty* debacle was now put behind them in the face of this senseless tragedy. The next day a queen of rock and a princess of hearts sat together in the Versace family pew. Elton John was devastated by the loss of his close friend and broke down. Diana felt genuine compassion for him, as she would have for all people in such painful circumstances. Nevertheless, as Patrick Jephson was later to remark, the Princess had a cool and calculating eye for a good photo opportunity and reviewing the photographs now; one can't help come to the opinion that this was just such an occasion. In that sense, perhaps both sides of Diana were sitting there – one doling out sincere comfort, the other milking it for all it was worth.

Four days later, on Saturday, 26 July, Diana travelled to Paris for a secret weekend with Dodi. She stayed at the Ritz Hotel on Place Vendôme, which is owned by Dodi's father, and was placed in the £6,000-a-night suite. She was picked up by Dodi at the heliport near the Eiffel Tower and taken to see the Windsor villa where the Duke and Duchess had lived in exile from 1953 until the Duke's death in 1972 – the very place where Prince Charles had visited his great-uncle over a quarter of a century before, but which was now also owned by Al Fayed.

The Princess reportedly slept alone before taking breakfast with Dodi and returning to London on Sunday 27, but not before accepting his invitation to join him on *Jonikal* on a six-day cruise to Corsica and Sardinia on 31 July. This time they would have the yacht to themselves, and they both understood it would be an imitate holiday in the full sense of the word. Nevertheless, it was clear to those who were close to the Princess at the time that Diana still hankered after Hasnat Khan. It was at about this time that Khan had reluctantly made the decision that a leopard never changes her spots and, despite her various tactics, had decided to end the relationship officially. By early August the relationship was over – in his mind at least. The Princess might have been devastated by such bad news, but it would appear that she by no means accepted it as final.

Kate Snell correctly points out that the press and many Diana biographers have always assumed that Diana and Hasnat parted either in the spring or the early summer. As a result her subsequent relationship with Dodi is seen as a new love affair in its own right – a real love at last. Such speculation is based on a fallacy. Hasnat Khan and Diana remained an item until the end of July, and Diana was to remain in touch with his family until her death a month later. This changes the way the last four weeks of her life should be viewed. Diana had never taken rejection lying down. She hadn't with Prince Charles, nor had she with Oliver Hoare. Hasnat Khan was to be no exception: she had already formulated a plan.

Khan had finished the relationship before, notably when Diana had leaked news of their relationship to the press. With the help of people like Joseph Sanders and Richard Kay she had talked him round. However, he seemed more adamant this time, and the Princess clearly thought that action rather than mere words was called for. Kate Snell records that, 'Any self-respecting Mills and Boon reader knows that to win her man back, the heroine must make him jealous, and jealousy was certainly a weapon in Diana's armoury that she had used before.' Diana went ahead with her plan to make Kahn jealous, despite advice from his uncle that such a course of action could not possibly succeed.

On Thursday, 31 July, Diana and Dodi departed for their cruise and by Saturday, 2 August they were being tracked down by a single member of the Italian paparazzi. His name was Mario Brenna, a respected photographer from Milan who was well known throughout Italian fashion and high-society circles. He had been Gianni Versace's personal photographer, and had met Diana at the designer's funeral a little over a week ago. Normally the paparazzi hunt in packs; often they share knowledge. But this was a secret assignment. Brenna had been instructed by a British photographer, Jason Fraser, who had apparently last seen Diana at her dress auction in New York earlier in the year.

Fraser had originally been a serious news and political photographer before switching to the more profitable world of celebrity. Diana had used him surreptitiously before, most notably during the period between 1989 and 1991 when James Coulthurst would tip him off at the Princess's command. Diana had long since learned that photographs can often say a lot more than words, and in this regard Fraser had served her well. Now she turned to him again.

She put the wheels in motion on or about 30 July when the thirty-three-year-old Fraser received a phone call from either someone very close to Diana, or possibly even Diana herself. Dodi was not himself aware at this moment of the plan for the proposed pictures that Brenna was subsequently to take.

Fraser was given the information that the Princess and Dodi were going away together on *Jonikal* and where the yacht was to be found. It was made abundantly clear to him that no complaints would be made if secret photographs of them were taken together, but on no account would they pose for them. Fraser came to the conclusion that it would be better to share both this information and the subsequent spoils with his friend Mario Brenna, whose expert knowledge of the Italian Riviera and access to power boats there meant that he was best placed to carry out the assignment.

On 2 August, Brenna spotted *Jonikal* moored off Cala di Volpe in north-east Sardinia. He noticed a blonde woman pacing the deck continually on her mobile phone, but despite observing her at a distance for six hours, she couldn't be certain that it was Diana. He returned the next day early in the morning and soon became sure the blonde was indeed the Princess. He was temporarily called away and he failed to take a photograph; when he returned, much to his horror, *Jonikal* had upped anchor and disappeared. Diana had only allowed minimal information to be leaked to Fraser. She knew that he and Brenna would earn a fortune from such photographs and therefore could be relied on to act upon the meagre facts being relayed and thus give the appearance of a real chase instead of the phoney tip-off job it really was. A crestfallen Brenna was forced to report to Fraser that he had lost the whereabouts of *Jonikal*. Fraser considered flying out himself, as to fail the Princess on this assignment would not only cause her extreme displeasure but also cost both men several hundred thousand pounds in fees.

Happily this wasn't necessary. Brenna received a call from a girlfriend to say that the Princess and Dodi had been seen window-shopping in Porto Cervo. On Monday, 4 August Brenna, now in his own powerboat, caught up with *Jonikal* as she set sail for Corsica. He followed and was on hand when the luxury yacht stopped on the southern tip of the island at Isola Piana and Dodi and Diana took a tender and headed for shallow waters and a swim. It was here that the first few photographs of the now famous 'kiss' collection were taken.

Howard Hodgson

The tender moved on to the Ile Cavallo and Brenna, who appeared to be minding his own business as he had some Italian friends on board, was able to get as near as twenty yards and shot a reel of film of the two of them sunbathing. Dodi was blissfully unaware of what was happening; Diana, on the other hand, was in her element and even managed to be looking into the camera while the straps of her bathing costume were provocatively dangling down around her elbows. She might not have known that he was actually taking the photographs at that very moment, but she knew that he would be at some point. This was Diana on parade – the consummate actress in love with her own image and self-needs, if not herself.

Later that day, after he had followed *Jonikal* to Punte de Sprono, Brenna climbed some rocks and, having fitted an ultra-powerful lens to his camera, waited for the couple to appear on deck. At around 5 p.m. they obliged and Brenna snapped more pictures, this time from around 500 yards. Diana, in a red floral swimsuit, had her arms around the hairy chest of the slightly tubby Dodi as the two locked in a tender embrace. Although the shots weren't of the finest quality because of the distance, the subject matter was sensational and worth a fortune.

Having done the job, Brenna developed the pictures and flew to London to share the fruits of his labour with Fraser. By Wednesday, 6 August, the media was in a frenzy as rumours circulated that photographs of Dodi and Diana kissing passionately were up for auction. Fraser's phone never stopped and picture editors with fat chequebooks were beating a path to his front door. A manic bidding war ensued. The eventual outcome was that the *Sunday Mirror* paid £250,000 for the right to be the first to run three quarters of the photographs, while the *Sun* and the *Daily Mail* paid £100,000 each for the second rights to run a full set.

On Sunday, 10 August, the *Sunday Mirror* launched its pictures that told a thousand words, and a new fairy-tale romance was born in the media. 'Locked in her lover's arms, the Princess finds happiness at last,' the paper enthused below the huge headline that simply proclaimed 'THE KISS'. The Princess, who was so often completely incapable of achieving the simplest form of happiness or self-control, had once again pulled off another amazing feat of deception, and once again fooled not only the nation but also the entire world in the process.

Later the same month, Fraser was again commissioned and in the last days of the Princess's life he achieved enough exclusive photographs to cover a further six front pages of the Princess and Dodi – this time sold exclusively to the British newspaper market. On the evening of 21 August, over a week after the kiss photographs had flashed around the world, Diana and Dodi arrived again in the South of France for their third time together on *Jonikal*. Once again the Harrods jet took them to Nice; once again *Jonikal* was waiting in the tiny port of St Laurent du Var.

The media was hungry for more photographs. The paparazzi would have been there in droves if they had known what was happening; but they didn't – only Fraser and two French photographers were allowed in on the secret, the latter to prevent the world from suspecting how Fraser repeatedly achieved such exclusivity. As usual he had been tipped off. There was genuine surprise on Dodi's face as their hush-hush holiday plans had been uncovered yet again. Over the next eight days Fraser got all the pictures he wanted as *Jonikal* cruised round the French Riviera before heading off to Portofino and Sardinia.

Whether it was Diana, using one of her disguised voices, or a source very close to her that tipped off Fraser for the original kiss sequence remains a matter of conjecture. What is not a mystery is that after three days on the latest trip, Diana dropped the pretence and started phoning Fraser openly from her mobile phone with instructions of what to shoot and when. She was clear that the nature of the photographs must still infer that they were taken without the subjects' knowledge and not appear to be posed. In Portofino, Fraser captured the couple on *Jonikal*'s deck as Dodi gently stroked Diana's shoulders and face. On the following morning, Monday, 25 August, Diana phoned the photographer in his hotel room, having surveyed his work in the newspapers, and complained that the quality wasn't good enough.

By now, Dodi also knew that Fraser was acting to Diana's orders; perhaps this was one reason why she had dropped the pretence and was now openly instructing him. How Dodi got to find out we will never know, but he was clearly happy to go along with the exposure of their relationship. It must have done his ego an enormous amount of good to see the global press proclaiming him as the lover of the world's most famous woman. He would also have been delighted with the vision of his father gleefully rubbing his hands together back at Harrods, mightily pleased with his eldest son.

For Diana's part she would have been revelling in all the attention.

Her addiction to this was just as great as it had been all those years ago when a courtier had discovered her crawling around the floor on her hands and knees reviewing pictures of her in that day's editions of the tabloid press. She also knew that Hasnat Khan couldn't help but be aware all of this media coverage. She probably took pleasure in his supposed pain and hoped that this would bring him to his senses.

This photographic procedure continued until Thursday, 28 August when Fraser suddenly received a call that told him that he had now taken enough photographs and his presence was no longer required. Naturally he obeyed, which is why he wasn't in Paris at the end of the week when the fatal accident occurred. Diana had controlled the whole Dodi affair from start to finish. She had manipulated the press and used photographs to send messages for years, but if she hadn't wanted any photographs taken throughout July and August, there wouldn't have been any. Given her ability and experience of how to avoid them, and the massive Al Fayed investment in security, there can be no doubting that.

Many commentators have taken another view and pointed out that perhaps the Princess had finally fallen in love with a man who really loved her and would give her all the undivided attention that dedicated men like the Prince of Wales and Hasnat Khan, or married ones like Oliver Hoare, couldn't. They believe that the media coverage was orchestrated by Diana as a celebration of this. To believe this is not to understand her at all. She only strove with blinkered determination for what she didn't have; if she eventually got it, it was never very long before she didn't want it any more. This was but a part of her character that was cruelly exaggerated by her medical condition, and is proved by her actions over and over again throughout her life.

I am supported in this view by the Princess's friend Lady Elsa Bowker. She claimed that before her death Diana had pursued Khan with such determination because he didn't appear to be under her spell and was therefore unobtainable – and the more distant he was, the more she wanted him. In the last weeks of her life, as he seemed to be slipping away from her forever, Lady Elsa became convinced that Diana's feelings had never been stronger and that she was doing everything to win the surgeon back.

On the other hand, the Princess was also supposed to have told Lady Bowker, as well as Rosa Monckton, Richard Kay and many others, that she adored Dodi and had never been happier. Moreover, the staff aboard *Jonikal* and Dodi's bodyguard, Trevor Rees-Jones, have all testified that the couple appeared to be very happy. Unfortunately, she also appears to have told most of them on different occasions that her affair with Dodi was nothing more than a holiday romance, and she often poked fun at the Al Fayed taste and their habit of always wanting to buy her expensive gifts behind his back. As a result some biographers like Lady Colin Campbell have bought the Dodi and Diana love; others like Kate Snell haven't. It is almost impossible to be certain given Diana's complex character. While no one can be really sure, it seems likely that the whole episode was not only motivated by Diana's constant need to live out her life in front of the media, but that this performance was directed towards Hasnat Khan. If she didn't win him back, she would at least get some satisfaction or even revenge by graphically showing him what a good time Dodi was giving her.

However, when this point was put to Diana's old friend and confidant Roberto Devorik by Kate Snell, he replied, 'If you are asking me if she went out with him [Dodi] to revenge herself on another relationship – no way. No way. It was not in Diana's mentality to be like that, and she never did that before.' I disagree. The Princess's life was littered, or perhaps cluttered, with acts of vindictive revenge. Ask Oliver Everett, Michael Colborne, Patrick Jephson, Barbara Barnes, James Gilbey, Tiggy Legge-Bourke, Raine Spencer, Victoria Mendham, Simone Simmons, Oonagh Toffolo, James Hewitt, Jane Atkinson, Elton John, Gianni Versace, Sarah Ferguson, Piers Morgan, Rosa Monckton, Julia Carling, Michael Gibbons, James Colthurst, Andrew Morton, Lady Susan Hussey, Oliver and Diane Hoare, Carolyn Bartholomew, Diana's own family, her husband and even the Queen. Loyalty and sorrow might have dimmed some of their memories and softened some of their comments, but they are but just a few who felt the effects of Diana's desire for revenge. Nevertheless, as a result Snell concludes, 'Although Diana was not the sort of person to take revenge, she knew from past experience that stories in the press could result in an emotional response from Hasnat: the report from Sydney in November 1996 when she had denied the relationship had upset Khan, and more pertinently the suggestion in the papers in June 1997 that there might be romance between her and Gulu Lalvani had caused Hasnat to cry foul.'

The probable truth is that the Princess hoped her action would win Khan back, but if it didn't, this was one hell of a face-saver. Either way she clearly approved of the pictures. On other occasions in her life when photographs had apparently invaded her privacy she had become emotional, upset and very angry. However, the kiss sequence, which was perhaps the greatest invasion of privacy that she had ever had to contend with, didn't raise a whimper of objection or even any sense of surprise – and as none showed her to have cellulite, there was no anger either.

In between her three holidays and one weekend in Paris with Dodi, which were crammed into a little over five weeks, the Princess flew to Bosnia on 8 August as part of her continuing campaign against landmines with the man who set her down the landmines road in the first place, Lord Deedes. While she was there, people noted that she appeared to be remarkably calm about the kiss photographs that had just exploded across the globe, although she did vaguely express some concern that the pictures had somewhat diverted attention from her Bosnian visit. She tried to make amends by having a photograph taken hugging a widow in a cemetery. The accompanying journalist reported that the Princess had seen the old woman from the road and simply had to stop in order to comfort her.

On 15 August, Diana flew to Greece for a cruise with her close friend Rosa Monckton. Ms Monckton is an intelligent and sensible woman and was one of the few remaining good influences in Diana's life. Married to newspaper editor Dominic Lawson, she is the granddaughter of Edward VIII's legal advisor, Walter Monckton, and sister of my colleague, the ex-Associated Newspapers man and Thatcherite eccentric Christopher Monckton. As a woman used to people in high places, she was never overawed by Diana, which is why her advice was so sound. She would tell the Princess what she thought she *should* hear rather than what she *wanted* to hear. At the request of Dodi, both women were flown to Greece in the Al Fayed jet. There, as a result of their private conversations, Rosa rather formed the opinion that while Diana seemed to be quite fond of Dodi, he was by no means the man she was destined to finish her days with. Unfortunately, in this regard, she was quite wrong.

On 21 August Diana returned to London only to fly straight out again on her final cruise with Dodi, knowing very well that Jason Fraser would be waiting at the quayside with his camera at the ready. On 23 August she called another of her close friends, Lana Marks, and told her that she was growing tired of cruising the Mediterranean and was looking forward to returning home. She added that Dodi would soon be a 'past chapter' in her life. On 25 August she called Elsa Bowker and told her that she had no plans to marry Dodi. The next day she called Hasnat but got his Uncle Jawad instead. She told him to tell Hasnat that she was looking forward to seeing him. Jawad told her that if she were trying to make Hasnat jealous with Dodi Al Fayed, it would not work. She replied that there was nothing in her relationship with Dodi. She repeated this comment to Roberto Devorik on 28 August, claiming that the relationship with Dodi was nothing more than 'a summer romance'. On 30 August she was even more explicit in a conversation with Lady Annabel Goldsmith when she claimed that she needed a new marriage like 'a bad rash on her face'.

In view of all the information available, it must be said that it seems highly unlikely that the Princess and Dodi Al Fayed would have become a permanent item. However, there can be little more hope for her relationship with Hasnat Khan. Even if she had lived and eventually won him back, it would never have lasted. His dedication to his work and her mental instability would have seen to that.

The inescapable truth, however unpalatable it might be, is that Diana was the common denominator in all of her failed relationships. If she couldn't make her fairy tale work with her true prince charming, her first love and only husband, she was unlikely to make it with anyone. She might have discovered the main reason for this by looking in the mirror, but her illness prevented her from any such honest acts of self-assessment. For Diana, happiness itself was a mirage – a place at the other end of the rainbow. The here and now was nearly always full of discontent, anxiety, imagined fear and very real anger – feelings of which she was rarely able to rid herself. There is absolutely no evidence that, had she lived, she would ever have been able to do so.

By now the press was tiring of the rash of 'exclusive' pictures. They started to criticise the relationship. It seemed that they didn't approve of a British princess, the mother of a future king, cavorting around the Mediterranean half-naked with the tubby son of a controversial and much despised – however unfairly or otherwise – Arab businessman. The Princess became alarmed. Her media campaign seemed to be backfiring. Her resurrection in the public's mind following Angola was in danger. She asked Richard Kay whether the media was anti-Dodi because he was rich. Kay replied that it was because he was Al Fayed's son. This response was reasonable and reflected a certain opinion in Fleet Street, which later gave rise to the infantile speculation in certain quarters that MI6 held the same opinion and acted upon it by having a hand in the couple's fatal car crash.

However, Kay didn't dare, for fear of losing his exclusive and special relationship with the Princess, add that there were by now many in the press who had knives out for her anyway. These journalists were fed up withbeing excluded or manipulated or both. They were fed up of her erratic behaviour that had them selling her as one thing before she made complete fools of them by becoming another. In short, they were fed up of being used. In addition, the seasoned among them suspected that the Princess had served her time as a heroine with the public and now, especially given the events of the last few days, which had offended British middle-class bigotry, there was more mileage in labelling her as spoiled, selfish, manipulative, vindictive and even mad. Many newspapers of Sunday, 31 August that had already gone to press before news of her death came through carried articles that bear witness to this view.

On the last full day of her life Diana seems to have started the day happily. She and Dodi had made plans to return to London via Paris so that they could collect a $205,000 ring that Diana had selected as a present from Dodi in the Monaco showroom of the renowned jeweller Alberto Repossi and which Dodi had arranged to pick up in Paris once it had been altered for Diana's finger. It was a cruel twist of fate: if Diana had stuck to her belief that Dodi shouldn't attempt to buy her love with gifts – as she had told both Elsa Bowker and Rosa Monckton – she would have never been in Paris at all that weekend. However, this was a seriously expensive gift, and even more costly than the $200,000 watch that Juan Carlos had reportedly bought her. Not even the Princess of Wales got offered presents like this all the time. It would have been very hard for any woman to resist – although it was somewhat dishonest if she intended to end the relationship on her return to London, as she had told so many of her friends. She clearly hadn't explained to Dodi that theirs was but 'a summer romance', or that she needed another marriage like 'a bad rash on my face'.

It is very hard not to think, if one assumes that she was being honest with her friends, that she was being extremely dishonest with Dodi. If this is not correct, the converse is true. Either way, Diana was misleading someone. Maybe she didn't know who. Perhaps she believed that if she couldn't get Hasnat Khan back, exquisite little gifts from Dodi like this were some compensation. Perhaps she even sensationally believed she could keep both affairs going. After all, fidelity had never mattered to her as long as it was her committing the infidelity, and she had run parallel affairs for most of her adult life. Extensive research by others and me has only served to fuel the speculation and proved that, as with many things that went on in the head of this beautiful but highly complex woman, we will never be certain.

The couple arrived mid-afternoon in the Harrods Gulfstream IV at Le Bourget Airport. It was supposed to be a secret location, and yet they were greeted by around thirty members of the paparazzi hungry to see their share of the cash that Jason Fraser and Mario Brenna had been enjoying. A surprised Dodi looked furious. The Princess just looked serene. Amid scenes reminiscent of Beatlemania, the couple were driven away in a black Mercedes. Behind them in a bottle-green Range Rover Henri Paul, Al Fayed's deputy director of security at the Ritz Hotel, carried the couple's luggage, which was destined for Dodi's flat near the Arc de Triomphe. Behind him came a posse of chasing paparazzi. Paul demonstrated his considerable driving skills by blocking them off and allowing the couple's car to escape to the former residence of the Duke and Duchess of Windsor.

Once at the Bois de Boulogne residence, Dodi, who was by now clearly in love with Diana and motivated by a lot more than just pleasing his father, showed her once more around the house. He had recently bought Julie Andrews' former Malibu home in California and had told friends that he hoped Diana and he could set up home there and also at the Bois de Boulogne house in Paris. Both ideas could have appealed to Diana – she loved California and she adored Paris. Moreover, in her mind the grass was always greener on the other side of the fence, and the idea of living in the same house as Edward VIII had would have no doubt appealed to her sense of the dramatic. Yet, as with her dreams of settling down in the country with Hewitt, she perhaps loved talking about them without ever having the intention to do any of it. We will never know.

For whatever reason, she showed an unusual interest in the property as she went round Prince Charles's great-uncle's former home – even inspecting the boiler and the refrigerator and asking questions about how many rooms were available for domestic and security staff. From there they were taken to the Imperial Suite at the Ritz. An excited Dodi made calls about the new Malibu house while the Princess telephoned Richard Kay in order to update him. He has since confirmed that she told him on that evening that she and Dodi were discussing a life together and that she would retire from public life in November but would still keep up some of her charity work. He later told Lady Colin Campbell, 'All was well in her world. She was as happy as I have ever heard her.'

There is no reason for Kay to lie. Nevertheless, what Diana had told him was in complete contrast to what she told Lady Annabel Goldsmith on the same day. Nor did she tell him that she intended to marry Dodi and that they intended to set up together a string of international hospices – which was what Dodi was telling his closest friends and family, one of who was his stepfather's brother, the diplomat Hassan Yassin, who happened to be staying at the Ritz at that time. Mr Yassin's credibility was later questioned when he repeated what Dodi had told him. The media immediately suspected that he was putting an Al Fayed spin on the story and taking advantage of the fact that the Princess was no longer able to contradict him. As happens so often with the British tabloid press, they had failed to do their homework before rushing into print. Not only was Hassan Yassin a respected and distinguished diplomat, but also he and Mohamed Al Fayed were in no way close to each other. The idea that he would assist either Mohamed's social aspirations or subsequent war with the House of Windsor following his son's death is frankly preposterous.

Yassin knew what Dodi had told him and had no reason to lie – just like Richard Kay, Lady Annabel Goldsmith, Lady Elsa Bowker, Lana Marks, Rosa Monckton, Jawad Khan or others. Again, the most likely explanation is that were all telling the truth as they knew it. Once again it was a deception, just as it had been with the Morton book and so many times since. Everybody, as they did at the time of Morton, seems to have concentrated on what they were told and assumed that that was the truth. Again the subject matter, the common denominator and the fountain of most of this information, directly or otherwise, was the Princess herself. It would appear that Dodi was making plans while Diana was only dreaming dreams, and in Dianaland the lines between fantasy and reality could become very blurred and hard for the rest of us to understand.

Having spoken to his step-uncle and arranged to meet up for a drink after dinner so that he might introduce him to the Princess, Dodi was then driven the short distance to the jeweller's to collect Diana's new ring. According to Alice Valentin, niece of the owner, 'The ring was from our collection of engagement rings called Tell Me Yes. It was in the window of their main showroom on Place Beaumarchais in Monte Carlo and they both came in to have a look. It was from the top of the range. The Princess said, "That's the one I want." Unfortunately it didn't fit and we had to send it away for alteration. At around 6.30 on Saturday, 30 August Mr Dodi Fayed's private secretary and bodyguard came in and checked over the shop to make sure everything was secure and make sure there were no photographers. Then Mr Fayed came over himself. He was only there a few minutes, but it was clear he was extremely happy. He was obviously very much in love and the ring meant an awful lot.'

Dodi then returned to the Ritz, collected Diana and took her to his apartment on the second floor of 1 rue Arsène Houssaye by the Arc de Triomphe. A table had been booked at the fashionable Chez Benoît close to the Pompidou Centre. However, by now the paparazzi had encircled the entrance to the apartment block. Dodi, who couldn't understand where they were getting their information from, cancelled the reservation at the restaurant and the couple retired to the relative security of the Ritz for dinner instead – arriving there not long before 10 p.m. to be greeted by around sixty photographers. The Princess's orchestrated media circus was getting out of hand and the conductor had by now lost control.

The couple decided to eat in the hotel's restaurant – the Espadan. However, as they entered a hush descended across the room as other open-mouthed diners just stared at them. Apparently Diana did not seem to mind, but Dodi found the experience unnerving and as a result they retired to have dinner in the privacy of the Imperial Suite instead. By now events appeared to be controlling Diana rather than the other way round. As they waited to be served, Dodi asked the management to call in Henri Paul – Al Fayed had devised a plan to get them back to his apartment after dinner. Dodi trusted Paul, who had done such a good job earlier in the day, and wanted him to drive them and Dodi's bodyguard, Trevor Rees-Jones, from the back of the hotel while his usual driver, Philippe Dourneau, would lead a decoy from the front of the hotel in his black Mercedes, with the bottle-green Range Rover following.

Paul had left the hotel for the night and had to be called back. As Dodi and Diana dined in the suite, he joined Trevor Rees-Jones and the other Al Fayed bodyguard for a drink in the hotel bar. In view of what was to happen later, it is significant that both bodyguards thought Henri Paul was completely sober when he joined them. This would appear to be confirmed by the security video footage taken of him moments before leaving the hotel, as he drops on his haunches to tie his shoelace with perfect balance before shooting up again and giving the impression that whatever drink or drugs he might have already consumed while off duty, they hadn't impaired his faculties, at least to the naked eye. At 12.20 a.m. the couple exited the hotel through the back door. Diana jumped into a back seat behind Trevor Rees-Jones while Dodi sat behind Henri Paul. Nobody put a seat belt on as the car roared away. At some point in the ensuing chase Rees-Jones, perhaps because he was neither intoxicated by drink, drugs or media obsession to the same degree as the others, had sensed the danger and belted up.

As the car pulled in to the rue Cambon it immediately became obvious that Dodi's plan had completely failed as a gaggle of paparazzi on motorbikes gave chase. As Henri Paul headed down the rue de Rivoli he decided to hit the accelerator and lose them. At Place de la Concorde he jumped a red light in a dangerous but successful attempt to put some distance between the Mercedes and the bikes. The Princess, as high as a kite on the excitement, hysterically roared her approval as the Mercedes hurtled at high speed towards the Pont d'Alma tunnel and took off over a slight ramp as the road gently curves to the right at the entrance. Paul had paid no attention whatsoever to the speed limit. Within seconds the car had struck a pillar within the tunnel. It was 12.24 a.m. in Paris, 11.24 in London, on the cusp of Sunday, 31 August 1997 – perhaps the most famous moment since the assassination of John F Kennedy.

In one tragic miscalculation, the media junkie had overdosed and cruelly, harshly and unnecessarily paid for it with her own life and that of her boyfriend and their driver. Is that a fair comment? After all, she wasn't driving the car and she wasn't riding the bikes. But the circus was only in town because of her media addiction. Moreover, she was only in Paris in the first place to collect a ring to celebrate a friendship that she had described in the last twenty-four hours as 'history' and 'a summer romance'. And it is highly probable that the paparazzi only knew she was there because she had wanted them to.

Of course she didn't cause the accident, but had it not been for her desire to manipulate, there would have been no car chase and therefore no accident. In addition, it has to be assumed that the car was travelling at high speed in an effort to shake off the paparazzi because the Princess wanted it to. Of course Henri Paul was driving, but he would have been acting on Dodi's orders. Given that Dodi was by nature a man keen to please, and was madly in love with Diana, it is quite unthinkable that he would have ordered Henri Paul to drive recklessly against the Princess's wishes. Moreover, there is irrefutable pictorial evidence to support this point. A traffic camera clearly captured the four occupants of the car just after it entered the tunnel and only a second or two before it crashed. It shows Henri Paul and Trevor Rees-Jones staring straight ahead and intently concentrating. Neither man is smiling. By contrast, Diana and Dodi are laughing hysterically in the back seat. The car was clearly being driven to their instruction, and to that extent they must posthumously accept their share of the responsibility for what happened.

That is the plain truth. And it is that truth that so many people find so completely unacceptable that they turn to outrageous and far-fetched conspiracy theories instead.

Only an arrogant and foolish biographer would now attempt to pre-empt the outcome of the various enquiries that still continue some nine years after the crash. Moreover, it is extremely unlikely that all the facts will ever be known. This is in itself a problem because it has opened up an opportunity for irresponsible theories of conspiracy to multiply. However, the facts and the theories don't sit comfortably with each other.

Several independent witnesses stated that there was a motorcycle approaching the tunnel as the Mercedes entered it. This is correct. It was being ridden by a twenty-eight-year-old chef named Eric Petel. As he entered the tunnel he noticed in his rear-view mirror a car approaching at high speed and flashing its headlights in warning as it roared passed him. Then he heard a deafening crash. As he entered the tunnel he realised that the car had smashed into a pillar, had spun round and was now facing the wrong way. The front was completely smashed in and there was smoke coming from the engine.

Petel rode up to the car and got off his bike. It was dark in the tunnel and he couldn't see much. As he peered into the car he noticed a woman with her head in between the two front seats and her back to him. He thought to pull her from the car in case it caught fire. He wiped her hair from her face as he rested her head on the rear armrest. It was only then that he realised that this injured woman was the Princess of Wales. Pushing the door closed again, he raced off on his bike to raise the alarm and within a minute had stopped at a pay phone and dialled the emergency services, but they refused to believe him. So he rode to the Avenue Mozart police station where he was laughed at until the news of the accident started to be reported over the police airwaves, whereupon he was handcuffed for half an hour before being questioned for two hours, during which time he was put under pressure to admit that he hadn't made a call in the first place.

Petel does not remember any other car being in the tunnel at the time of the accident. However, other witnesses did. This might be explained by the fact that it could have gone through and out the other side by the time Petel pulled up. Gary Hunter, a London solicitor on a weekend break with his wife, told Scotland Yard that he had seen a small car, possibly a Fiat Uno, coming out of the tunnel only moments after the accident. A Parisian couple, who wished to remain nameless, were on the slip road into which the tunnel exits when they claim that they also saw a Fiat Uno. It was white, battered and backfiring as it came out of the tunnel. They didn't think that the driver, who had a large dog on the back seat, noticed them, as he appeared to be too busy looking into his rear-view mirror to see what was happening back inside the tunnel. They thought that he was in his early forties, had short brown hair and was wearing a bomber jacket. They believed that the car was about ten years old and had a Paris plate – perhaps 92, which would mean that the car came from the relatively poor and densely populated Hauts-de-Seine region. According to them this happened at 12:25 a.m. – surprisingly a full minute after we know the accident occurred and when Petel would have been attending to the Princess. Alternatively, their watch may have been slightly fast.

Martine Monteil, the chief superintendent of the Paris Criminal Brigade, headed up the subsequent investigation into the accident. She painstakingly collected several other witness statements from people who came forward to say that they had also seen a small car come out of the tunnel after the crash. In addition, there was one from a man who had been apparently walking above the entrance when he noticed a small car enter the tunnel in the slow right-hand lane, while a black Mercedes was bearing down at speed in the fast left-hand lane just moments before the crash.

Despite their best efforts, Monteil's team failed to find this car until they appeared to have stroke of good fortune. A man went into a police station in the suburb of Clichy, which is about five kilometres from the scene of the accident, to pay a traffic fine. He was driving his brother's Fiat Uno, which had recently been sprayed red despite being twelve years old. In November 1997, the police in Clichy tipped off Monteil and she sent six officers at 6 a.m. the next morning to arrest the owner – a second-generation Vietnamese immigrant by the name of Le Van Thanh. Immediately he admitted having bought the wreck in the summer and that his brother, who worked in a Citroen garage, had offered to respray it for him. It had originally been a white car when he had bought it. According to Thanh, the fact that his brother had resprayed the car on the same Sunday that Diana had been killed was purely coincidental.

This seemed to be correct when tests on the car's original white paint proved to be different to samples found at the scene of the accident. Nevertheless, it seemed premature to many when Madame Monteil ruled out Thanh and other suspects and closed her investigation shortly after. However, other sources, including Mohamed Al Fayed's own team of investigators, kept an open mind on Thanh and other Fiat Uno owners who had cropped up during their own investigations.

James Andanson not only owned a white Fiat Uno of similar age but was also a member of the paparazzi and rumoured to be linked to the French secret services. A conspiracy theory quickly evolved that suggested that upon the orders of the secret services, Andanson had swerved in front of the Mercedes and caused it to crash before escaping unhurt. The fact that two years later he was found dead, locked inside his burned-out car only served to dignify the theory as believers claimed that he had been eliminated in order to prevent him from ever selling his story. All very compelling Ian Fleming stuff at first sight – until closer examination, that is, when the theory doesn't stand up to too much scrutiny. There is absolutely no evidence to suggest that Andanson's Fiat was the one in the tunnel. It would have been a simple comparison to make between his car's paint and that found in the tunnel after the crash. The fact that Al Fayed's own investigation team made no such comparison or even requested that the official team did, despite Al Fayed's insistence that Dodi and Diana had been murdered, suggests that they were able to eliminate the vehicle anyway. There is absolutely no evidence whatsoever that Andanson had ever been a member of the French secret services. Even if he had been, why would he wish to commit murder by using his own car? Who does that? Cars used in criminal acts are always stolen, as everybody knows. Why would the French secret services want to murder the member of the British Royal Family most popular with the French public? Even if they did, and Andanson was a member, it would be highly unlikely that such a part-time amateur would be given the assignment. And just as with the Mannakee accident over a decade earlier, why would any professional assassination squad want to employ such a messy, public and extremely unreliable form of execution? Remember Trevor Rees-Jones was in the front seat and survived because he was wearing a seat belt. Dodi might have survived if he had been, and Diana would almost certainly have done. Who would ensure that they didn't wear the seat belts? Trevor Rees-Jones? Henri Paul? The idea that they could have is ridiculous. The idea that they would want to is idiotic. The idea that they would do this and then crash the car while being in the front is completely preposterous.

Nevertheless, supporters of this theory are keen to point out Andanson's horrible death as corroborating evidence, claiming that he was eliminated along with his car by French secret services to prevent him from selling his part in the assignation to the world's press. They ignore the fact that this was two years later, which gave the photographer more than ample time to make the financial killing that they would have us believe caused his eventual murder. They also forget that any admission to having played a part in the same would have undoubtedly led to Andanson having to endure a lengthy prison sentence.

Had Andanson ever made the vaguest of claims that he was involved, or had there been any evidence to point the finger of suspicion in his direction, these people might have had a point worthy of further investigation?. But he didn't and there is none, which is why the Al Fayed investigation team, keen as they were to find a culprit, nevertheless ruled him out.

An even more ridiculous conspiracy theory is that Henri Paul was himself an MI6 operative who had been ordered to assassinate the

Princess. Supporters of this theory point to the fact that he had over £100,000 in thirteen different bank accounts. This theory ignores that there is absolutely no evidence linking Paul with MI6 or any other secret-service operation. Secondly, if he was with MI6, why would Tony Blair order Diana's assassination? These believers argue that he didn't but that it was either Prince Charles or Prince Philip. They forget that the government and not the monarchy control MI6. Mr Blair may have been panic-stricken at the thought of the Princess wandering over to Northern Ireland 'to sort out people's heads', but that would hardly be a reason to have her murdered. He may be many things, but the Princess's assassin? I think not. Moreover, even if the Royal Family had direct access to MI6, which it doesn't, it is both preposterous and insulting to think they would use such power to order the elimination of anyone. In addition, the Princess's death was bound to make her a martyr, and that would certainly cause the monarchy trouble. Prince Charles above all others understood this and said as much not long after her death. And as with Mannakee's death and the Andanson theory, why would any secret-service operation want to engage such an unreliable method of disposal? Lastly, why on earth would Henri Paul select a method of assassination that put his own life in danger and actually killed him?

As for the £100,000 that Henri Paul had stashed away – might this not have been saved from undeclared gratuities? After all, Arab princes, restricted in their own countries by religious piety, stayed at the Ritz in Paris to have a really good time. Henri Paul would have been ideally placed to lay on a week's worth of varied pleasures and might expect more than a £1,000 tip in return. Thirteen bank accounts would be needed to fool the French Inland Revenue, especially as the French have one of the world's highest rates of informing on each other.

Then there are those who claim that Henri Paul's blood samples were switched. Again, there is no evidence that they were. Nevertheless, the investigating judge Hervé Stephan went back to the morgue and had additional samples of blood, hair and skin tissue taken in the presence of the police, and photographed the whole procedure as a result of Mohamed Al Fayed having disputed the findings of the original samples. The high levels of alcohol and carbon monoxide in Henri Paul's blood are naturally a cause for concern, as they would have impaired his faculties sufficiently to prevent him from standing up, never mind driving a car at high speed. This point remains unexplained but that in itself does not prove foul play.

Another theory suggests that someone was stationed just inside the tunnel and shone a blinding light in Henri Paul's eyes, which caused him to lose control of the vehicle. But this wouldn't even guarantee an accident let alone the deaths of those inside the car. Moreover, who would have known where and when the Mercedes was going? The answer to that question is Dodi, Diana, Henri Paul, Trevor Rees-Jones and a very small number of Al Fayed staff back at the Ritz, who would have had less than four minutes to get from the hotel, park up and be in position.

Is it not much more likely that the Fiat Uno just happened to be in the wrong place at the wrong time? Maybe it entered the tunnel in the slow right-hand lane just before the Mercedes took off at four times the speed limit as it hit the ski-jump curve in the left fast lane. Perhaps the Fiat Uno wasn't far enough over to the right? Perhaps Paul had already lost control of his vehicle? For whatever reason, the vehicles brushed against each other and the Mercedes' front bumper grazed the backlight of the Fiat as it flew past. Skid marks made by the Mercedes clearly indicate that Paul, a man described by Al Fayed as a better driver even when drunk than many others sober, was struggling to control the vehicle and it slammed into pillars in the centre of the tunnel.

The driver of the other car panics. Perhaps he is over the alcohol limit. Perhaps he isn't insured. Perhaps he thinks the accident was his fault. Perhaps he's worried about losing his no-claims bonus. He might have a criminal record, have no driving licence, be an illegal immigrant or be frightened of the police – who knows? People leave the scene of an accident every day of the week for numerous and often not decent reasons, but implausible assassination is rarely one. Nevertheless, he melts away into the night. The following day he realises that the Princess of Wales was killed in the Mercedes that he had had a collision with. Is he going to come forward and risk becoming the fall guy? It would take an uncommonly decent man, or one with the deepest religious conviction, to do that. Given the facts we know, this is the most likely explanation of what happened; it is certainly the only theory that stands up to all the evidence.

So in the end, was it a masterful assassination or just a tragic and terrible accident? Remember, it was a surprise visit to Paris and assassinations, especially those requiring split-second timing, surely take some planning. Moreover, nobody could have known what route the car was going to take. This would have made it impossible to guarantee staging a crash with another car requiring precision timing. In addition, if Dodi and Diana had been wearing seat belts they might have lived. Which secret service or assassin would organise a hit with so many variables, opportunities for things to go wrong and possibilities for the intended victim to survive?

If anyone had intended to murder the Princess, there had been ample opportunity as she wandered around London unprotected for the previous two years. If anyone had wanted to murder her as a result of her association with the likeable Dodi Al Fayed – an outrageous suggestion that hints at a racist dislike of his Arabic origin – a hastily devised hit on a surprise visit to Paris was hardly the answer when the previous seven days had provided numerous perfect opportunities to kill the Princess while she was swimming. A couple of trained frogmen could have grabbed her foot and held her underwater long enough to drown her before releasing her body – nice and clean and certain, and easily put down to a swimming accident, probably due to cramp.

Eventually, the police investigation came to the conclusion that the evidence overwhelmingly pointed towards an accident and that all the conspiracy theories were fanciful. It remains to be seen, but it is highly likely, that the British coroner's investigation underway at the time of writing will reach the same conclusion. In the absence of any new evidence, the facts must lead people with an open mind to the conclusion that what happened at 12.24 a.m. on 31 August 1997 was an awful and tragic accident. A perfectly decent young man was fighting for his life. Three people were dead: a trusted, popular and loyal Al Fayed staff member, the charming, kind and extremely likeable heir to the Al Fayed fortune and perhaps the best-loved, most beautiful princess history had ever known. Whatever her flaws, the world was a poorer place as a result.

Chapter Eighteen
The Funeral (1997)

The first call alerting the Royal Family to Diana's accident came when Sir Robin Janvrin, the Queen's deputy private secretary, was called at 1 a.m. BST, 2 a.m. CET. He had been asleep in a house assigned to him on the Balmoral estate. The call was from the British Ambassador in Paris, Sir Michael Jay. News was vague. Apparently there had been a car accident. Dodi Al Fayed was reported as dead. Diana, who had been travelling with him, was injured but no one knew how badly. Their car had smashed into the support pillars of a tunnel that runs by the side of the River Seine. It had been trying to escape a group of paparazzi. It was a notorious black spot and there had been many previous fatalities there.

Janvrin immediately had the Queen, the Prince of Wales, the Queen's equerry and several protection officers woken. An emergency operations room was set up in one of the castle's many offices. Meanwhile in London, the Prince's press secretary Sandy Henney and his deputy private secretary Mark Bolland were being alerted to the situation by the media, who were perhaps better informed than Sir Michael Jay as they had established direct contact with the French emergency services. Mark Bolland immediately rang Stephen Lamport, the Prince's principal private secretary, at his London home. Now everyone was awake and either attempting to discover further news or making plans as to how to react to it.

Then Prince Charles called Bolland. The Prince was shocked, upset and yet obviously trying his hardest to rise to the occasion and be the leader that he felt he ought to be. He wanted information. Bolland didn't have it. Nevertheless, that didn't prevent the Prince asking the same questions over and over again. How badly hurt was Diana? What had caused the accident? Where had it happened? Who was driving? The conversation went round in a circle for almost an hour. It seemed to Bolland that the Prince was desperately searching for comfort that things would turn out all right – that the Princess, the mother of his sons and a woman to whom he remained attached despite everything, would survive. Naturally, Bolland did what he could, but it was impossible to give the Prince the good news that he craved. Indeed, it was hard to give him any news – there simply wasn't any reliable information. One minute her injuries were serious but not fatal, the next she had walked away relatively unhurt.

Meanwhile, in Paris the Princess was losing her desperate struggle for life. She had been tended to before the emergency services arrived by a Dr Mailliez who had happened upon the accident not long after Eric Petel. The doctor later recalled that the Princess was semiconscious and muttering, but her words understandably made no sense before she fell into a state of deep unconsciousness from which she never recovered. The claim by Mohamed Al Fayed that she had left a dying message to someone and that this had been passed on is almost certainly fanciful. The doctor tried to reassure the Princess in a soothing manner that the ambulance was on the way as he cleared her airways to help her breathing and put a resuscitation mask over her mouth. He was later to state that he had not been impeded in this superficial treatment by the massed ranks of the paparazzi, who had by now caught up with their target and were photographing the dying Princess, as claimed by some British newspapers. Then the ambulance arrived and Dr Mailliez left the scene of the accident unaware of whom he had been treating.

Subsequently, the French emergency services were lambasted, and while their initial response to Eric Petel's first call was hardly impressive, thereafter they were exemplary and any criticism is most unfair. The truth is that the Princess never had a chance. Her internal injuries were catastrophic. The blood vessels in her heart were so badly ruptured that survival was impossible. A tear of the pulmonary artery was not the only internal injury, which is the assumption of those who have since claimed that her life might have been saved if she had been taken to hospital quickly enough. Had the emergency serves moved her suddenly, she would have almost certainly died there and then. Moreover, most medical opinion now accepts that she would have died within twenty minutes of the accident if it hadn't been for the tremendous efforts of the emergency services, who kept her alive in the vain hope that if they could do so until she reached hospital, perhaps a miracle could be performed. In fact they managed to extend her life by over an hour and a half, and it wasn't their fault that divine providence didn't intervene during that time. Dr Mailliez was amazed when he learned that she had survived that long. His assessment was, 'Nothing could have saved her. She didn't stand a chance.'

Despite the expert and tireless efforts of the emergency services, the Princess suffered a cardiac arrest around the time she arrived at the

Pitié-Salpêtrière Hospital. The medical team fought furiously to save her life, but their task was impossible. The Princess had suffered a heart attack as she was being cut out of the car. Her superior left pulmonary artery was ripped and her pericardium ruptured. In other words, a main artery that draws blood from the lungs and back into the heart had been torn off and was pumping blood into her internal cavity instead of her heart, while her heart's protective membrane had also been ripped, which allowed more blood to pour into the right side of her chest cavity. Such injuries meant that Diana was mortally wounded at the moment of impact. In addition, she had also suffered many other superficial injuries such as a fractured right arm, two large gashes on her right thigh, wounds to her forehead and left ankle and some severe bruising to her body and hands.

Now it was the turn of the hospital staff. They also made a superhuman effort to save her. For two hours they attempted to revive this beautiful woman with adrenalin injections and hand massage of her heart. Finally, they were forced to accept failure and that Diana, Princess of Wales was dead.

Unaware of his ex-wife's fate the Prince, between agonised telephone calls, prayed for her deliverance. He determined to assist with her recovery and even confided that he had always known that she would return to him and that he would look after her. He seemed vague and almost distant – as though in shock and clinging to hope.

Then the news eventually came through that she was dead. 'They are all going to blame me, aren't they?' he announced with a characteristic note of self-pity. 'The world's going to go completely mad, isn't it? We're going to see a reaction that could destroy the monarchy?' Self-pity maybe, but most perceptive. Naturally the Prince of Wales immediately considered his children. The Queen had advised from the moment that they had become aware of the accident that the princes should not be woken. Charles went along with this, but had radios removed from their rooms and the television taken from the nursery so that they could only be told the atrocious news by their father when they awoke. Unfortunately, this was to be one of the only points that the Prince and the Queen were able to agree on. For the first time ever, war broke out between them. The Prince revolted against the Queen's will in the raw emotion that he felt to the Princess's death, his different reactions to those of his mother to it and what was needed in order to present the Royal Family in the best possible light given the

The King and Di

spotlight that this tragedy would throw them under.

Mother and son avoided addressing each other face to face. No doubt it would have been more natural and certainly more efficient if they had, but that was not the Windsor way. The Queen sat in her suite of rooms on the first floor of the castle. Her son sat next door in his. They talked to each other through their staff, some of whom – like Mark Bolland for the Prince or Sir Robert Fellowes, who was on holiday in Norfolk, for the Queen – weren't even in the castle. It soon became obvious that St James's Palace and Buckingham Palace were in complete and utter disagreement with each other over what action should be taken and what respect accorded to the Princess of Wales. Charles held the softer attitude, perhaps because of his continued sensitivity to his sons' mother and the monarchy's situation as much as the shrewd judgement of Mark Bolland, who was a skilled media manipulator.

Even before it was announced that the Princess had died, a disagreement had erupted. The Prince had decided that he must rush to her side and see her in hospital. Bolland telephoned Robin Janvrin and told him as much, and pointed out that the Prince did not intend to debate the point. He was going whatever the Queen thought. Janvrin was completely taken aback by the Prince of Wales's wilfulness, and questioned his wisdom before declaring that an airplane from the Queen's flight couldn't just be commandeered. The Prince would need the Queen's consent and he would be unlikely to get it. Relations were frosty but Bolland, confident of the Prince's backing, declared that if that was the case, the Prince would take a scheduled flight from Aberdeen.

It is at this point that courtiers and close friends of the Prince of Wales are unanimous in pointing out that he still held the Princess in deep affection, prayed for her every night and accepted as being every bit as much a part of his family as the children, in spite of the cruel blows that she had dealt him with her fabrication of their life together. Their assertions are held up by his actions over the next few hours and days, which proved this beyond doubt and are subject to numerous independent accounts.

Charles had considered taking William and Harry to Paris with him, but had put off making a final decision until he knew the extent of her injuries in case they were upset by them. At about 3.30 a.m. Mark Bolland again rang Robin Janvrin to find out if anything had been resolved regarding the Queen's plane. At 3.45 a.m. they were interrupted and Bolland had to hold on as Janvrin took another call. He talked to Nick Archer, who was with Janvrin as he waited. Archer broke the news that he had just taken a call from the British Ambassador in Paris and was now on the phone to the Prince regrettably to inform him that the Princess of Wales had died a short time ago. The announcement that went out at 4.30 a.m. said that she had died at 4 a.m. This was not correct – she had actually died earlier. Mark Bolland, who has become somewhat bitter following his removal from St James's Palace some time later, was nevertheless doing an excellent job for the monarchy in general and the Prince in particular at this time. He immediately phoned Camilla Parker Bowles and informed her of the sad news. He warned her to be guarded against press intrusion, advised her to speak to Alan Kilkenny, her own PR advisor, and told her to expect a call from a very distressed Prince of Wales at any time.

The Prince had already spoken to Camilla several times, but had been hopeful that Diana was not too seriously injured, so Bolland's announcement of her death was a tremendous shock – as a mother she was devastated for William and Harry, and as a lover she was terrified what the public's reaction would be to the Prince.

The announcement of the Princess's death had only hardened Charles's resolve to go to Paris. But the Queen remained against the idea and was strongly supported by Sir Robert Fellowes who agreed that it would be wrong to make too much fuss. However, not all of her staff agreed with her and some became increasingly convinced by the Prince's argument. In the end, Robert Janvrin won the day by changing his mind and asking the Queen, 'What would you rather, ma'am – that she came back in a Harrods van?' That did the trick: the mere thought was enough to secure the Queen's assent to send Operation Overlord live.

This plan had been in existence for years, but happily had never been needed. It was designed to bring the body of a deceased royal back to London. It had always been believed that the Queen Mother would be the first unfortunate passenger, which given her remarkable age was not unreasonable. Naturally no one had ever thought it would be Diana, still young, beautiful, fit and full of vitality. There was a BAe 146 on standby for this purpose. The plane left Northolt at 10 a.m. on a convoluted route to Paris. On board were Stephen Lamport, Mark

Bolland and Sandy Henney. First stop was RAF Wittering in Rutland, where Diana's two sisters were collected. Sir Robert Fellowes had been given the task of breaking the bad news to the Spencers, but then the Prince had phoned Sarah and suggested that she and her sister Jane might like to accompany him on the flight.

From there it was on to Aberdeen to collect the Prince of Wales. Charles had wisely decided that the trip was no place for his sons. He had accompanied them with the Queen and the rest of the family to church before leaving them in the care of Tiggy Legge-Bourke, who had fortunately just arrived in Scotland to collect the boys and return them to their mother. She and their cousin Peter Phillips were utterly amazing with William and Harry that day and for the rest of the coming week. Their actions made an awful time just slightly more bearable.

On the flight, Diana's sisters understandably spent most of the time in tears. The Prince was sober and controlled, but underneath clearly very emotional. Stephen Lamport explained to everyone what would happen when they arrived and how they might have to meet Mr Al Fayed if he was at the hospital. The Prince acknowledged that he would have to, as he couldn't run the risk of the press turning a refusal into a typical tabloid scandal. Moreover, he understood that whatever else Al Fayed stood for that the Prince didn't like, the man had just lost his eldest son and must also be grief-stricken. However, both sisters were adamant that they wouldn't even meet him, never mind speak to him. In the event, he wasn't there. By the time the Prince arrived, Mohamed Al Fayed had already collected his son's body and returned to England so that a Muslim burial could be effected before sundown, as is the custom of Islam. Instead the Prince was greeted at the hospital by President Chirac who had come in person to express France's great sorrow. Then Charles, accompanied by Diana's two sisters, was taken to a small room by a doctor. A priest also accompanied them at the request of the Prince and led them in prayer.

The royal party were not prepared for what they saw. Diana had already been embalmed by French embalmers. The London funeral directors, Levertons, approved of their French counterparts' work when they arrived. She had been dressed in a dress and shoes donated by Sylvia Jay, the wife of the British ambassador, as her own luggage had already been collected from the Ritz Hotel by Al Fayed and flown back to London in his private jet. She had been placed in a coffin that Levertons had prepared and which had been flown out from RAF Brize

Norton in Oxfordshire. Neither Levertons nor the French embalmers had done a bad job, nor had her butler Paul Burrell arranged her hair in an inappropriate way; it was just that her body lay so still, appeared so cold and marble-like – nothing like the Diana they all knew. Moreover, her head had been badly damaged in the crash and they didn't like the distorted look on her face. This can be a common reaction to first seeing a deceased loved one, especially one lost suddenly rather than following a long and taxing illness, when the reaction is often different as the presentation appears to be an improvement rather than a shock.

They stayed with the Princess for seven minutes. As they reappeared, Sarah and Jane were sobbing from the depths of inner despair that only the loss of a much-loved family member can conjure up. They were immediately ushered into another room for a moment of privacy. Prince Charles was not crying, but he obviously had been. He was visibly distressed; his eyes were red and his face contorted as he attempted to hold back his emotion. He closed his eyes, bit his lip and regained some composure before shaking hands with the doctors and nurses who had fought so hard to save Diana's life. One who was present was later to remark; 'He went from human being to Windsor.' He had been trained all his life to do nothing else. The parents of the accident's only survivor, Trevor Rees-Jones, were also in the hospital. On learning this, the Prince asked if he might meet them.

Then the coffin was closed and draped with the Royal Standard. The Princess was about to start her long and sombre journey home. Pall-bearers carried her down the corridor. People parted and bowed their heads in silence as the coffin passed them en route to the hearse waiting outside. There were thousands in the street. Everyone was silent. As the motorcade made its way through the city towards the airport, heads bowed as it passed. People in pavement cafés stood up. Still everyone was silent. Prince Charles was deeply moved and grateful for this mark of respect. Once on the plane, he seemed to comfort himself by saying several times, 'Wasn't it wonderful that everyone stood up?'

However, it wasn't too long before his mood changed when he discovered what had been planned upon their arrival at Northolt. He asked who would meet them there – Tony Blair and the Lord Chamberlain, Lord Airlie. That was fine. How many RAF pall-bearers would carry the coffin? There would be eight. That was fine. Would the flowers he had ordered be there? Yes. Where was Diana's body to be taken from the airport? The Fulham mortuary, commonly used by the Royal Coroner. That was not the answer he wished to hear. 'Who decided that?' the Prince exploded. 'Nobody asked me. Diana is going to the Royal Chapel at St James's Palace. Sort it. I don't care who has made the decision, she is going to the Royal Chapel.' This is how the Prince's biographer Penny Junor reports the Prince's words to Sandy Henney, who spent the remainder of the flight ensuring that the Prince's instructions were carried out.

Andrew Morton, in his book *Diana: In Pursuit of Love*, launches into an attack on Junor and disputes the accuracy of her statement, claiming, 'In the coming weeks and months, however, the impression was given by Prince Charles' staff and his literary apologists, notably Penny Junor, that it was only his decisive intervention in the critical first few hours and his subsequent mastery of the funeral details that saved the monarchy. While the Queen and her courtiers dithered about whether Prince Charles should go to Paris in the first place and, if he did, whether he should be authorised to use the royal flight, Charles, it was said, showed a steely resolve, determined that he should go to France to bring his ex-wife home. If a royal flight were not forthcoming, his assistant private secretary and spin-doctor, Mark Bolland, declared, the Prince would get a scheduled flight from Aberdeen. Again, when they returned to Britain, the Prince was so horrified that Diana was going to the mortuary in Fulham – a strict legal requirement – that he insisted that she should be laid to rest in the Chapel Royal at St James's Palace. Using the vernacular of an East End gangster, the Prince, according to Junor, told a hapless aide: "Sort it. I don't care who has made the decision." In touch, compassionate and strong minded, the busy Prince was subsequently credited with virtually every innovation in the funeral week … this, however was not the way senior courtiers remembered the funeral week … "Charles was like a wet weekend at Balmoral … he was poleaxed with guilt, and any suggestion that he was taking charge was ridiculous."

As is his habit, Andrew Morton does not name his source. I have spent two years trying to unmask this courtier and have been unable to do so, despite exhaustive enquiries. Instead, I have discovered universal support for Penny Junor's version of these events. Firstly, Princess Margaret confirmed before her death that Prince Charles's behaviour at Balmoral was both robust and determined, and even though she was sympathetic with the point of view of her sister, she made it clear that she thought he had been admirable and had been accurately described by Junor.

Secondly, Sandy Henney, who was the 'hapless aide' unfairly referred to by Morton, has since confirmed that those were indeed the Prince's instructions on the plane. She can't remember if they were the exact words, but the tone was spot on. Moreover, at no time did he then or later in the week appear like a wet weekend in Balmoral, nor racked with guilt.

Thirdly, Jon Snow, the experienced Channel 4 news reporter, known as a socialist sympathiser and an unlikely monarchy propagandist, has stated that a member of the royal entourage confirmed to him, 'I was told by two sources, one inside the royal circle, one ministerial, that an almost immediate breakdown appeared within hours of the discovery of Diana's death. The Queen did not want the body anywhere near a royal palace, anywhere near a royal chapel. She wanted her left at an undertaker's on the Fulham Road [actually a mortuary in Fulham] ... The whole thing deteriorated into the most appalling slanging match which at one point found Charles shouting at Sir Robert Fellowes ... On the flight-deck of the plane that Charles did eventually take to Paris ... a place which effectively became his office because denied royal protocol he now had to find some way of getting all the things which protocol would normally have provided ... such minute details as the flowers that were to be put on the coffin had to be called up.'

Fourthly, a cabinet minister then told Snow that, 'Charles had been unable to call on the royal protocol in any form ... he had no alternative but to call on the government and see what they could do. And I think Number 10, conscious of the public reaction, already realised that they would have to do whatever could be done.'

Fifthly, Clayton and Craig's well-researched book confirms Junor's version of events, as does Lady Colin Campbell, Jonathan Dimbleby and all other serious biographers – as opposed to those, like Andrew Morton, with a particular axe to grind.

Sixthly, despite extensive efforts, I have been completely unable to find a single person from the Queen's household who admits ever speaking with Mr Morton.

Only Andrew Morton knows from where he received his information. His version of the events on the plane on its way back from Paris is fanciful and designed to show the Prince up in a less favourable light. In an obsessive sort of a way Charles must never appear to be anything but weak and selfish in any Morton description. But it is the other versions of the story that are correct.

The initial decision to use the Fulham mortuary had almost certainly been made by Sir Robert Fellowes, doing what he thought that the Queen would have wanted (Morton is incorrect to state that it was a legal requirement for the body to be deposited there). There can be little doubt that Prince Charles felt genuine grief for the loss of his former wife, the mother of his children and a woman for whom, in a fatherly sort of way, he was still very fond. On the other hand, his mother and father were so heartily fed up with their erstwhile daughter-in-law that their true feelings of dislike for a girl they believed to be spoiled, self-obsessed and devious and who had done so much damage to the monarchy and thus undermined their years of dedicated hard work, could hardly be concealed. In their opinion she had caused so much trouble while she was alive and was now beginning to create mayhem on her death. Sir Robert was well aware of Her Majesty's feelings and would have taken them into account when naming the mortuary. It has been suggested that he took the decision due to his personal dislike of the Princess. There is no evidence to support this and he would never have dreamed of making such a personal decision, whatever his feelings towards Diana might have been.

After Prince Charles's intervention, via Sandy Henney's heated phone calls from the aircraft's flight deck, things were changed. The Princess would have outriders and she would go to the Royal Chapel at St James's.

After the plane landed at Northolt, it taxied to the airport building where it was met by the Prime Minister, the Lord Chamberlain, pall-bearers and about 150 journalists and photographers. In an eerie silence, the coffin was removed from the plane and placed in a waiting hearse. The only sound was that of the Royal Standard flapping against the side of the coffin in the evening breeze. Having brought his former wife and tormentor dutifully home, the Prince climbed back aboard the plane for the return journey to Balmoral to be with his sons, while the hearse started its slow journey down the A40 into west London. The mood of the nation, which had been whipped up by continual television coverage on all channels, now became apparent. Shock and disbelief had turned into dismay and growing mass hysteria. The route into the city was lined with cars and people who had come out on this late summer's evening to watch the coffin pass.

World leaders were recording glowing tributes as flowers started to appear at every building that the Princess had ever lived in. Self-publicists queued up to get on the television to grab their moment of fame by recounting their Diana experience for grateful producers who were struggling to fill the time as twenty-four-hour television on just one subject became a reality. This need to keep the programme going and hopefully make it more interesting than the other channels' version of the same thing quite naturally led the conversations on air to become more sensational and fanciful as every angle was explored time and time again. This not only increased the public's grief – even sucking in anti-monarchists and people who had disliked Diana only twenty-four-hours before – but also fomented an antipathy the public felt towards the monarchy and the press.

The main targets were the tabloid press and their paparazzi friends for hounding the Princess, the Prince of Wales for having driven his beautiful wife away by his affair with Camilla Parker Bowles, and the Queen for being a cold and heartless mother-in-law. In all three cases the public were responding to misleading information that had been created on purpose by Diana herself.

The initial finger was pointed at the media by Charles Spencer. He ignored the fact that he had previously warned his sister to stop playing the publicity game and seek psychiatric help for her mental disorder, and accused the press of having 'blood on their hands'. But like his sister he was a keen player of the game himself. He claimed to be either a journalist or a celebrity when it suited him, but reverted to being a private citizen when it didn't. Like Diana, he had completely forgotten that people were only interested in either of them because of her royal connection and not because they came from the Spencer family – which had never sparked any interest in the public mind, except for the occasional society scandal. While not being in the same league as his sister, Spencer is nevertheless a capable press manipulator himself. He knew his 'blood on their hands' comment would grab the headlines and place him at the centre of the stage. However, not only were such comments quite unfair as the press were in Paris at the Princess's invitation and it was her and not them who had decided to travel at high speed and without a seat belt, they were also unwise. The tabloid press squirmed as the visual media repeated his comments over and over again. They would bide their time and then pay him back – many times over.

However, the British media's initial position wasn't helped by a rash of Sunday newspaper articles that were highly critical of Diana and had hit the streets before news of her death had broken. The press had begun increasingly to question the Princess's conduct during the last two months of her life. She had subjected her sons to Dodi and, even worse, his father, and the whole episode had reeked of her manipulation and self-obsession. Many editors had obviously decided that in future Diana might be more valuable to them in news terms as an object of criticism rather than hero worship, and her current erratic and selfish behaviour had made that decision all the easier. Even the normally loyal *Daily Mail* had been joining in. On 27 August, just four days before her death, their renowned correspondent the late Lynda Lee-Potter had written, 'The sight of a paunchy playboy groping a scantily dressed Diana must appal and humiliate Prince William ... As the mother of two young sons she ought to have more decorum and sense.'

Then, on the same morning that people were waking up to the shocking news of the Princess's death, Bernard Ingham had written in the *Sunday Express*, 'Princess Diana's press relations are now clearly established. Any publicity is good publicity ... I'm told she and Dodi are made for each other, both having more brass than brains.'

Over the same breakfast table a *Sunday Mirror* reader would have been told rather pompously by Chris Hutchins, 'Just when Diana began to believe that her current romance with likeable playboy Dodi Fayed had wiped out past liaisons, a new tape recording is doing the rounds of Belgravia dinner parties. And this one is hot, hot, hot! I must remember to take it up with Diana next time we find ourselves on adjacent running machines at our west London gym.'

Even the broadsheets were at it. The *Sunday Times* had decided to serialise Oliver James's book *Britain on the Couch* and lead with his daring royal psychoanalysis that majored on Diana, her childhood and her failed relationship with both of her parents. It was largely accurate and thus extremely unflattering to all three of them. It exposed the real Diana in a fashion that would be considered to be heresy once the world realised she was dead. Even the photograph alongside the headline 'DIANA ON THE COUCH' was unflattering – she was red-eyed, tearful and jowly. I have never seen the print reproduced since.

When these journalists had put pen to paper some time during the previous week, Diana was alive, well and making a fool of herself while apparently embarrassing the nation. The press appeared to have caught the mood of the people – many on the tube or in a bus queue seemed to be expressing these opinions. But her death had brought Diana instant purification and pity, and the very people who would have agreed with every word they had written just a day earlier suddenly rounded on those same columnists. In many people's eyes she may have been a sinner when the articles had been written, but by the time they were published she had become a saint and the people had apparently always thought so – having erased any earlier opinions from their minds.

Such criticism, which of course would never have been written by any of the columnists if they had known what was going to happen, was immediately seized upon by an angry public as proof that Charles Spencer was right, and the national hysteria grew. The media needed to respond quickly and change direction. It immediately decided on a two-pronged attack. It would firstly join in the glorification of the Princess and thus be seen to be at one with the people by writing what they wanted to read. Ross Benson, who in real life had had little time for Diana, wrote in the *Daily Express*, 'She was the butterfly who shone with the glamour which illuminated all our lives.' Simon Jenkins commented in *The Times*, 'A comet streaked across the sky of public life and entranced the world.' Paul Johnson in the *Daily Mail* called her 'A gem of purest ray serene.' Such bloated expressions of virtue were but a sample of the general tone from the newly converted Diana devotees who had been ordered to make amends and clear the media's name.

The second part of the strategy was as typical of the British media as it was unsavoury. It would seek to deflect any further criticism by finding another scapegoat and running a bruising campaign against them. As usual, the Royal Family was an easy target that wouldn't hit back. Prince Charles's prediction that he and his family would be blamed and criticised was about to come true.

So in the week between her death and the funeral, the press desperately tried to get rid of the initial public perception that they had the Princess's blood on their hands. The finger of blame and the fist of frustration were increasingly shaken in the direction of the Royal Family by a profession keen to wriggle out of the suggestion that this tragedy was in any way their doing. One senior employee at Associated

Newspapers, who can't be named as he still works there, told me, 'The word was all over the place – not just here but at the *Sun*, everywhere – that we should dig up every possible positive and lovely story about Diana, while we should really dish the dirt on the other royals and portray them as callous. My editor actually said at the morning meeting that he wanted to see the public pumped up like the Frogs had been during the French Revolution.'

He and his media colleagues nearly got their way. In the days following Diana's death, the future of the monarchy was seriously tested as a combination of public grief and media manipulation that would have amazed Diana herself by developed and fed off each other. Meanwhile the Royal Family stayed in Scotland and remained silent. This only seemed to increase public anger: it was perceived that the Queen didn't care about the people's grief – if she did then she would return to London and address the nation. The vast majority of people seemed to forget in their act of mass hysteria that Prince William and Prince Harry had just lost a mother and that their father and their grandmother deserved a little privacy in order to comfort their loved ones. Every family deserves that. Grief is the price that we must all pay for close and deep love. It cannot be compared to a sense of loss felt for someone only ever known through daily pictures in the press.

So the British public, manipulated by a guilt-ridden press, behaved with massive self-indulgence and demanded that the Royal Family return to London so that it might see their grief. This was quite the lowest piece of national behaviour experienced in the nation's modern history. It was not only monstrously unkind and selfish, it was amazingly hypocritical. The public had started the week blaming the media for not allowing Diana privacy in her love life (completely unaware that it was indeed Diana who had been manipulating the coverage), but by midweek they were demanding that the nation should be allowed to invade the Royal Family's private bereavement and healing process.

A groundswell of opinion forced the Royal Family to take political decisions instead of the domestic ones to which it was entitled. By Thursday, after a set of wounding headlines – 'SHOW US YOU CARE' (the *Daily Express*), 'WHERE IS OUR QUEEN?' (the *Sun*), and 'YOUR PEOPLE ARE SUFFERING, SPEAK TO US MA'AM' (the *Daily Mirror*) – the Queen was forced back to London in order to address the nation from Buckingham Palace on Friday, while it was announced that Princes

Andrew and Edward would go on a walkabout in the Mall and talk to the grieving crowds. Earlier in the day Prince Charles and his two sons mingled with the hundreds of mourners piling up the thousands of floral tributes outside Kensington Palace. At Buckingham Palace and St James's Palace, the Queen and Prince Philip did the same. Unlike Charles and the boys who did so freely, I am told that the Queen and the Duke did so under duress and then purely out of a sense of duty. Nevertheless, it countered the charge that they didn't care and, given the uncertain mood of the people, it must have taken some courage. These gestures saved the day and calmed the situation before the funeral the following day. In particular, the Queen's well-delivered live television address appeased the public. She had recognised their grief and they seemed satisfied.

The public reaction had been extraordinary, not just in Britain but also in America and to a lesser extent around the rest of the globe. The image of Diana had been young, beautiful, a princess, a mother, a rebel, a saint. Her beauty had captivated the world, while her charm and manipulative skills had kept her face on every magazine cover for years. The result was that the public identified with her as a major icon in a world increasingly impressed by pop culture; people had become accustomed to her and almost felt that they knew her. The idea that she was also vulnerable – just like the rest of us – simply made identification with her all the easier.

There had also been a lot of criticism of her, especially of late, as the mirage faded and exposed the real woman behind the vision, but this was washed away by the public's tears and the media's desire to make amends: a saint had been born. Her good deeds were exaggerated and her bad deeds forgotten as the mirage passed into history as if the real woman never existed.

Due to her divorce the Princess wasn't entitled to a state funeral, and the Queen's initial reaction was that she wasn't going to get much more than a semi-public service at St George's Chapel in Windsor Castle. The funeral she got – the cortège, the pageantry, Westminster Abbey and a semi-state occasion watched by millions around the world – was the doing of Prince Charles. He alone initially argued for it, and he was eventually supported by Tony Blair. Together they talked the Queen into it. This has been confirmed to me both by royal courtiers and by people then working at 10 Downing Street.

The funeral was just like a state occasion, and was brilliantly organised by the Earl Marshall's office. Ironically the British, who find it so very hard to run a decent railway service, always excel at this. The cortège made its way from Kensington Palace via Buckingham Palace, where it paused for members of the Royal Family to pay their respects; as it passed St James's Palace and Clarence House, it was joined by Prince Charles, Prince William, Prince Harry, the Duke of Edinburgh and Charles Spencer. The boy princes behaved like men as they walked behind their mother's coffin accompanied by their father, grandfather and uncle. Prince Charles looked the most emotional – his face racked with grief, which was uncharitably put down to guilt by certain journalists. We now know, of course, that he had nothing to be guilty about. Rather, he had lost someone with whom he had at one time hoped to spend his life and who was the mother of his sons. These two boys, whom he has always loved dearly, would now bravely have to face the future without her. He above all others could feel their pain, and it showed.

The guest list for the actual service in Westminster Abbey represented Diana well. It was more about pop culture than royalty. Indeed, apart from the British Royal Family, which was together for the first time since 1992 and included the Duchess of York, other royalty was particularly thin on the ground. Instead, there were charity colleagues, friends from the aristocracy, former lovers like Hasnat Khan, movie stars like Tom Cruise, Nicole Kidman, Steven Spielberg, Tom Hanks and Arnold Schwarzenegger, pop stars Elton John, George Michael and Sting, designers like Donatella Versace, Karl Lagerfeld, Christian Lacroix and Sandro, and there were scores of fashion editors and photographers.

Charles Spencer gave the eulogy. He ruined what would have otherwise been a moving and in some ways accurate tribute to his sister by an unfair and inaccurate attack on the Royal Family and an amazing swipe at his own mother. Lady Sarah Spencer-Churchill later remarked, 'Was it really necessary to allude to the lonely train journeys he and Diana had made between their divorced parents, in Frances's presence? What did he hope to accomplish by accusing the Royal Family of treating Diana badly? And what rubbish was he jabbering on about when he said Diana needed no royal title to wield her particular brand of magic. Did he think anyone would have heard or cared about her if she remained Lady Diana Spencer? Is the title Princess of Wales not a royal title? His speech, for speech is what it was, was more suited to the political hustings than a sister's funeral.'

This is fair comment, and Lady Sarah Spencer-Churchill might have gone further: there was no mention of the Earl's rows with his sister; no mention that he had at times been less than supportive of much of her conduct. He was rightly not prepared to wash his dirty linen in public, so to flag up Diana's difficult relationship with her former husband, his family and their mother was one-sided, selfish and irresponsible. Nevertheless, given that so few of the public understood what Diana's life beyond the mirage was really like, his cheap shots enjoyed public acclaim and even a round of applause in the Abbey, which must have been extremely hurtful to the young princes.

He had also made the point that Diana's family, her blood relatives, would play a major part in bringing up her sons the way she would have wanted – an inference being that their father was incapable of doing so. Apparently he feared they would become stifled by duty and tradition if their upbringing were left to the Royal Family alone. But the Royal Family must live on a staple diet of duty and tradition if it is to fulfil its function and survive. In exchange for such a shackled life, it lives in splendour and privilege. That is its pact with the people. Diana never understood this and always confused monarchy with celebrity. Apparently her brother was equally confused. However, her sons weren't; nor were they in any doubt about who they wished to bring them up. In the years after the funeral they grew even closer to their father. This was entirely their own decision based on a deep love of their father.

Charles Spencer's acclaim was very short-lived. His own marriage was in trouble, and he wanted a divorce. He was keen that this be heard in South Africa, where he had a home, as the settlement would be much lower than in the UK.

Suddenly Spencer knew what it was like to be on the receiving end of a hostile media. They had been waiting to avenge his attack on their virtue by accusing them of having 'blood on their hands': now they were eager to expose him as an arrogant, cruel and hypocritical bully; that he had actually admitted as much in a letter to his mistress; that he believed he was entitled to treat her badly as he accused her of being a devious and cunning liar. She was allegedly all the things that he had also accused his sister of being – a chronic symptom of their shared condition.

As the case was heard, the British tabloids reported how Spencer had allegedly mistreated Victoria, recounting the moment he announced his intention to divorce her, and cited a speech he gave while she had been in hospital, that had apparently alluded jokingly to how mentally thick and yet physically thin she was.

On agreeing to settle with Victoria shortly before she was due to give evidence, a somewhat bruised Charles Spencer returned to Althorp and set about using Diana's memory to raise money for the Diana Memorial Fund. Having refused her permission to have a house on the estate while she was alive due to the intrusion it might cause, he converted a stable block into a permanent museum to his sister, provided a resting place after her demise, and from 1998 happily watched bucket loads of cash roll in. By 2004 the public interest had waned and the numbers fallen so drastically that he announced its closure at the end of the annual two-month season of July and August.

In addition to Spencer's barbed address, the prime minister read the lesson. It was a ridiculously over-emotional reading. Then there was the pure syrup of an old Elton John hit written in honour of another mentally frail celebrity – Marilyn Monroe – which had quickly had new lyrics cobbled together to dedicate it to the dead Princess. And of course there were more hymns and prayers, 'Cwm Rhondda' and the Commendation. Then the Welsh Guards shouldered the coffin out of the Abbey to 'Flights of Angels' and placed Diana in a remarkably old hearse for such an occasion. It set off for Althorp along a route lined with thousands of genuinely grieving people.

The nation, with true twentieth-century excess, had been caught up in mass hysteria one minute but was back at work the next. By the first anniversary of the Princess's death, the vast majority of people asked by a television channel to comment on the significance of the date had no idea; only a handful of flowers marked the occasion outside Kensington Palace, in complete contrast to the mountains of floral tributes that had been laid down by a inconsolable public just one year before.

Perhaps this is telling of modern emotion and a star's relationship with the public. It had all been seen before. In the twentieth century, girls who craved stardom as a result of their own insecurities and had the looks to do something about it – Marilyn Monroe, Jayne Mansfield, Diana Dors, Natalie Wood and countless others – achieved what they wanted partly because of their vulnerability, with which the public could identify. Their addiction to fame did not bring them happiness, but it caused those close to them much unhappiness. They all were unable to sustain personal relationships and had a tendency to press the self-destruct button again and again. They all wanted the public's adoration, but they blamed the public for the pressure of it; and yet they were suicidal when fickle fans looked elsewhere

In many ways Diana was no different. It is perhaps true to say that if she had just stayed cleaning her sister's flat until some suitable Sloane Ranger asked her to marry him, she would have been better off. Of course she would have still suffered from her mental condition and, as a result, her husband and children would have had as tough a time as her. But she would never have been exposed to the addictive drug of public acclaim – the addiction that increased her unhappiness and, in the end, caused her to be racing to her death through a Paris underpass.

In the year that immediately followed the Princess's death, the Royal Family appeared to return to the serenity that had existed in those pre-Diana and Fergie days. In particular the Prince of Wales, freed from the constant attention-seeking and negative briefing of the press by the Princess, enjoyed a considerable renaissance. Mark Bolland's media guidance helped, as did the media's anger at Charles Spencer. Stories of what Diana could really be like started to surface, and there was a genuine sympathy from the public as they watched a single parent bringing up two boys. But the most important reason was the one that Diana had always tried to submerge and was petrified of being revealed: the simple fact that Prince Charles was a loving father and was adored by his sons. Public perception was changed in a matter of months. Indeed, by the end of 1998, Prince Charles had overtaken Tony Blair in the BBC Radio 4 poll as Man of the Year. Perhaps, finally, the public had been allowed to see beyond the mirage.

Conclusion
'They who would rule in this kingdom'

'Remember that there will be difficult times in the last days. People will be selfish, greedy, boastful and conceited; they will be insulting, disobedient to their parents, ungrateful and irreligious; they will be unkind, merciless, slanderers, violent and fierce; they will hate the good; they will be treacherous, reckless and swollen with pride; they will love pleasure rather than God …'
1 Timothy 3: 1–4

Much has changed on these islands known as the United Kingdom of Great Britain since the end of the Second World War. As a people we have become financially much better off. Our comfortable life bears no comparison with the harsh realities of having a terrifying war nearby, often fought in the very skies above the nation's head; nor to the spartan economy of the bankrupt victor once the bombing had stopped. And yet, as our monetary wealth has grown, it would seem that we have become poorer in human spirit and religious spiritualism. Our shallow lives lack a certain direction as we have become distracted, even blinded, by the need to follow instant popular fashion and acclaim.

Perhaps our lives have not changed altogether for the better. Indeed, a number of opinion polls conducted since the millennium have indicated that a majority of British people believe that the quality of life was better fifty years ago than today, despite our increased material wealth. A similar percentage would prefer to live abroad if they could. This would have been a quite unthinkable thought half a century ago, when the British, from all walks of life, saw themselves as the custodians of goodness, at the head of the world's greatest empire, quite superior to any other nation and living in a 'green and pleasant land'.

The monarchy has been a rare stable feature in this new quick-fire, all-changing, media-driven, image-conscious, fashion-obsessed Britain; but even the monarchy has been forced to play catch-up, as have many other British institutions and similar holders of traditional values. Perhaps it had become a little too comfortable. Nevertheless, as things changed after the War, it survived, and indeed remained very popular. This popularity was centred upon a young queen, her husband and their children playing the role of the nation's model family. In the 1950s this seemed to work, as press deference still existed and the Royal Family was always kept a carefully calculated distance from the Queen's subjects. However, this disguised the fact for some time that she was presiding over a realm where what she ruled was moving on and the monarchy, its values and all that it stood for was being left behind.

Understandably, working people, having had to put up with much hardship in defence of the realm, relished a future without having to pay so much deference to what many saw as an insufferably arrogant and self-righteous middle class. After all, the War had been a great leveller and now the common man expected his reward. He had voted for change in 1945. This brought to power a Labour government that promised equality and a land 'fit for heroes'. As a result, anything that was middle class or better in post-war socialist Britain was seen as standing for an 'old order' and was therefore stuffy, old-fashioned and to be tolerated rather than revered as respect for such values gradually disappeared. This idea gained momentum in the 1960s when this passive working-class revolution obtained a fashionable status and being part of it was 'cool' while being part of the old order was 'square'. And although this revolution made a virtue of peace, its abandonment of moral attitudes was to sow the seeds of much social unrest and violence, which later exploded in British cities. It ignored the fact that attacking and ridiculing the middle classes for their values invited the young born to lower-income families to become lawless and to accept no responsibility. It wasn't their fault. How could it be? The new thinking told them that they had been born unfairly to the 'have nots' of this life. It was an accident of low-income birth, and that was the fault of a class society. Politically correct sentiments perhaps, but sentiments that provided a perfect excuse for the villain to portray himself as the victim of British society.

Such a cancer, having manifested itself in our cities and towns, became evident as early as the 1980s before growing into a disease that today threatens to endanger the future of many parts of the country if not checked. Streets are awash with violent crime that is more often than not motivated by drug addiction; in housing estates the elderly are terrorised by children who roam with the arrogance of those who know the police will not arrive. A more complete contrast to the financially poorer but morally richer Jarrow marchers of some sixty years earlier would be hard to imagine.

However, throughout the 1960s and 1970s, few seemed to understand that you can't pull an order down without erecting a new one. The human needs more rules than any other animal on the planet. As a result, playwrights, singers, actors and artists lined up to play the working-class hero who stood for these fashionable principles. Indeed some, like John Lennon, even concealed a very real middle-class background in an effort to invent a working-class past. This self-indulgent period, having guaranteed so much future misery, was not to last permanently.

By 1979 the economy, which had been brought to its knees as a result of more than thirty years of this popular but unrealistic thinking, demanded a change as the nation's future prospects began to look humiliatingly bleak. And so a second post-war social revolution occurred as the nation decided on a lurch to the right and the introduction of a Thatcher meritocracy, which strove to undo much of what had occurred politically since 1945. And by the time her Conservative Party was replaced in 1997 by a New Labour government, things had moved on yet again. Now it was footballers, singers, actors and even television chefs who made up a new 'celebrity royalty' and, with materialism back in fashion, it was these stars, fuelled by greed, self-absorption and the need for public acclaim, that fizzed across our media galaxy and were burned out in no time as adoration turned to vilification, humiliation and nervous breakdown. The rest of us had a nervous breakdown just seeking to copy, keep up and meet the monthly payments on our credit cards as a most irresponsible consumer-credit boom took off.

Perhaps the resulting 'here today, gone tomorrow' society is not the right setting for an institution that seeks long-term survival. The 'old royalty' of the monarchy has always needed the long-lasting qualities of mystique and respect in order that its star might continue to shine brightly in the public's mind. For whether the British have enjoyed good sovereigns or endured bad ones, the institution of monarchy has been part of the system of government for over a thousand years – a system that sought to allow the monarchy to evolve between the eighteenth and twentieth centuries, when so many European neighbours were eliminating their own royal families, sometimes violently. So why did the British seek to redefine and retain theirs?

The thinking was that a constitutional monarchy provided

democracy, unity and continuity. It was later realised that it also provided a huge commercial boost to the tourist industry and was a lot more cost-effective than many republics. For example, the upkeep of the French presidency is higher annually than that of the British monarchy. Democracy is assured because the monarch holds the power of the judiciary (the application of the law), while the elected government of the people holds the legislative power (the making of the law). Therefore the people's government makes the laws that the people have elected it to make, but with the Crown controlling the legal system (as opposed to the government), it is still possible for the individual to take the government to court. Thus democracy is preserved by a constitutional monarchy retaining a power that it cannot use but which prevents any government from seizing it and using it against the people.

Moreover, it is recognised that any form of government needs to have a head of state. The British constitutional monarchy has a certain advantage over other heads of state because its role is non-political. In many republics this is not the case. For example, if an American votes for a Republican candidate but gets a Democrat as president, his head of state is not the person he chose or wanted. In Britain, there are thousands of people who would hate the very idea of Tony Blair being head of state, and thousands others who would have preferred to live abroad rather than see Margaret Thatcher as president. However, nearly all readily stand to attention for the playing of 'God Save the Queen'. The thinking has always been that anyone could vote for whichever political party they wanted, but still unite behind a monarchy not tarnished by political policy, a symbol of undiluted patriotism.

Through the monarchy, continuity and unity are assured, along with a strong tie to our history and traditions in order that we know who we are. However, in the last thirty years there have been those concerned with political correctness, many of them secretly favouring a republic, who would seek to undermine that continuity, believing that ethnic minorities, immigrant workers and asylum seekers don't feel part of this history and that British people should play it down, apologise for our imperial past and perhaps even scrap the monarchy. As a result, many children in school have not been taught to be proud of their history or of being British, and this has given rise on the one hand to low national esteem and an unhealthy backlash from some rather unsavoury racists on the other. Moreover, if you seek to

The King and Di

downgrade the nation's patriotism, you must start by diminishing its most important focus – the monarchy. In such a climate, the Crown has been relegated from a figurehead of national pride to the object of cheap tabloid gossip. Nevertheless, however much the politically correct brigade and closet republicans don't like to admit to it, there is a frustrated patriotism that bursts on to the streets each time there is an opportunity. The Queen's Golden Jubilee in 2002 was one such occasion; England winning the Rugby World Cup in 2003 was another. Both times a million people took to the streets of central London in a mass celebration of national pride.

Originally, the sovereign was all-powerful and ruled autocratically with the assistance of a handful of ministers. Parliament, which needed to be called in order to raise taxes, began to flex its muscles in the seventeenth century and this led to the Civil War between it and Charles I, who believed in the divine right of kings. Charles lost, was executed and Britain became a republic. After eleven years the monarchy was restored amid much rejoicing, and on his death Charles II left the throne firmly re-established. His brother James II was forced to abdicate only four years later due to his Roman Catholic faith, but despite this nobody wanted to go back to having another harsh and colourless republic. In order that he might obtain the crown, William III, James's son-in-law, had to agree to a limitation of his powers. From then on the sovereign's powers were to go on reducing until the reign of George V in the early part of the twentieth century, since which time they have remained largely unaltered.

As a result of its survival, while other monarchies were ousted, the British Crown has developed an almost unique nature and this has provided a major financial bonus for the economy. Ever since the rise of mass tourism in the 1960s, the monarchy has emerged as the nation's foremost tourist attraction. It is this living connection with the country's famous history, as demonstrated by daily events like the Changing of the Guard, that brings tourists in their droves to this otherwise wet and, in places, uninspiring island. It is precisely because Britain is a sceptred isle and can demonstrate an ongoing link with history and genuine majesty that tourists choose to come here. Hollywood invests millions to create make-believe kingdoms, but Great Britain still has the real thing. As a result the British economy gratefully accepts billions in foreign currency each year. This alone, according to its supporters, is a good reason why the nation should preserve the Crown.

It might be that the ingredients needed to do this are love and respect from the people, deference from the media and a life of distance, duty and example from the monarchy locked away behind large palace gates in order to protect the mystique and stop the inevitable domestic squabbles from getting out. Perhaps this is the only way that the dream might be preserved. But today this is a very hard thing to achieve. Respect and deference are apparently insults to our human rights, and the press pick the flesh off any 'celebrity' in a frenzied attack before discarding the bones and moving on in search of a new hero to worship for a week or two.

This has all proved to be a very difficult problem for the monarchy to deal with. When the monarch was our political leader, with power and no intense and disrespectful media to worry about, his or her job was in many ways much easier and the outcome never really in doubt. Imagine if the Tudors were suddenly to replace the Windsors at the head of today's constitutional monarchy and be placed in the full spotlight without the power they wielded in the sixteenth century. The tabloid press would be running ten-page scandal specials daily as the domestic and political antics of Henry VIII, Mary I and Elizabeth I would completely eclipse any mess Princess Margaret, Diana or the Duchess of York may have got themselves into.

But in the late 1970s, the Queen's advisers didn't appear to understand this and decided that the crown must swim with the tide and modernise. So the monarchy began to flirt with mass-media exposure by seductively removing some of its royal veils of mystique, in an attempt to appear to be thoroughly modern and enter (and indeed win) the international celebrity stakes. It turned up the heat on its less noble competition by producing, in 1981, a spectacular fairy-tale wedding. There was a handsome prince, resplendent in his naval uniform; his beautiful, young and innocent bride, in a wonderful, long, flowing ivory gown; a golden coach pulled by a magnificent fanfare of trotting horses; a real palace, that even the smallest child knew was not artificially created in some corner of a film lot; a cathedral made famous across the world by Charles Dickens and the London blitz; actual heads of state from every corner of the globe; and a cast of thousands – the happiest and proudest subjects in the universe, or so it seemed.

The fairy tale became the story of a small, shy, artistic boy who had no say in being born the Prince of Wales but who, despite his shortcomings, set out to help his countrymen rather than live the life of a playboy while waiting for his mother to die. It also became the story of a shy young girl who, while delighted to have been born an aristocrat, was sad to have endured what she saw as an unhappy childhood, dreamed of marrying a prince, did so, and went on, despite her flaws, to become an icon with the four attributes the western world has become so keen to worship: fame, beauty, youth and wealth. As a result of these qualities, which she had in abundance, and her early and untimely death, it is hard to think of a more famous or better-loved heroine in recent history.

Some people saw it as a tale of a boy from the old order marrying a girl from the new, separated by twelve years. But that is too simple: to make any sense of these characters, this has also to be a story of a society – a society that has shown little desire to prevent its recent moral decline and doesn't seem to want to be saved, especially if salvation takes the form of self-discipline and acts of selflessness, responsibility and deference. It also has to be a story of us, a people who perhaps, having lost an empire and its status, were destined to be placed in a key position to let the lunatics run the asylum and be in the vanguard of a western movement to fulfil St Paul's predictions as the war-weary old could only watch as powerless, unfashionable and unheard spectators. It is most important to understand the changing face of Britain since the Second World War in order to comprehend how the monarchy's fairy-tale wedding became a Greek tragedy before turning into a 'What the Butler Saw' farce. This is because without the vehicle of tabloid journalism, the Princess of Wales would never have been able to circulate such damaging fantasy, and that kind of press only exists because we want it to.

Over the last twenty years, such a cacophony of speculation, lies and farce has been dished up that it is only when one can understand the motives of some of the major players that one can start to pick out the truth from the half truths, the fanciful, the misrepresentations, the spin and the lies. During this period, media frenzy has splashed in the shallow waters of tabloid trash, celebrity addiction and self-obsession in order to satisfy the public's unquenchable thirst for gossip. As a result, it is only natural to wonder how much more of a pounding the monarchy can take before the lies begin to be believed and its future is put into real doubt, or at the very least a highly controversial movement gains momentum for Prince Charles to stand aside in favour of his son – even if there is no justification for this whatsoever.

So life was always going to be difficult for twentieth-century monarchy, whether born to it or thrust into it by marriage; but the Prince of Wales has had a particularly tough time of it. What is the correct course for him? His ancestors were political rulers, but he will be a constitutional monarch. He cannot captain one political team and then change sides when it is defeated at the polls to captain another, so not only can he not take sides, he mustn't allow his political beliefs to be known or cross the political line, even when something he cares about passionately needs to be said. The Prince of Wales sometimes finds this very difficult and has, in the past, come close to jumping over the line with both feet. He must learn to refrain from making this mistake, for while his good intention should not be doubted, it is not his job to be so engaged and it would weaken the monarchy even further once he is crowned king if he continued down this path.

However, his current position is almost impossible. If he does nothing, he stands accused of being a parasite; if he acts, for every supporter there will always scores of others saying that he shouldn't interfere. If he speaks of a desire to be a 'defender of faith, he is condemned for not accepting his responsibility as Defender of *the* Faith; if he talks of his own Christian beliefs, he is reminded that he is to be the next constitutional monarch of a multi-faith nation. If his pronouncements in the 1980s were modern and forward-thinking, as some of his statements were on the environment, inner cities, religion and architecture, the tabloid press, offended professionals and those who stood to lose financially as a result of his comments were all only too quick to mock him and dismiss his opinions as the ramblings of the Loony Prince; if his opinions were conservative and longed for a sense of spiritualism, family values and a clear understanding of right and wrong, he was out of touch with modern society and, as an old relic of a bygone age, had little in common with his subjects, and should remain silent.

And yet if such avant-garde opinions had been made by John Lennon, or conservative ones by Margaret Thatcher, they would have been received in many quarters as pearls of wisdom. For the Prince it is different: speak out and he is damned, stay silent and he is a waste of space and money. Either way he is born into a lifelong job that remains permanently in the media spotlight and needs to be sustainable, while all other celebrities are jettisoned by a press that builds people up in order to destroy them.

Maybe, in this valueless era that celebrates the short term, it was only ever possible for him to have been a hero for a short time. Perhaps that time was twenty-five years ago when, as a young bachelor prince he had a reputation for being a bit of an action man. Over his thirty-five years as Prince of Wales, only a few people have managed to stay alive and survive the media onslaught. The four pop knights of Paul McCartney, Cliff Richard, Elton John and Mick Jagger have managed it at a cost of being demoted from sixties superstars to tabloid court jesters. Politicians are washed down the media toilet as soon as possible. Honeymoons are usually short and only death brings on an attack of revisionism. When Mrs Thatcher eventually passes away, remember to buy a copy of the *Daily Mirror*'s tribute to her as proof of this point. So it is possible that Prince Charles had reached the peak of his popularity, with the tabloid press if not the nation, when he married. After all, that is where Hollywood might have finished the film.

But once the shy Princess Diana had found her media feet and realised that the press could be a huge emotional comfort as well as a violent weapon with which she might damage, if not destroy, her enemies, the Prince of Wales had no chance. She was young, photogenic and very beautiful, and the media's growing love affair with her made him, at times, both jealous and depressed as they stopped reporting his serious speeches in favour of photographing her at lunch. Worse, they were to cast her as a thoroughly modern princess, an icon fit for the pages of *Hello!*, while he was suddenly recast as a scatty, big-eared, balding, middle-aged man who talked to his plants. Having given him this image, they refused to take anything he said seriously.

Charles was born to be the king of a grand, famous and much-admired but fast-fading and nearly bankrupt empire that was looking for a lifeline and a new image at the time of his birth. He, like the rest of us, would have to get used to that, as he would to great political, social, spiritual and moral change as his realm struggled to adapt to such upheavals and re-invent itself as the home of the swinging sixties, free love, socialism, nationalisation and the Beatles, before standing on its head and becoming the custodian of right-wing Thatcherism. And as we have seen, he would also have to learn to cope with absent parents, a formal home life, a hard and demanding father, a hateful and bullied school existence, constant media scrutiny and in time, a wife who posed him many problems. She struggled at home to cope with life and yet could snap out of such deep depression, in a second, to strut the world stage as an amazing and truly adored superstar of the Hollywood mould. In time she would delight in upstaging her husband while attempting to bring down everything that he had been brought up to protect. He was supposed to uphold the discipline and mystique that allows a dynasty to last a thousand years. She, like her famous Hollywood counterparts, didn't seem to mind letting the veil slip to prove that she, and indeed the Windsors, could be as domestically troubled as the rest of us. Worse, as we have seen, she only remembered to give one side of that story, and even then it does not always stand up to too much scrutiny.

The role of Prince of Wales has always been a hard one. It has never been harder than now. If it were not for an accident of birth, perhaps Charles would not have been an automatic candidate; I'm sure he would never have put himself forward for the job. He has had to overcome many personal deficiencies to get this far, and he still has some to overcome – most of which, now that he is in his fifties, he never will. He is only human, after all. But he had no say in being born into this role, and to date has shown a remarkable sense of duty and love towards everyone, both in his family and in the country, where his tireless work and bravery should single him out for special praise and a place in our hearts. Although he is no longer the pin-up prince of his youth, there is a great deal that deserves our respect in this kind and intelligent man. Prince Charles has shown us all a great deal of love and devotion because he loves Britain selflessly. In such an imperfect world, perhaps he should be forgiven his minor failings as a result. Moreover, he is commercially one of the most successful ambassadors this country has ever sent abroad, and at home has done more to resolve the plight of children born into the dysfunctional ghettos of Britain's housing estates than anyone, while protecting us all from some of the selfish excesses of big business and government. Have we really the right to expect him to have done better? Has any previous holder of the title done as well?

And while the late Princess of Wales may not have always acted in a way that put country, or even family, before herself, there were reasons for this that were beyond her control, and probably go back to her youth, as we have seen. She was more of a victim than a villain; even then, she was not so much a victim of the Windsors as of her own problems. Nevertheless, the book has attempted to correct some elements of her story that have often been incorrectly reported and for which she often appears to be responsible.

This is important. It is only right and proper, in this increasingly gullible world of twenty-four-hour media, that the correct version of these events is told for the benefit of those who have been unfairly maligned, as well as for history and for truth itself. There will be those who will not want to hear this truth. This is increasingly a problem in a world where people assume that their beliefs are sacrosanct and any actual evidence to the contrary is angrily rejected. But the truth has to be preserved all the same. This book does not seek to be one of revelation, but one of accurate fact.

Moreover, this work rejoices, without reservation, in the good that both the Prince and Princess of Wales have achieved, and recognises the pressures they both had to endure, not for personal financial gain but in service of the nation. Naturally both made mistakes and weren't always perfect – no human being is. But his dedication cannot be questioned, and in the case of the Princess one marvels at how she brightened up so many poor, ill and dying people's lives during her short life.

Nevertheless, the mischief that the Princess had sewn by her false accusations and vindictive lies were not to die with her; they haunted the House of Windsor, kept alive by men keen to use her memory either to line their own pockets or further their ambition, or both. As a result, some eight years after her death, over eighty per cent of the British public still believed that Prince Charles had only married Diana in order to produce a son and heir; that he never loved her and continued to see his mistress Camilla Parker Bowles throughout his marriage. The vast majority of these people viewed Diana as a victim of a cruel and cold Windsor family, and many even believed that her death was ordered by the British Establishment in order to rid them of this troublesome young woman. It was even suggested that the Prince of Wales had a hand in such business. In 2005, one national tabloid even reported that over ninety per cent of its readership was convinced that the Princess's accident was staged and that she was really murdered.

On 10 February 2005, the Prince of Wales announced his engagement to Camilla Parker Bowles. The Sky Television News Channel was inundated with emails denouncing the couple and refusing to wish them well as they had made Diana's life miserable; some even implied that they had caused her death. It was much the same on all the other channels who recorded the couple's longstanding relationship and showed the *Panorama* interview: one could either bless the marriage of a couple that obviously loved one another despite the damage their affair had created, they seemed to be saying, or one could refuse to do so on the grounds that they had been responsible for causing the Princess of Wales so much unhappiness. There was hardly a hint that Camilla Parker Bowles had been absent from the Prince's life for years; there was absolutely nothing about the fact that the Princess of Wales had been a serial adulterer for the greater part of her marriage; and it was not mentioned that she found it quite impossible to sustain a monogamous relationship to anyone, ever. The result was that most phone-in polls conducted by the television stations on the day of the announcement recorded that sixty per cent of people were against the marriage.

The following day the newspapers were largely supportive of the Prince and his bride to be. Only the *Daily Mail* said that it had mixed feelings, having apparently now forgotten that a few months earlier it had admitted that it was the Princess of Wales who had been the first to commit adultery. The *Daily Mirror* wished the couple well, but also printed a two-page article that was perhaps the most pompous and flatulent ever to appear in a British tabloid. Its author, Paul Burrell, told his former boss that he could either be king or marry Camilla, but he 'couldn't have his cake and eat it'. As a result of the polls, however, the media changed tack and, in the weeks leading up to the wedding, the Prince and his bride to be were forced cruelly and most unjustly to run a gauntlet of tabloid bile and bitterness. Instead of the time being one of happy anticipation for the couple, it was turned into one of public humiliation that reflected poorly upon the British press and its apparent readership. Such was the nasty and wholly unwarranted nature of such attacks that the ex-editor of the *Daily Mirror* Piers Morgan seriously admonished his media colleagues on television for their malicious attacks. Nevertheless, even he stopped short of telling the truth, as to do so would no doubt have been considered to be heresy.

Nevertheless, the Prince, often wrongly considered by many to be something of a wimp, had stood firm and eventually done the right thing by a woman who had never done anything but selflessly devote herself to him during the nineteen years that she had been invited to do so. In this he was loyally supported by his sons who wished for nothing more than their father's happiness. Prince William had grown up to be a tall and handsome young man with more than passing resemblance to Diana. His 2:1 in Geography from University must have made his father very proud, as it no doubt would have done his mother. He remains shy and reluctant to take on the official duties that were forced on his father at the same age, but those who know him don't doubt that he will rise to the challenge when eventually called upon.

Prince Harry, perhaps a more typical Spencer, was not as academically gifted as his elder brother, and certainly inherited his mother's penchant for fun and excitement. This caused his teenage years to be occasionally marred by press stories of underage drinking and illegal drug taking. However, most of this was blown up out of all proportion by the media and was dealt with sensitively by his father. It should never be forgotten that Harry lost his mother just as he was entering puberty, and since then has had his every move since spied on by a cruel and devious media. All in all he has coped rather better than might have been expected. He is now at Sandhurst, and is expected to take rather well to army life.

Both boys' love and devotion to their father was more than apparent on his wedding day, as was his tenderness to them and his new bride. As the television coverage unfolded, this came across clearly, as did the support of the much larger than expected crowd. The television figures were excellent as the nation once more turned up and, despite the best efforts of the tabloid press, supported the monarchy. The next day the tabloids once more stood on their heads and declared the event a great success.

And what of Great Britain? If it wishes to retain its constitutional monarchy in the future and one day see a Charles III and a William V, it will have to learn to question the motives of the closet republicans. It will have to demand more privacy and deference for the crown. It will have to find champions in the media to endorse this cause. Above all, it will have to rediscover its spiritual base and core values, or the winner in the next reality TV show might just as well be king for a week.

This was the real story of the Prince and Princess of Wales. If you are British, it was also yours.

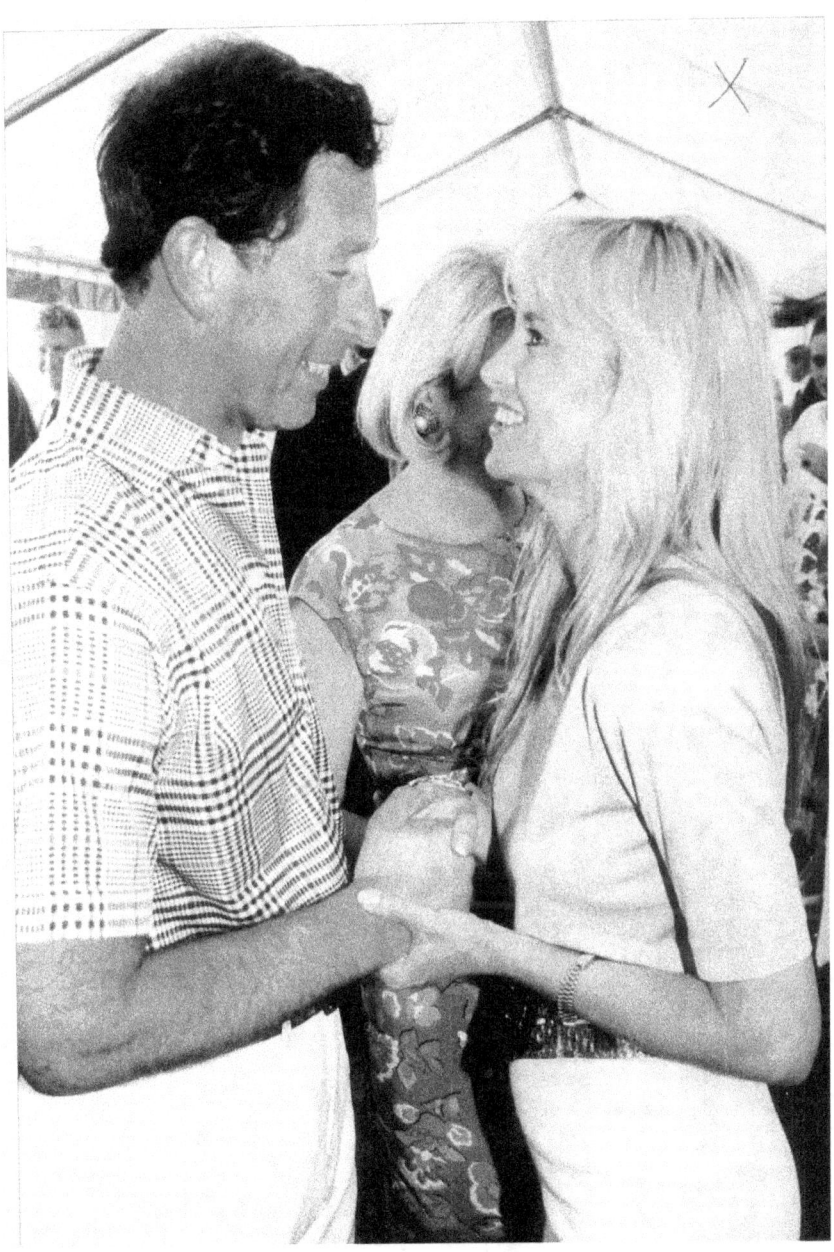

The Prince of Wales with a very special friend, actress Susan George. All eyes are on them(except for the royal mistress Kanaga, in the centre), but the prince and Ms George only have eyes for each other.

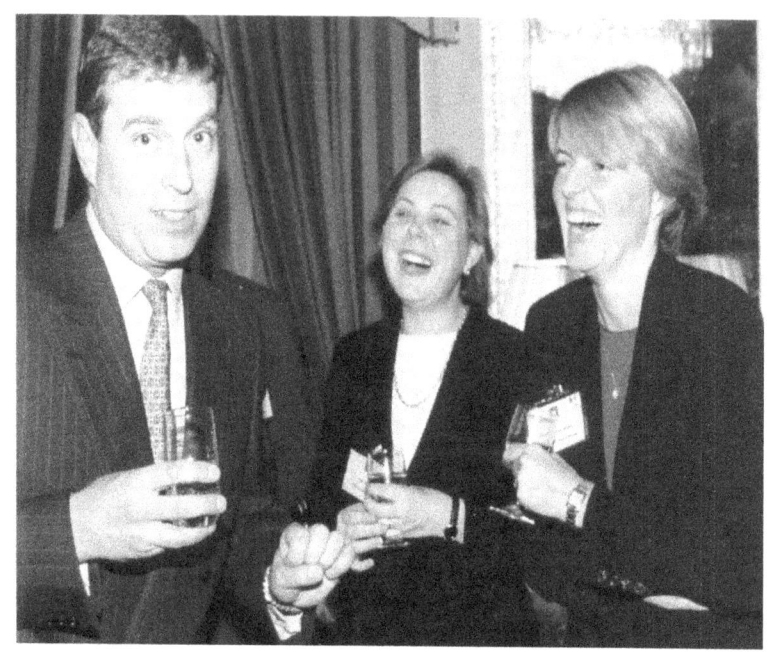

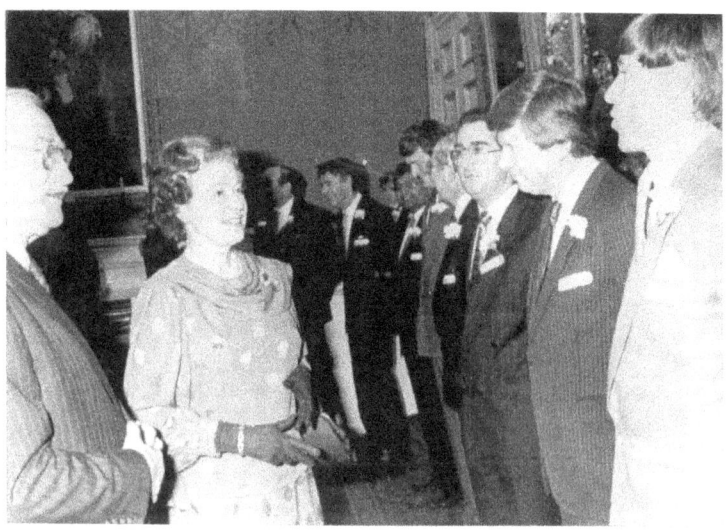

Top: My wife Christine (right) with Prince Andrew, 2005.
Bottom: I am honoured to be presented to Her Majesty the Queen, 1988.

Howard Hodgson

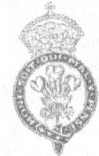

19th August, 1991

Dear Mr. Hodgson,

I am afraid it has taken me a very long time to find your kind letter, for which I heartily apologize, but with so much going on at present I can never get to my letters! I was very touched you should have bothered to write and I have since seen you at Highgrove when I could see for myself that you were a new man! However, my back is now considerably better, owing to endless exercises recommended by the physiotherapist, and I will do anything to avoid an operation!

Yours sincerely,

Charles

A letter received from HRH the Prince of Wales in 1991 following my advice for the Prince to consider a back operation.

The King and Di

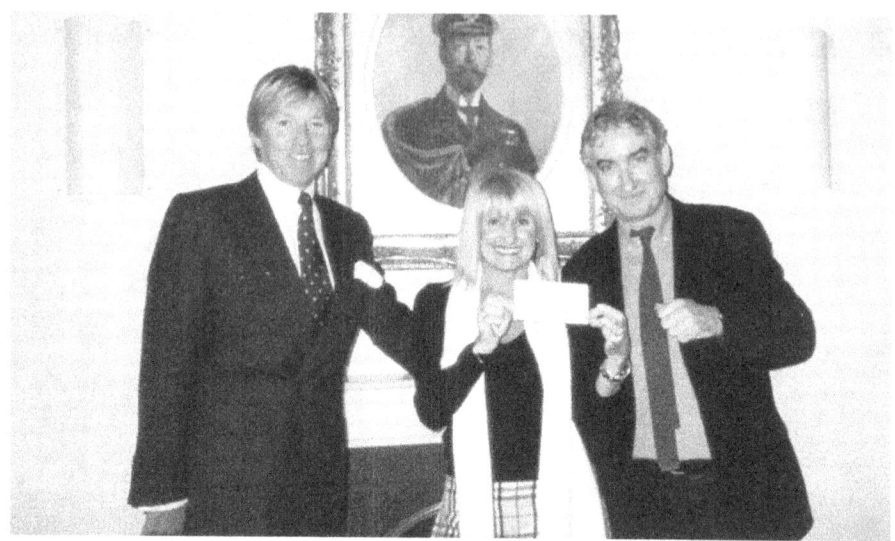

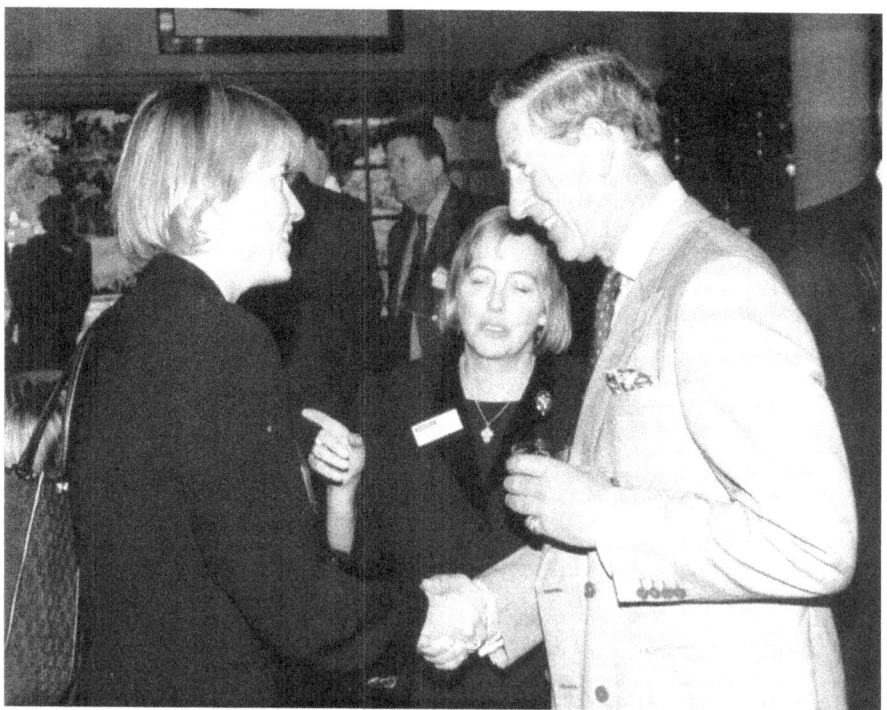

Top: Howard and Marianne Hodgson presenting a cheque from Charles Hodgson Foundation For Children to Tom Shebbeare at the Prince's Trust Headquaters, 2004. Shebbare is a well valued man by Charles.
Bottom: My wife Christine with Julia Cleverdon and Prince Charles, 2003

Howard Hodgson

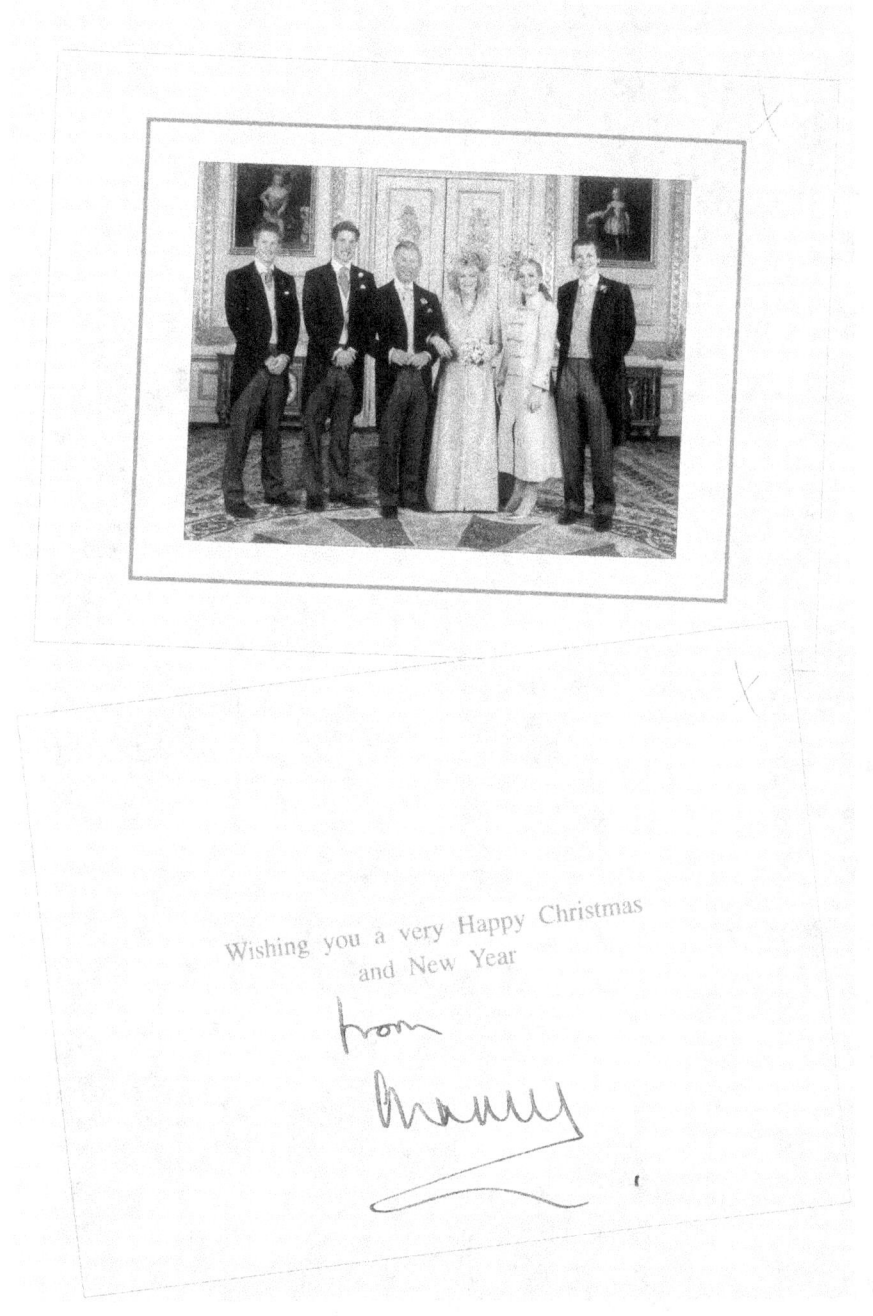

Our card from the Prince of Wales for Christmas 2005.

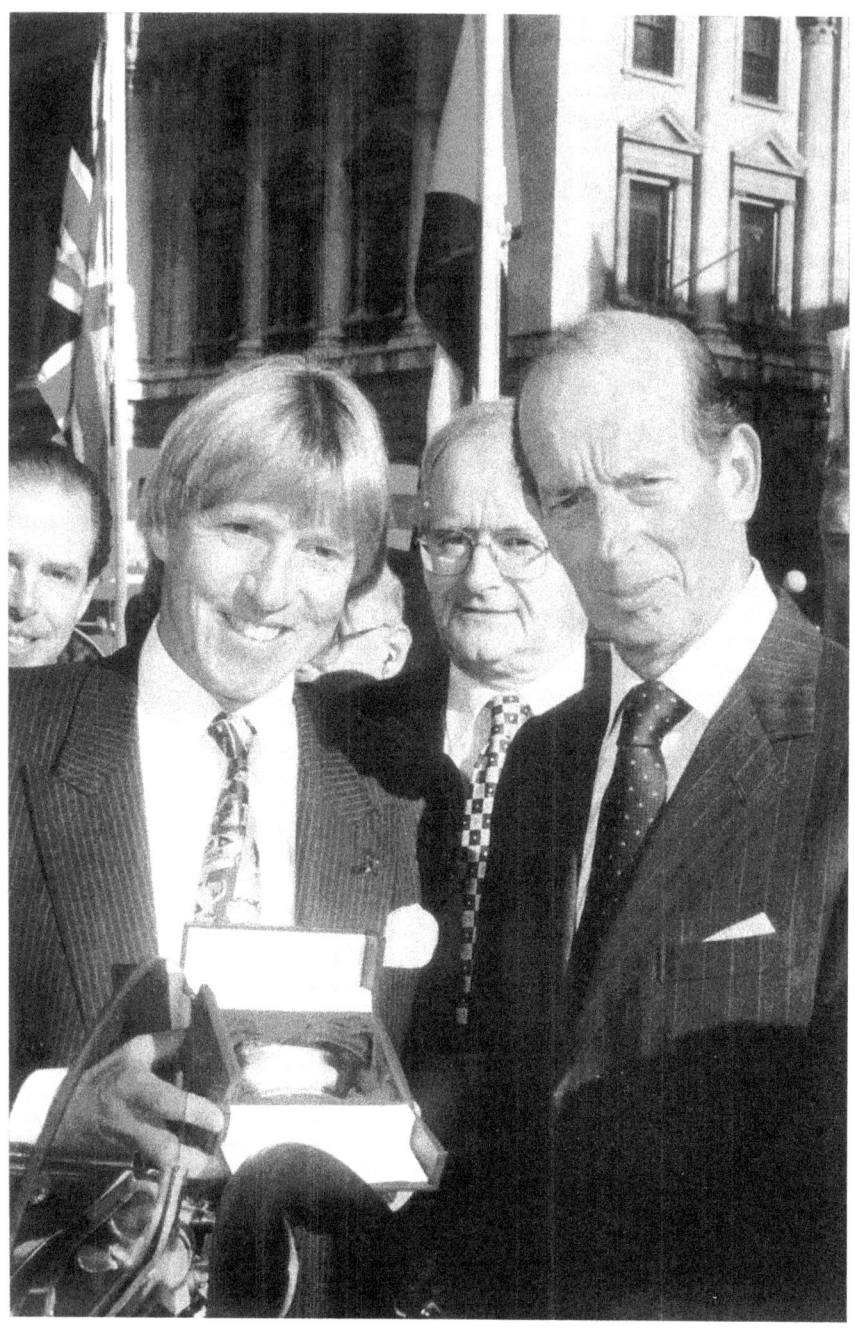

Me with the Duke of Kent at the start of the London to Jordan car rally, 1997.

Bibliography

Below are some of the reference books I have used either as a source of information or to compare with what I have discovered myself.

When it is uncertain who is correct, I usually repeat all versions of events and let the reader decide. I am also generous in mentioning other author's works, including:

Beddell Smith, Sally, *Diana: The Life of a Troubled Princess*, Aurum Press, 1999
Burchill, Julie, *Diana*, Weidenfeld & Nicolson, 1998
Burrell, Paul, *A Royal Duty*, Penguin, 2004
Campbell, Beatrix, *Diana: How Sexual Politics Shook the Monarchy*, The Women's Press Ltd, 1998
Campbell, Lady Colin, *The Real Diana*, Arcadia Books, 2005
Clayton, Tim, and Craig, Phil, *Diana: Story of a Princess*, Simon & Schuster, 2001
Delorm, René, *Diana & Dodi: A Love Story*, Pocket Books, 1998
Graham, Caroline, *Camilla: Her True Story*, Blake Publishing, 2003
Hastings, Max, *Editor: A Memoir*, Pan, 2003
Hewitt, James, *Moving On*, Blake Publishing, 2005
Holden, Anthony, *Charles: A Biography*, Weidenfeld & Nicolson, 1988
Hodgson, Howard, *How to Become Dead Rich*, Pavilion, 1992
Hoskyns, John, *Just in Time: Inside the Thatcher Revolution*, Aurum Press, 2000
Hurd, Douglas, *Memoirs*, Abacus, 2004
Patrick Jephson, Patrick, *Portraits of a Princess: Travels with Diana*, St Martin's Press, 2004
Dimbleby, Jonathan, *The Prince of Wales*, Little, Brown, 1994
Junor, Penny, *Charles: Victim or Villain?*, Harper Collins, 1998
Morgan, Piers, *The Insider*, Ebury Press, 2005
Morton, Andrew, *Diana: Her True Story*, Michael O'Mara, 1992
— *Diana: Her True Story in Her Own Words*, Michael O'Mara, 2003
— *Diana: In Pursuit of Love*, Michael O'Mara, 2004
Rees-Jones, Trevor, *The Bodyguard's Story*, Little, Brown, 2000
Snell, Kate, *Diana: Her Last Love*, Andre Deutsch, 2000
Spoto, Donald, *Dynasty*, Simon & Schuster, 1995

Wharfe, Ken, and Jobson, Robert, *Diana: Closely Guarded Secret*, Michael O'Mara, 2002

Wilson, Christopher, *The Windsor Knot*, Citadel Press, 2003

Index

Aberystwyth 90, 91, 98, 101
Adam, Brian 163
Adeane, Honourable Edward 246
Adler, Mike 571, 572
Afro-Caribbean youth 162, 163
Agincourt 34
Ahrends, Peter 562
Aids, Aids Crisis Trust 343, 363, 398, 398, 403, 444, 523, 571, 572, 589, 599, 600
Aiglon 67, 68, 69
Airlie, Lord 638
Airy, Sir Christopher 393, 491
Albert, Prince 166, 167
Alexander, Professor Christopher 569
Alexandra, Princess, of Kent 36
Alice, Princess 103
Allen, Clive 549
Allibar (racehorse) 207, 239
Allison, Ronald 197
Althorp, Lady Frances *see* Shand Kydd, Frances
Althorp, John, Viscount *see* Spencer, 8th Earl
Althorp House, Northamptonshire 49, 57
American Psychiatric Association Board of Trustees 271
American Red Cross 588
Americans, view of Great Britain xvii, xviii
Andanson, James 627
Anderson, Eric 75, 436
Anderson, Mabel 32
Andrew, Prince 189, 194, 202, 263, 295, 372, 375, 382, 389, 463, 486, 488
Angola 388, 575, 576, 577, 580 581, 584, 588, 59, 598, 604, 607, 619
Angry Brigade 119
Annabel's 418, 420, 547
Anne, Princess 32 41 44, 108, 131, 137, 230, 424, 487, 488, 575
Anne, Queen 48
Annenberg, Walter 143
anorexia nervosa 241, 242, 269, 270, 271

Anson, Charles 463, 553
Archer, Nick 636
Aristocracy 42, 48, 61, 67, 362, 372, 404, 450, 647
Armstrong-Jones, Sarah 238
Arnold, Harry 195, 206, 292
Ashcombe, Baron 130
Asian youth 163-4
Associated Newspapers 475 531, 618, 644-645
Aston Villa Football Club 419
Atkinson, Jane 561, 571, 572, 599, 617
Attlee, Clement 24,323
Australia 137
   Charles at school in 54, 71, 76
   official visits to 80-84, 88 100, 101, 102, 108, 111, 115, 139, 142, 153, 154, 175, 237, 238, 239, 244, 246, 283, 311, 312, 313, 339
Avon, Lord (Anthony Eden) 111
Aylard, Richard 385, 476, 487, 491, 515, 525, 553, 554, 558

Bailey, Christian 89
Baldwin, Stanley 29
Balmoral 40 41, 42, 76 , 82 , 89 , 113 , 116 , 117 , 132 , 134 , 138, 139, 144, 170, 199, 200, 201, 202, 204, 207, 214, 244, 266 267, 268, 274, 292, 306, 373, 374, 431, 485, 486, 511, 602, 606, 610, 632, 639, 640, 641
Barber, Anthony (later Lord) 104
Barnes, Barbara 297, 440 617
Barrow Green Court, Oxted 603
Barry, Stephen 207, 253,,307
Bartholomew, Carolyn 396, 451, 467, 470, 500, 617
Bartholomew, William 467
Bashir, Martin 549
Bastille Day 608
BBC 34, 170, 221, 230, 260.420, 454, 548, 549, 550, 551, 554 555, 575, 578, 594, 650
BDP *see* borderline personality disorder 271, 272, 273, 299, 300, 301, 312, 367, 369, 499, 519
Beatles 64, 65, 72, 206, 311, 324, 659
Beatrice, Princess 508
Beaufort, Duke of 103

Beaufort Hunt 207-208, 305
Beck, Peter 42
Beckham, David 28
Beckwith-Smith, Anne 281, 309, 380, 385, 554
Benn, Anthony Wedgwood 218
Benson, Ross 70, 536, 544
Berni, Mara and Lorenzo 396
Berry, Simon 190
Bevan, Anthony 416
Birmingham 160, 220, 222, 303, 320, 336, 419
BITC *see* Business in the Community
Black Prince 166
Blair, Cherie 583
Blair, Tony 8, 15, 105, 333, 348, 360, 361, 364, 458, 582, 583, 588, 589, 590, 598, 604, 629, 638, 646, 650, 654
  attitude to Diana 397, 647-8, 700
  at death of Diana 713, 722
Blarney Castle 450
BLF *see* Business Leaders Forum
Bolland, Mark 632, 635, 636, 639, 650
Bond, Jennie 578
Bonnington, HMS 149
borderline personality disorder (BPD) 290-3, 322-5, 337, 401, 533, 551, 591, 271, 272, 273, 299, 300, 301, 312, 367, 369, 499, 519
Bosnia 506, 575, 595, 618
Boston, Massachusetts 331, 335
Bow Group 350
Bowker, Lady Elsa 616, 622
Bowler, Hamoush 536
Boyd, William 70, 71
Brabourne, Lady (mother) 181
Brenna, Mario 612, 613, 621
Britain:
  after Second World War 49-51
  changes in xviii-xix, 734
  economy 49-51, 95, 96, 97-8, 99-101, 229-30, 232-4, 327-9, 349-51, 360, 363-4, 384, 388, 389-91, 729-30
  in First World War 4
  life in 727-30

meritocracy 352-3
patriotism in 731-2
post-war problems 4-6
in Second World War 3
values 662-3
Britain on the Couch 643
Britannia, Royal Yacht 37, 181, 200 ,309 ,433
British Coal 351
British Medical Association 298
British Sub Aqua Club 154
Broadlands 125, 129, 148, 201, 249, 264
Brocket, Charles, Lord 378-79
Brooke, Peter 493
Brown, Carolan 504, 523-24, 539, 543
Brown, Gordon 564, 590
Brown, Harold 497
Brown, Tina 319 ,Brundtland Report 352
Bryan, John 487
Buckingham Palace, residence at 13, 16, 23, 251-2, 254-5, 268, 272
bulimia 240-42, 265, 268-71, 273, 275, 283-84, 368, 395, 451, 455-56, 479, 504
Burchill, Julie 228
Burrell, Paul 315, 362, 363, 406, 408, 432, 438, 480, 490, 497, 585 638, 662
Burrell, Mrs Paul 363
Business in the Community (BITC) 328, 329, 331, 333-39, 343-45,360, 496, 515, 570, 591
Business in the Environment 591
Business Leaders Forum (BLF) 340, 591
Butler, Lord Rab 85, 86 87, 101
Buxton, James 85

Caernarfon Castle 93
Callaghan, James 154, 218, 221, 222
Cambridge University 153
Cameron, Lady Cecil 251
Campbell, Beatrix 228

Campbell, Lady Colin 58, 193, 194, 202, 288, 316, 382, 391, 405, 461, 462, 463, 486, 502, 512, 513, 525, 529, 537, 538, 542, 553, 560, 617, 622, 640
Canada, visits to 33, 108, 283, 309, 433, 575, 590, 593
Cannes Film Festival 380
Cardiff 45, 89, 95, 98, 419
Carling, Julia 539-41, 544, 553, 617
Carling, Will 538, 539
Cartland, Barbara 55, 262
CBI 221
CBS 260
Ceausescu, President 346, 347
Centrepoint 571
Chalker, Lynda 505
Channel 4 TV 549, 640
Charles I 655
Charles II xv, 15, 48, 224, 225, 655
Charles, Prince:
  academic ability 64-5, 73-4, 93
  acting 63-4, 69, 80-1
  affairs 209, 218-19
  affairs with Camilla 248, 270, 314, 535, 717
    Diana's lies and delusions about 218, 243, 248, 265-7, 269-70, 305, 310, 313, 339, 343, 400, 446-7, 482, 492, 506, 610
    first affair 126-9
    nicknames 265, 266
    second affair 129-30, 203, 209
    third affair 208, 343, 410, 439-40, 442, 443-4, 490, 560-7, 574, 655
  affairs of state 347-97
  appearance 47
  artistic ability 72
  in Australia 65-71, 73
  author's personal relationship with 455-67
  as baby 7
  baptism 6
  becomes Prince of Wales 28-9
  birth 3, 6-7, 12-13
  birthday party for Camilla 675

character 18, 29, 91, 103, 140-1
'cherry brandy' incident 62
childhood 13-17, 18-30
comparison with Edward VIII 9-10
concern for energy conservation 381-3
concern for environment 381-3, 385-9, 631
controversial interests 92-3
counsellor of state 78
and death of Djana 700-1, 706, 708-16, 719, 721, 722, 726
dedication 18
depression 437-9
described as visionary 570
desire for family life 247
developing relationship with Diana 204-28, 252-3
divorce 614, 615-21
   improved relationship after 648, 665, 666, 667-8
early impressions of Diana 204-5
education 19, 21-3, 25-30, 49, 53-74, 94
as employer 395-6
engagement to Camilla 626, 739-40
engagement to D 234-8, 248-75
feelings of inadequacy 63
first meeting with Camilla 126
first meeting with Diana 46-7, 49
girlfriends 46-7, 48, 124-7, 138, 178-82, 192-3, 202-3, 257-60, 281
health 22
hit by boomerang 69
homosexuality lies 616-17
honeymoon with Diana 281-6
in House of Lords 92
investiture as Prince of Wales 81, 84-90
journals 118, 119, 142, 143-4, 144, 174
knight of the garter 79
lack of jealous feelings in 257
letters 120, 506-7
   from school 59, 60-1, 64, 65
love of acting 29
love for Camilla 126-9
love of literature 94, 281-2

love of siblings 246-7
married life with D 299-326, 329-46, 399-403, 404-54, 437-8, 440-8, 491, 520-1, 526-7, 529
medals 143
memory of grandfather 15
military career 47, 105-20, 128, 131-2, 133-8, 140-51, 153
  in Fleet Air Arm 145-6
  RAF training at Cranwell 109-12
  in Royal Navy 105-7, 112-20, 128, 131-2, 133-8, 140-51, 153
musical ability 62-3, 72-3
official events in year 659-60
overseas tours 79, 93, 101-5, 251, 337, 394, 441, 492-4, 539-42
parachute jumps 110-11
parascending 135
paying taxes 545
people's support for 567
as pilot 109-10, 145-6
political interests 76-7, 156-7
presents to 27
proposal to D 228
radio interview 81-2
relationship with father 14, 18-59, 89, 90, 94, 106-7, 149, 530
relationship with grandmother 14, 18, 19, 63, 94, 226
relationship with media 47, 48, 62, 78, 80-1, 333-4, 339, 358, 371, 387, 487, 491, 572, 574-6, 726
relationship with mother 13, 14, 437
relationship with sons 119-20, 319-21, 340, 400, 437, 442, 464-5, 473, 475-7, 555, 560, 670, 724, 726, 741
religion and mysticism 60, 70, 94, 171-7, 394
  interest in Islam 660-3
representing Queen 9, 78, 104, 135-6, 659
role 735-6, 737-8
rows with D 267, 283-4, 285, 293
rural pursuits 24
sailing 61
search for purpose 153-63
search for wife 126-7, 130-1, 139-40, 159, 179-82, 206-7, 209
  requirements 206-7, 244-5
self-confidence 67-8, 71, 75, 90, 102, 136, 138, 147-8, 437

self-deprecation 17-18, 63, 91, 117
self-pity 177, 655, 708
selfishness 183-4, 200, 212, 214, 301
sense of humour 93
separation from D 530-48
shyness 18, 26, 76
skiing, sport, accident 450-3
sport 29, 30, 61, 71, 79, 104
   polo 47, 79, 92, 104, 135, 203-4, 438, 442-3, 485, 493
   skiing 484
   swimming 61
   wrestling and boxing 27
state functions 92
support for alternative medicine 321
support for 'loony' ideas 321-2
temper 91, 113, 135, 170-1, 212, 294, 333
titles 16, 28-9
tonsilectomy 22-3
on tour with parents 19-21
TV interview 87
TV programme on life 568-72, 574-6
unfashionable ideas 352-3
university 74-8, 80-1
views on architecture 623-6, 657-8
views on education 626-32
views of marriage 130-1, 244-6
wedding to Camilla 741
wedding to D 275-81
   fireworks preceding 270-1
   memorabilia 265
work with young people, unemployed and inner cities 160-7, 318, 351-2, 354-77, 491, 568-9, 631, 655-7
   see also Prince's Trust; Prince's Youth Business Trust
workload 394-5

Charles and Diana: Portrait of a Marriage 477
Charles: Victim or Villain 54, 229, 512
Charteris, Lord 530
Cheam School, Berkshire 42, 286
Checketts, David 77, 149

Checketts family 79
Chelsea Harbour club *see* Harbour Club 495, 539, 540, 542, 543, 544, 573
Chequers 583
Chew, Robert 70, 82
Chipp, David 471
Chirac, President Jacques 637
Chopp, Nicola 376, 377, 378
Christian, Fletcher 15, 228
Church of England: 40, 72, 76, 102, 131, 169, 172, 222, 224, 232, 510
  admission to 26
Churchill, Lord Randolph 42
Churchill, Winston 17, 23, 28, 30, 58
Churchill, HMS 123
Citizens Service 339
Civil List 166, 494
Civil War 48, 655
Clarence House 31, 207, 237, 240, 244, 253, 259, 260, 601, 647
Clarke, Kenneth 567
Clarke, Mary 186
Classiebawn Castle 181
Clayton, Tim 61, 209
Clegg Commission 222
Cleverdon, Julia 496
Clifford, Max 502-503
Clinton, Bill 15, 583
Co-operative Wholesale Society 601
Coal Board 320-321
Cojean, Annick 588
Colborne, Michael 168, 238, 246, 247, 250, 251, 256, 274, 284, 308, 309, 399, 617
College of Heralds 47
Collins, Phil 163
Colthurst, James 190, 227, 450, 455, 462, 500, 617
Colville, Sir Richard 38
Combermere Barracks, Windsor 393
Commission on Social Justice 339, 590
Commonwealth 26, 28, 29, 33, 34, 37, 45, 111, 113, 148, 155, 236, 254, 420

Community Service by Offenders 159
Community Venture 338-9
Conservative government 28, 105-6, 159, 217-9, 221, 226, 322, 329, 457, 564-5, 582, 598
Conservative Party 103, 219, 220, 352, 588, 653
Constantine, King, of Greece 475
Cook, Robin 583
Cornish, Francis 246, 256
Cornwall, Duchy of 154, 158, 165, 563, 592
Costner, Kevin 604
Cowes Regatta 200
Craig, Phil 61
Craig-Harvey, Lucinda 190
Cranwell 113-5
Crawford, Geoffrey 526
crime 25, 159, 161, 254, 327, 515, 582, 596, 652
Cripps, Sir Stafford 24
Crockard, Mr 417, 420
Cruise, Tom 647

Dagley, Evelyn 308
Daily Express 502, 644, 645
Daily Mail 155, 158, 173, 216, 229, 317, 341, 374, 378, 408, 434, 443, 451, 459, 463, 464, 479, 486, 522, 525, 527, 531, 534, 535, 536, 541, 542, 545, 547, 573, 583, 586, 587 614, 643, 644, 662
Daily Mirror 213, 249, 253, 293, 408, 467, 490, 508, 645, 659, 662
Daily Star 205, 292, 318, 467
Daily Telegraph 224, 249, 523, 565
Dalton, Hugh 25
Daly, Barbara 259
Darenth Park 58
Dartmouth, Raine, Countess of *see* Spencer, Raine
Dartmouth, Royal Naval College 84, 117
David, Prince *see* Edward VIII
Davies, Dr Michael 273, 534
Davies, Steve 386
de Gaulle, Charles, funeral 111
de Pass, Commander Robert 195
Dear, Geoffrey 336

Debrett's Peerage 224
Deedes, Bill 574
Demarchelier, Patrick 469, 493
Dempster, Nigel 155, 156, 216, 317
devaluation 24, 64, 90
Devorik, Roberto 687
Diana, Princess of Wales (formerly Lady Diana Spencer) xvi-xvii, 140
  abortion 594
  affairs:
    after divorce 678-88, 690, 691-6
    before marriage 201, 202
    during marriage 243, 343, 401, 402-3, 405, 406-11, 415, 416-19, 425-35, 442-4, 448-50, 491-2, 498-9, 527-8, 531-5, 561, 579, 592-8, 600-6, 609
  anti-landmines work 424, 637-45, 648, 653, 665, 688
  attempts to change accession 474-5, 583-4, 606, 611, 612
  attitude to Thatcher 355-6
  author's encounters with 467-70
  background 32, 263
  at Balmoral 23
  birth 35
  birth of sons 319-21, 339, 340, 342, 407, 419, 447
  boyfriends 201, 202
  bullying others 40
  Charles as hero to 47, 48-9
  car chases 588-9, 695-6
  charitable work 167, 397, 420, 488-90, 580-2, 633-45
  claiming fitness to be C's wife 131
  claims about Camilla 209, 218, 243, 248, 265-7, 269, 269-70, 305, 310, 313, 339, 343, 400, 446-7, 482, 492, 506, 610
  'classless' claims 37
  communication skills 45, 198-9
  comparison with Edward VIII 9-10
  confidante of stepmother 669, 671
  consulting alternative medical practitioners 172, 535, 556, 557, 636
  criticisms of 104, 209-10, 330
  death 696-703, 705-10
    body brought back to England 710-13
    media coverage 716-20

delight in title 42-3
descriptions of C 69, 119
determination to marry C 197, 272
distancing C's friends and staff 329-37
divorce 612, 614, 615-21
   improved relationship after 648, 665, 666, 667-8
early years 31-49
eating disorders 255-6, 283, 286-90, 304, 306, 496-7, 517-18, 556-7, 610, 651
education 40-1, 45-6, 48-9, 59, 191-2, 193, 306-7
effect on men 335
employment 196, 198-200, 201
engagement 234-8, 249-75
at father's death 494
first meeting with C 46-7, 49
flirting 343, 344-5, 417
friendship with Sarah Ferguson 252, 254
funeral 722-4
getting drunk 282
hatred of stepmother 44, 195, 253, 547, 671
helping handicapped 44-5
helping people in crisis 450-3
honeymoon 281-6
image 353-4, 487-8
inaccuracies about 31-2
insecurities 35-6, 258, 265-6
interests 262
jealousies 257-8, 259-60, 265-9, 274, 283, 304, 310, 313, 410, 420, 422, 442, 481, 482-3
lack of discipline 262-3, 268, 589
London apartment 198
losing virginity 195-6
low self-esteem 45-6
making nuisance phone calls 594-5, 611, 666
making threatening phone calls 421-2
married life 299-326, 329-46, 399-403, 404-54, 491, 526-7, 529
medical consultations 292, 294-5, 322

mental problems 41, 42, 46, 213, 236-7, 240, 252, 255-8, 290-3, 300, 322-5, 337, 342-3, 401, 497, 500, 533, 551, 553, 556-7, 591, 598, 611
mood swings 207, 256-7, 260-1, 274, 420-1, 491
musical tastes 434
narcissism 591
obsession with individuals 403-4
official engagements alone 304, 544
official engagements with Charles 299, 302-3, 304, 337, 338, 441, 492-4, 539-42, 553
in operating theatre 603, 611
personality 39-40, 42
pregnancies 299, 304-5, 309-13, 314-17, 319, 339
proposal from Charles 228
public engagements 557-8, 577, 653-4
public infatuation with 302-3, 307, 337, 353-4, 614, 653, 716, 719, 721-2, 725
relationship with Charles 204-38
relationship with Camilla 217-18, 259
relationship with grandmother 37-8
relationship with media 52, 178, 214-16, 222-3, 308, 315-16, 333, 426, 427-8, 436, 450, 477, 490, 492, 493-4, 520, 572, 575, 578-9, 585-92, 662, 690, 717-18, 720-1, 736
  collusion with 473-4, 515, 579, 582, 589, 598, 673-6, 694, 695-6
  obsession with 317, 487-8
  paparazzi 585, 587-9, 591-2, 611, 673, 682-6, 694, 695-6, 706, 717
  TV interview 610-11
relationship with mother 39, 44, 619, 671
relationship with political leaders 647-8
relationship with Queen Mother 216-17, 255, 276, 620
relationship with sons 39, 325-6, 437, 442, 446, 474-86, 511, 522, 543, 550, 614, 675
retiring from public life 580-2, 584-5
returning to public life 598
rows 283-4, 285, 293, 309-12, 344
royal connections 263
Royal Family shocked by 536
royal role for 306
search for career 193, 194, 196

search for husband 193-4
self-justification 39
selling dresses for charity 654
separation 530-48
  agreement 582-3
skiing 196-7, 451
stripped of HRH title 619-20
"suicide" attempts 309-12, 337, 402, 416, 502, 512, 553, 557, 610
suspicious nature 300
temper and tantrums 41, 260-1, 274, 284, 285, 307, 313, 332-3, 421
treatment of staff 330, 422-5
trying to control C 329-30
TV interviews 87, 607-14, 666
two sides of nature 200-2, 268, 402-3, 644-5
unsuitability to be C's wife 220-1, 274-5
vengeful nature 201-2, 583-4
visit to astrologer 521
voting for abolition of monarchy 326
wedding 275-81
  fireworks preceding 270-1
  memorabilia 265
wish to be roving ambassador 636-7, 647-8, 676

Diana: Her New Life 474
Diana: Her True Story 19, 209, 227, 452, 459, 521, 570
Diana: Her True Story - In Her Own Words 463
Diana: In Pursuit of Love 229, 231, 452, 639
Diana Memorial Fund 385, 649
Diana in Private: The Princess Nobody Knows 461
Diana: Story of a Princess 61, 229
Dimbleby, Jonathan 30, 33, 95, 229, 265, 288, 425, 516, 520, 640
Dimbleby, Richard 34, 36
Dole, Elizabeth 588
Donovan, Terence 469
Dorchester 361, 563
Dors, Diana 649
Douglas-Home, Sir Alec 109
Dourneau, Philippe 623
Dryden Society 89
Duchy of Cornwall *see* Cornwall, Duchy of

Duchy Originals 593
Dunne, Philip 389, 391, 410, 453

Earth in Balance (film) 354
Eating Disorders Association 469
Ebbw Vale 97, 107
Edinburgh, Duke of *see* Philip, Prince
education and business partnerships 335-6
Edward III 166
Edward VI 40
Edward VII 27, 130, 133, 153, 166, 233
Edward VIII (later David, Duke of Windsor) 28, 30, 33, 125, 126, 127, 153, 179, 181, 232, 233, 258, 526, 618, 621
Edward, Prince 49
Edwards, Arthur 195, 205, 206, 289, 292, 312, 516
Edwards, Bob 212, 216
Eleuthera 135, 179, 180, 292
Elizabeth I 15, 656
Elizabeth II (formerly Princess):
   accession to throne 25, 26, 50
   agreeing to Andrew and Sarah's separation 510
   'annus horribilis' speech 545
   attending Earl Spencer's wedding 35
   attitude to Diana 314, 316, 330, 715-16
   attitude to Duke of Windsor 121, 123
   Commonwealth tours 15, 19-20
   coronation 5, 17
   creates Charles Prince of Wales 28-9
   on Charles's education 21
   at Charles's investiture 87-8
   at Charles's wedding to Diana 276, 279
   and death of Diana 708-9, 710, 713, 714-15, 717, 720, 721, 722
   doubts on Charles's marriage 226
   Diana's opinion of 550
   godson 263
   and grandchildren 319
   household 34
   marriage 11-12
   and media 223, 308

as mother 13-14
organising choice of university for C 74-5
overseas tours 93
paying taxes 545
receptions before C's wedding 268-9
refusal to interfere in C's marriage 445, 500
requesting C and D divorce 614, 615
Silver Jubilee 158
taking action over C's marriage 529-30, 535
taking C to school 25
Elizabeth, Queen (later Queen Mother) 72, 710
attending Earl Spencer's wedding 35
attitude to Duke of Windsor 14-15, 121, 122, 124
attitude to Mountbatten 106
birthday celebrations, 70th 95-6
at C's wedding to D 276, 279
marriage 246
prank 87
relationship with C 14, 18, 19, 63, 94
relationship with D 216-17, 255, 276, 620
in wartime 3
Elliott, Commander 151
Ellis, 'Deadly' Doug 419
Elton John AIDS Foundation 599
Emanuel, David and Liz 259
Emily 372
English, Sir David 434, 527, 531
English Heritage 592
English National Ballet 571
environment 7, 31, 42, 70, 89, 100, 154, 159, 164, 167, 169, 190, 237, 324, 332, 339, 340, 346, 347, 349, 350, 351, 352, 354, 355, 356, 360, 361, 364, 434, 442, 446, 507, 568, 569, 570, 572, 591, 592, 594, 658
Eton 50, 66, 68, 75, 436, 437, 535, 585, 587, 588, 599
Eugenie, Princess 461
European Economic Community (European Common Market) 109, 154
Everett, Oliver 246, 307, 385, 617
Expo '70 101

Falklands War 122, 296, 352

Farrer & Co. 558
Fayed, Dodi 534, 535, 547, 623, 643
Fayed family 547, 604, 606
Fellowes, Robert 186, 189, 297, 375, 439, 468, 470, 476, 478, 530, 635, 636, 637, 640, 641
Ferguson, Sarah *see* York, Duchess of
Fermoy, Lord 49
Fiji, visit to 110, 145, 172
Filderman, Janet 297, 316, 473, 504
Financial Times 106, 596
Fincher, Jayne 249, 256, 317, 433, 529
First magazine 359
Fisher, Kelly 610
Fitzgerald, Chryssie 504
Flannery, Bernie 497
Fleet Air Arm 60, 122, 146
food rationing 24-5
Foot, Michael 97, 107, 590
Foreign Office 109, 110, 119, 307, 346, 372, 375, 575, 595
Four Seasons restaurant, New York 589
Fowler, Norman 335
Fox, HMS 136
Frank, Debbie 607
Fraser, Lady Antonia 260
Fraser, Jason 612, 618, 621
Free Wales Army 90
Frescobaldi, Marchesa Bona 371
Frost, Sir David 549

Gailey, Dr 437
Galtieri, General 320
Gandhi, Mahatma, centenary of birth 99
Gardener, Jim 343
Garnett, Thomas 76
Gavin, Kent 468
General Electricity Generating Board 354
George I 48
George III 160
George IV 153

George V 27, 48, 160, 655
George VI 23, 29, 30, 33, 34, 49, 233, 295
George, Prince, of Denmark 202
George, Richard 418, 422
George, Susan 209
Ghana, President of 249
Gibbons, Michael 585, 587, 599, 617
Gilbey, James 193, 194, 228, 366, 392, 453, 465, 478, 483, 484, 501, 508, 617
Glenconner, Lord 440
Gloucester, Duke and Duchess of 297
Goldsmith, Lady Annabel 409, 619, 622
Goldsmith, Sir James 426
Good Morning America 317
Goodman, Lord 481
Goons 80, 83, 115, 129, 160, 437
Gordonstoun 46, 62, 66-72, 74, 76, 77, 78, 80-85, 91, 101, 149, 152, 159, 167, 186, 197, 199, 338, 399, 436
Graham, Katherine 588
Granville, Lady 26
Great Ormond Street Children's Hospital 571
Green, Donald 73
Green Belt 352
Green Party 353
Grosvenor, Gerald 62
Guardian 38, 344, 431
Guinness, Sabrina 174
Guinness Housing Trust 592
Gulf States 595
Gulf Wars 110
Gummer, John 358

Hackney, Rod 341
Hahn, Dr Kurt 68
Haines, Joe 108
Hair 65
Halifax, regeneration scheme 331, 332
Hall, Jerry 440
Halo Trust 579

Hamilton, Willie 226
Handsworth 160-1, 336
Hanks, Tom 7647
Hanson, Brian 570
Harbour Club, Chelsea 539
Harris, Kenneth 231
Harrods 191, 465, 601, 603, 610, 615, 621, 636
Harry (Henry), Prince:
   birth 339, 340, 407, 419, 447, 741
   as child 461, 464-6
   and death of mother 709, 711, 720, 722
   holiday with mother 670, 671-2, 673-5, 678, 679
   parentage 448, 555
   polo 485
   promoted as next monarch 475
   relationship with father 119-20, 319-21, 340, 400, 437, 442, 464-5, 473, 475-7, 555, 560, 670, 724, 726, 741
   relationship with mother 39, 325-6, 437, 442, 446, 474-86, 550, 614
Harvey, Glenn 532
Haskins, Chris 335
Hastings, Max 9, 158, 464, 470, 515, 519, 523, 551
Hatchards 465
Headway 526
Healey, Denis 57, 16, 218, 335
Heart of the Hunter 170
Heath, Edward 78, 86, 95-6, 97-8, 99, 101, 103, 104, 160, 229, 231, 232, 347, 348, 390, 646
Hello! 242, 281, 417, 671, 737
Help the Aged 467-8, 577, 633
Henney, Sandy 612, 705, 713, 714, 716
Henry V 16
Henry V (Shakespeare) 63-4
Henry VII (Henry Tudor) xv, xvi, 32
Henry VIII xvi, 23, 237, 733
Herbert, Harry, 17th Earl of Pembroke 202, 406-7, 433
Hermes, HMS 145-6
Hermione, HMS 118
Heseltine, Sir William 84, 85, 86, 254

Hewitt, James 415, 419, 427, 428-31, 432-5, 440, 442-3, 446, 481, 491, 498-9, 506, 528, 534-5, 600, 604, 610, 612, 687, 692
Higgins, Stuart 514-15, 531, 539, 650
Higgs, John 396
Highgrove 217, 320, 396, 419, 421, 438, 442, 461-3, 465-6, 468, 485, 658, 675
Hill House 22
HIll-Norton, Sir Peter 113
Hirohito, Emperor 93
History of King Richard III xvi
Hitchens, Christopher 489, 645
Hoare, Diane (née Waldner) 592, 594, 598, 602, 611, 687
Hoare, Oliver 419, 448, 491, 499, 579, 592-4, 595, 606, 686, 687
Hodge, Barry 594
Hodgson, Christine 468-9
Hodgson Holdings plc 458, 462-3, 467, 669
Holden, Anthony 277, 345, 549-51, 560, 613
Holdgate, Sir Martin 385
Hollywood xvii
Holt, Harold 78
Holyhead 548
Hong Kong 93, 542, 648
Hope, Bob 142
Hoskyns, Sir John 327-8
House of Commons 456
House of Fraser 669
House of Lords 92
Howard, Michael 655
Howard, Philip 627
Howe, Sir Geoffrey 327, 328, 378
Humphrys, John 608
Hunter, Gary 697
Hussein, Saddam 660-1
Hussey, Marmaduke 607
Hussey, Lady Susan 254, 262, 271, 272, 607, 687
Hutchins, Chris 718
Hyde, Anne 217
Hyde Park Barracks 430-1

ICI 233
I'm a Celebrity Get Me Out of Here 413
Independent 627
India 492-3
Ingham, Bernard 718
Inner City Aid 371-4
Inner-City Action 657
inner-city 'compacts' 364-5
Insider 648
Institut Alpin Videmanette 191-2, 193
International Red Cross 558, 598, 633, 637
Invincible, HMS 478-9
IRA 108, 114, 185-6, 223, 559
Islam 660-3
ITN 518
ITV 512, 607

Jackson, Michael 609, 610
Jagger, Mick 165, 484, 736
James I 3, 32
James II 217, 732
James, Oliver 718
Janvrin, Sir Robin 525, 705, 709, 710
Japan, official visit to 93
Jay, Margaret 488-9, 490
Jay, Sir Michael 705
Jay, Sylvia 712
Jenkins, Roy 95
Jenkins, Simon 658, 719
Jephson, Patrick 49, 241-2, 343-4, 421, 435-6, 488, 492, 497, 507-8, 525, 537-8, 544, 557, 558, 580, 584, 598, 612-13, 615, 617, 680, 687
John, Elton 165, 450, 460, 598, 667-8, 680, 687, 723, 725, 736
Johns, Dick 109
Johnson, Lyndon 78, 96
Johnson, Paul 719
Johnstone, Sir Johnnie 254, 272
Joint Jubilee Trusts 155
Jones, Hywel 76-7
Jones, Jack 100-1

Jonikal (motor yacht) 670, 672, 676, 676-9, 680-5, 684-5, 686-7
Joseph, Sir Keith 231-2
Juan Carlos, King, of Spain 417-18, 680, 691
Julius, Anthony 618
Jung, Carl 174, 175
Junor, Penny 40, 219, 220, 242, 244, 250, 409-10, 418, 421, 526, 565, 713-14
Jupiter, HMS 137, 138, 142-4

Kalahari Desert 172-4
Kay, Richard 201, 477, 586, 590-2, 599, 605, 606, 636, 681, 686-7, 690, 692-3
Kennedy, John, Jnr 649
Kennedy, Nigel 460
Kensington Palace 309, 320-1, 365, 407-9, 411, 418-19, 421, 427, 428, 429, 433, 442, 468, 528, 547, 593, 596, 597, 610, 618, 636, 648, 725
Kent, Duke of 263
Kenya 174
Keppel, Alice 126, 130
Kerr, Lady Cecily 178
Keswick, Lady Susan 267
Khalid, King of Saudi Arabia 264
Khan, Hasnat 593, 601-6, 609, 649, 654, 678, 681, 685, 686, 687-8, 689, 691, 723
Khan, Imran 468, 604
Khan, Jawad 689, 693
Khan, Jemima 468, 605
Kidman, Nicole 723
Kinnock, Neil 504-5, 646, 655
Kissinger, Henry 614
Klosters 450-3, 484-5
Knatchbull, Amanda 133, 139-40, 179-82, 184, 185, 196, 203, 207, 210, 225, 247, 263, 273
Knatchbull, Nicholas 185
Knatchbull, Timothy 185
Knevitt, Charles 372
Knight, Andrew 511, 518, 519-20, 524, 526, 532, 534-5
Knopfler, Mark 165
Korea 539-42, 553

Korean War 50
Krier, Leon 625, 632

Labour government 4, 5, 50-1, 81, 95, 98-101, 161, 162, 229-30, 231,
  234, 347, 380, 728
Labour Party 504-5, 646, 655
Lacroiz, Christian 723
Lagerfeld, Karl 723
Lalvani, Gulu 605, 647, 688
Lamb, Christina 642-3, 644
Lamport, Stephen 705-6, 711
landmines 397, 424, 637-45, 648, 665, 688
Lanesborough Hotel, Knightsbridge 482-3
Last Word 649
Latsis, John 535
Lawson, Dominic 688
Lawson, Nigel 389-90, 391
Lech, Austria 494
Lee-Potter, Lee 718
Legge-Bourke, Alexandra (Tiggy) 421-2, 442, 480-1, 482-3, 598, 611,
  621, 650, 652-3, 666, 670, 675, 687, 711
Lennon, John 51, 352, 729, 736
Lennox, Ken 214-15, 315-16, 515-16
Leprosy Mission 577, 634
Leslie, Ann 76
Levertons (funeral directors) 712
Lewis, Sergeant Ron 253
Lightbody, Helen 13, 24
Lindsay, Alice 453
Lindsay, Hugh 450, 452, 453
Lindsay, Sarah 453
Linley, David, Viscount 252
Liverpool 516, 567
Liverpool, Lord 95
Lloyd George, David 351
London:
  Mansion House 624
  Ménage à Trois restaurant 425
  Paternoster Square 624, 657

swinging capital 52
London Stock Exchange 99, 349
Lost World of the Kalahari 172-3
'love-in' of 60s 51
Ludgrove school 479
Ludlow Races 217
Luxemburg, Duke of 430
Lyle, Felix 521, 552

Macbeth (Shakespeare) 64
McCartney, Paul 9, 51, 165, 736
McCorkindale, Simon 219
Macdonald, Sir Roderick 119
McGlashan, Dr Allan 322
McGregor, Ian 348, 349
McGregor, Lord 513, 518-19, 520, 523
McKay, Lord 519
Mackie, Philip 525, 612
Macmillan, Harold 5, 104, 105
Macmillan Nurses 461
McNee, Sir David 163
Mail on Sunday 590
Mailliez, Dr 706, 707
Major, John 363, 393, 504-5, 530, 547, 558, 583, 646, 647, 655, 657-8, 668
Malibu, California 692
Malta 19-21, 79
Mandelson, Peter 512, 666
Mangold, Tom 608
Mannakee, Barry 403, 407-17, 418, 425, 427, 428, 429, 430, 433-4, 442, 446, 491, 499, 701
Manners, Lady Theresa 204
Mansfield, Jayne 725
Margaret, Princess 276, 320, 484, 537, 714, 733
Margaret, Princess, of Hesse and the Rhine 258, 331, 342, 620
Marks, Lana 324, 689, 693
Marks, Dr Neville 324
Mary I xv, 733
Mary, Queen (wife of George V) 122

Mary Rose 394, 631-2
Mary Rose Trust 631-2
Mass Observation 12
Max, Prince, of Baden 56
Maxwell, Robert 224
Mazzucchelli, Roberto 672
media 52, 66
  campaign with 85
  coverage of D's death 716-20
  C's relationship with 47, 48, 62, 78, 80-1, 333-4, 339, 358, 371, 387, 487, 491, 572, 574-6, 726
  D's relationship with 52, 178, 214-16, 222-3, 308, 315-16, 333, 426, 427-8, 436, 450, 477, 490, 492, 493-4, 520, 572, 575, 578-9, 585-92, 662, 690, 717-18, 720-1, 736
    D's obsession with 317, 487-8
    paparazzi 585, 587-9, 591-2, 611, 673, 682-6, 694, 695-6, 706, 717
  relationship with 144-5, 178-9
Mellor, David 657
Ménage à Trois restaurant 425
Mendham, Victoria 423-5, 621, 644, 666, 687
Menzies, Kate 427, 433
Menzies, Sir Robert 65
MI5 415, 565, 609
MI6 415, 690, 700
Michael, Prince, of Kent 19
Michael, George 165, 723
Middle East 377
Milligan, Spike 69
Minerva, HMS 128, 132, 135, 136, 137, 247
Mischon de Reya 618
Mitchell, Dr David 322
Mitterand, François 544
monarchy 728-36
  attitude to 3, 8, 12, 17, 728-9
  cost of 730
  democracy and 730-1
  dissatisfaction with 545-6
  fairy tale of 733-4
  functions 237, 261, 274

as head of state 731
　　losing mystique 733
　　powers of 732
　　threat to 10, 614
　　tourism and 732
　　votes for abolition of 326
Monckton, Christopher 688
Monckton, Rosa 201, 553, 686-7, 688-9, 691, 693
Monckton, Sir Walter 49, 688
Le Monde 653, 676
Monroe, Marilyn 725
Monteil, Martine 698
Mooney, Bel 326, 480
Moore, Sir Philip 155, 217
More, Sir Thomas xvi
Morgan, Piers 447-8, 648, 650-3, 687, 740
Morrison, Peter 381-2
Morton, Andrew 239-44, 245, 265, 301, 316, 345, 368, 400, 410, 423, 453, 474, 494, 494-5, 497-8, 503, 509-11, 516, 521, 522-3, 546, 577, 713-14
　　awards 523
　　C's friends and family reactions to book 529-30
　　D turning against 244, 509, 521, 553, 598, 687
　　D's attitude to 590
　　information from D 35, 41, 219, 239-40, 248, 255, 256, 266, 309-11, 340-1, 342, 343, 397, 400-1, 423, 495, 497, 499-503, 505-8, 536, 539, 571, 666
　　sources xx, 477, 512, 514-15, 715
Mountbatten, Lord Louis 9, 20, 27, 74, 132
　　birthday celebrations 95-6
　　correspondence with C 66-7, 79, 89-90, 117, 118-19
　　death 185-7, 223
　　feelings for Duke of Windsor 121-2, 123-4
　　importance to Royal Family 105-6
　　relationship with C 63, 66-7, 89-90, 94, 105-6, 120-2, 124-5, 137, 138-9, 146-9, 159, 171, 172, 180, 182, 183-5, 186-7, 206
　　in Royal Navy 141
Mountbatten, Philip *see* Philip, Prince, Duke of Edinburgh
Mugabe, Robert 577

Murdoch, Rupert 66, 224, 308, 504, 511, 512-13, 515, 531, 538, 545-6, 574, 577, 589, 599, 614, 669
Museum for Women in the Arts, Washington, DC 653-4
Mustique 484

Nadir, Asil 592
Nadir, Ayesha 592
narcissism 591
Nassau 135-6
National Aids Trust 488-9, 490, 634
National Association of Teachers 629
National Enquirer 528
National Exhibition Centre 160
National Fruit Collection campaign 394
National Heritage Memorial Fund 657
National Lottery 658
National Union of Mineworkers (NUM) 98, 99, 348, 349
National Westminster Bank 99
nationalisation 5, 6
NATO exercises 115-16, 118-19
NBC 277
Neil, Andrew 511, 512, 514, 518, 525, 575, 576, 578
Nepal 558
New Labour 506, 646, 647
New York 654
New York Times 5
New Yorker 654
New Zealand, visits to 93, 337
News International 511, 532, 541
News of the World 293, 535, 594, 601, 602
Newsnight 613
Newspaper Proprietors Association 21
Nicholls, Michael 608
Nixon, Richard 96, 102-3
Norfolk, HMS 113-18, 137-8, 170
Northern Ireland 559
Northfield, Lord 384

Oborn, Sarah 626

O'Brien, Stephen 356-7, 358, 359, 365-7, 373, 375, 377
Observer 375
Officer, Paul 332
Ohshima, Tatsuo 291
'Old Man of Lochnagar' 137
Oldfield, Bruce 430
O'Mara, Michael 501-2, 507, 517, 521
O'Neill, Eva 403
Open University 160
Operation Overlord 710-13
Orbach, Susie 556
organic farming 658-9
Orwell, George 100
O'Sullivan, Gilbert 129

Palmer, Marie-Pierre 39
Palmer, Sonia 406
Palmer-Tomkinson, Charles 208, 450-1
Palmer-Tomkinson, Patty 208, 212, 439, 447, 450-2, 453
Palumbo, Peter 47-8, 264, 399, 522, 610, 613, 623-4, 637
Panorama 45, 326, 584, 607-14, 633, 666, 739
Pantycelyn Hall 82
Panzer, Dr Basil 584
paparazzi 585, 587-9, 591-2, 611, 673, 682-6, 694, 695-6, 706, 717
Papua New Guinea 69-71
Parachute Regiment 111
parascending 135
Paris 544, 680, 691-703
   Chez Benoît 694
   Pitié-Salpêtrière Hospital 707-8
   Ritz Hotel 680, 692-3, 694, 694-5, 701
Paris Match 80, 544
Park House, Sandringham 34
Parker Bowles, Andrew 127, 128-9, 136, 208, 217, 219-20, 257, 269, 280, 439, 442, 443, 567
Parker Bowles, Camilla (née Shand):
  affairs with C 248, 270, 314, 535, 717
    D's lies and delusions about 218, 243, 248, 265-7, 269-70, 305, 310, 313, 339, 343, 400, 446-7, 482, 492, 506, 610

letters 506-7
nicknames 265, 266
second affair 129-30, 203, 209
third affair 208, 343, 410, 439-40, 442, 443-4, 490, 560-7, 574, 655
affairs with C first affair 126-9
ancestry 33
birthday party at Highgrove 675
at Charles and Diana's wedding 278
Charles's present to 266
and death of Diana 710
early relationship with Charles 126-9
engagement to Charles 626, 739-40
family background 126
first meeting with Charles 126
marriage to Parker Bowles 128-30, 134, 136, 209, 219-20, 257
messages from Diana 421
present to Charles from 283
relationship with Diana 217-18, 259, 449
wedding to Charles 741
Parker Bowles, Laura 129
Parker Bowles, Tom 129, 278, 479
Parkinson, Mary 468, 469
Parkinson, Michael 468, 469
Parry, Vivienne 420-1, 551, 610
Pasternak, Anna 554
Paterson, Tony 382
Patten, Chris 385, 386, 387
Patten, John 631
Paul, Henri 692, 694-5, 696, 699-700, 701, 702
Peat, Sir Michael 431-2, 544, 617
Peat, Stephen 411, 412, 413
Peebles, Catherine (Mispy) 19, 21, 22
Pembroke, Henry Herbert, 17th earl of 202, 406-7, 433
Perahia, Murray 659
Percival, Allan 612
permissive society 51-2
Petel, Eric 696-7, 698, 706, 707
Philip, Prince, Duke of Edinburgh (formerly Philip Mountbatten):

attending Spencer's wedding 35
attitude to Mountbatten 105, 106
and C's education 21, 53, 65-6, 68, 69, 73
C's friends prompt action over marriage 530
at C's wedding to D 279, 628
and death of D 715-16, 721, 722
decision on C's university 74, 75
education 25, 60
letters to D 541
marriage 11-12
overseas tours 93
pressure on C to marry 224-5
relationship with children 14, 18-19, 59, 89, 90, 94, 106-7, 149, 224-5, 248, 530
relationship with D 217, 314, 620
in Royal Navy 13, 106
taking C to school 25
teaching C rural pursuits 24
view of C and D's marriage 445-6
Phillips, Mark 134-5, 136, 537
Phillips, Peter 711
PHKI 455, 458
Pike, Charlotte 620
Pilgrims of Great Britain 103
Pinta (ketch) 61
Pitchford Manor 657-8
Planet Hollywood 559
Plumptre, Honourable George 202
Podgorny, President 105
Police 162-3
polo 79, 92, 104, 135, 203-4, 438, 442-3, 485, 493
Pompidou, Georges 105
Pompidou, Madame 105
Poundbury, Dorset 394, 625-6, 631, 632, 657
Prague Heritage Fund 659
Pratt, George 160-1, 162, 163
press 52, 66
press *see* media
Press Complaints Commission (PCC) 513, 518, 520, 524, 561, 578

Press Council 223
Prince of Wales Committee 656
Prince of Wales Community Venture 368-9
Prince of Wales (Dimbleby) 242, 572-4, 575, 576-7
Prince of Wales Environment Committee for Wales 155
Prince of Wales Institute of Architecture 632-3, 657
Prince's Scottish Youth Business Trust 656
Prince's Trust 155, 160-7, 170, 177, 354, 368, 383, 459-61, 462-4, 490, 548, 568, 633, 655
  Volunteers programme 369, 655
Prince's Youth Business Trust (PYBT) 354-5, 356, 357, 368, 371, 372, 463, 655-6
Princess in Love 554
Prior, Jim 327, 349
Prior, Lady 327
Priory Clinic, Roehampton 286, 650-1
Private Eye 218, 227, 343
privatisation 350-1
Psychejam.com 290
Psychiatry and Clinical Neurosciences 292
public schools, principles behind 54-5
Puttnam, David, Lord 400, 401, 432, 522, 610

Queen's Jubilee Trust 161

RAF 109-12
Raine, Kathleen 176-7
Ramsey, Michael, Archbishop of Canterbury 74, 77, 80
Random House 672
Rapp, Lieutenant 149-50, 151
Rather, Dan 277
rationing 4, 5, 6
Reagan, Nancy 142
Reagan, Ronald 142
Real Diana 44, 595
Recorder of London 6
Red Cross 13, 26, 558, 598, 633, 653, 654
  anti-landmines work 637-43, 665
Reenan, Cyril 531

Rees-Jones, Trevor 686-7, 694-5, 696, 699-700, 701-2, 712
Reid, Sue 409, 413
Rendall, John 417
Repossi, Alberto 691
Retail Candy Stores Institute of America 26
Rice, Tim 468
Richard, Cliff 736
Richard III xv, xvi
Riddell, John 357, 372, 373, 374, 395
Riddlesworth Hall prep school 40
Ridley, Nicholas 385, 386, 388-9
Rippon, Angela 277
Rivett, Jenny 556
Robertson, Geoffrey, QC 579
Robertson, Mary 199-200
Robertson, Patrick 199-200
Roche, Frances *see* Shand Kydd, Frances
Rock and Royalty 667-8, 680
Rock, Tessa 602
Rogers, Richard 624-5
Rogers, Rita 556
Rolls Royce 96
Romsey, Norton 210, 226, 272, 281, 315, 316, 330, 524, 526
Romsey, Penny 209-10, 226, 272, 281, 293, 316, 524
Rothermere, Lord 523-4
Rowan, Dr Peter 286-7, 289-90
Royal Anthropological Institute 155
Royal Ascot 559
Royal Berkshire Hospital 476
Royal Brompton Hospital 601-2, 606
Royal Collection Trust 659
Royal Duty 341, 447-8
Royal Family 220-1, 400
   attitude to 8, 12, 17
   criticised at D's death 719-21
   jealousy of family members' popularity 300
   modernising 84-5
   PR mistakes by 558
   problems of belonging to 300-1

Royal Family (TV) 86-7
Royal Institute of British Architecture 336
Royal Jubilee Trusts 368
Royal Marriages Act (1772) 245
Royal Marsden NHS Trust 634
Royal Navy, C's service in 105-8, 112-20, 128, 131-2, 133-8, 142-51, 153
Royal Regiment of Wales 86
Royal Scots Guards 34
Royal Train 222-3
Runcie, Robert, Archbishop of Canterbury 237, 279-80

Sadat, President Anwar 282, 283
St James's Palace 560, 710
St John of Fawsley, Lord 512
St Thomas's Hospital 496
Sakara (schooner) 679
San Lorenzo restaurant 219, 333, 433
Sanders, Joseph 547, 551-2, 579, 583, 595, 600, 602, 603, 604, 681
Sandhurst 34, 741
Sandringham 14, 15, 23, 34, 196, 309-10, 543, 544
Sandringham (labrador) 329-30, 331
Sandro 723
SANE 325, 395
Santa Cruz, Lucia 76, 125-6
Saudi Arabia, King of 661
Saunders, Mark 588-9
Save the Children 638
Scapa Flow 143-4
Scargill, Arthur 347-8, 349
Scarman, Lord 371
Schwarzenegger, Arnold 723
Scott, Rory 202
Scottish Business in the Community 656
Secombe, Harry 69, 161
'Seeing is Believing' campaign 367
Sellers, Peter 69
Serota, Angela 511
Seth-Smith, Kay 199

Settelen, Peter 38, 469, 549, 556, 570
Shackleton, Fiona 618
Shadows of a Princess 435
Shakespeare, William xvi, 628, 642
Shakespeare Birthday Speech 628
Shand, Bruce 126
Shand, Camilla *see* Parker Bowles, Camilla
Shand, Rosalind 126
Shand Kydd, Frances (formerly Lady Althorp, née Roche) (mother of Diana) 514, 619, 671, 723
  divorce 37-8, 281
  eating disorders 255
  losing custody of children 37
  marriage to Althorp 35
  marriage to Shand Kydd 38
  meeting Althorp 34-5
  as mother 38-9
  problems 39
  relationship with D 39, 44, 619, 671
  relationship with mother 37-8, 223
  second divorce 39
  self-justification 39
Shand Kydd, Janet 36
Shand Kydd, Peter 35, 38, 39
Sharples, Sir Richard 132
Shaw, George Bernard 13
Shea, Michael 223, 308
Shebbeare, Tom 165-6, 177, 369, 373, 377, 457, 458, 459, 464, 490
Sheffield, Davina 47, 178
Shrewsbury, Earl of 359-60
Silver Jubilee 158
Simmons, Simone 556, 649-50, 666, 687
Simpson, John 657
Simpson, Wallis 10
Sinatra, Frank 142
Six-Day War 50
Sky News 541, 739
Smith, George 616-18
Smith, John 505, 646

Smith, Julia *see* Carling, Julia
Snell, Kate 675, 681, 687
Snow, Jon 714-15
Snowdon, Earl of 86, 537
Soames, Sir Christopher 122
Soames, Nicholas 104, 209-10, 226, 272, 544, 613
Soames, Rupert 425
soccer violence 52
Sofia, Queen, of Spain 417, 418
Spencer, 1st Lord 32
Spencer, 6th Earl 33
Spencer, Albert Edward John (Jack), 7th Earl 33-4, 35, 42
Spencer, Charles, 9th Earl 42, 191, 448, 553, 598, 609, 671
   birth 35
   and death of D 719, 722, 723-4
   divorce 724
   hatred of stepmother 44, 195
   and media 717, 719, 724
   sets up Diana Memorial Fund 724-5
Spencer, Lady Cynthia 34
Spencer, Lady Diana *see* Diana, Princess of Wales
Spencer, Jane 44, 198, 254, 320, 553, 598, 671
   birth 35
   and death of D 711, 712
   marriage 193
Spencer, John, 8th Earl (formerly Viscount Althorp):
   army record 34
   concealing D's mental problems 42, 227, 235-6
   death 44, 494
   divorce 37-8
   on D's engagement 235
   at D's wedding 276-7, 278, 279
   family 35
   as father 38
   illness 194-5
   marriage to Frances 35-6
   marriage to Raine 43
   meeting Frances 34-5
   serving royal family 34

Spencer, Raine (formerly Countess of Dartmouth) 43-4, 194-5, 235, 236, 253, 669, 671, 687
Spencer, Robert 202, 268
Spencer, Sarah 210, 269, 448
  birth 35
  bulimia 255
  dating C 46-7, 48, 178, 192-3
  and death of D 711, 712
  hatred of stepmother 44
Spencer, Victoria 724
Spencer family:
  ancestry 32-3
  attitude to Windsors 32
  coat of arms 32
  false genealogy 32
  finances 33-4
Spencer House, London 33, 34
Spencer-Churchill, Lady Caroline 427
Spencer-Churchill, Lady Sarah 44, 193, 195-6, 201, 342, 444-5, 723
Spice Girls 662
Spielberg, Steven 723
spin xv-xvii
Sprecher, Bruno 451, 452
Squidgygate telephone tapes 531-5, 539, 561, 566, 567, 582, 633
Stanley, Kevin 276
Stark, Koo 406
Status Quo 165
Stephan, Hervé 701
Stevens, Sir John 413
Stewart-Wilson, Blair 254, 272
Sting 723
stock market crash 388, 389
Stott, Richard 515, 561
Stratford-upon=Avon 628
Sun 144, 224, 270, 293, 308, 309, 311, 315, 358, 384, 387, 388, 418, 452, 476, 487, 504-5, 505, 509, 515, 527, 531-2, 538-9, 545, 561, 576, 649-50, 684, 721
Sunday Express 520, 718
Sunday Mirror 222-3, 227, 387, 604, 605, 627, 684, 718

Sunday Pictorial 17
Sunday Times 402, 511, 512-13, 515, 517, 518, 524, 525, 526, 529, 573-4, 575, 576-7, 578, 584, 627, 633, 642, 718
Swan theatre, Stratford-upon-Avon 628
Symonds, Nathalie 602

Taj Mahal 493, 494
Tang, David 648, 673
Taylor, Bryce 578, 579, 580
Te Kanawa, Kiri 277, 659
Tebbit, Norman 349, 388, 389
TECs *see* Training Enterprise Councils
telephone calls:
  tapes of:
    Camillagate 560-7, 574, 582, 584, 633
    Squidgygate 531-5, 539, 561, 566, 567, 582, 633
Teresa, Mother 654, 666
Tesco 513
Testino, Mario 649-50
Tetbury 264
Thanh, Le Van 698-9
Thatcher, Margaret 5, 51, 100, 165, 229, 232-3, 236, 278, 306, 319, 326-9, 347, 348, 349-51, 354-5, 357-8, 359, 360-1, 363-4, 368, 373, 374, 377, 378-9, 381, 386, 387-8, 389, 390, 391-3, 437, 490, 645-6, 647, 655, 730, 731, 736
  attitude to C 154, 355, 363, 377, 379, 395
  downfall 391-2, 393
  D's view of 397
  opinion of D 355, 398
Thin, James 513
Thomas, George 82
Thomas Cranmer Schools Prize 626
Thompson, John 362
Thorpe, Jeremy 99
Tickell, Sir Crispin 387
Timbertop (school) 65-6, 67-71
Times 6-7, 12, 237, 513, 584, 627, 719
Today newspaper 505, 526
Toffolo, Joseph 601

Toffolo, Oonagh 556, 601, 649, 666, 687
Townend, Henry 22
Trade Union and Labour Relations Act (1975) 100
trade unions 49-50, 97, 98, 99-101, 326, 329, 347-9
Training Enterprise Councils (TECs) 364
Travels with a Princess 435-6
Trinity College, Cambridge 75-8
Tryon, Dale (Kanga), Lady 218, 219, 266, 267, 343
TUC 100-1, 230
Turner, Tina 165
TVam 608
Twigg, Stephen 520

UNICEF 637
United Cerebral Palsy Fund 599, 614
United Kingdom *see* Britain
United World Colleges 155, 179
University College of Wales, Aberystwyth 81, 82-4
University of Wales 155
Upper Clyde Shipbulders 96
Urdd National Eisteddfod 83-4
USA:
   economy 6-7
   post-war 5
      help to former enemies 4
   repayment of debt to 4
   visits to 101-3, 141-2

Vacani, Madame Betty 196
Valentin, Alice 693-4
Valetta, Malta 19-20
van Cutsem, Hugh 109-10
van der Post, Lauren 172-4, 175, 176, 182, 281-2, 283, 285, 322
Vanity Fair 345, 487, 549, 550, 648
Venables, Terry 608, 609
Versace, Donatella 723
Versace, Gianni 450, 667-8, 678, 680, 682, 687
Victoria, Queen 8, 23
Vietnam War 96

Villalonga, Jose Luis de 418
Vision of Britain 394
Vogue 654

Waddell, Robert 72-3
Wakeham, John 382-3, 519
Wakeham, Lord 519
Waldner, Diane *see* Hoare, Diane
Waldner, Baroness Louise de 592
Wales 81-90, 299, 302-3, 478
Walker, Penny 42-3
Walker, Peter 349
Wallace, Anna 178, 202-3, 426
Walsh, Helen 422-3
Walters, Alan 327-8
Walters, Barbara 277, 606
Ward, Tracy 426
Warner rothers 672
Washington, DC 653-4
Washington Post 653
Waterhouse, David 427-8, 429, 430, 433, 442, 446, 528
Welch, Raquel 484
Wellesley, Lady Jane 47, 178
West, Hazel 430
West Heath School 40-1, 44, 48
Westmacott, Peter 540-1, 542
Westminster Abbey 17
Westminster Hall 16
Whalley, Christopher 600, 605
Wharfe, Ken 241-2, 403, 443, 578, 593
What Is Our Heritage? 43
Wheatley, John 467
Whitaker, James 214-15, 222, 269-70, 315, 447, 448, 515, 516, 540-1, 542
Whitehead, Philip 101
Whitlam, Mike 598, 637-9, 641, 653
Wiessler, Christian 609
Wiggin, Daniel 195
Wiggin, Sir John 195

Willcocks, Sir David 277
William I (the Conqueror) 32
William III 32, 732
William, Prince 654, 740-1
  accident with golf club 476-7
  birth 319-21, 342
  as child 461, 464-5
  and death of mother 709, 711, 720, 722
  holiday with mother 670, 671-2, 673-5, 677, 679
  overseas visit with parents 337
  polo 485
  promoted as next monarch 474-5, 478, 611
  relationship with father 119-20, 319-21, 340, 400, 437, 442, 464-5, 473, 475-7, 560, 670, 724, 726, 741
  relationship with mother 39, 325-6, 437, 442, 446, 474-86, 522, 543, 550, 614, 650, 675, 718
  suggests D sell dresses for charity 654
Williams, Reverend Harry 77-8
Williams, Robbie 662
Wilson, Sir Charles 74
Wilson, Christopher 177
Wilson, Harold 50, 74, 78, 81, 95, 99, 101, 104, 160, 229, 390
Windsor, Duke of *see* Edward VIII
Windsor, Wallis, Duchess of 123-4
Windsor Castle 23, 309, 543, 544-5, 547
Windsor Great Park 432-3
Winfrey, Oprah 606
Wintour, Anna 654
Wood, Natalie 725
Woods, Edward 76
Woods, Robin, Dean of Windsor 74-5
Worcester, Marquis of 426
World in Balance 394
World Cup (football) 51-2
World War I 4
World War II 3, 20
  Britain after 49-51
Worsthorne, Peregrine 53-4
Writing on the Wall 101

Wyatt, Steve 508, 536, 537
Wyatt, Woodrow 227

Yacoub, Sir Magdi 602, 603
Yassin, Hassan 693
Yom Kippur War 97
York, Sarah, Duchess of (née Ferguson) 17, 492, 598, 722, 733
   affairs 508, 536, 537, 539
   ancestry 33
   betrayed by D 536
   commercial activities 619
   D's jealousy of 408, 435, 687
   engagement 419-20
   friendship with D 252, 254, 418-19, 510
   popularity 408
   relationship with media 420
   rivalry with D 425
   Royal Family shocked by 536
   separation 510, 536-7, 538, 582
   skiing 451
   undisciplined behaviour 589
Young, David (later Lord) 165
Young, Paul 165
Young England Kindergarten 198-9, 215-16
Yu, Lily Hua 556

Zetland, Lord and Lady 461
Ziegler, Philip 158
Zimbabwe 577